UNDERSTANDING BIPOLAR DISORDER

UNDERSTANDING
BIPOLAR
DISORDER

A Developmental Psychopathology Perspective

Edited by
David J. Miklowitz
Dante Cicchetti

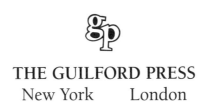

THE GUILFORD PRESS
New York   London

© 2010 The Guilford Press
A Division of Guilford Publications, Inc.
72 Spring Street, New York, NY 10012
www.guilford.com

Printed in the United States of America

This book is printed on acid-free paper.

Last digit is print number: 9   8   7   6   5   4   3   2   1

The authors have checked with sources believed to be reliable in their efforts to provide
information that is complete and generally in accord with the standards of practice that
are accepted at the time of publication. However, in view of the possibility of human
error or changes in medical sciences, neither the authors, nor the editor and publisher,
nor any other party who has been involved in the preparation or publication of this work
warrants that the information contained herein is in every respect accurate or complete,
and they are not responsible for any errors or omissions or the results obtained from the
use of such information. Readers are encouraged to confirm the information contained in
this book with other sources.

Library of Congress Cataloging-in-Publication Data

Understanding bipolar disorder : a developmental psychopathology perspective /
edited by David J. Miklowitz, Dante Cicchetti.
    p. ; cm.
  Includes bibliographical references and index.
  ISBN 978-1-60623-622-2 (hardcover)
  1. Manic–depressive illness. 2. Developmental psychobiology. I. Miklowitz, David
Jay, 1957– II. Cicchetti, Dante. III. Title.
  [DNLM: 1. Bipolar Disorder—etiology. 2. Adaptation,
Psychological. 3. Developmental Disabilities—psychology. 4. Risk Factors.
WM 207 U55 2010]
  RC516.U53 2010
  616.89′5—dc22
                                                                        2009039177

About the Editors

David J. Miklowitz, PhD, is Professor of Psychiatry in the Division of Child and Adolescent Psychiatry at the University of California, Los Angeles, School of Medicine, and Senior Clinical Research Fellow in the Department of Psychiatry at Oxford University. His research focuses on family environmental factors and family psychoeducational treatments for adult-onset and childhood-onset bipolar disorder. Dr. Miklowitz is a recipient of the Distinguished Investigator Award from the National Alliance for Research on Schizophrenia and Depression and the Mogens Schou Award for Research from the International Society for Bipolar Disorders, among other honors. He has published over 200 articles, book chapters, and books.

Dante Cicchetti, PhD, is McKnight Presidential Chair and Professor of Child Psychology and Psychiatry at the University of Minnesota. His research focuses on developmental theory as well as science, policy, and practice related to child maltreatment, depression, mental retardation, and other domains of development. Dr. Cicchetti has received awards including the three highest honors of the Developmental Division of the American Psychological Association: the G. Stanley Hall Award for Distinguished Contribution to Developmental Psychology, the Urie Bronfenbrenner Award for Lifetime Contribution to Developmental Psychology in the Service of Science and Society, and the Mentor Award in Developmental Psychology. He has published over 400 articles, books, and journal special issues, and is the founding and current Editor of *Development and Psychopathology*.

Contributors

Lyn Y. Abramson, PhD, Department of Psychology, University of Wisconsin, Madison, Wisconsin

Caleb M. Adler, MD, Division of Bipolar Disorders Research, Center for Imaging Research, Department of Psychiatry, University of Cincinnati College of Medicine, Cincinnati, Ohio

Lauren B. Alloy, PhD, Department of Psychology, Temple University, Philadelphia, Pennsylvania

Andy C. Belden, PhD, Department of Psychiatry, Washington University School of Medicine, St. Louis, Missouri

Boris Birmaher, MD, Department of Psychiatry, University of Pittsburgh Medical Center, Pittsburgh, Pennsylvania

Gabrielle A. Carlson, PhD, Department of Child and Adolescent Psychiatry, Stony Brook University School of Medicine, Stony Brook, New York

Michael A. Cerullo, MD, Division of Bipolar Disorders Research, Department of Psychiatry, University of Cincinnati College of Medicine, Cincinnati, Ohio

Dante Cicchetti, PhD, Institute of Child Development and Department of Psychiatry, University of Minnesota, Minneapolis, Minnesota

Melissa P. DelBello, MD, Division of Bipolar Disorders Research, Department of Psychiatry, University of Cincinnati College of Medicine, Cincinnati, Ohio

Rasim Somer Diler, MD, Department of Child and Adolescent Psychiatry, Western Psychiatric Institute and Clinic, University of Pittsburgh Medical Center, Pittsburgh, Pennsylvania

David E. Fleck, PhD, Division of Bipolar Disorders Research, Center for Imaging Research, Department of Psychiatry, University of Cincinnati College of Medicine, Cincinnati, Ohio

Mary A. Fristad, PhD, ABPP, Departments of Psychiatry and Psychology, Ohio State University Medical Center, Columbus, Ohio

Rachel K. Gerstein, MA, Department of Psychology, Temple University, Philadelphia, Pennsylvania

Joseph F. Goldberg, MD, Department of Psychiatry, Mount Sinai School of Medicine, New York, New York; Affective Disorders Research Program, Silver Hill Hospital, New Canaan, Connecticut

Tina R. Goldstein, PhD, Department of Child and Adolescent Psychiatry, Western Psychiatric Institute and Clinic, University of Pittsburgh Medical Center, Pittsburgh, Pennsylvania

Stephen P. Hinshaw, PhD, Department of Psychology, University of California, Berkeley, Berkeley, California

Shari Jager-Hyman, MA, Department of Psychology, Temple University, Philadelphia, Pennsylvania

Jessica Keyser, MA, Department of Psychology, Temple University, Philadelphia, Pennsylvania

Robert A. Kowatch, MD, PhD, Division of Child and Adolescent Psychiatry, Cincinnati Children's Hospital Medical Center, Cincinnati, Ohio

Joan L. Luby, MD, Department of Psychiatry, Washington University School of Medicine, St. Louis, Missouri

Erin B. McClure-Tone, PhD, Department of Psychology, Georgia State University, Atlanta, Georgia

Matt McQueen, ScD, Institute for Behavioral Genetics, University of Colorado, Boulder, Colorado

Amy N. Mendenhall, PhD, MSW, School of Social Welfare, University of Kansas, Lawrence, Kansas

Stephanie E. Meyer, PhD, private practice, Los Angeles, California

David J. Miklowitz, PhD, UCLA Semel Institute for Neuroscience and Human Behavior, David Geffen School of Medicine, University of California, Los Angeles, California; Department of Psychiatry, Oxford University, London, United Kingdom

Jayasree Nandagopal, MD, Division of Bipolar Disorders Research, Department of Psychiatry, University of Cincinnati College of Medicine, Cincinnati, Ohio

Robin Nusslock, PhD, Department of Psychology, Northwestern University, Evanston, Illinois

Nick C. Patel, PharmD, PhD, Department of Psychiatry and Health Behavior, Medical College of Georgia, Augusta, Georgia; Corphealth Incorporated, Fort Worth, Texas

Robert M. Post, MD, Department of Psychiatry, George Washington University School of Medicine, Washington, DC; Bipolar Collaborative Network, Bethesda, Maryland

Stephen M. Strakowski, MD, Division of Bipolar Disorders Research, Center for Imaging Research, Department of Psychiatry, University of Cincinnati College of Medicine, Cincinnati, Ohio

Jeffrey R. Strawn, MD, Department of Psychiatry, University of Cincinnati College of Medicine, Cincinnati, Ohio

Mini Tandon, DO, Department of Psychiatry, Washington University School of Medicine, St. Louis, Missouri

Michael E. Thase, MD, Department of Psychiatry, University of Pennsylvania School of Medicine and Philadelphia Veterans Affairs Medical Center, Philadelphia, Pennsylvania; Department of Psychiatry, University of Pittsburgh Medical Center, Pittsburgh, Pennsylvania

Snezana Urosevic, PhD, Department of Psychology, University of Minnesota, Minneapolis, Minnesota

Patricia D. Walshaw, PhD, Department of Psychiatry and Biobehavioral Sciences, University of California, Los Angeles, School of Medicine, Los Angeles, California

Erik Willcutt, PhD, Institute for Behavioral Genetics and Department of Psychology and Neuroscience, University of Colorado, Boulder, Colorado

Eric A. Youngstrom, PhD, Department of Psychology, University of North Carolina at Chapel Hill, Chapel Hill, North Carolina

Preface

Bipolar disorder (BD) is both a common and highly disabling condition. It affects as many as one in 25 adults and between 420,000 and 2,072,000 children in the United States alone (Post & Kowatch, 2006). BD takes an enormous toll on an individual's quality of life and causes considerable stress and hardship for the family. People with the disorder spend as much as half of their lives in states of illness, mostly in states of depression rather than mania (Judd et al., 2002). As many as one in every six persons with BD dies by suicide, and almost half attempt suicide one or more times (Harris & Barraclough, 1997; Jamison, 2000). By 2020, the World Health Organization estimates that BD will be the sixth leading cause of disability among all medical disorders (Murray & Lopez, 1996).

In the 1970s and 1980s, with the advent of lithium, antidepressants, and later the anticonvulsant medications, many in the psychiatric community believed that the problem of BD had been solved. Advances in behavioral genetics offered incontrovertible evidence that the disorder was heritable, even if the phenotype varied from person to person or from generation to generation (Smoller & Finn, 2003). Early findings with positron emission tomography, structural neuroimaging, and neuropsychology studies suggested changes in the brain, particularly in frontal lobe functioning (e.g., Powell & Miklowitz, 1994). Thus, the disorder was seen as genetic and biological in origin, and its developmental origins commanded little attention. Moreover, psychotherapy was relegated to a supporting role relative to drug treatment and was seen primarily as a means to keep people on their medications. Nonetheless, patients continued to have frequent recurrences, residual symptoms between episodes, and decrements in functioning and quality of life (Gitlin, Swendsen, Heller, & Hammen, 1995).

Fortunately, there has been a shift in our thinking about BD in the past two decades. First, many more patients report a childhood onset than we originally thought: Recent studies have found that between 15 and 28% of adults with BD reported that the onset occurred before the age of 13, and between 50 and 66% reported onset before the age of 19 (Leverich et al., 2002; Perlis et al., 2004). Sec-

ond, an early onset has been found to be associated with a host of negative outcomes in adulthood, including lengthy episodes, multiple "polarity switches," a
continuously cycling course, and a preponderance of mixed episodes, psychosis,
and suicidal behaviors (Birmaher et al., 2006; Brent, Baugher, Bridge, Chen, &
Chiapetta, 1999; Geller et al., 2002). Third, although at times seeming to appear
overnight, BD has a lengthy prodrome, with behavioral and emotional dysregulation observable even in toddlerhood (Correll et al., 2007; Luby, Tandon, & Belden,
2009; Post & Kowatch, 2006; Radke-Yarrow, Nottelmann, Martinez, Fox, & Belmont, 1992). These findings have helped refocus our attention on BD as a neurodevelopmental disorder, much like schizophrenia.

The purpose of this book is to bring together what is known about the development of BD from the genetic, neurobiological, cognitive, and psychosocial perspectives. We have asked each of the authors, all of whom are highly regarded
experts in the field, to consider BD from a *developmental psychopathology* perspective (Cicchetti & Rogosch, 2002; Cicchetti & Toth, 1998). What do we know
about how BD symptoms emerge at different developmental stages? How do mood
symptoms unfold in the context of dynamic interactions between risk or protective factors in the genetic, biological, psychological, familial, or sociocultural
contexts? How do we explain the variability in outcomes among children who
initially look very similar (multifinality)? In contrast, how do we explain why
children with many different initial presentations can all develop into adults with
the same disorder (equifinality)? Finally, how do we modify our pharmacological and psychosocial treatments to address the unique needs of persons with the
disorder at different stages of development?

We begin the book with an overview of the developmental psychopathology framework and its application to BD (Cicchetti). This chapter explains the
terminology and key assumptions used throughout the book. Cicchetti discusses
the nature of person × environment interactions; the complex interplay among
genetic, biological, psychological, and social factors as they unfold across development; and the multifactorial nature of BD.

The book is divided into five sections. Part I (Chapters 2–4) is devoted to
the phenomenology and diagnosis of BD in children. Considerable disagreement
exists on how to define the boundaries between pediatric BD and other childhood-onset disorders or even its boundaries with normal development. Meyer
and Carlson offer an historical overview of the BD concept in children, urging the
field to take a critical eye toward the premises of DSM-IV (American Psychiatric
Association, 1994) in making diagnostic differential decisions. They review the
developmental discontinuities between childhood and adult BD; the role of age at
onset and puberty; and the distinctions among childhood, adolescent, and adult
mania. Youngstrom, in applying key concepts of developmental psychopathology,
encourages a highly scientific approach to determining what is and is not BD.
One comes away impressed with the ease by which he moves back and forth from
the scientific to the clinical-observational level. Both of these chapters will be of
considerable value to clinicians and researchers who struggle with how to define
BD in children.

Luby, Belden, and Tandon address the highly controversial issue of BD during the preschool years. Many readers will go into the chapter doubting the validity of bipolar diagnoses in very young children, but will be surprised at how their opinions change once acquainted with the considerable progress in this area.

Part II (Chapters 5–7) addresses the onset, prognosis, and course of BD in children, adolescents, and adults. Diler, Birmaher, and Miklowitz describe several longitudinal investigations of the course of BD in children and shed light on the continuities and discontinuities in symptom presentations across the lifespan. Their discussion of the Course and Outcome of Bipolar Youth study, the largest longitudinal study of bipolar spectrum disorders to date, answers many questions (and formulates many others) about the progression of the disease over time. Moving to late adolescence, Alloy, Abramson, Urosevic, Nusslock, and Jager-Hyman examine a cohort of college students who were deemed at risk for BD. Together with their later chapter in the etiology section (Alloy, Abramson, Walshaw, Keyser, and Gerstein), Alloy and colleagues present a cognitive vulnerability–stress formulation for understanding the onset and course of BD, as informed by their earlier work on unipolar depression. In many ways, their work provides the most direct test of a developmental psychopathology formulation, given their continuous measurement of cognitive predisposition, temperament, family history, and stress in students at risk for BD spectrum disorders.

Finally, Goldberg persuasively argues that the predictors of the course of BD in adulthood provide a window for understanding the development of the illness itself. His analysis of risk and protective factors includes personality structure; locus of control; resilience to stress; temperamental traits; and genetic, neurotrophic, and environmental considerations. Goldberg reminds us that symptoms comprise only one domain of outcome. Work functioning, social functioning, family relationships, and quality of life, while harder for us to measure, are often the most important outcome variables to patients.

Part III, on etiology (Chapters 8–12), discusses the many causes of BD from a multiple-levels-of-analysis perspective. In their methodologically rigorous chapter on genetic vulnerability, Willcutt and McQueen make clear what can and cannot be concluded from behavioral genetic and gene-mapping studies. The approach of parsing the effects of heritability, shared environments, and nonshared environments suggests directions for future research, notably the importance of identifying environmental variables with prognostic significance in genetically vulnerable samples. Fleck, Cerullo, Nandagopal, Adler, Patel, Strakowski, and DelBello review the rapidly growing area of neuroimaging (structural and functional neuroimaging, magnetic resonance spectroscopy, positron emission tomography, and diffusion tensor imaging). Although no diagnostically specific biological markers have yet been found, it is likely that these methods will increasingly be used to map the pathophysiology of BD and identify children at risk for the disorder.

Deficits in social cognition and response flexibility are discussed in a particularly erudite chapter by McClure-Tone, who explores how bipolar children and adults understand social relationships (e.g., why they view neutral faces as negative) and the neural correlates of these cognitive and interpersonal processes. Post and Miklowitz address the interactive roles of life events, neuropathophysiology, family stress, and the onset of BD with reference to the "kindling" and stress-sensitization models. The role of childhood adversity (notably physical and sexual abuse) in the background of persons with BD is becoming increasingly apparent, with its downstream effects observable well after the onset of the disorder.

Part IV (Chapters 13–16) concerns the treatment of BD in youth and adults. As is true throughout the book, we asked the authors to approach treatment from a biopsychosocial perspective, whether the topic is psychopharmacology (Kowatch, Strawn, and DelBello; Thase), family-focused therapy or dialectical behavior therapy (Miklowitz and Goldstein), or multifamily or individual family psychoeducation (Mendenhall and Fristad). The evidence base for individual medications and psychosocial approaches is limited at this stage. Nonetheless, practice guidelines for the pharmacological and psychosocial management of early-onset BD are being articulated (Kowatch et al., 2005). It is likely that future guidelines will combine various forms of pharmacotherapy and psychotherapy at different phases of the illness or even during the prodrome. It is hoped that future investigations will use early intervention and prevention paradigms to elucidate the role of environmental/contextual and individual resilience variables in the onset of bipolar spectrum disorders.

We are fortunate to be able to conclude the book (Part V, Chapter 17) with a first-person account by Stephen Hinshaw, a clinical psychologist whose father suffered from BD. Growing up with the disorder, along with his own training in developmental psychopathology, gives Hinshaw a unique view of the development of the illness, its risk and protective factors, and its effects on family members. His recommendations on how to address the stigma of BD in our treatments are quite timely.

We hope that the reader will come away from the book with an appreciation of BD as an evolving, dynamic process. As we learn more about this disorder, the nature of the interactions among genetics, biology, cognition, and the psychosocial context becomes more complex than originally believed. We hope that this book will encourage new researchers and clinicians to take on the challenges of understanding and effectively treating this fascinating condition.

DAVID J. MIKLOWITZ
DANTE CICCHETTI

REFERENCES

American Psychiatric Association. (1994). *Diagnostic and statistical manual of mental disorders* (4th ed.). Washington, DC: Author.

Birmaher, B., Axelson, D., Strober, M., Gill, M. K., Valeri, S., Chiappetta, L., et al. (2006). Clinical course of children and adolescents with bipolar spectrum disorders. *Archives of General Psychiatry, 63*(2), 175–183.

Brent, D. A., Baugher, M., Bridge, J., Chen, T., & Chiapetta, L. (1999). Age- and sex-related risk factors for adolescent suicide. *Journal of the American Academy of Child and Adolescent Psychiatry, 38,* 1497–1505.

Cicchetti, D., & Rogosch, F. A. (2002). A developmental psychopathology perspective on adolescence. *Journal of Consulting and Clinical Psychology, 70*(1), 6–20.

Cicchetti, D., & Toth, S. L. (1998). The development of depression in children and adolescents. *American Psychologist, 53*(2), 221–241.

Correll, C. U., Penzner, J. B., Frederickson, A. M., Richter, J. J., Auther, A. M., Smith, C. W., et al. (2007). Differentiation in the preonset phases of schizophrenia and mood disorders: Evidence in support of a bipolar mania prodrome. *Schizophrenia Bulletin, 33*(3), 703–713.

Geller, B., Zimerman, B., Williams, M., Bolhofner, K., Craney, J. L., Frazier, J., et al. (2002). DSM-IV mania symptoms in a prepubertal and early adolescent bipolar disorder phenotype compared to attention deficit hyperactive and normal controls. *Journal of the American Academy of Child and Adolescent Psychopharmacology, 12,* 11–25.

Gitlin, M. J., Swendsen, J., Heller, T. L., & Hammen, C. (1995). Relapse and impairment in bipolar disorder. *American Journal of Psychiatry, 152*(11), 1635–1640.

Harris, E. C., & Barraclough, B. (1997). Suicide as an outcome for mental disorders: A meta-analysis. *British Journal of Psychiatry, 170,* 205–208.

Jamison, K. R. (2000). Suicide and bipolar disorder. *Journal of Clinical Psychiatry, 61*(Suppl. 9), 47–56.

Judd, L. L., Akiskal, H. S., Schettler, P. J., Endicott, J., Maser, J., Solomon, D. A., et al. (2002). The long-term natural history of the weekly symptomatic status of bipolar I disorder. *Archives of General Psychiatry, 59,* 530–537.

Kowatch, R. A., Fristad, M., Birmaher, B., Wagner, K. D., Findling, R. L., Hellander, M., et al. (2005). Treatment guidelines for children and adolescents with bipolar disorder. *Journal of the American Academy of Child and Adolescent Psychiatry, 44*(3), 213–235.

Leverich, G. S., McElroy, S. L., Suppes, T., Keck, P. E. J., Denicoff, K. D., Nolen, W. A., et al. (2002). Early physical and sexual abuse associated with an adverse course of bipolar illness. *Biological Psychiatry, 51,* 288–297.

Luby, J. L., Tandon, M., & Belden, A. (2009). Preschool bipolar disorder. *Child and Adolescent Psychiatric Clinics of North America, 18*(2), 391–403.

Murray, C. J. L., & Lopez, A. D. (1996). *The global burden of disease: A comprehensive assessment of mortality and disability from diseases, injuries, and risk factors in 1990 and projected to 2020.* Boston: Harvard University Press.

Perlis, R. H., Miyahara, S., Marangell, L. B., Wisniewski, S. R., Ostacher, M., DelBello, M. P., et al. (2004). Long-term implications of early onset in bipolar disorder: Data from the first 1000 participants in the Systematic Treatment Enhancement Program for Bipolar Disorder (STEP-BD). *Biological Psychiatry, 55,* 875–881.

Post, R., & Kowatch, R. A. (2006). The health care crisis of childhood-onset bipolar illness: Some recommendations for its amelioration. *Journal of Clinical Psychiatry, 67*(1), 115–125.

Powell, K. B., & Miklowitz, D. J. (1994). Frontal lobe dysfunction in the affective disorders. *Clinical Psychology Review, 146*(6), 525–546.

Radke-Yarrow, M., Nottelmann, E., Martinez, P., Fox, M. B., & Belmont, B. (1992). Young children of affectively ill parents: A longitudinal study of psychosocial development. *Journal of the American Academy of Child and Adolescent Psychiatry, 31*(1), 68–77.

Smoller, J. W., & Finn, C. T. (2003). Family, twin, and adoption studies of bipolar disorder. *American Journal of Medical Genetics, Part C: Seminars in Medical Genetics, 123*(1), 48–58.

Acknowledgments

David J. Mikowitz: I would first like to acknowledge support from the National Institute of Mental Health (Grant Nos. R01MH073781 and R34MH077856) and the National Association for Research on Schizophrenia and Depression (NARSAD Distinguished Investigator Award). I was also fortunate to receive a Council on Research and Creative Work Faculty Fellowship from the University of Colorado for the 2006–2007 academic year, which allowed me to work and study at Oxford University, where the majority of this book was conceptualized. My graduate students and postdoctoral fellows at the University of Colorado were instrumental in directing my research efforts and offering hypotheses about the role of psychosocial factors in bipolar disorder. I would especially like to acknowledge Elizabeth George, PhD, Dawn Taylor, PhD, Tina Goldstein, PhD, Chris Schneck, MD, and Eunice Kim, PhD. I feel very fortunate for the mentorship, friendship, and collaboration I have enjoyed through the years with Ellen Frank, PhD, David Kupfer, MD, David Axelson, MD, and Boris Birmaher, MD, at the University of Pittsburgh. I owe much of my development as a researcher and clinician to Michael J. Goldstein, PhD, of UCLA (1930–1997), my mentor in graduate school. My thanks go to my wife, Mary Yaeger; my daughter, Ariana; my brother, Paul Miklowitz, and his family; and my mother, Gloria Miklowitz, a children's author who has published over 60 books. They have all been a source of warmth and inspiration during the writing of this book. My late father, Julius Miklowitz, a professor of mechanical engineering, has been a source of inspiration throughout my life.

Dante Cicchetti: I appreciate the support of my assistant, Jeanne Cowan, and my close friends and colleagues Fred A. Rogosch, PhD, and Sheree L. Toth, PhD. During my work on this volume, I was supported by grants from the National Institute on Drug Abuse (Nos. DA12903 and DA17741), the National Institute of Mental Health (Nos. MH45027 and MH067792), and the Spunk Fund, Inc. Finally, words cannot fully express the depth of my gratitude to Jules Bemporad, MD, Norman Garmezy, PhD, Marianne Gerschel, Kenneth Kaplan, MD, Paul Meehl, PhD, Robert Post, MD, and Alan Sroufe, PhD. They have been ongoing sources of support and inspiration in my life.

Finally, we both would like to express our sincere thanks to Executive Editor Kitty Moore at The Guilford Press, who provided her considerable editorial talents to the development of this book, and to the staff at Guilford who assisted in its production.

Contents

PART III. ETIOLOGY/RISK AND PROTECTIVE MECHANISMS

PART IV. TREATMENT

PART V. A FIRST-PERSON ACCOUNT

CHAPTER 1

A Developmental Psychopathology Perspective on Bipolar Disorder

Dante Cicchetti

The thesis proposed in this chapter is that the principles and tenets inherent to a developmental psychopathology perspective can serve to elucidate the understanding of bipolar disorder (BD) across the life course. A developmental psychopathology approach espouses the conviction that comprehending the genesis (i.e., origins) and epigenesis (i.e., the development of new, different abilities across each stage of the life span) of adaptation and maladaptation in their full complexity necessitates that we possess an understanding of the organization and integration of diverse biological, psychological, and social systems at multiple levels of analysis within individuals across different contexts and varying developmental periods (Cicchetti, 2006, 2008).

Developmental psychopathology represents a movement toward comprehending the causes and determinants, course, sequelae, and treatment of mental disorders through its synthesis of knowledge from multiple disciplines (Cicchetti, 1990; Cicchetti & Posner, 2005; Masten, 2006, 2007). The undergirding developmental orientation impels researchers to pose new questions about the phenomena they study. For example, with regard to bipolar illness, it becomes necessary to move beyond identifying features that differentiate children, adolescents, and adults who have and who do not have BD (e.g., affect dysregulation, attributional distortions) to articulating how such differences have evolved developmentally within a multilevel and dynamic social ecology (Miklowitz & Cicchetti, 2006b). Likewise, rather than being concerned with merely describing the symptoms of BD in children, adolescents, and adults (as would be the focus of the DSM-IV), the emphasis shifts to ascertaining how similar and different biological and psychological organizations contribute to the expression of depressive, hypomanic, or manic outcomes at each specific developmental level. Because psychopathology unfolds over time in a dynamically developing organism, the adoption of a developmental perspective is critical in order to comprehend the processes underlying individual pathways to adaptive and maladaptive outcomes in persons with BD.

Although abnormalities in the broad domains of genetics, neurobiology, cognition, emotion, and interpersonal relations are present to varying degrees among individuals with BD (Goodwin & Jamison, 2007; Miklowitz & Cicchetti, 2006a), these diverse areas do not exist in isolation. Rather, they are complexly interrelated and mutually interdependent (Cicchetti & Cannon, 1999; Cicchetti & Tucker, 1994; Gottlieb, 1991, 1992; Gottlieb & Halpern, 2002; Thelen & Smith, 1998). Consequently, it is essential for researchers to strive to comprehend the interrelations among the biological, psychological, and social systems in order to delineate the nature of BD, including the discovery of ways in which the organization and integration of these systems may promote resilient functioning (Charney, 2004; Curtis & Cicchetti, 2003). Relatedly, because there are myriad risk factors associated with BD and its comorbid forms of psychopathology (Goodwin & Jamison, 2007), it is critical for researchers and clinicians to acquire a firm grasp of the multilevel biological and psychological processes and mechanisms that contribute to the emergence, maintenance, and recurrence of BD. Because of the continuities and divergences from normal functioning that are manifested in BD, empirical research on pathways to BD as well as prospective longitudinal investigations of its developmental course and sequelae also hold promise for advancing understanding of the relation between normality and psychopathology.

In this chapter, I begin by explicating why a developmental psychopathology perspective can be usefully applied toward enhancing our understanding of BD. Next, I discuss the parameters of developmental psychopathology, including the core principles of the discipline. Throughout this presentation, I highlight aspects of a developmental psychopathology approach that are especially relevant to the investigation and treatment of BD. I conclude by suggesting future directions for studying BD within a developmental psychopathology framework; moreover, I address social policy implications that emanate from investigating BD through the lens of developmental psychopathology.

WHAT IS DEVELOPMENTAL PSYCHOPATHOLOGY?

The integrative nature of a developmental approach to psychopathology was articulated by Eisenberg (1977), who stated that development "constitutes the crucial link between genetic determinants and environmental variables and between physiogenic and psychogenic causes" (p. 225). Development thus encompasses "not only the roots of behavior in prior maturation as well as the residual of earlier stimulation, both internal and external, but also the modulations of that behavior by the social fields of the experienced present" (p. 225). Not surprisingly, given the intimate link between the study of normality and psychopathology, similar depictions of normative developmental processes have been espoused in the literature.

Whereas the term *developmental psychopathology* has frequently been equated with the study of mental disorders among children and youth, this perspective encompasses a much broader approach to studying development, normal and abnormal, across the life span (Cicchetti, 1990, 1993). A developmental analysis is necessary for tracing the roots, etiology, and nature of maladaptation so that interventions may be sensitively timed and guided as well as developmentally appropriate (Toth & Cicchetti, 1999). Moreover, a developmental perspective will prove useful for uncovering the compensatory mechanisms, both biological and psychological, that may be used in the face of significant adversity (Curtis & Cicchetti, 2003).

Developmental psychopathology is an integrative scientific discipline that strives to unify, within a life span framework, contributions from multiple fields of inquiry with the goal of understanding the mutual interplay between psychopathology and normative adaptation (Cicchetti, 1990, 1993; Cicchetti & Toth, 1991). A developmental analysis presupposes change and novelty, highlights the critical role of timing in the organization of behavior, underscores multiple determinants, and cautions against expecting invariant relations between causes and outcomes. A developmental analysis is as applicable to the study of the gene or cell as it is to the investigation of the individual, family, or society (Cicchetti & Pogge-Hesse, 1982; Davies & Cicchetti, 2004; Miklowitz, 2004; Werner & Kaplan, 1963).

Developmental psychopathologists seek to engage in a comprehensive evaluation of biological, psychological, and social processes and to ascertain how the transaction among these multiple levels of analysis may influence individual differences, the continuity or discontinuity of adaptive or maladaptive behavioral patterns, and the pathways by which normal and pathological outcomes may be achieved (Cicchetti & Schneider-Rosen, 1986). In practice, this entails comprehension of and appreciation for the developmental transformations and reorganizations that occur over time; an analysis of the risk and protective factors and mechanisms operating within and outside the individual and his or her environment over the course of development; the investigation of how emergent functions, competencies, and developmental tasks modify the expression of a disorder or lead to new symptoms and difficulties; and the recognition that a particular stressor or set of stressful circumstances may eventuate in different biological and psychological difficulties, depending on when in the developmental period the stress occurs.

Developmental Analysis

There are two interrelated goals inherent to a developmental analysis. First, a developmental analysis strives to investigate the specific evolving biological and psychological systems that are characteristic of individuals at varying developmental stages across the life span. This requires formulating questions about a phenomenon in terms of what capacities are characteristic of an individual during a particular developmental period and how a given process or mechanism becomes manifested in view of those developmental capacities and attainments of the individual. Age-appropriate limitations in children's cognitive, emotional, and social development may make the expression of specific manic and depressive symptoms beyond their capabilities. Thus, the delineation of those characteristics relevant to the overt manifestation of BD at different ages can probably only be accomplished by means of longitudinal prospective studies that measure skills and capacities in a variety of biological and psychological domains. Consequently, to comprehend BD fully, researchers must consider developmental variations in cognitive, social cognitive, and emotional capacities, in addition to other psychological and biological domains of functioning, to ascertain how particular outcomes—normal, psychopathological, or resilient—are exhibited during varying periods of development. One would not predict that the developmental variations in internal cognitive structures would enable individuals with BD of different ages to use similar strategies to interpret, express, or defend against their affective experiences or internal emotional states. Likewise, cognitive difficulties associated with BD can lead to impairments in regulatory processes that affect, and are affected by, attention networks and executive functions (Dickstein et al., 2004; Klimes-Dougan, Ronsaville, Wiggs, & Martinez, 2006; Meyer et al., 2004). Thus, a developmental analysis is needed to highlight the processes most likely to contribute to vulnerabilities or strengths at each developmental level in persons with BD.

Second, a developmental analysis seeks to examine the prior sequences of adaptation or maladaptation in development that have contributed to an outcome in a particular developmental period. In order to achieve this goal, it is essential that the current status of an individual's functioning be examined in the context of how that status was attained across the course of development. For example, given the multiplicity of biological and psychological processes affected by BD, directing attention to examining early developmental functioning (i.e., prior development) that may be theoretically related to later appearing BD organizations may prove to be very fruitful (Cicchetti & Sroufe, 2000; Cicchetti & Tucker, 1994; Sroufe, 2007). Accordingly, to obtain an understanding of the abnormalities in emotion regulation, close interpersonal relations, or the core negative attributions about the self that often exist in BD, researchers may begin by investigating the early development of these features, their developmental course, and their interrelations with other psychological and biological systems of the individual (Cicchetti & Sroufe, 2000; Leibenluft, Charney, & Pine, 2003; McClure-Tone, Chapter 11, this volume).

Normal and Abnormal Development

The field of developmental psychopathology is concerned with expanding its knowledge base by focusing on the extremes of adaptation and nonnormative processes of development rather than on central tendencies and uniformities in normative processes of growth and development emphasized in classic developmental psychology. As such, developmental psychopathology underscores and highlights the dialectic between normal and abnormal development (Cicchetti, 1984, 1993, 2006; Cicchetti & Toth, 2009; Rutter, 1986; Rutter & Garmezy, 1983; Rutter & Sroufe, 2000). By virtue of its emphasis on comparing and contrasting abnormal development with normative developmental patterns, and investigating the similarities as well as differences between normality and psychopathology, the strengths and weaknesses associated with atypical development are underscored (Cicchetti, 1993; Karmiloff-Smith, 2007).

The central focus of developmental psychopathology is the elucidation of developmental processes and how they function as indicated and elaborated by the examination of extremes in developmental outcome. Such extremes contribute substantial diversity to the possible outcomes in development, thereby enhancing the understanding of developmental processes. Research in the field of developmental psychopathology is not limited to the investigation of mental disorders. Scientists working in the discipline of developmental psychopathology are interested in examining the entire range of developmental processes and functioning. Not only are the disordered extremes the subject of study, but also the subclinical range of functioning is viewed as being important to the goal of understanding the organization of normal and abnormal development. Individuals in the subclinical range of adaptation (e.g., children with cyclothymic moods) may be vulnerable to the subsequent emergence of psychopathology (e.g., the onset of bipolar I disorder) on the basis of the developmental organization of their biological, psychological, and social systems (e.g., negative attributional styles in the context of adverse family environments in which one or more parents have bipolar spectrum disorders). The investigation of processes that contribute to the later emergence of a disorder, such as BD, as well as processes that mitigate against disordered outcomes provides further insight into the full range of developmental phenomena.

Developmental psychopathology is especially applicable to the investigation of transitional turning points in development across the life span. This is due to its acknowledgment that disorders may appear for the first time in later life and because of its advocacy for the examination of the course of disorders once manifest, including their phases and sequelae (Goodwin & Jamison, 2007; Post, Weiss, & Leverich, 1994; Zigler & Glick, 1986).

Research Approaches within Developmental Psychopathology

The nature of the developmental process elucidates a clear perspective on how to conceptualize empirical research on the origins and course of later emerging psychopathology. Researchers conducting investigations aimed at identifying early precursors of later emerging BD face numerous conceptual and methodological challenges. Because of developmental changes in neurobiological and physiological systems, as well as parallel developments in cognitive, social cognitive, socioemotional, and representational systems, investigators cannot presume phenotypic similarity between early precursors and later impairments (Carlson & Meyer, 2006; Youngstrom, Meyers, Youngstrom, Calabrese, & Findling, 2006). Consequently, studies of the early precursors of later psychopathology should conceptualize and measure features of early development that are theoretically related, but not necessarily behaviorally identical, to the emergence of subsequent BD.

Given the importance of a life span view of developmental processes and an interest in delineating how prior development influences later development, a major issue in developmental psychopathology involves how to determine continuity in the quality of adaptation across developmental time. Sroufe (1979) has articulated the concept of coherence in the organization of behaviors in successive developmental periods as a means of identifying continuity in adaptation despite changing behavioral presentations of the developing individual. Crucial to this concept is a recognition that the same behaviors in different developmental periods may represent quite different levels of adaptation. Behaviors indicating competence within a developmental period may indicate incompetence when evidenced within subsequent developmental periods. Normative behaviors early in development may indicate maladaptation when exhibited later in development. Thus, the manifestation of competence in different developmental periods is rarely indicated by isomorphism in behavioral presentation (i.e., *homotypic continuity*).

Additionally, it must be recognized that the same function in an organized behavioral system can be fulfilled by two dissimilar behaviors, whereas the same kind of behavior may serve two different functions (Werner & Kaplan, 1963) and that the same behavior also may play different roles in different systems. As a result, it is especially important to distinguish between similarities and differences in higher order organization of symptomatology (*molar level*) and component behavioral manifestations of symptomatology (*molecular level*) during different developmental periods. The reorganization of biological and psychological systems that takes place at each new level of development means researchers could not expect to see, for any symptom, behavioral isomorphism at the molecular level, even if there is isomorphism at the molar level. For example, individuals who experience recurrent bipolar depressions during the transition from preoperational to concrete operational thought may display excessive and inappropriate guilt, a loss of self-esteem, and a decrease in activity throughout the episode. Consequently, at a molar level, the depressive symptoms at the latter period (i.e., concrete operational) will be isomorphic to those of the earlier period (i.e., preoperational). Nonetheless, the particular manifestation of the guilt feelings, loss of self-esteem, and psychomotor retardation may change and develop during the transition, when the child's cognitive, representational, socioemotional, and behavioral competencies undergo a rather radical development across these developmental periods. In this way, there may be noteworthy differences at the molecular level.

Because development typically involves the organization through integration of previously differentiated behaviors, we can predict that the expression of bipolar illness may indeed be characterized by molar continuities but additionally by molecular discontinuities and changes. At the molar level, continuity will be preserved by an orderly development in the organization of behaviors; however, at the molecular level, the behaviors that are present at different periods may vary but the meaning may remain coherent (i.e., heterotypic continuity). Thus, a child who exhibits attention-deficit/hyperactivity disorder (ADHD) symptoms at age 7 and develops a bipolar, mixed episode at 15 may have the same molar organization but different molecular behaviors at different phases of development. We believe that the study of the development of the mood disorders over the life course is likely to be fruitful and to reveal the relationship between pathological processes and normal development only if the behavior of individuals with an affective disorder is examined simultaneously at the molar and molecular levels.

Furthermore, examining the course of adaptation once an episode of BD has remitted would benefit from the utilization of a developmental perspective. For example, the examination of the functioning characteristics of individuals previously diagnosed with BD who have returned to a nondisordered condition would provide additional valuable information about BD. It may be possible to identify core characteristics of functioning that remain stable but that no longer give rise to BD because of compensatory factors in the environment, within the individual, or through gene × environment (G × E) interactions that promote resilient adaptations (Cicchetti & Curtis, 2006, 2007). It is conceivable that research such as this might reveal that certain functioning characteristics that were causally relevant to BD in an earlier environment have become positively adaptive in a new context. They not only may not detract from but may actually facilitate successful adaptation. An example might be the personality trait of "novelty seeking" or "exuberance," which before the onset of BD might be associated with abusing drugs, keeping chaotic sleep–wake schedules, or conflict in family relationships. After multiple episodes, a person high in novelty seeking might be more willing to try innovative treatments, to use his or her high energy states in artistic and other creative endeavors, or to experiment with new social contexts that might provide protection against recurrences.

It also may be erroneous to assume that normalized behavior necessarily reflects improvements in processes that were once causal to the development of BD. Accordingly, a developmental psychopathology perspective encourages us to remain open to the possibility that at least some of the characteristics we typically view as functioning deficits in fact may be neutral or even advantageous. Stated differently, they may translate into assets or deficits depending on other characteristics of the individual or the environment. For example, in some contexts acting on impulse may lead individuals with BD to noteworthy and creative achievements, whereas in other contexts impulsive acts may result in persons with BD behaving in a dangerous fashion, resulting in self-destructive outcomes.

PRINCIPLES OF DEVELOPMENTAL PSYCHOPATHOLOGY

In this section, the major principles that are central to elucidating the understanding of both normal and atypical patterns of development are discussed and their relevance to the study of BD is highlighted. It is asserted that the incorporation of these principles into the design and implementation of longitudinal investigations from their inception will proffer a powerful framework for guiding and informing the future research agenda on the causes, sequelae, course, and treatment of BD.

The Mutual Interplay between Normal and Abnormal Development

A focus on the boundary between normal and abnormal development is central to a developmental psychopathology analysis (Cicchetti, 1984, 1989, 1993; Cicchetti & Toth, 1991, 2009; Rutter & Garmezy, 1983). Such a perspective emphasizes not only how knowledge from the study of normal development can inform the study of high-risk conditions and psychopathology but also how the investigation of risk and pathology can enhance our comprehension of normal development.

The study of BD from a developmental perspective can make many significant contributions to theories of normal development, primarily by contributing greater precision to existing theory and by forcing us to examine theories of development critically in relation to our knowledge about psychopathology. The results of such empirical and theoretical investigations may be the description of alternative developmental pathways that lead to the same or different outcomes of the developmental sequence and a weighting of the respective roles of biological, social, emotional, and cognitive factors in mental growth. Furthermore, before one is capable of identifying deviances that exist in a system, one must possess an accurate description of the system itself. Only when we understand the total ongoing development of normal systems can we fully comprehend developmental deviations as adaptational irregularities of those systems (von Bertalanffy, 1968). Because developmental change may be rapid or gradual, it is necessary to consider normative trends of developing skills in the social, emotional, and cognitive domains so as to be in a better position to evaluate deviation or maladjustment. In addition, it is critical to consider intraindividual variation in the overt manifestations of an episode of BD and individual protective factors or stressors that may inhibit or potentiate bipolar illness.

Thus, the application of knowledge of normal biological, cognitive/social cognitive, representational, and socioemotional development to the understanding of bipolar illness results in an articulation of how components of individual functioning in persons with BD contribute to their symptomatic presentation. For example, many of the internal processes implicated in existing theories of BD do not exist in isolation. Deficits in neurobiological, neurochemical, social cognitive, emotion regulatory, parent–child attachment, impulse control, executive functions, neuropsychological development and functioning, and other systems tend to covary significantly in children and adults with BD (see, e.g., Goodwin & Jamison, 2007; Miklowitz & Cicchetti, 2006a). This covariance, in turn, often renders difficult the important task of disentangling causal processes (Richters, 1997). In some instances, suspected causal processes actually may be the products of other covarying systems and only spuriously related to BD. In other cases, a process may indeed influence depressive, hypomanic, or manic behavior; however, the nature and extent of its causal influence may be masked or clouded by the influence of other interacting systems.

One strategy that could be used to help disentangle causal influences among multiple, interactive systems would be to identify and examine the functioning of individuals with BD who possess particular functioning deficits and not others. For example, individuals who have ongoing depressions between bipolar episodes could be compared and contrasted with individuals who have periods of complete remission between their bipolar breaks. Multiple processes investigated individually in this manner may provide significant insights into the distinctive roles they play in normal adaptation and into how those roles might change and require reconceptualization within a broader matrix of functioning deficits among persons with bipolar illness. Conversely, the examination of aberrations in the biological, cognitive, social cognitive, socioemotional, and other biological and psychological domains in individuals with BD contributes to a more complete comprehension of how these systems function in normal development (Cicchetti, 1984, 1993, 2006).

The Importance of a Life Span Perspective

Development extends throughout the entire course of life, and adaptive and maladaptive processes emerge over the life span. From infancy through senescence, each period of life has its own developmental agenda and contributes in a unique fashion to the past, present, and future organization of individual development, normal or abnormal. Thus, individuals with a mood disorder, such as BD, may move between pathological and nonpathological forms of functioning. Moreover, even in the midst of a disordered period, individuals may display adaptive as well as maladaptive processes so that it becomes possible to delimit the presence, nature, and boundaries of the underlying psychopathology.

With respect to the emergence of psychopathology, all periods of life are consequential in that the developmental process may undergo a pernicious turn toward psychiatric disorder at any phase. Many disorders have several distinct phases. The factors that are associated with the onset of a disorder may be very different from those that are associated with the cessation of a disorder or with its repeated occurrence. For example, a positive family history of BD is strongly associated with a higher risk of BD onset. In contrast, a positive family history of BD predicts a good response to lithium once an individual has developed the disorder (Grof, Alda, Grof, Fox, & Cameron, 1993).

In contrast to the often dichotomous world of mental disorder/nondisorder depicted in the extant literature, a developmental psychopathology perspective recognizes that normality often fades into abnormality. Thus, because individuals with BD can have extended periods of normal functioning and also can move into a disordered period unexpectedly, being cognizant of the boundary between normal and atypical functioning is particularly relevant for persons with bipolar illness. For example, it is quite likely that during an acute episode individuals with BD may not recognize that they are in an illness phase. Therefore, strategies for helping them to detect signals of deteriorating functioning during the wellness stage is critically important. Family members, friends, and significant others also can be enlisted and may be helpful in the "detection" process.

Moreover, in developmental psychopathology, "adaptive" and "maladaptive" may assume differing definitions depending on whether one's time referent is immediate circumstances or long-term development, and processes within the individual can be characterized as having shades or degrees of psychopathology. With respect to bipolar illness, such a life span perspective suggests that, even when recurrent depression, hypomania, or mania have occurred, future remission and more adaptive functioning are possible (cf. Jamison, 1993, 1995; Jamison, Gerner, Hammen, & Padesky, 1980; Kraepelin, 1921).

Rutter (1989) has conjectured that key life "turning points" may be times when the presence of protective mechanisms are especially likely to help individuals redirect themselves from a risk trajectory onto a more adaptive developmental pathway. Likewise, Toth and Cicchetti (1999) have suggested that these periods of developmental transition may also afford opportunities when individuals are most amenable to profiting from therapeutic interventions. Whereas change in functioning remains possible at each transitional turning point in development, prior adaptation does place constraints on subsequent adaptation. In particular, the longer an individual continues along a maladaptive ontogenic pathway, the more difficult it is to reclaim a normal developmental trajectory (Cicchetti & Tucker, 1994; Sroufe, 1989). Furthermore, recovery of function to an adaptive level of developmental organization is more likely to occur after a period of pathology if the level of organization before the breakdown was a competent and adaptive one (Sroufe, Egeland, & Kreutzer, 1990).

Developmental Pathways: Diversity in Process and Outcome

Since the emergence of developmental psychopathology as an interdisciplinary science, diversity in process and outcome has been among the hallmarks of its perspective. As Sroufe (1990, p. 335) has asserted, "One of the principal tasks of developmental psychopathology is to define families of developmental pathways, some of which are associated with psychopathology with high probability, others with low probability." Even before a psychiatric disorder emerges, certain pathways signify adaptational failures that probabilistically forebode subsequent psychopathology (Gottlieb, 2007). An example comes from a 40-year follow-up of children who showed mild or moderate externalizing behavior, as rated by teachers when they were ages 13 to 15. By middle adulthood, these children had shown greater rates of alcohol abuse, marital failure, occupational impairment, and psychiatric disorder than comparison children rated low in externalizing behavior (Colman et al., 2009).

It is expected that (1) there are multiple contributors to BD outcomes in any individual, (2) the contributors vary between individuals with BD, (3) there is heterogeneity among persons with BD in the features of their biological and psychological disturbances and underlying dysfunctions, and (4) there are numerous pathways to BD. Moreover, it is believed that there is heterogeneity among individuals who possess many of the risk factors for BD but who do not develop the disorder. In this regard, the principles of equifinality and multifinality, derived from general systems theory (Cicchetti & Rogosch, 1996; von Bertalanffy, 1968), are germane.

Equifinality refers to the observation that a diversity of paths may lead to the same outcome. This alerts us to the possibility that a variety of developmental progressions may eventuate in BD rather than positing a singular primary pathway to disorder. In contrast, *multifinality* suggests that any one component may function differently depending on the organization of the system in which it operates (Cicchetti & Rogosch, 1996; Wilden, 1980). Multifinality states that the effect on functioning of any one component's value may vary in a different system; thus, the same risk factor or starting point may eventuate in a wide dispersion of outcomes. Actual effects will depend on the conditions set by the values of additional components with which it is structurally linked. Consequently, the pathology or health of the system must be identified in terms of how adequately its essential functions are maintained. Stated differently, a particular adverse event should not necessarily be seen as leading to the same psychopathological or nonpsychopathological outcome in every individual with BD. Likewise, individuals with BD may begin on the same major pathway and, as a function of their subsequent "choices," exhibit very different patterns of adaptation or maladaption (Cicchetti & Tucker, 1994; Sroufe, 1989; Sroufe et al., 1990).

For example, it is common for individuals with BD who were maltreated to become engaged in alcohol and drug use (Post & Leverich, 2006). These individuals with BD may engage in alcohol and substance use as a means of self-medicating and escaping from their traumatic experiences and their mood fluctuations. However, not all individuals with BD who were maltreated embark on a substance use pathway and instead will be able to engage in more direct competent means of dealing with their trauma histories, especially if they have the benefit of social supports and appropriate treatment.

Because of the diversity in processes and outcomes that characterize development, the developmental psychopathology approach to BD does not proffer a simple unitary etiological explanation. Although commonalities in pathways in different clusters of persons with BD may be delineated, it also is possible that BD is not the only outcome associated with each pathway. Although pathways may be discovered that are specific to BD in some individuals, there also are likely to be a range of dysfunctions and comorbid dysfunctions and disorders (e.g., anxiety disorders, ADHD, substance abuse disorders, personality disorders), of which an affective disorder (e.g., BD) may be one. Thus, the empirical investigation of BD must be conceptualized within a larger body of inquiry into the developmental patterns promoting adjustment difficulties and psychopathology.

A pathways approach builds on knowledge gained from variable-oriented studies; however, attention is shifted to exploring the common and the uncommon outcomes as well as alternative routes by which outcomes are achieved by different individuals (cf. Cicchetti & Schneider-Rosen, 1986). Thus, what might be considered error variance at the group level must be critically examined for understanding diversity in process and outcome. The emphasis on person-centered observation highlights the transition from a focus on variables to a focus on individuals, and this transition is essential for demonstrating equifinality and multifinality in the developmental course.

The growing knowledge that subgroups of individuals manifesting similar problems arrived at them from different beginnings and that the same risk factors may be associated with different outcomes has proven to be critical not only because it has the potential to bring about important refinements in the diagnostic classification of mental disorders, but also because it calls attention to the importance of continuing to conduct process-oriented studies (Bergman & Magnusson, 1997; Richters & Cicchetti, 1993; von Eye & Bergman, 2003). The examination of patterns of commonality within relatively homogeneous subgroups of individuals and concomitant similarity in profiles of contributory processes becomes an important data analytic strategy. Moreover, the need to examine the totality of attributes, psychopathological conditions, and risk and protective processes in the context of each other rather than in isolation is seen as crucial for understanding the course of development taken by individuals. For example, the presence of BD in a child, adolescent, or adult would have different developmental implications depending on whether it occurs alone or in conjunction with other types of psychopathology. The meaning of any one attribute, process, or psychopathological condition needs to be considered in light of the complex matrix of individual characteristics, experiences, and social contextual influences involved, the timing of events and experiences, and the developmental history of the individual.

This attention to diversity in origins, processes, and outcomes in understanding developmental pathways does not suggest that prediction is futile as a result of the many potential individual patterns of adaptation (Sroufe, 1989). There are constraints on how much diversity is possible, and not all outcomes are equally likely (Cicchetti & Tucker, 1994; Sroufe et al., 1990). Nonetheless, the appreciation of equifinality and multifinality in development encourages theorists and researchers to entertain more complex and varied approaches to how they conceptualize and investigate development and psychopathology. Researchers on BD should increasingly strive to demonstrate the multiplicity of processes and outcomes that may be articulated at the individual, person-oriented level within existing longitudinal data sets. Ultimately, future endeavors must conceptualize and design research on BD at the outset with these differential pathways concepts as a foundation (Richters, 1997). In so doing, progress toward achieving the unique goals of developmental psychopathology—to explain the development of individual patterns of adaptation and maladaptation—will be realized (cf. Sroufe & Rutter, 1984).

Individuals Play an Active Role in Their Own Development

There has been a growing recognition of the role of the developing person as a processor of his or her experiences. The environment does not simply create individuals' experiences; rather, individuals also choose and create their experiences and their own environments in a changing world (Scarr & McCartney, 1983). Individuals select, integrate, and actively affect their own development and the environment in a dynamic fashion (Cicchetti & Tucker, 1994; Wachs & Plomin, 1991). The principle of contextualism conceptualizes developmental processes as the ongoing interaction between an active, changing individual and a continuously unfolding, dynamic context (Cicchetti & Aber, 1998). Thus, maladaptation and psychopathology are considered to be products of the transaction among an individual's intraorganismic characteristics, adaptational history, and the current context (Boyce et al., 1998; Sroufe, 1997).

Various difficulties will constitute different meanings for an individual depending on cultural considerations (Garcia Coll, Akerman, & Cicchetti, 2000) as well as an individual's experiential history and current level of psychological and biological functioning. The integration of the experience, in turn, will affect the adaptation or maladaptation that ensues. Moreover, we now know that social contexts exert effects not only on psychological processes but also on biological structures, functions, and processes (Boyce et al., 1998; Cicchetti, 2002; Cicchetti & Tucker, 1994; DeBellis, 2001; Eisenberg, 1995; Nelson & Bloom, 1997). For example, persons at risk for developing BD who experience traumatic environmental adversity will possess a greater likelihood that their genetic vulnerability will get expressed and that the neural circuitry associated with aspects of BD will be activated (see Post & Miklowitz, Chapter 12, this volume).

Multiple Levels of Analysis

A "systems view" conceives development as being hierarchically organized into multiple levels that mutually influence each other (Gottlieb, 1992; Thelen & Smith, 1998). "Top-down" as well as "bottom-up" bidirectional effects are theorized to occur among the various levels. Accordingly, genetic activity ↔ neural activity ↔ behavior ↔ environment can serve as a schematic representation of this systems view. These bidirectional effects among levels of the system result in a probabilistic conceptualization of epigenetic development in all individuals, including those with a mental illness, such as persons with BD (Cicchetti & Tucker, 1994; Gottlieb, 1992). The probabilistic epigenesis perspective thus implies that individuals are neither unaffected by earlier experiences nor immutably controlled by them. Change in developmental course is thought to be possible as a result of new experiences, reciprocal interactions between levels of the developing person, and the individual's active self-organizing strivings for adaptation (see also Cicchetti & Tucker, 1994). Thus, epigenesis is viewed as probabilistic rather than predetermined, with the bidirectional and transactional nature of genetic, neural, behavioral, and environmental influences over the life course capturing the essence of probabilistic experiences. Because development is a dynamic process, assertions about causality must include a temporal dimension that specifies and describes when the experience or coactions occurred (Gottlieb & Halpern, 2002).

Different levels of analysis—genetic, biological, social, psychological, familial, or cultural—constrain other levels. As scientists investigating BD learn more about multiple levels of analysis, researchers conducting their work at each level will need to develop theories that are consistent across all levels. When scientists in different disciplines function in isolation, they run the risk of formulating theories that will ultimately prove to be incorrect because vital information from other disciplines has either been ignored or is unknown. Just as is the case in systems neuroscience (Cowan, Harter, & Kandel, 2000), it is critical that there be an integrative framework that incorporates all levels of analysis about complex systems in the development of BD. As Miklowitz and Cicchetti (2006b) stated, "An interdisciplinary multiple-levels-of-analysis approach has the potential to become the guiding light in the next generation of studies on bipolar disorder" (p. 937).

It is now widely understood that individual risk factors seldom are powerful enough to exert sufficient influence to result in psychopathology (Sameroff & Chandler, 1975; Willcutt & McQueen, Chapter 8, this volume). Moreover, when they appear to have such effects, it is highly likely that they are surrogates for multiple, unobserved influences. Much more commonly, adequate prediction of either disturbance or resilience necessitates the consideration of multiple risk and protective factors and their interplay (Cicchetti & Rogosch, 1999). Moreover, the consequences of any risk factor depend on myriad other aspects embedded in the developmental context. For example, even abused and neglected children, who generally are confronted with an array of difficulties in addition to their maltreatment experiences, differ in their functioning depending on the level of community violence present in their lives; abused and neglected children who resided in settings high in extrafamilial violence exhibit the highest level of behavioral problems (Lynch & Cicchetti, 1998).

In addition, a particular vulnerability may not pose risk in the context of a protective condition. For example, Suomi (2000) has discovered that, relative to the long (l) allele, the short (s) allele in the serotonin transporter gene promoter region confers no detectable liability for rhesus monkeys reared by nurturant foster mothers; in fact, such animals become leaders of the group. Yet the same gene polymorphism may confer vulnerability for anxiety and behavioral pathology in monkeys raised without adults. In another interesting example, Baldwin, Baldwin, and Cole (1990) found that in high-risk families from low-socioeconomic backgrounds, levels of restriction and control in parenting (i.e., authoritarian par-

enting practices) were related to successful child outcomes, and that such parenting practices were more frequent in high-risk than in low-risk families showing
child success. Accordingly, controlling forms of parenting may be a protective
factor for one group but not for another. These examples also illustrate the probabilistic rather than the causal status of risk factors. Knowledge of the differential
mechanisms that underlie disparate subgroups of disorders (i.e., equifinality) can
help to enhance the specificity of prediction from risk factors to developmental
outcome.

Over the course of the past several decades, there has been a growing
acknowledgment that the investigation of developmental processes, both normal
and abnormal, necessitates that scientists must utilize different methods and levels of analysis depending on the questions being addressed in their research. One
of the most dramatic examples of this is the work on experience-dependent brain
development (Black, Jones, Nelson, & Greenough, 1998; Greenough, Black, &
Wallace, 1987). The viewpoint is now widely shared that neurobiological development and experience are mutually influencing (Cicchetti & Tucker, 1994; Eisenberg, 1995; Nelson & Bloom, 1997). Rather than adhering to a unidimensional
belief in the deterministic role that unfolding biology exerts on behavior, it is
now widely believed that brain function and its subsequent influence on behavior
possesses self-organizing functions that can, in fact, be altered by experiences
incurred during sensitive periods of development. Specifically, it has been demonstrated that social and psychological experiences can modify gene expression and
brain structure, functioning, and organization, including patterns of neuronal
and synaptic connections (Kandel, 1998, 1999). Such experiential conditions may
interact with an individual's genetic makeup to alter processes, such as the timing
of the initiation of transcription for a specific gene, the duration for which it does
so, or whether the gene will be translated or expressed. These changes not only
contribute to the biological bases of individuality but also play a prominent role
in initiating and maintaining the behavioral anomalies that are induced by social
and psychological experiences (Kandel, 1998).

The mechanisms of neural plasticity are integral to the very anatomical structure of cortical tissue and cause the formation of the brain to involve an extended
malleable process that presents developmental psychopathologists with new ave-
nues for understanding the vulnerability of the brain as a basis for the emergence
of mental disorder. Perturbations that take place in the developing brain can trigger a cascade of growth and function changes that lead the neural system down
a path that deviates from that usually taken in normal neurobiological development, resulting in the development of aberrant neural circuitry that contributes to
these early developmental abnormalities, eventuating in relatively enduring forms
of psychopathology (Black et al., 1998; Cicchetti & Cannon, 1999; Cicchetti &
Thomas, 2008; Courchesne, Chisum, & Townsend, 1994; Nowakowski & Hayes,
1999).

To comprehend BD in its full complexity, all levels of analysis must be examined and integrated. Research in the area of resilience has begun to follow this

interdisciplinary, multiple-levels-of-analysis perspective (Cicchetti & Blender, 2006; Cicchetti & Rogosch, 2007; Curtis & Cicchetti, 2007; see also papers in Cicchetti & Curtis, 2007).

Resilience

Developmental psychopathologists are as interested in individuals at high risk for the development of psychopathology who do not manifest it over time as they are in individuals who develop an actual mental disorder (Cicchetti & Garmezy, 1993; Luthar, 2006; Luthar, Cicchetti, & Becker, 2000; Masten, 1989; Masten, Best, & Garmezy, 1990). Moreover, researchers in developmental psychopathology emphasize the importance of understanding the functioning of individuals who, after having diverged onto deviant developmental pathways, resume normal functioning and achieve adequate adaptation (Cicchetti & Rogosch, 1997; Masten et al., 1990).

Resilience has been operationalized as the individual's capacity for adapting successfully and functioning competently despite experiencing chronic adversity or after exposure to prolonged or severe trauma. Resilience is a dynamic developmental process; it is multidimensional in nature, exemplified by findings that individuals who are at high risk for or who have a mental disorder may manifest competence in some domains and contexts, whereas they may exhibit problems in others.

Research on the determinants of resilience also highlights the need to examine functioning across multiple domains of development. An example from BD is provided by Keck and colleagues (1998), who found that, after a manic or mixed episode, 48% of adults with bipolar I disorder had symptomatically recovered by 1 year. When recovery was defined as "functional," meaning the regaining of preepisode level of social–occupational status, the rate was only 24%. To provide a further example, consider a school-age child with BD who was formerly categorized as resilient based solely on an examination of his or her cognitive abilities. If that child manifests subsequent poor peer relationships over time, many would assume that the child is evidencing discontinuity from his or her earlier resilient cognitive functioning. In fact, we may be observing evidence of maladaptation that would have been observed much earlier had his or her peer relations been previously examined. Furthermore, the ability to function in a resilient fashion in the presence of biological, psychological, environmental, and sociocultural disadvantage may be achieved through the use of developmental pathways that are less typical than those negotiated in usual circumstances. Thus, an important question for researchers to address is whether the employment of alternative pathways to attaining competence renders individuals more vulnerable to manifesting delays or deviations in development. Although only prospective longitudinal investigations can fully address this issue, it is critical to ascertain whether these individuals are more prone to developing maladaptation or psychopathology in later life. Given the nonstatic nature of the construct, we do not expect children identified as resilient to be immune to declines in functioning at each subsequent developmental period.

Investigations aimed at discovering the processes leading to resilient outcomes and on the processes underlying recovery of adaptive function offer great promise as an avenue for facilitating the development of prevention and intervention strategies (Luthar et al., 2000; Toth & Cicchetti, 1999). Through the examination of the proximal and distal processes and mechanisms that contribute to positive adaptation in situations that more typically eventuate in maladaptation, researchers and clinicians will be better prepared to devise ways of promoting competent outcomes in individuals at high risk for developing BD (Beardslee & Podorefsky, 1988; Luthar & Cicchetti, 2000).

Despite the attention paid to discovering the processes through which individuals at high risk do not develop maladaptively, the empirical study of resilience has focused primarily on detecting the psychosocial determinants of the phenomenon (Charney, 2004; Curtis & Cicchetti, 2003). For research on resilience to grow in ways that are commensurate with the complexity inherent to the construct, efforts to understand underlying processes will be facilitated by the increased implementation of multidisciplinary investigations designed within a developmental psychopathology framework. Research of this nature would entail a consideration of biological, psychological, and environmental/contextual processes from which varied pathways to resilience (equifinality) might eventuate as well as those that result in diverse outcomes among individuals who have achieved resilient functioning (multifinality) (see Cicchetti & Curtis, 2007). Along these lines, the investigation of multiple aspects of the processes underlying resilience can shed light on the nature of the interrelation among various developmental domains in individuals with BD. For example, how do cognition, affect, and neurobiological growth relate with one another at various developmental periods? When an advance or a lag occurs in one biological or psychological system, what are the consequences for other systems?

It is important that these issues receive focused attention from researchers, because the presence of capacities of one of these systems may be a necessary condition for the development or exercise of capacities of another system. For example, certain cognitive skills may be necessary for the development of particular affective expressions and experiences (Hesse & Cicchetti, 1982). Lags in these systems may then result in compensatory development, which may, in some instances, leave the child vulnerable to psychopathology. Over time, difficulty in the organization of one biological or psychological system may tend to promote difficulty in the way in which other systems are organized as hierarchical integration between the separate systems occurs. The organization of the individual may then appear to consist of poorly integrated component systems. As the converse of the effects of early competence, early incompetence will tend to promote later incompetence because the individual arrives at successive developmental stages with less than optimal resources available for responding to the challenges of that period. Again, however, this progression is not inevitable but probabilistic. Changes in the internal and external environment may lead to improvements in the ability to grapple with developmental challenges, resulting in a redirection in the developmental course.

The role of biological factors in resilience is suggested by evidence on neurobiological and neuroendocrine function in relation to stress regulation and reactivity (Cicchetti, Rogosch, Gunnar, & Toth, in press; Gunnar & Vazquez, 2006), by behavioral genetics research on nonshared environmental effects (Rende & Waldman, 2006), and by molecular genetics research that may reveal the genetic elements that serve a protective function for individuals experiencing significant adversity (Cicchetti & Blender, 2006). To provide an example gleaned from the field of molecular genetics, research suggests that it is conceivable that the gene encoding high monoamine oxidase A (MAOA) activity and the l/l genotype of the serotonin transporter gene (5-HTT) gene may confer protection against the development of antisocial behavior in males who have been maltreated and against the development of depression in individuals who have been maltreated, respectively (Caspi et al., 2002, 2003). Consequently, the negative developmental sequelae associated with child maltreatment are not inevitable but appear to be the result of G × E interactions between risk (i.e., low-activity MAOA; the s/s genotype of 5-HTT) or protective (i.e., high-activity MAOA; the l/l genotype of 5-HTT) genes and maltreatment (see Cicchetti, Rogosch, & Sturge-Apple, 2007).

Several studies of early childhood adversity and the subsequent development of early-onset BD have suggested that adults with bipolar illness who had been physically or sexually abused during childhood not only displayed an earlier onset of BD than did nonabused adults with BD but also experienced a more severe and treatment-resistant course once the illness became manifest (Post & Leverich, 2006). In addition to the experience of early child abuse, it would be important to investigate whether the presence of risk alleles of genes implicated in BD were interacting with physical and sexual maltreatment to produce the severe outcomes (Hayden & Nurnberger, 2006; Serretti & Mandelli, 2008; Willcutt & McQueen, Chapter 8, this volume).

Children who develop in a resilient fashion despite having experienced significant adversity play an active role in constructing, seeking, and receiving the experiences that are developmentally appropriate for them. To date, research investigations that search for mechanisms of G × E interaction have yet to address the role that genetic factors may play in influencing how children who are developing in a resilient fashion have actively transformed their social environment (known as evocative gene–environment correlation) (Rende & Waldman, 2006; Scarr & McCartney, 1983). At the neurobiological level, different areas of the brain may attempt to compensate; on another level, individuals may seek out new experiences in areas where they have strength (Black et al., 1998; Cicchetti & Tucker, 1994). The effects of social experiences, such as child abuse and neglect, on brain biochemistry and microstructure may be either pathological or adaptive. With respect to the experience of child maltreatment, depending on how the individual interprets and responds to the abuse, as well as the genetic elements that are expressed, the effects either may be pathological (the typical outcome) or may not preclude normative development (a resilient outcome) (Cicchetti & Rogosch, 2009; Cicchetti & Valentino, 2006). Thus, neither early neurobiological anomalies nor aberrant experiences should be considered as determining the ultimate fate of the individual with BD (the notion of probabilistic epigenesis).

A multilevel approach to resilience also affords an additional avenue for examining the biological and social constraints that may operate on aspects of the developmental process throughout the life course. Moreover, through investigating the multiple determinants of resilient adaptation, we are in a position to discover the range and variability in individuals' attempts to respond adaptively to challenge and ill fortune.

Translational Research

In recent years, the National Institute of Mental Health has emphasized the importance of translational research in the biological, behavioral, and social sciences (Cicchetti & Toth, 2006; Gunnar & Cicchetti, 2009). In the National Advisory Mental Health Council's (2000) report *Translating Behavioral Science into Action*, strategies for enhancing contributions of behavioral science to society more broadly were proposed. In this report, "translational research is defined as research designed to address how basic behavioral processes inform the diagnosis, prevention, treatment, and delivery of services for mental illness, and, conversely, how knowledge of mental illness increases our understanding of basic behavioral processes" (p. iii). Research examining basic biological processes, such as in genetic and neuroscience investigations on mental illness, also can be translated into preventive interventions and treatment initiatives (Cicchetti & Gunnar, 2009; Cicchetti & Thomas, 2008). The formulation of translational research in the behavioral and biological sciences is in direct accord with three of the key tenets of a developmental psychopathology perspective, namely the reciprocal interplay between basic and applied research, between normal and abnormal development, and a multiple-levels-of-analysis perspective (Cicchetti & Toth, 1991, 1998; Pellmar & Eisenberg, 2000). Research on resilience from a multilevel perspective is an excellent example of translational research because it also lends itself to informing prevention and intervention initiatives.

The principles of developmental psychopathology lend themselves to fostering translational research that has implications for society, policymakers, and individuals with BD and their families. The very subject matter of the field of developmental psychopathology necessitates thinking clearly about the implications of the work and devising strategies that will help to remedy the problems associated with BD. By developing relationships between researchers from different disciplines and policymakers, social policy initiatives also can build upon empirical evidence. Furthermore, if basic research on individuals with BD is designed with clinical and policy questions at the forefront, rather than as a post hoc afterthought, a true research-informed policy agenda would be achieved that could benefit the welfare of persons suffering from BD and their families.

For example, at what phases of development will psychosocial interventions have a maximal preventive effect among children at risk for BD and by what mechanisms? Basic neurobiological research could inform our understanding of when children at risk for BD develop facial emotion recognition errors (e.g., viewing neutral faces as negative) and the neural structures and circuitry with which these errors are correlated (i.e., amygdala/ventromedial prefrontal cortex circuits) (Rich et al., 2006). Results of such studies may suggest that certain forms of psychosocial intervention (e.g., psychoeducation, cognitive-behavioral therapy, or interpersonal therapy) can effectively teach emotion labeling skills, but only among children who have shown an ability to mentalize or infer emotional states in others. In turn, demonstrating that such interventions influence aberrant neural pathways and result in symptom improvement, in part mediated by improved emotion recognition, would inform our understanding of developmental pathways in the onset of BD.

Prevention and Intervention

The major objective of the field of prevention science is to intervene in the course of development in order to reduce or eliminate the emergence of maladaptation and mental disorder as well as to promote resilient adaptation in individuals at high risk for psychopathology (Ialongo et al., 2006). To achieve this laudable goal, it is essential that prevention scientists possess a complex, multilevel understanding of the course of normality to formulate an in-depth portrayal of how deviations in normal developmental processes can eventuate in maladaptation and mental disorder. Because of its focus on the mutual interplay between the investigation of normal and abnormal development, the field of developmental psychopathology is well poised to provide the theoretical foundation for prevention and intervention initiatives (Institute of Medicine, 1994).

Developmental psychopathologists believe that efforts to prevent the emergence of psychopathology or to ameliorate its effects also can be informative for understanding processes involved in psychopathological development (Hinshaw, 2002; Kellam & Rebok, 1992). For example, if the course of development is altered as a result of the implementation of randomized controlled prevention trials and the risk for negative outcomes is reduced, then prevention research helps to specify processes that are involved in the emergence of psychopathology or other maladaptive developmental outcomes (Ialongo et al., 2006). As a consequence, if randomized controlled prevention trials examine mechanisms of intervention action, then they can be conceptualized as true experiments in modifying the developmental course, thereby providing insight into the etiology and pathogenesis of disordered outcomes (Cicchetti & Hinshaw, 2002; Hinshaw, 2002; Howe, Reiss, & Yuh, 2002; Kellam & Rebok, 1992). Thus, prevention research not only leads to support or lack of support for theoretical formulations accounting for the development of psychopathology, but it also can contribute to the knowledge base of strategies that can be implemented to reduce psychopathology and promote positive adaptation. Knowledge of developmental norms, appreciation of how developmental level may vary within the same age group, sensitivity to the changing meaning that problems have at different developmental levels, attention to the effects of developmental transitions and reorganizations, and understanding of the factors that are essential features to incorporate into the design and implementation of preventive interventions all may serve to enhance the potential for optimal intervention efficacy (Noam, 1992; Toth & Cicchetti, 1999).

Whereas much of the work on BD and other types of psychopathology is, of necessity, naturalistic and correlational in nature, given ethical constraints on randomly assigning developing persons to key environmental or psychobiological conditions, the gold standard for clinical intervention and prevention research is the randomized clinical trial. The experimental nature of such investigations provides an unprecedented opportunity to make causal inferences in the field (Kraemer, Wilson, Fairburn, & Agras, 2002). The types of independent variables manipulated in clinical or prevention trials may be several steps removed from crucial, underlying etiological factors, given that such trials are primarily concerned with the practical, clinical goals of alleviating suffering and promoting competence rather than isolating primary causal variables. Nonetheless, careful research design and assiduous measurement of ancillary, psychological, and biological process variables through which intervention effects may occur can shed light on theory-driven mechanisms underlying healthy and pathological development (Cicchetti & Gunnar, 2008; Hinshaw, 2002; Howe et al., 2002; Kraemer et al., 2002).

Research on BD has directed too little effort toward developing and evaluating psychosocial models of prevention that can be adjunctive to pharmacological treatment (for an exception, see Miklowitz & Chang, 2008). (For examples of efficacious preventive interventions for mothers with major depressive disorder and their young offspring, see Cicchetti, Rogosch, & Toth, 2000; Toth, Rogosch, Manly, & Cicchetti, 2006.) Rather than awaiting a full-blown disorder to emerge, risk markers that portend possible illness could be identified. Early identification and possible prevention could minimize the magnitude of the disease process and possible impairment. Prevention strategies become particularly relevant to the increasing diagnosis of the disorder in early childhood. As we progress with the ability to detect genetic and neurobiological markers of disease, prevention again emerges as an important future avenue to pursue. Such prevention strategies also could minimize the likelihood of the brain circuitry for BD becoming hardwired and increasingly recalcitrant to potential neuroplastic changes.

CONCLUSION AND FUTURE DIRECTIONS

Although it is evident that research on BD has engendered greater clarity with respect to clinical description, etiology, pathogenesis, psychosocial and drug treatment, and development, there remains much to examine in the future. I discuss several empirical and practical issues that require greater attention as well as areas in need of enhanced theoretical integration (see Table 1.1 for illustrative examples).

To begin, a developmental psychopathology perspective underscores the importance of conducting ongoing prospective multiwave longitudinal studies that are properly designed and methodologically rigorous and that can provide an accurate portrayal of the life course trajectories of those afflicted with the varying subtypes of BD. Moreover, there is a strong need to be able to investigate BD before it emerges. What populations should be targeted to enhance the likelihood of observing BD at greater than population prevalence rates? What are the earlier precursors to BD across multiple levels of analysis? How can prodromal abnormal signs be identified within the framework of developmental psychopathology? A developmental perspective also would help to articulate and understand those factors that may contribute to the maintenance of BD over the life course, quite separate from those that might contribute to its etiology. In particular, a fuller comprehension of the role played by child physical and sexual abuse and child neglect in the development of BD is needed (Post & Leverich, 2006).

Another area that merits attention is the need to resolve the underlying structure and natural organization of BD. The DSM approach to diagnosing BD yields a phenotype that is characterized by considerable heterogeneity. Consequently, there exists great variability across the population of individuals diagnosed as having BD. This heterogeneity may reflect our flawed efforts to conceptualize a

---

TABLE 1.1. Future Research and Practical Issues on Bipolar Disorder: A Developmental Psychopathology Approach

- Research in the interdisciplinary field of developmental psychopathology examines processes underlying the interrelation between adaptive and maladaptive development over the life course. The principles of this discipline can be used to augment the understanding and treatment of BD.
- A multiple-levels-of-analysis perspective and an interdisciplinary developmental psychopathology approach must be incorporated into the research armamentaria of investigators studying BD.
- Investigations conceived within a developmental psychopathology framework must incorporate a multilevel perspective in the study of the processes leading to resilient adaptation in individuals with BD.
- Theory and empirical research on basic biological and psychological developmental processes must increasingly be used to inform prevention and intervention initiatives in BD.
- Scientific discoveries emanating from developmental psychopathology must be translated into practical social policy applications that contribute to reducing the stigma that exacerbates the burden of mental illness for individuals with BD and their families.

complex phenotype, variability in the underlying pathological process, the DSM decision to dichotomize a collection of dimensional symptom and trait variables, or all three. It is important to undertake latent structure statistical analyses of the BD phenotype; sophisticated data analytic methods now exist that enable researchers to sort individuals efficiently into meaningful relatively homogeneous clusters (e.g., finite mixture modeling; latent-class analysis).

Clinical features that run in families may aid in the categorization of more homogeneous phenotypes of BD. One such feature is polarity at illness onset, which is related to severity and course of BD. Kassem and colleagues (2006) discovered that sibling pairs with BD who were concordant for mania at illness onset were, on average, older, less likely to exhibit panic attacks or alcoholism, and more likely to display genetic linkage to chromosome 16p but no linkage to chromosome 6q. Thus, polarity at onset may be useful in the delineation of homogeneous subtypes of BD that may have distinct developmental courses.

Research in the area of endophenotypes also should be conducted. The endophenotype is a measurable component, unseen by the unaided eye, along the pathway between distal genotype and disease (Gottesman & Gould, 2003; Gottesman & Shields, 1972). Endophenotypes may be neurophysiological, endocrinological, neuroanatomical, cognitive, or neuropsychological in nature. Furthermore, the endophenotype is thought to represent a simpler clue to genetic underpinnings than the disease syndrome itself. The incorporation of endophenotypes will be extremely useful to advancing genomic, neuroimaging, neurobiological, and psychological investigations of BD.

Investigators and practitioners with a developmental perspective are interested not only in the differences between individuals with and without mental disorders but also in their similarities (Cicchetti, 1993; Zigler & Glick, 1986). Indeed, there are striking similarities between persons with bipolar illness and their well counterparts. For example, children and adults with BD, just as with persons who are nondisordered, experience a range of feelings, possess a need for connectedness with others, seek a sense of order in their worlds, strive for autonomy, and attempt to find meaning in their life experiences (Hinshaw & Cicchetti, 2000).

Individuals with BD typically shift from phases of normality to psychopathology and back. Almost all such individuals experience stages and phases of remission and relapse throughout the life span. Moreover, not only do persons with BD have periods of remission, but also an appreciable number manage to function in an adaptive and productive manner for prolonged periods of their lives. Accordingly, individuals with BD should not be reduced to their psychiatric diagnoses. Those persons with BD who have been successfully treated and those whose illnesses are in remission may be strikingly similar to persons who are without mental disorder. Unlike other psychotic spectrum disorders where impairment may be more chronic, individuals with BD may lead productive and fulfilled lives (see Hinshaw, 2005). As such, the stigma that commonly accompanies major mental disorders might be minimized if the public were sufficiently educated about the resilience that is possible. The processes that promote resilience in BD should be a central focus of the next generation of research in BD.

In contrast to the viewpoint that mental disorders are "brain disorders" or "brain diseases," developmental psychopathologists conceptualize mental disorders in a more complex, dynamic systems fashion (Cicchetti & Cannon, 1999; Cicchetti & Thomas, 2008; Cicchetti & Tucker, 1994). Although the brain is clearly involved in all mental disorders, many other systems contribute and transact with the brain in dynamic fashion over the life course to bring about experience-dependent brain development (Greenough et al., 1987). The motivation underlying the promotion of the viewpoint that mental disorders are "brain diseases" may, in part, be to help reduce personal and family blame for aberrant behavior and emotion (Hinshaw & Cicchetti, 2000). Nonetheless, it is essential that researchers convey scientific truth to the lay public regarding the complex, multilevel, and dynamic processes that undergird the development of psychopathology in general and BD in particular. Whereas we believe that there are strong psychobiological predispositions to many forms of mental disorder, the concept of "brain disorder" may connote primacy or exclusivity for the biology and fail to underscore transactional processes. The increased emphasis on a multilevel, dynamic systems approach to psychopathology and resilience (Cicchetti & Blender, 2006; Cicchetti & Curtis, 2007; Masten, 2007), the growing attention paid to G × E investigations in the development of psychopathology and resilience (Cicchetti, 2007; Moffitt, Caspi, & Rutter, 2006; Rutter, 2006), and the application of a multilevel developmental psychopathology perspective to mental illnesses that have traditionally been studied nondevelopmentally (such as BD) will contribute to educating the public about the causes and consequences of mental disorder. The reduction of stigmatization toward persons with mental disorder, which can actually be exacerbated by simplified attributions like "brain disorder," will contribute to reducing the burden of mental illness for persons with BD and their families (Hinshaw, 2006).

Research in developmental psychopathology has enhanced our understanding of risk, disorder, and resilience across the life course (see, e.g., Cicchetti & Cohen, 1995a, 1995b, 2006a, 2006b, 2006c). Advances in genomics, G × E interactions, and epigenetics, growth in the understanding of neurobiology and neural plasticity, and progress in the development of methodological and technological tools, including brain imaging, hormone assays, and statistical analysis of developmental change, pave the way for multiple-levels-of-analysis research programs aimed at elucidating the development and course of BD (Cicchetti & Curtis, 2006; Masten, 2006). Moreover, the information that is emanating from the field of developmental psychopathology can be integrated into the conceptual base and measurement armamentaria of scientists from diverse disciplines, even if they do not consider themselves to be developmental psychopathologists. These knowledge gains not only will benefit the scientific study of BD but will also permit translation to informing developmentally based preventive strategies and interventions that will contribute to reducing the individual, familial, and societal burden of BD.

REFERENCES

Baldwin, A., Baldwin, C., & Cole, R. (1990). Stress-resistant families and stress-resistant children. In J. Rolf, A. Masten, D. Cicchetti, K. Nuechterlein, & S. Weintraub (Eds.), *Risk and protective factors in the development of psychopathology* (pp. 257–280). New York: Cambridge University Press.

Beardslee, W. R., & Podorefsky, M. (1988). Resilient adolescents whose parents have serious affective and other psychiatric disorders: Importance of self-understanding and relationships. *American Journal of Psychiatry, 145,* 63–69.

Bergman, L. R., & Magnusson, D. (1997). A person-oriented approach in research on developmental psychopathology. *Development and Psychopathology, 9,* 291–319.

Black, J., Jones, T. A., Nelson, C. A., & Greenough, W. T. (1998). Neuronal plasticity and the developing brain. In N. E. Alessi, J. T. Coyle, S. I. Harrison, & S. Eth (Eds.), *Handbook of child and adolescent psychiatry* (pp. 31–53). New York: Wiley.

Boyce, W. T., Frank, E., Jensen, P. S., Kessler, R. C., Nelson, C. A., Steinberg, L., et al. (1998). Social context in developmental psychopathology: Recommendations for future research from the MacArthur Network on Psychopathology and Development. *Development and Psychopathology, 10,* 143–164.

Carlson, G. A., & Meyer, S. E. (2006). Phenomenology and diagnosis of bipolar disorder in children, adolescents, and adults: Complexities and development issues. *Development and Psychopathology, 18,* 939–969.

Caspi, A., McClay, J., Moffitt, T., Mill, J., Martin, J., Craig, I. W., et al. (2002). Role of genotype in the cycle of violence in maltreated children. *Science, 297,* 851–854.

Caspi, A., Sugden, K., Moffitt, T. E., Taylor, A., Craig, I. W., Harrington, H. L., et al. (2003). Influence of life stress on depression: Moderation by a polymorphism in the 5-HTT gene. *Science, 301,* 386–389.

Charney, D. (2004). Psychobiological mechanisms of resilience and vulnerability: Implications for successful adaptation to extreme stress. *American Journal of Psychiatry, 161,* 195–216.

Cicchetti, D. (1984). The emergence of developmental psychopathology. *Child Development, 55,* 1–7.

Cicchetti, D. (Ed.). (1989). *Rochester Symposium on Developmental Psychopathology: The emergence of a discipline* (Vol. 1). Hillsdale, NJ: Erlbaum.

Cicchetti, D. (1990). A historical perspective on the discipline of developmental psychopathology. In J. Rolf, A. Masten, D. Cicchetti, K. Nuechterlein, & S. Weintraub (Eds.), *Risk and protective factors in the development of psychopathology* (pp. 2–28). New York: Cambridge University Press.

Cicchetti, D. (1993). Developmental psychopathology: Reactions, reflections, projections. *Developmental Review, 13,* 471–502.

Cicchetti, D. (2002). The impact of social experience on neurobiological systems: Illustration from a constructivist view of child maltreatment. *Cognitive Development, 17,* 1407–1428.

Cicchetti, D. (2006). Development and psychopathology. In D. Cicchetti & D. Cohen (Eds.), *Developmental psychopathology* (2nd ed., Vol. 1, pp. 1–23). New York: Wiley.

Cicchetti, D. (Ed.). (2007). Gene–environment interaction [Special issue]. *Development and Psychopathology, 19*(4).

Cicchetti, D. (2008). A multiple-levels-of-analysis perspective on research in development and psychopathology. In T. P. Beauchaine & S. P. Hinshaw (Eds.), *Child and adolescent psychopathology* (pp. 27–57). New York: Wiley.

Cicchetti, D., & Aber, J. L. (Eds.). (1998). Contextualism and developmental psychopathology [Special issue]. *Development and Psychopathology, 10*(2).

Cicchetti, D., & Blender, J. A. (2006). A multiple-levels-of-analysis perspective on resilience: Implications for the developing brain, neural plasticity, and preventive interventions. *Annals of the New York Academy of Science, 1094*, 248–258.

Cicchetti, D., & Cannon, T. D. (1999). Neurodevelopmental processes in the ontogenesis and epigenesis of psychopathology. *Development and Psychopathology, 11*, 375–393.

Cicchetti, D., & Cohen, D. J. (Eds.). (1995a). *Developmental psychopathology: Risk, disorder, and adaptation* (Vol. 2). New York: Wiley.

Cicchetti, D., & Cohen, D. J. (Eds.). (1995b). *Developmental psychopathology: Theory and method* (Vol. 1). New York: Wiley.

Cicchetti, D., & Cohen, D. (Eds.). (2006a). *Developmental psychopathology: Developmental neuroscience* (2nd ed., Vol. 2). New York: Wiley.

Cicchetti, D., & Cohen, D. (Eds.). (2006b). *Developmental psychopathology: Risk, disorder, and adaptation* (2nd ed., Vol. 3). New York: Wiley.

Cicchetti, D., & Cohen, D. (Eds.). (2006c). *Developmental psychopathology: Theory and method* (2nd ed., Vol. 1). New York: Wiley.

Cicchetti, D., & Curtis, W. J. (2006). The developing brain and neural plasticity: Implications for normality, psychopathology, and resilience. In D. Cicchetti & D. Cohen (Eds.), *Developmental psychopathology* (2nd ed., Vol. 2, pp. 1–64). New York: Wiley.

Cicchetti, D., & Curtis, W. J. (Eds.). (2007). A multilevel approach to resilience [Special issue]. *Development and Psychopathology, 19*(3).

Cicchetti, D., & Garmezy, N. (1993). Prospects and promises in the study of resilience. *Development and Psychopathology, 5*, 497–502.

Cicchetti, D., & Gunnar, M. R. (2008). Integrating biological processes into the design and evaluation of preventive interventions. *Development and Psychopathology, 20*, 737–743.

Cicchetti, D., & Gunnar, M. R. (Eds.). (2009). *Meeting the challenge of translational research in child psychology: Minnesota Symposium on Child Psychology* (Vol. 35). New York: Wiley.

Cicchetti, D., & Hinshaw, S. P. (Eds.). (2002). Prevention and intervention science: Contributions to developmental theory [Special issue]. *Development and Psychopathology, 14*(4).

Cicchetti, D., & Pogge-Hesse, P. (1982). Possible contributions of the study of organically retarded persons to developmental theory. In E. Zigler & D. Balla (Eds.), *Mental retardation: The developmental difference controversy* (pp. 277–318). Hillsdale, NJ: Erlbaum.

Cicchetti, D., & Posner, M. I. (2005). Cognitive and affective neuroscience and developmental psychopathology. *Development and Psychopathology, 17*, 569–575.

Cicchetti, D., & Rogosch, F. A. (1996). Equifinality and multifinality in developmental psychopathology. *Development and Psychopathology, 8*, 597–600.

Cicchetti, D., & Rogosch, F. A. (1997). The role of self-organization in the promotion of resilience in maltreated children. *Development and Psychopathology, 9*, 799–817.

Cicchetti, D., & Rogosch, F. A. (1999). Psychopathology as risk for adolescent substance use disorders: A developmental psychopathology perspective. *Journal of Clinical Child Psychology, 28*, 355–365.

Cicchetti, D., & Rogosch, F. A. (2007). Personality, adrenal steroid hormones, and resilience in maltreated children: A multi-level perspective. *Development and Psychopathology, 19*, 787–809.

Cicchetti, D., & Rogosch, F. A. (2009). Adaptive coping under conditions of extreme stress:

Multi-level influences on the determinants of resilience in maltreated children. In E. Skinner & M. J. Zimmer-Gembeck (Eds.), *Coping and the development of regulation: New directions in child and adolescent development* (pp. 47–59). San Francisco: Jossey-Bass.

Cicchetti, D., Rogosch, F. A., Gunnar, M. R., & Toth, S. L. (in press). The differential impacts of early abuse on internalizing problems and diurnal cortisol activity in school-aged children. *Child Development.*

Cicchetti, D., Rogosch, F. A., & Sturge-Apple, M. L. (2007). Interactions of child maltreatment and 5-HTT and monoamine oxidase A polymorphisms: Depressive symptomatology among adolescents from low-socioeconomic status backgrounds. *Development and Psychopathology, 19,* 1161–1180.

Cicchetti, D., Rogosch, F. A., & Toth, S. L. (2000). The efficacy of toddler–parent psychotherapy for fostering cognitive development in offspring of depressed mothers. *Journal of Abnormal Child Psychology, 28,* 135–148.

Cicchetti, D., & Schneider-Rosen, K. (1986). An organizational approach to childhood depression. In M. Rutter, C. E. Izard, & P. B. Read (Eds.), *Depression in young people: Developmental and clinical perspectives* (pp. 71–134). New York: Guilford Press.

Cicchetti, D., & Sroufe, L. A. (2000). The past as prologue to the future: The times they've been a changin.' *Development and Psychopathology, 12,* 255–264.

Cicchetti, D., & Thomas, K. M. (2008). Imaging brain systems in normality and psychopathology. *Development and Psychopathology, 20,* 1023–1027.

Cicchetti, D., & Toth, S. L. (1991). The making of a developmental psychopathologist. In J. Cantor, C. Spiker, & L. Lipsitt (Eds.), *Child behavior and development: Training for diversity* (pp. 34–72). Norwood, NJ: Ablex.

Cicchetti, D., & Toth, S. L. (1998). Perspectives on research and practice in developmental psychopathology. In W. Damon (Ed.), *Handbook of child psychology* (5th ed., Vol. 4, pp. 479–583). New York: Wiley.

Cicchetti, D., & Toth, S. L. (Eds.). (2006). Translational research in developmental psychopathology [Special issue]. *Development and Psychopathology, 18*(3).

Cicchetti, D., & Toth, S. L. (2009). The past achievements and future promises of developmental psychopathology: The coming of age of a discipline. *Journal of Child Psychology and Psychiatry, 50,* 16–25.

Cicchetti, D., & Tucker, D. (1994). Development and self-regulatory structures of the mind. *Development and Psychopathology, 6,* 533–549.

Cicchetti, D., & Valentino, K. (2006). An ecological transactional perspective on child maltreatment: Failure of the average expectable environment and its influence upon child development. In D. Cicchetti & D. J. Cohen (Eds.), *Developmental psychopathology* (2nd ed., Vol. 3, pp. 129–201). New York: Wiley.

Colman, I., Murray, J., Abbott, R. A., Maughan, B., Kuh, D., Croudace, T. J., et al. (2009). Outcomes of conduct problems in adolescence: 40 year follow-up of national cohort. *British Medical Journal, 338,* 2981.

Courchesne, E., Chisum, H., & Townsend, J. (1994). Neural activity-dependent brain changes in development: Implications for psychopathology. *Development and Psychopathology, 6,* 697–722.

Cowan, W. M., Harter, D. H., & Kandel, E. R. (2000). The emergence of modern neuroscience: Some implications for neurology and psychiatry. *Annual Review of Neuroscience, 23,* 343–391.

Curtis, W. J., & Cicchetti, D. (2003). Moving research on resilience into the 21st century: Theoretical and methodological considerations in examining the biological contributors to resilience. *Development and Psychopathology, 15,* 773–810.

Curtis, W. J., & Cicchetti, D. (2007). Emotion and resilience: A multilevel investigation of hemispheric electroencephalogram asymmetry and emotion regulation in maltreated and nonmaltreated children. *Development and Psychopathology, 19,* 811–840.

Davies, P. T., & Cicchetti, D. (Eds.). (2004). Family systems and developmental psychopathology [Special issue]. *Development and Psychopathology, 16,* 477–797.

DeBellis, M. D. (2001). Developmental traumatology: The psychobiological development of maltreated children and its implications for research, treatment, and policy. *Development and Psychopathology, 13,* 539–564.

Dickstein, D. P., Treland, J. E., Snow, J., McClure, E. A., Mehta, M. S., Towbin, K. E., et al. (2004). Neuropsychological performance in pediatric bipolar disorder. *Biological Psychiatry, 55,* 32–39.

Eisenberg, L. (1977). Development as a unifying concept in psychiatry. *British Journal of Psychiatry, 131,* 225–237.

Eisenberg, L. (1995). The social construction of the human brain. *American Journal of Psychiatry, 152,* 1563–1575.

Garcia Coll, C., Akerman, A., & Cicchetti, D. (2000). Cultural influences on developmental processes and outcomes: Implications for the study of development and psychopathology. *Development and Psychopathology, 12,* 333–356.

Goodwin, F. K., & Jamison, K. R. (2007). *Manic-depressive illness: Bipolar disorders and recurrent depression* (2nd ed.). Oxford, UK: Oxford University Press.

Gottesman, I., & Shields, J. (1972). *Schizophrenia and genetics: A twin study vantage point.* New York: Academic Press.

Gottesman, I. I., & Gould, T. D. (2003). The endophenotype concept in psychiatry: Etymology and strategic intentions. *American Journal of Psychiatry, 160,* 636–645.

Gottlieb, G. (1991). Experiential canalization of behavioral development: Theory. *Developmental Psychology, 27,* 4–13.

Gottlieb, G. (1992). *Individual development and evolution: The genesis of novel behavior.* New York: Oxford University Press.

Gottlieb, G. (2007). Probabilistic epigenesis. *Developmental Science, 10,* 1–11.

Gottlieb, G., & Halpern, C. T. (2002). A relational view of causality in normal and abnormal development. *Development and Psychopathology, 14,* 421–436.

Greenough, W., Black, J., & Wallace, C. (1987). Experience and brain development. *Child Development, 58,* 539–559.

Grof, P., Alda, M., Grof, E., Fox, D., & Cameron, P. (1993). The challenge of predicting response to stabilizing lithium treatment: The importance of patient selection. *British Journal of Psychiatry, 163,* 16–19.

Gunnar, M. R., & Cicchetti, D. (2009). Meeting the challenge of translational research in child psychology. In M. R. Gunnar & D. Cicchetti (Eds.), *Meeting the challenge of translational research in child psychology: Minnesota Symposia on Child Psychology* (Vol. 35, pp. 1–27). New York: Wiley.

Gunnar, M. R., & Vazquez, D. (2006). Stress neurobiology and developmental psychopathology. In D. Cicchetti & D. Cohen (Eds.), *Developmental psychopathology* (2nd ed., Vol. 2, pp. 533–577). New York: Wiley.

Hayden, E. P., & Nurnberger, J. I. (2006). Molecular genetics of bipolar disorder. *Genes, Brain and Behavior, 5,* 85–95.

Hesse, P., & Cicchetti, D. (1982). Perspectives on an integrative theory of emotional development. *New Directions for Child Development, 16,* 3–48.

Hinshaw, S. P. (2002). Intervention research, theoretical mechanisms, and causal processes related to externalizing behavior problems. *Development and Psychopathology, 14,* 789–818.

Hinshaw, S. P. (2005). *The years of silence are past: My father's life with bipolar disorder.* Cambridge, UK: Cambridge University Press.

Hinshaw, S. P. (2006). Stigma and mental illness: Developmental issues and future prospects. In D. Cicchetti & D. Cohen (Eds.), *Developmental psychopathology* (2nd ed., Vol. 3, pp. 841–882). New York: Wiley.

Hinshaw, S. P., & Cicchetti, D. (2000). Stigma and mental disorder: Conceptions of illness, public attitudes, personal disclosure, and social policy. *Development and Psychopathology, 12,* 555–598.

Howe, G. W., Reiss, D., & Yuh, J. (2002). Can prevention trials test theories of etiology? *Development and Psychopathology, 14,* 673–694.

Ialongo, N., Rogosch, F. A., Cicchetti, D., Toth, S. L., Buckley, J., Petras, H., et al. (2006). A developmental psychopathology approach to the prevention of mental health disorders. In D. Cicchetti & D. Cohen (Eds.), *Developmental psychopathology* (2nd ed., Vol. 1, pp. 968–1018). New York: Wiley.

Institute of Medicine. (1994). *Reducing risks for mental disorders: Frontiers for preventive intervention research.* Washington, DC: National Academy Press.

Jamison, K. R. (1993). *Touched with fire: Manic–depressive illness and the artistic temperament.* New York: Free Press.

Jamison, K. R. (1995). *An unquiet mind: A memoir of moods and madness.* New York: Free Press.

Jamison, K. R., Gerner, R. H., Hammen, C., & Padesky, C. (1980). Clouds and silver linings: Positive experiences associated with primary affective disorders. *American Journal of Psychiatry, 137,* 198–202.

Kandel, E. R. (1998). A new intellectual framework for psychiatry. *American Journal of Psychiatry, 155,* 457–469.

Kandel, E. R. (1999). Biology and the future of psychoanalysis: A new intellectual framework for psychiatry revisited. *American Journal of Psychiatry, 156,* 505–524.

Karmiloff-Smith, A. (2007). Atypical epigenesis. *Developmental Science, 10,* 84–88.

Kassem, L., Lopez, V., Hedeker, D., Steele, J., Zandi, P., NIMH Genetic Initiative Consortium, et al. (2006). Familiality of polarity at illness onset in bipolar affective disorder. *American Journal of Psychiatry, 163,* 1754–1759.

Keck, P. E. J., McElroy, S. L., Strakowski, S. M., West, S. A., Sax, K. W., Hawkins, J. M., et al. (1998). Twelve-month outcome of patients with bipolar disorder following hospitalization for a manic or mixed episode. *American Journal of Psychiatry, 155,* 646–652.

Kellam, S. G., & Rebok, G. W. (1992). Building etiological theory through developmental epidemiologically based preventive intervention trials. In J. McCord & R. E. Tremblay (Eds.), *Preventing antisocial behavior: Interventions from birth through adolescence* (pp. 162–195). New York: Guilford Press.

Klimes-Dougan, B. Ronsaville, D., Wiggs, E. A., & Martinez, P. E. (2006). Neuropsychological functioning in adolescent children of mothers with a history of bipolar or major depressive disorders. *Biological Psychiatry, 60,* 957–965.

Kraemer, H. C., Wilson, G. T., Fairburn, C. G., & Agras, W. S. (2002). Mediators and moderators of treatment effects in randomized clinical trials. *Archives of General Psychiatry, 59,* 877–884.

Kraepelin, E. (1921). *Manic-depressive insanity and paranoia.* Edinburgh, UK: Livingston.

Leibenluft, E., Charney, D. S., & Pine, D. S. (2003). Researching the pathophysiology of pediatric bipolar disorder. *Society of Bipolar Psychiatry, 53,* 1009–1020.

Luthar, S. S. (2006). Resilience in development: A synthesis of research across five decades. In D. Cicchetti & D. Cohen (Eds.), *Developmental psychopathology* (2nd ed., Vol. 3, pp. 739–795). New York: Wiley.

Luthar, S. S., & Cicchetti, D. (2000). The construct of resilience: Implications for intervention and social policy. *Development and Psychopathology, 12,* 857–885.

Luthar, S. S., Cicchetti, D., & Becker, B. (2000). The construct of resilience: A critical evaluation and guidelines for future work. *Child Development, 71,* 543–562.

Lynch, M., & Cicchetti, D. (1998). An ecological-transactional analysis of children and contexts: The longitudinal interplay among child maltreatment, community violence, and children's symptomatology. *Development and Psychopathology, 10,* 235–257.

Masten, A., Best, K., & Garmezy, N. (1990). Resilience and development: Contributions from the study of children who overcome adversity. *Development and Psychopathology, 2,* 425–444.

Masten, A. S. (1989). Resilience in development: Implications of the study of successful adaptation for developmental psychopathology. In D. Cicchetti (Ed.), *Rochester Symposium on Developmental Psychopathology: The emergence of a discipline* (Vol. 1, pp. 261–294). Hillsdale, NJ: Erlbaum.

Masten, A. S. (2006). Developmental psychopathology: Pathways to the future. *International Journal of Behavioral Development, 31,* 47–54.

Masten, A. S. (Ed.). (2007). *Multilevel dynamics in developmental psychopathology: The Minnesota Symposia on Child Psychology* (Vol. 34). Mahwah, NJ: Erlbaum.

Meyer, S. E., Carlson, G. A., Wiggs, E. A., Martinez, P. E., Ronsaville, D. S., Klimes-Dougan, B., et al. (2004). A prospective study of the association among impaired executive functioning, childhood attentional problems, and the development of bipolar disorder. *Development and Psychopathology, 16,* 461–476.

Miklowitz, D. J. (2004). The role of family systems in severe and recurrent psychiatric disorders: A developmental psychopathology view. *Development and Psychopathology, 16,* 667–688.

Miklowitz, D. J., & Chang, K. D. (2008). Prevention of bipolar disorder in at-risk children: Theoretical assumptions and empirical foundations. *Development and Psychopathology, 20,* 881–897.

Miklowitz, D. J., & Cicchetti, D. (Eds.). (2006a). A developmental perspective on bipolar disorder [Special issue]. *Development and Psychopathology, 18*(4).

Miklowitz, D. J., & Cicchetti, D. (2006b). Toward a life span developmental psychopathology perspective on bipolar disorder. *Development and Psychopathology, 18,* 935–938.

Moffitt, T. E., Caspi, A., & Rutter, M. (2006). Measured gene–environment interactions in psychopathology: Concepts, research strategies, and implications for research, intervention, and public understanding of genetics. *Perspectives on Psychological Science, 1,* 5–27.

National Advisory Mental Health Council. (2000). *Translating behavioral science into action: Report of the National Advisory Mental Health Council's behavioral science workgroup* (No. 00-4699). Bethesda, MD: National Institutes of Mental Health.

Nelson, C. A., & Bloom, F. E. (1997). Child development and neuroscience. *Child Development, 68,* 970–987.

Noam, G. (1992). Development as the aim of clinical intervention. *Development and Psychopathology, 4,* 679–696.

Nowakowski, R. S., & Hayes, N. L. (1999). CNS development: An overview. *Development and Psychopathology, 11,* 395–418.

Pellmar, T. C., & Eisenberg, L. (Eds.). (2000). *Bridging disciplines in the brain, behavioral, and clinical sciences.* Washington, DC: National Academy Press.

Post, R. M., & Leverich, G. S. (2006). The role of psychosocial stress in the onset and progression of bipolar disorder and its comorbidities: The need for earlier and alternative modes of therapeutic intervention. *Development and Psychopathology, 18,* 1181–1211.

Post, R. M., Weiss, S. R. B., & Leverich, G. S. (1994). Recurrent affective disorder: Roots in developmental neurobiology and illness progression based on changes in gene expression. *Development and Psychopathology, 6*, 781–814.

Rende, R., & Waldman, I. (2006). Behavioral and molecular genetics and developmental psychopathology. In D. Cicchetti & D. Cohen (Eds.), *Developmental psychopathology* (2nd ed., Vol. 2, pp. 427–464). New York: Wiley.

Rich, B. A., Vinton, D. T., Roberson-Nay, R., Hommer, R. E., Berghorst, L. H., McClure, E. B., et al. (2006). Limbic hyperactivation during processing of neutral facial expressions in children with bipolar disorder. *Proceedings of the National Academy of Sciences USA, 103*, 8900–8905.

Richters, J. E. (1997). The Hubble hypothesis and the developmentalist's dilemma. *Development and Psychopathology, 9*, 193–229.

Richters, J. E., & Cicchetti, D. (1993). Mark Twain meets DSM-III-R: Conduct disorder, development, and the concept of harmful dysfunction. *Development and Psychopathology, 5*, 5–29.

Rutter, M. (1986). Child psychiatry: The interface between clinical and developmental research. *Psychological Medicine, 16*, 151–160.

Rutter, M. (1989). Pathways from childhood to adult life. *Journal of Child Psychology and Psychiatry, 30*, 23–51.

Rutter, M. (2006). *Genes and behavior: Nature–nurture interplay explained.* Malden, MA: Blackwell.

Rutter, M., & Garmezy, N. (1983). Developmental psychopathology. In E. M. Hetherington (Ed.), *Handbook of child psychology* (4th ed., Vol. 4, pp. 774–911). New York: Wiley.

Rutter, M., & Sroufe, L. A. (2000). Developmental psychopathology: Concepts and challenges. *Development and Psychopathology, 12*, 265–296.

Sameroff, A. J., & Chandler, M. J. (1975). Reproductive risk and the continuum of caretaking casualty. In F. D. Horowitz (Ed.), *Review of child development research* (Vol. 4, pp. 187–244). Chicago: University of Chicago Press.

Scarr, S., & McCartney, K. (1983). How people make their own environments: A theory of genotype–environment effects. *Child Development, 54*, 424–435.

Serretti, A., & Mandelli, L. (2008). The genetics of bipolar disorder: Genome "hot regions," genes, new potential candidates and future directions. *Molecular Psychiatry, 13*, 742–771.

Sroufe, L. A. (1979). The coherence of individual development: Early care, attachment, and subsequent developmental issues. *American Psychologist, 34*, 834–841.

Sroufe, L. A. (1989). Pathways to adaptation and maladaptation: Psychopathology as developmental deviation. In D. Cicchetti (Ed.), *Rochester Symposium on Developmental Psychopathology: The emergence of a discipline* (Vol. 1, pp. 13–40). Hillsdale, NJ: Erlbaum.

Sroufe, L. A. (1990). Considering normal and abnormal together: The essence of developmental psychopathology. *Development and Psychopathology, 2*, 335–347.

Sroufe, L. A. (1997). Psychopathology as an outcome of development. *Development and Psychopathology, 9*, 251–268.

Sroufe, L. A. (2007). The place of development in developmental psychopathology. In A. Masten (Ed.), *Multilevel dynamics in developmental psychopathology pathways to the future: The Minnesota Symposia on Child Psychology* (Vol. 34, pp. 285–299). Mahwah, NJ: Erlbaum.

Sroufe, L. A., Egeland, B., & Kreutzer, T. (1990). The fate of early experience following developmental change: Longitudinal approaches to individual adaptation in childhood. *Child Development, 61*, 1363–1373.

Sroufe, L. A., & Rutter, M. (1984). The domain of developmental psychopathology. *Child Development, 55*, 17–29.

Suomi, S. J. (2000). Gene–environment interactions and the neurobiology of social conflict. *Annals of the New York Academy of Sciences, 1008*, 132–139.

Thelen, E., & Smith, L. B. (1998). Dynamic systems theories. In W. Damon & R. Lerner (Eds.), *Handbook of child psychology* (Vol. 1, pp. 563–634). New York: Wiley.

Toth, S. L., & Cicchetti, D. (1999). Developmental psychopathology and child psychotherapy. In S. Russ & T. Ollendick (Eds.), *Handbook of psychotherapies with children and families* (pp. 15–44). New York: Plenum Press.

Toth, S. L., Rogosch, F. A., Manly, J. T., & Cicchetti, D. (2006). The efficacy of toddler–parent psychotherapy to reorganize attachment in the young offspring of mothers with major depressive disorder. *Journal of Consulting and Clinical Psychology, 74*(6), 1006–1016.

von Bertalanffy, L. (1968). *General system theory.* New York: Braziller.

von Eye, A., & Bergman, L. R. (2003). Research strategies in developmental psychopathology: Dimensional identity and the person-oriented approach. *Development and Psychopathology, 15*, 553–580.

Wachs, T. D., & Plomin, R. (Eds.). (1991). *Conceptualization and measurement of organism-environment interaction.* West Lafayette, IN: Purdue University Press.

Werner, H., & Kaplan, B. (1963). *Symbol formation.* New York: Wiley.

Wilden, A. (1980). *System and structure.* London: Tavistock.

Youngstrom, E., Meyers, O., Youngstrom, J. K., Calabrese, J. R., & Findling, R. L. (2006). Diagnostic and measurement issues in the assessment of pediatric bipolar disorder: Implications for understanding mood disorder across the life cycle. *Development and Psychopathology, 18*, 989–1021.

Zigler, E., & Glick, M. (1986). *A developmental approach to adult psychopathology.* New York: Wiley.

PART I

PHENOMENOLOGY AND DIAGNOSIS

CHAPTER 2

Development, Age of Onset,
and Phenomenology in Bipolar Disorder

Stephanie E. Meyer and Gabrielle A. Carlson

> [Phenomenology] refers to the study of psychopathology, broadly defined, including signs, symptoms, and their underlying thoughts and emotions. When used in this way, phenomenology provides the basis for nosology, or the development of disease definitions, diagnostic categories, or dimensional classifications.
>
> —ANDREASEN (2007, p. 108)

The impact of development on phenomenology is an interesting but complicated issue. Manifestations of a disorder at different ages may be, in part, a window into how the brain is functioning (Blumberg et al., 2006) and how the organism deals with change. From a clinical standpoint, however, we want to know the meaning and diagnostic significance of the symptoms a child is expressing and whether the meaning is the same at age 5 as it is at age 10, 15, 20, and beyond. It goes without saying that certain phenomena are normal at one age and not at another or that they mean one thing at one age and another at a different age.

In mania, one of the important questions is the degree to which the symptoms and behaviors that appear to be occurring in children, or at least are elicited during psychiatric evaluations, are continuous with those problems in adulthood. We are trying to short-circuit a long wait. The assumption is that if we know a child with manic behaviors at age 8 will continue to have those behaviors at age 28 (an example of homotypic continuity), then clinicians and researchers interested in bipolar disorders (BD) in youth can apply what we know about BD in adults and perhaps prevent the condition from worsening by offering therapies that have proven efficacy in adult samples. Of course, this perspective assumes that the causal agents underlying manic symptomatology across the life span are the same. On the other hand, if the behaviors at varying stages have a different significance (i.e., the continuity is heterotypic), it will be imperative to understand that a different diagnostic outcome will likely unfold, requiring a different approach.

DEFINITION

The recurrent or episodic nature of mania and depression has been the age-old hallmark of BD. The DSM (American Psychiatric Association, 2000) for the past 30 years has tried to capture this by defining an episode as a "distinct period," different from the person's "usual self" during which specific symptoms co-occur. For mania, these include an "abnormally and persistently elevated, expansive, or irritable mood" accompanied by at least three additional symptoms (four if mood is irritable), including inflated self-esteem or grandiosity, decreased need for sleep, pressured speech, flight of ideas, distractibility, increased involvement in goal-directed activities or psychomotor agitation, and excessive involvement in pleasurable activities with a high potential for painful consequences. In order to meet full criteria for mania, symptoms must last at least a week, or 4 days for hypomania. However, before the disorder fully expresses itself, episodes may be briefer than 4 days. Episodes of depression, which must last a minimum of 2 weeks, are characterized in children by sad, empty, or irritable mood along with other symptoms of feeling worthless, preoccupation with death or suicide, agitation/feeling slowed down, and changes in appetite, sleep, and energy level.

For prepubertal children especially, the devil has been in the details in defining episode, euphoria, grandiosity, decreased need for sleep, and distinguishing the other symptoms of BD from various childhood conditions, especially attention-deficit/hyperactivity disorder (Carlson & Meyer, 2006). Further complicating matters is the probability that mania may look very different among prepubescent youth than members of well-characterized adult samples. Some researchers have identified as bipolar those symptom patterns in youth that do not resemble the episodic nature of BD in adults as it has been classically described (Biederman et al., 2000). According to McClellan, Kowatch, and Findling (2007), this presentation has been adopted in community settings where BD is characterized by "outbursts of mood lability, irritability, reckless behavior, and aggression." Shifts in mood state are short-lived, and irritability, rather than euphoria, tends to be the predominant and most impairing mood state.

The criteria used to diagnose BD in children and adolescents vary markedly across sites, and even where there is agreement regarding definitional parameters, there may be differing ways in which the criteria are applied or interpreted. Efforts have been made to adapt adult mania criteria for prepubertal children, adjusting for developmental differences (Geller, Zimerman, Williams, DelBello, Bolhofner, et al., 2002). However, these modifications are difficult to interpret, given the paucity of data regarding the normative range of mood variability and changes in self-esteem among young children as well as developmental, clinical, and contextual factors that may moderate the long-term significance of these characteristics. To encourage diagnostic consistency across sites, Leibenluft's laboratory at the National Institute of Mental Health (NIMH) has identified another syndrome, severe mood dysregulation (SMD), which they distinguish from pediatric BD (Leibenluft, Charney, Towbin, Bhangoo, & Pine, 2003). SMD is characterized by chronic, rather than episodic, mood symptoms (anger and sadness), and there is no evidence of euphoria or grandiosity, although other symptoms of mania may be present. Most important to this condition is the markedly increased reactivity to negative emotional stimuli that is manifest verbally or behaviorally (e.g., response to frustration with extended temper tantrums, verbal rage, or aggression toward people or property). In its most rigorous definition, these must occur on average three or more times per week for the past 4 weeks and be present in one setting but with some evidence in another (Leibenluft et al., 2003).

HISTORY

Interest in examining the relation between childhood behaviors and adult-onset BD can be traced back to Kraepelin's (1921) monograph on manic–depressive insanity. Following its publication, child psychiatrists began looking for similar presentations among their young patients. Although subsequent case studies suggested that mania was rare in children, there was some suggestion that early-onset manic depression was being overlooked because of its overlap with other childhood diagnoses and normative childhood behavior (Harms, 1952). Efforts to characterize childhood-onset mania were temporarily stalled in 1960 after the publication of an influential article in which the authors reviewed the psychiatric literature from 1884 to 1954 and concluded that "the occurrence of manic-depression in early childhood as a clinical phenomenon has yet to be demonstrated" (Anthony & Scott, 1960).

In the 1960s, evidence regarding the efficacy of lithium for treating adults with manic depression led to efforts to identify lithium-responsive behavioral profiles in children. Initial studies suggested that lithium was most effective in treating early-onset presentations closely resembling classic manic depression and less effective in treating children with broader behavioral dysregulation (Youngerman & Canino, 1978). After the establishment of standard symptom criteria for diagnosing mania in adults, there were attempts to adapt these criteria for use with children (Weinberg & Brumback, 1976). In 1979, Davis introduced the concept of a "manic-depressive variant syndrome of childhood," which characterized children and adolescents exhibiting heightened reactivity to seemingly minor events, hyperactivity, and disruptions in interpersonal relationships, frequently with a family history of manic depression.

By the 1980s, there was growing acceptance of the diagnosis of manic depression, or bipolar disorder as it was now called, in youth, with the belief that symptoms were continuous with the adult form of the illness. However, a lack of longitudinal data has limited any conclusions that can be made regarding the continuity of symptoms across the life span.

The Impact of DSM Decision Making on Understanding Development in Bipolar Disorder

In recent decades, the exploration of phenomenology in bipolar illness across the life span has largely been reduced to the application of DSM-based checklists. As Andreasen (2007) has pointed out, "[DSM criteria] were never intended to provide a comprehensive description. Rather, they were conceived of as 'gatekeepers'—the minimum symptoms needed to make a diagnosis." Thus, they are most useful for determining whether a given person "meets the criteria" for a given diagnosis, but do not allow us to flesh out the broader developmental, behavioral and environmental context in which symptoms are being expressed.

DSM's "atheoretical" approach limits opportunities to account for circumstances that may be important to understanding the child and his or her behavior. Indeed, "distinct periods" of mood change and increased energy may occur for a variety of reasons. For example, school is often a significant stressor for children. If a child is manageable at home, or has not encountered any significant cognitive challenges, and then has difficulty negotiating the demands of kindergarten with resulting rebelliousness, some might say that this is the start of an episode of mania because it is the "onset" of irritability. This is especially true in a child with attentional difficulties who may be significantly stressed in school but whose frustration tolerance and mood lability are more manageable over the summer. It may be that these stressors have no relevance to diagnosing mania, but we cannot research the question in children because the DSM-based interviews have not afforded us a way to study it.

Limitations of Assessment Measures

Insofar as assessment measures of mania focus on the presence of symptoms, there is little opportunity to truly understand phenomenology. Even in semistructured interviews, where the interviewer has latitude to elicit symptoms, what ultimately gets recorded for research purposes is the presence, absence, or possibly the severity of the symptoms that determine that the criteria are met. Descriptive notes that provide examples of specific behaviors do not get recorded. What we want to know from a developmental perspective is not only whether, but how, euphoria or grandiosity, or goal-directed hyperactivity, or excessive involvement in pleasurable activities, manifest and change with age, IQ, environmental context, cognitive development, and puberty. We cannot know these things if the only information that is recorded is the higher level construct that is endorsed in the interview.

Interviews used to diagnose bipolar illness in children vary somewhat in how they elicit information and from whom they obtain it (Galanter, Goyal, Jenna, & Fisher, 2008). If the key feature to a manic episode is its discreteness as a phenomenon, there should be a clear onset, offset, and return to a premorbid level of functioning. Otherwise, disentangling episode onset from developmental shifts (onset of terrible 2s or 3s, stressful transitions to school in a child with other problems) becomes difficult. Some interviews (e.g., the Washington University version of the Kiddie Schedule for Affective Disorders and Schizophrenia for School-Age Children [WASH-U-K-SADS; Geller, Zimerman, Williams, DelBello, Frazier, et al., 2002]) request extensive descriptive information regarding each symptom, including onset and offset, but do not require that symptoms co-occur within an episode in order to meet criteria for BD. Determining whether criteria for a disorder are met is done post hoc by reassembling the symptoms. That means that symptoms are often counted twice and that a symptom, like irritability, from one condition (i.e., depression) is counted in another disorder too. The K-SADS Present and Lifetime Version (K-SADS-PL; Kaufman et al., 1997) emphasizes that symptoms in common with other psychiatric disorders (e.g., distractibility) should be not rated as a mania symptom unless they have intensified with the onset of abnormal mood (e.g., Birmaher et al., 2009). Lifetime comorbid diagnoses are not assigned if they occur exclusively during a mood episode.

A problem more specific to studies of BD in children and adolescents has been the lack of consensus regarding definition and assessment practices in young people. Some researchers require euphoria or grandiosity to be present (Geller, Zimerman, Williams, DelBello, Frazier, et al., 2002; Leibenluft et al., 2003); others feel that severe irritability/explosiveness is the defining feature of very early-onset BD (Mick, Spencer, Wozniak, & Biederman, 2005; Wozniak et al., 2005).

Parents are always interviewed, but some researchers do not directly interview children younger than age 12 (Wozniak et al., 1995); others interview all youth. When both parent and child are interviewed, criteria may be met if symptoms are endorsed by parent, child, some from each (the *or* rule), or both parent and child (the *and* rule). Some groups weigh parent report more heavily if parent and child responses differ. Whenever attempts have been made to decide on the best informant, the results are confounded because there is no gold standard against which to determine veracity.

Decisions about informants need more than a simplistic "and/or" rule (Jensen et al., 1999). When there are informant differences, there needs to be an understanding about what is occurring rather than dismissing one or the other (Carlson et al., 2009). The importance of informant source is highlighted in genetic studies in which heritability estimates in children may change depending on informant source (Thapar & Rice, 2006). The result of these differences in symptom ascertainment is that we do not know how to interpret the differences obtained between investigators and thus cannot reflect on phenomenological and developmental data. Finally, although careful attention has been paid to symptom ascertainment in interviews like the K-SADS-PL, the phenomenology present at worst episode rather than first episode is collected. There is no guarantee that these are the same, and they probably are not (Birmaher et al., 2009).

Pathways to Bipolar Illness

A developmental psychopathology perspective has the potential to greatly enrich our understanding of the phenomenology of bipolar spectrum conditions across the life span by going beyond simple symptom counts and description toward examining the various factors within and outside of an individual that play a role in shaping pathways to illness. There are emerging clues within the existing literature suggesting that children at risk for BD are hindered by a broad range of challenges when faced with salient developmental tasks (Cicchetti & Toth, 1995). In particular, studies have shown that before full manifestation of illness, high-risk youth frequently manifest neuropsychological deficits (Meyer et al., 2004), temperamental difficulties (West, Henry, & Pavuluri, 2007), and broad-ranging behavioral symptoms (Carlson & Weintraub, 1993; Meyer et al., 2004). Moreover, children at heightened risk for bipolar illness are less likely to receive optimal parenting (Miklowitz & Chang, 2008; Schenkel, West, Harral, Patel, & Pavuluri, 2008) and adequate social supports (Pellegrini et al., 1986). Thus, they are more likely to face the challenges of each developmental period with inadequate resources and coping strategies.

Genetic and Environmental Factors

At this point, there is little doubt that genetic influences are important in the onset and course of BD across the life span; however, precise etiological mechanisms have yet to be elucidated. With advances in molecular genetic studies, sufficient evidence has accumulated to rule out a major bipolar locus (Berrettini, 1998). On the other hand, researchers have realized for some years that susceptibility chromosomal loci of smaller effect likely contribute to the presence and variability of BD (Craddock & Sklar, 2009; Gershon et al., 1998). There have been a number of molecular genetic studies within the adult literature, but many promising findings have not been replicated. Within the pediatric bipolar literature, preliminary results point to a possible linkage to chromosome 9q34 (Faraone, Lasky-Su, Glatt, Van Eerdewegh, & Tsuang, 2006) as well as an association between early-onset BD and the Val66 allele of the BDNF gene (Geller, Badner, et al., 2004).

Although susceptibility loci are thought to increase the risk for BD, they do not appear to be necessary or sufficient for its development (Berrettini, 1998). Indeed, etiological models suggest the importance of gene × environment interactions in shaping the onset, course, and recurrence of BD (Mendlewicz, 1998; Staner et al., 1997; Stefos, Bauwens, Staner, Pardoen, & Mendlewicz, 1996). Growing evidence suggests a number of psychosocial factors that appear to play a pathogenic role in the development of BD. Specific findings suggest that parenting styles characterized by low levels of warmth and high negativity and irritability represent a risk factor for early age at onset of BD, as well as poor illness course (Geller, Tillman, Craney, & Bolhofner, 2004; Meyer et al., 2006). Physical and sexual abuse have also been identified in several studies as a risk factor for early-onset bipolar illness (Leverich et al., 2002) and have been linked to a variety of negative course indicators, including rapid cycling, elevated risk of suicidal behavior, and high comorbidity rates, including substance use disorders (Leverich et al., 2002). Other psychosocial variables that have been linked to early-onset BD include poor social supports (Pellegrini et al., 1986; Petti et al., 2004), parental divorce and conflict (Davenport, Zahn-Waxler, Adland, & Mayfield, 1984; Geller, Craney, et al., 2002; Pellegrini et al., 1986), low levels of family cohesion and organization (Chang, Blasey, Ketter, & Steiner, 2001; Romero, DelBello, Soutullo, Stanford, & Strakowski, 2005), insecure attachment relationships, and increased familial conflict (Chang, Blasey, Ketter, & Steiner, 2001). Perinatal risk factors may also increase risk for early-onset BD, with preliminary data pointing to prenatal exposure to prescribed medications and nonprescribed substances (O'Connor et al., 2002; Pavuluri, Henry, Nadimpalli, O'Connor, & Sweeney, 2006).

Behavioral and Neurobiological Indicators of Risk

An important question in bipolar research is, what is inherited? Researchers have begun to search for phenotypes that are thought to represent etiologically homogeneous forms of, or precursors to, BD (Depue et al., 1981; Leboyer et al., 1998). In addition to providing insight into the genetic mechanisms involved in the transmission of BD, these phenotypic markers are potentially valuable in the study of developmental and environmental contributions to bipolar illness. Promising areas of inquiry include temperament, neurocognitive profiles, and neurobiological differences.

Temperament

The idea that full-blown BD may be preceded by a particular premorbid temperament dates back to the beginning of the century. In 1921, Kraepelin wrote, "There are certain temperaments which may be regarded as rudiments of manic-depressive insanity. They may throughout the whole of life exist as peculiar forms of psychic personality without further development; but they may also become the point of departure for a morbid process which develops under peculiar conditions and runs its course in isolated attacks" (Akiskal, Djenderedjian, Rosenthal, & Khani, 1977, p. 1227). More recently, Akiskal (1996) has introduced the term *affective temperament* to describe dispositions "that are closest to the biological underpinnings of drive, affect, and emotion" and that play a major role in determining the type and intensity of developmental experience. Furthermore, these temperaments, which have been termed *cyclothymic, hyperthymic, irritable,* and *dysthymic,* are considered to be on a continuum with BD. This model hypothesizes a reciprocal relationship between affective temperament and negative life experiences. Early caregiving experiences are thought to interact with constitutional vulnerability, thus making an individual more susceptible to the effects of later negative life events. Negative life events are believed to occur with greater frequency among individuals with temperamental dysregulation. In turn, such life experiences are thought to be responsible for triggering the onset of BD (Akiskal, 1996).

Early data regarding temperament and adult-onset BD suggest that approximately one-third of individuals who manifest an affective temperament will eventually develop BD (Akiskal et al., 1977; Depue et al., 1981). More recent studies using temperament rating scales have similarly found children at high risk for BD to exhibit underlying temperamental vulnerability. One study of 2- to 6-year-old offspring of parents with BD found that these children had higher rates of behavioral disinhibition than offspring of parents with panic disorder, major depression, or no history of psychiatric illness, while another study found that high-risk offspring between 6 and 18 years who already met criteria for a major psychiatric diagnosis were less flexible and exhibited more negative affect and poorer task orientation than unaffected offspring (Chang, Blasey, Ketter, & Steiner, 2003). Notably, one retrospective study of infant and toddler temperament in children with early-onset BD indicated that these children could be differentiated from children with ADHD and healthy controls in terms of severity of early temperamental characteristics. Specific areas in which the children with early-onset BD were more impaired included difficulty sleeping, difficulty nursing, excessive crying, difficulty being consoled, separation distress, and being slow to warm up following separation. In toddlerhood, these children were described as less adaptable, more emotionally intense, more negative, and less well regulated compared with both nonbipolar groups. These characteristics of difficult temperament were stable from infancy to toddlerhood and were predictive of increased residual mood symptoms after the onset of the disorder (West et al., 2007).

Neurobiological Markers

Emerging findings from neurobehavioral studies have identified a number of atypical cognitive and affective processes associated with bipolar spectrum conditions, including poor frustration tolerance (Rich et al., 2007), deficits in executive functioning (Meyer et al., 2004; Pavuluri, Schenkel, et al., 2006), working memory (Doyle et al., 2005; Pavuluri, Schenkel, et al., 2006; Rucklidge, 2006), decreased attentional capacities (Doyle et al., 2005; Pavuluri, Schenkel, et al., 2006), particularly during emotional challenges (Rich et al., 2007), and cognitive inflexibility (Dickstein et al., 2007).

Recent neuroimaging studies have begun to shed light on underlying structural and functional correlates of these behavioral markers as they manifest in bipolar illness. Across the life course, BD has been found to be associated with abnormalities in cortical and subcortical brain regions thought to be involved in the regulation of emotion (Chang et al., 2004; Dickstein et al., 2005; Frazier et al., 2005; Soares & Mann, 1997; Strakowski, DelBello, & Adler, 2005). Although not well understood, these structural abnormalities are generally believed to result from transactional influences of genetic, environmental, and developmental processes (Soares & Mann, 1997).

The two most replicated morphological findings in the early-onset BD literature are the presence of white matter hyperintensities (WMH) and atypical amygdala volume. Findings regarding WMH have been well replicated among patients with BD throughout the life span; however, these abnormalities have also been found in a number of other neuropsychiatric disorders and, therefore, do not appear to be specific to bipolar illness. Discoveries regarding amygdala size vary across the life course. In children and adolescents with BD, results have revealed decreased amygdala size (Blumberg et al., 2003; Chang et al., 2005; Del-Bello, Zimmerman, Mills, Getz, & Strakowski, 2004), whereas most adult studies have reported increased amygdala volume or no differences between patients and controls (Strakowski et al., 2005).

A number of additional structural abnormalities have been reported in the early-onset literature but require replication. Two studies have reported enlarged basal ganglia regions (Wilke, Kowatch, DelBello, Mills, & Holland, 2004), including the putamen (DelBello et al., 2004), whereas other studies have found reductions in hippocampal size (Blumberg et al., 2003; Frazier et al., 2005) and decreased total cerebral volume among children (DelBello et al., 2004; Frazier et al., 2005) but not adults. In general, existing studies have been limited by small sample sizes, cross-sectional design, and the fact that most have not been able to control for medication effects, comorbid conditions, or variations in mood state. Most have pooled together children and adolescents without taking into account varying stages of brain development (Pavuluri, Birmaher, & Naylor, 2005).

The Effect of Puberty

Puberty is an important biological/age-related marker of development. Both the psychoses of schizophrenia and major depressive disorder show a steep increase in onset around puberty (e.g., Angermeyer & Kühn, 1988; Angold, Costello, Erkanli, & Worthman, 1999). In depression, the increase occurs in women. If early-onset depression is more likely to be bipolar in nature, some of that increase will include bipolar depression. We would then expect to see a gender-specific rise in females with BD at puberty. There is emerging evidence that this is the case.

Birmaher and colleagues (2009), comparing childhood-onset with adolescent-onset BD in a well-characterized, research-acquired clinical sample, found depression to be the more common type of onset in teens and the gender association to change from male preponderance in children to female preponderance in adolescents. Although numbers of symptoms did not differ by age, the quality of symptoms changed at least as far as could be ascertained by the K-SADS-PL. Teens appeared to have more severe and more adult-like symptoms of mania and depression. Explanations for this were not possible from this data set for some of the methodological reasons described earlier.

Data from a large insurance database of more than 1.2 million claims revealed that new diagnoses of BD tripled for males between childhood and adolescence but increased sixfold for girls (Olfson, Crystal, Gerhard, Huang, & Carlson, 2009). It was not possible to determine what percentage of this increase was due to depression versus mania, but judging by the increase in antidepressant prescriptions in this bipolar sample we speculate that many of the teens were depressed. Clearly, the impact of puberty on the phenomenology of BD needs further study.

Findings from the NIMH Bipolar Genetics Initiative (Blehar et al., 1998) suggest a possible role for reproductive hormones on the onset and course of bipolar illness. Sixty-six percent of women in this study reported regular mood changes during the menstrual or premenstrual phase of their cycle. Of this group, the majority of women described increased irritability, anger outbursts, and mood lability, while some reported only depressive symptoms.

Alloy, Abramson, Walshaw, Keyser, and Gerstein (2006) have proposed an etiological model of BD that takes into account the various cognitive, genetic, cultural, social, and environmental risk factors that come into play with onset of puberty, making this a time of heightened risk for emergence of bipolar illness, particularly among girls (see Alloy et al., Chapter 10, this volume). The model is based on the cognitive-vulnerability-transactional stress perspective that has been applied to the study of unipolar depression, similarly emphasizing the transactional relationship among emerging negative cognitive styles and life stress. The authors postulate that cognitive vulnerability may be heightened as normal adolescent brain development sets the scene for the manifestation of maladaptive cognitive biases and self-regulatory strategies. Girls, in particular, show a tendency toward rumination and negative cognitive styles, possibly accounting for a predominantly depressive course among adolescent females with bipolar illness.

At the same time, adolescence is a time of increased exposure to stressful life events as well as maximal social and academic pressures and increased biological and behavioral reactivity to stressful experiences, with females exhibiting these changes more than males (Alloy et al., 2006; Papadakis, Prince, Jones, & Strauman, 2006; Shibley Hyde, Mezulis, & Abramson, 2008). Heightened stress sensitivity, and therefore vulnerability to the development of mood symptoms, appears to be shaped through the interaction of genetic endowment and early experience. In particular, negative parenting and maltreatment are associated with maladaptive levels of stress reactivity (Alloy et al., 2006) and have also been linked to risk for early-onset bipolar illness (Leverich et al., 2002; Meyer et al., 2006).

AGE AT ONSET

In order to understand how development might impact the phenomenology of BD, we need to know what we mean by "development." The answer to the question of impact will depend on whether we simply compare symptom manifestations of different age groups or use cognitive development or biological maturity to decide. We speculate that symptom manifestation at the *actual age* at which the patient is presenting is important, but that the duration of illness may also change phenomenology. In other words, the symptoms presenting as the illness is unfolding may be different from those that present when the disease is fixed. Thus, information needs to be collected in ways that allow for multiple types of comparisons.

Another pertinent question is the age or ages at which we would expect changes in phenomenology. Child and adolescent psychiatrists traditionally separate preschool, school-age, and adolescent children. These are important time frames in brain maturity. Most of the controversy surrounding BD in youth has focused on children younger than age 12, and the younger the child, the greater the controversy.

Finally, age at onset, the age at which the person first becomes recognizably ill, may confer a different impact on phenomenology than current age at which the illness is occurring. Age at onset may be associated with different etiological factors and different outcomes (Bellivier, Golmard, Henry, Leboyer, & Schurhoff, 2001; Bellivier et al., 2003).

There are also data suggesting that different outcomes in BD are predicted by whether onset is depressive or manic in nature. Thus, it may be relevant to know whether having a mania onset changes the phenomenology of the disorder, not just the age at which it is said to have occurred. For instance, mania onset may predict a predominantly manic course, which may have a better outcome (Forty et al., 2009; Perris & d'Elia, 1966; Stephens & McHugh, 1991). Conversely, a depressive onset may presage a depressive course (Perugi et al., 2000), and mood episodes starting with depression are worse (Turvey et al., 1999). If very early onset is worse than later onset, is it because of the early age of onset? Or are those with early onsets more likely to have a depressive or mixed episode onset, which is predictive of a more chronic course?

Cognitive Age

Although age and cognition are usually closely associated, understanding the impact of cognition on phenomenology is also potentially meaningful. These variables are disassociated in people with developmental disabilities. An interesting question is whether the phenomenology of mania in an intellectually disabled adult more closely resembles that of his or her chronological age counterpart or developmental age counterpart. When this question was specifically examined a number of years ago in adults with mental retardation (Carlson, 1979, 1981), the data suggested that puberty predicted recognizable motor/vegetative aspects of mania and depression. Cognitive development was reflected in the content of what the patient said. Thus, even severely intellectually disabled adults had definable mood episodes that resembled their chronological age mates, not their cognitive/developmental age mates.

Whether cognition is defined in Piagetian terms (preoperational, concrete, and formal operations) or by language age, we might speculate that symptom manifestations are likely to be different. We certainly might speculate that how a child is able to describe what he or she is experiencing or whether he or she understands the questions being asked will change significantly with cognitive and language maturity. For instance, a 6- or 7-year-old who thinks he can swim across a lake because his dad says he can "swim like a fish" may be manifesting very literal thinking rather than classical manic grandiosity (Carlson & Meyer, 2006).

Age at First Manic Episode

Because we would maintain that the phenomenology of mania is the defining aspect of BD, it may be important to distinguish between age of onset (which may be a depressive episode) and the age at which a *first syndromal manic episode* occurred. A person who appeared in retrospect to be depressed at age 7 or 8 and then has a manic episode at age 16 will have, we suspect, an episode that more closely resembles adult mania than child mania. An example is the case of a child referred at age 13 for a schizophrenia study (Calderoni et al., 2001). At age 10 he was angry and assaultive; by age 13 he was depressed; by age 15, he was psychotic and manic, at which time he was treated with lithium and antidepressants; and by age 21 he was functioning fairly well. The diagnosis of BD was made long after the illness onset. Should onset be determined by age 10 when he was angry and assaultive but not clearly manic; at age 13, when he became depressed; or at age 15, when he was clearly manic? In our opinion, the clearest designation for age of onset is the age at which the first clear manic or hypomanic episode occurs. That may be some years after other psychopathology is observed.

Adult psychiatrists are chagrined by the long period of time between apparent illness onset and final illness recognition. It is much easier to make these judgments retrospectively when you know what the disorder has become than to make prospective predictions when you do not know how the illness will evolve.

Decreasing Age of Onset

With growing interest in childhood-onset BD over the past 10 to 15 years, each new study of adult-onset BD appears to find earlier and earlier age of onset. Beginning with the survey of the then-titled National Depressive and Manic-Depressive Association membership (Lish, Dime-Meenan, Whybrow, Price, & Hirschfeld, 1994), patient recollection of when their symptoms first began has become the standard in determining illness onset. In that survey of 500 members, in which only 4% of subjects were younger than age 25, 17% said they thought their illness onset was age 9 or younger. The majority of patients said that their symptomatology and recurrences were depressive or mixed. Compared with those who recalled the onset as older, the younger onset members had more school dropout (55% vs.

23%), more financial difficulty (70 vs. 54%), and more relational problems, sub-stance abuse, self-injury and minor crime. In other words, although not recorded as such, rates of childhood psychopathology and psychosocial impairment were much higher in the early-onset compared to the older onset group.

Other recent adult bipolar studies also describe much earlier age of onset than seen in previous generations. For the Stanley Center studies the median age of registrants born before 1940 (1900–1939) was 63 and their median age of onset was 23; for those born between 1940 and 1959, the median age at registry was 48 and the median age of onset was 19 years (Chengappa et al., 2003; Kupfer et al., 2002). Not emphasized, however, is that the 20 years covered from 1940 to 1959 included 1,080 subjects, compared with only 138 subjects from the earlier 40 years. The question is whether age of onset has truly dropped or if the smaller number of surviving, chronically ill older people are as interested in signing up for studies as the larger numbers of younger people who do so. Also relevant is how accurately patients recall much more distant time points. Type of onset in this sample was depressed in 60%, manic in 20%, and mixed in 20%.

In the Systematic Treatment Enhancement Program (STEP-BD) study, 1,000 patients with bipolar spectrum disorder (71.6% with bipolar I) had a median age at study registration of 41 years. In this study, 28% of people with bipolar I said they had had their first episode before the age of 13. Similar to the Stanley Center study registrants, only 24.3% had mania as their initial episode. Rates of anxiety comorbidity were highest in the patients who recalled earliest onset (any anxiety disorder 69.2% vs. 44.7% in the remainder of the sample of adolescent- and adult-onset patients). The same was true for ADHD, for which rates were 20.4% versus 6.5%. Not surprisingly, substance/alcohol use was more problematic in 18-year and under versus over 18-year onsets, with drug abuse being more significant in the younger onset group (33% vs. 15.1%) (Perlis et al., 2004).

Curiously, in the National Comorbity sample (Kessler et al., 2005), lifetime rates of BD were higher in those younger than 30 than those older than 30. It is dif-ficult to understand how an early-onset disorder, with onsets that occur through senescence, should have a declining lifetime prevalence with age. Although not usually considered, it is possible that there is a developmental phenocopy of mania spectrum symptoms seen in the general population that is not continuous with true BD. Alternatively, declining rates of reported illness may be accounted for by recency effects in the younger group (i.e., greater likelihood of reporting symptoms that occurred more recently).

Goodwin and Jamison (2007) suggest a number of reasons for the decreas-ing age of onset: (1) changes in nosology and treatment definition; (2) genetic anticipation; (3) use of stimulants and antidepressants; and (4) use of recreational drugs. What is not clear, of course, is whether the adults in the STEP-BD and Stanley Center studies, who were now in their 40s, were remembering childhood behavior or anxiety disorder or early-onset BD. Because child and adolescent psy-chiatrists have been unable to agree on defining and diagnosing BD when the child and his or her parent are actually sitting in the office providing information, it is doubtful that patient recall of 20 to 30 years will be more discriminatory or accurate. Moreover, the need for stimulant or antidepressant use suggests that the child was already ill, thus calling into question the explanation that these medications lowered the age of onset. We conclude that early age of onset and widespread symptomatology remain confounds in samples at any age.

Bipolar Phenomenology across the Life Span

Teen versus Later Adult Onset of Mania

Recognized since Kraepelin's extensive observations of patients hospitalized with severe psychopathology is the fact that manic–depression onset with manic episodes (mixed or otherwise) can be a phenomenon of youth. Although Kraepelin treated adults, he found that "first attacks" of 903 cases of manic–depressive insanity showed a few cases beginning at ages 10 and 15 years and a steep increase around age 20. The high rate of first onset decreased around age 35 and gradually declined. Interestingly, mixed attacks prevailed at ages 15 to 30 and depressive attacks were more prevalent thereafter.

Winokur, Clayton, and Reich (1969) reported that one-third of their patients were already ill with mania by age 20, and new onsets declined after age 30. Loranger and Levine (1978) recorded age of first symptoms, treatment, and hospitalization in 200 adults hospitalized for mania at Cornell's Payne Whitney Clinic based on patient charts from 1957 to 1977. No one had been treated for mania before age 13, although five people had had symptoms and a history of other psychiatric pathology. A steep rise at ages 15 to 19 was evident, and one-third of the patients had been hospitalized before their 25th birthday.

More recent studies have used a sophisticated statistical approach called *admixture analysis*, a method for identifying the model that best fits the observed distribution of a continuous variable. They have found rather consistently that embedded within the pattern of a steep rise and gradual fall of age of onset are two, possibly three, age groups: an early-onset group, which peaks in midadolescence; a young adult group, with a mean age of onset in the mid-20s; and an older onset group, whose mean age seems to vary but ranges from about 40 to 50 (Table 2.1). The implications of this, of course, are that different age groups may have varying genetic and developmental underpinnings. It is not far-fetched to assume that there is another age of onset group starting prepubertally, but children have not been included in these large studies of age of onset.

One small study used nonreferred adults with BD from a family study of youth with and without ADHD to compare those with child-onset BD with those with adult onset. The former had a longer duration of illness, more irritability than euphoria, a mixed presentation, a more chronic or rapid-cycling course, and increased comorbidity with childhood disruptive behavior disorders and anxiety disorders (Mick, Biederman, Faraone, Murray, & Wozniak, 2003).

There have been numerous studies of phenomenology comparing adolescents/young adults with older patients. These have included comparisons using age of

TABLE 2.1. Studies Examining Distributions of Age of Onset

Study	Sample	Mean age, years (SD)		
		Young	Adult	Older
Kennedy et al. (2005)	First episode of mania; 1965–1999; 57% female; 22% prior depression; 61% white; 17% by age 20; 56% by 30; 9% > 60 years; n = 246		25.56 (5.96) n = 192	51.01 (16.26) n = 54
Bellivier et al. (2003)	Consecutive patients in France, Switzerland, Germany; n = 368	17.6 (1.8) 21.4%	24.6 (6.1) 57.3%	39.2 (9.6) 21.2%
Bellivier et al. (2001)	Consecutive inpatients and outpatients in France meeting DSM-IV criteria for BPAD; DSM-IV criteria for either a major depressive episode or mania; AAO mania or depression from medical records and interview; n = 211	< 18 16.9 (2.7) 41.4%	26.9 (5.0) 41.9%	> 40 46.2 (8.0) 16.6%
Schürhoff et al. (2000)	Consecutive inpatients and outpatients in France meeting DSM-IV criteria for BPAD; DSM-IV criteria for either a major depressive episode or mania; AAO mania or depression from medical records and interview; n = 211	< 18 15.5 (1.9) n = 58		> 40 48.5 (7) n = 39
Manchia et al. (2008)	181 outpatients from a lithium clinic in Sardinia; n = 76 men, 105 women	≤ 21 18.1 (2.3) 36%	22–33 24.3 (5.3) 39%	> 33 41 (11.5) 25%
Lin et al. (2006)	211 probands with BD, with 1,856 family members self-reported AAO mania or depression	≤ 21 16.6 (5.1) 79.7%	22–28 26.0 (1.4) 7.2%	> 28 34.7 (6.6) 13.1%

Note. BPAD, bipolar affective disorder; AAO, age at onset; BD, bipolar disorder.

onset as well as the age at presentation for treatment. Teen/young adult samples generally have more complex episodes of mania compared with onset later in adulthood. Psychosis is more common and severe (i.e., delusions, hallucinations, and first-rank symptoms) (Carlson, Bromet, Driessens, Mojtabai, & Schwartz, 2002; Kennedy et al., 2005; McGlashan, 1988; Schürhoff et al., 2000), and there is more rapid cycling and more intermixed depressive features, or mixed episodes (McElroy, Strakowski, West, Keck, & McConville, 1997; Schürhoff et al., 2000). Suicidal behavior may be associated with earlier age of onset, although suicidality may simply be associated with depressive/mixed features that characterize episodes. Some recent data suggest that irritable rather than elated mood is more of a feature of younger onset (Birmaher et al., 2009; Kennedy et al., 2005), although again irritability may simply be another way of identifying the episode as dysphoric and mixed.

Teen/young adult onset is also associated with higher rates of comorbidity, with general and anxiety disorder (Schürhoff et al., 2000) and substance abuse

(Carlson et al., 2002; Kennedy et al., 2005; Lin et al., 2006) in particular. When studied, disruptive behavior disorders (ADHD and conduct disorder) also occur at higher rates in younger onset subjects (Carlson, Bromet, & Jandorf, 1998; Carlson, Bromet, & Sievers, 2000; Kessler et al., 2005; Perlis et al., 2004).

Some studies find that people with teen-onset BD have a more protracted course with poorer functional outcome compared with adults (Birmaher et al., 2006; Carter, Mundo, Parikh, & Kennedy, 2003). However, very few studies have tried to disentangle the separate impact of earlier age of onset, longer time ill, and co-occurring comorbidities, which themselves confer poor outcome. Carlson and colleagues (2002) found that comorbidity of childhood psychopathology was a greater contributor to poorer functional outcome at 4-year follow-up than early age of onset in patients with bipolar I (predominantly manic/psychotic). This continued to be true at the 10-year follow-up, although there were few early-onset patients without other childhood-onset disorders (Ruggero, Carlson, Kotov, & Bromet, in press).

Not everyone finds early (at least adolescent) onset associated with comorbidity and a refractory course, however. Researchers in Canada and India appear to have selected a sample of more classic manic–depressive teens with a somewhat more benign clinical picture and course (Duffy et al., 2002; Jairam, Srinath, Girimaji, & Seshadri, 2004; Kutcher, Robertson, & Bird, 1998).

Child versus Adolescent Onset of Mania

Very few studies have compared child- and adolescent-onset mania, and among those that have, the inconsistencies across studies, strict adherence to DSM-based description, and lack of distinction between age of onset versus current age make findings difficult to interpret. Thus, we are hard-pressed to compare child versus adolescent onset of mania with any degree of confidence. Nevertheless, one of the most consistent psychopathological features in age comparisons is the co-occurrence of ADHD and male preponderance in preadolescents diagnosed with BD. When investigators have used *age at clinical presentation* as the point of reference for age, rates of ADHD were highest in children but still relatively high in teens (Biederman et al., 2005; Findling et al., 2001; Geller et al., 2000). When *age of onset* was the object of study, rates of ADHD were much lower in teens (Birmaher et al., 2009; Faraone et al., 1997; Masi et al., 2006).

Using data from the Course and Outcome of Bipolar Youth study, Birmaher and colleagues (2009) employed the lifetime worst episode to distinguish between child and teen onset. Although age of onset and current age were described, the actual age of the worst episode was not explicitly stated because the K-SADS does not elicit that information. It appears that symptoms of mania in childhood-onset cases were, in fact, milder in this study than they were in teen-onset patients. BD not otherwise specified, the symptoms of which were found to be milder and briefer than bipolar I and II disorders, was more common among individuals with childhood-onset manic symptoms. Ratings of elation were lower in the younger cohort, but level of irritability was higher, which is also consistent with Masi and colleagues' (2006) data.

THE DILEMMA OF DIAGNOSTIC STABILITY

Few disorders appear to carry a "lifetime sentence." If one meets criteria for ADHD at age 10 and not at age 20, it is considered "outgrown." If one has a depressive episode at age 15 and 5 years later there have been no further episodes, the disorder is considered remitted. If the patient remembers having had the episode, it is considered a lifetime episode, but one is not considered "depressed" for the rest of one's life. With BD, the prevalent notion is that if one ever has had a manic episode, the patient is branded for life because, at least in adult psychiatry, the viewpoint is that there is a high likelihood that another episode will occur at some point. Hence, the field has no qualms about calling a person "bipolar" as opposed to saying he or she has had an episode of mania or depression. The questions to be addressed are, does the same certitude hold for children, and at what age should there be this level of certainty?

The issue inherent in diagnostic stability is how valid diagnosis is over time. As Schwartz and colleagues (2000) stated:

> Since the introduction of DSM III, psychiatric clinicians and psychiatric epidemiologists have used a common set of diagnostic criteria but application of these criteria differs. Clinicians observe patients' phenomenology longitudinally, integrating multiple sources of information before making a firm diagnosis. . . . Regardless of how diagnoses are formulated, they can shift over time because of changes in patients' clinical state, clarity stemming from treatment response, emergence of significant, previously unrevealed clinical information, or reinterpretation of previously gathered information. (p. 593)

The Suffolk County Mental Health Study (Schwartz et al., 2000) used a sample of patients ages 15 to 60 with a first hospitalization for psychosis. The most temporally consistent diagnoses between baseline and 2-year follow-up were schizophrenia (92%), BD (83%), and major depression (74%). Diagnoses were made using the combination of highly reliable semistructured interviews, other informants, medical records, and a team of experienced psychiatrists assembling the data without knowledge of consensus diagnoses from the earlier assessments. Neither age at onset nor age at index episode appreciably changed diagnostic stability.

Perhaps not surprisingly, by 10 years, diagnostic consistency had dropped compared with baseline. Of 193 respondents on whom there were data for most evaluation time points between baseline and 10 years, only 51% retained their original diagnosis. Child psychopathology in general (odds ratio = 2.6, confidence interval = 1.3–5.3) and childhood externalizing disorders in particular (odds ratio = 4.3, confidence interval = 2.3–8.0) were associated with inconsistent diagnosis. Of those respondents who had a bipolar diagnosis and were given a differ-ent diagnosis at 10 years, most developed schizophrenia or were considered to have a schizoaffective condition (i.e., they may have had mood swings but their interepisode course was predominantly either psychotic or marked by negative symptoms). There were a number of respondents whose course of illness and sub-sequent symptoms defied diagnostic classification. In three patients whose initial presentation appeared to be manic but expressed within the context of severe drug use, the subsequent course indicated no further episodes of mood disorder (Ruggero et al., in press).

There has been, however, a presumption that the diagnosis of BD, whenever it is made, trumps anything else a patient can develop. It may be that some patients allegedly with BD and a poor outcome in fact have something other than BD.

The Suffolk County mental health data describe adolescents and young adults. Although there are several longitudinal studies of children and adolescents that now stretch to late adolescence, these articles describe percentage of time ill rather than diagnostic consistency among young people with mania. In fact, there are no data of which we are aware that have addressed the question of long-term (from childhood into young adulthood) diagnostic stability in prepubertal BD. It would be remarkable if there were no diagnostic shifts. It will be necessary to rediagnose children over time to determine what course changes occur, how fre-quently, and with what implications. The notion that, once made, a diagnosis of BD should prevail in perpetuity requires solid data, especially given the treatment implications, which often point to complex combinations of mood stabilizers and atypical antipsychotics.

Equally important, too, is what other conditions or situations develop when the straight path from child to adult BD is not taken. Whereas there is consider-able stability between adolescent and adult depression (homotypic continuity), heterotypic continuity would appear to characterize prepubertal depression. Prepubertal onset cases were predicted by psychosocial adversity, family psy-chopathology, anxiety, and behavior disorders (Rutter, Kim-Cohen, & Maughan, 2006). Although there was some continuity between child and adult depression, substance abuse and conduct disorder were also frequent outcomes (Harrington, Fudge, Rutter, Pickles, & Hill, 1990; Weissman et al., 1999). It would be surpris-ing if childhood-onset BD did not have equally heterogeneous outcomes.

MULTIFINALITY AND EQUIFINALITY

An extension of the question of diagnostic stability is the concept of multifinal-ity and equifinality. Equifinality implies that a given disorder can emerge from a variety of developmental pathways, and multifinality indicates that high-risk situ-ations or a particular set of behaviors can diverge toward a multitude of quite dis-parate paths (Cicchetti & Rogosch, 1996). Although we cannot yet reflect on this issue regarding long-term outcome of behaviors that are called bipolar, there are some data that allow us to look at harbingers of what becomes BD at least in children, adolescents, and young adults. Several longitudinal studies allow a glimpse into the question of what behaviors are present before symptoms of mania and BD occur in syndromal form. Three of these are high-risk studies: a study examining offspring of lithium responsive and nonresponsive adults with BD (Duffy, Alda, Crawford, Milin, & Grof, 2007), the National Institute of Mental Health (NIMH) high-risk study (Radke-Yarrow, 1998), and the Stony Brook high-risk study (Carlson & Weintraub, 1993). Unfortunately, the study of Amish offspring with BD, which has the potential of providing the best offspring data because there are no substance abuse and antisocial comorbidities to complicate course, has used unconventional and unreplicatable methods to describe the offspring at risk (Shaw, Egeland, Endicott, Allen, & Hostetter, 2005). Finally, the Dunedin study (Kim-Cohen et al., 2003) followed a community sample into adulthood and provides data on adults who met structured interview criteria for mania and factors that prefaced that outcome.

Using data from the NIH high-risk study, the long-term diagnostic trajectories of youth who met criteria for the Child Behavior Checklist juvenile bipolar phenotype (CBCL-JBD; n = 16) during childhood and/or adolescence were examined. The CBCL-JBD phenotype is characterized by elevated scores on the CBCL Attention Problems, Anxious/Depressed, and Aggressive Behavior subscales and was named as such because it has been found to be common among children with a diagnosis of BD. Participants in this study are part of a larger 23-year longitudinal prospective study of offspring of mothers with unipolar depression, bipolar illness, or no history of psychiatric illness (Radke-Yarrow, 1998) who were followed from early childhood through young adulthood at regular intervals. There have been no previous studies examining the relationship of the CBCL-JBD profile to BD in adulthood. Results of this high-risk study revealed that fewer than one-third of offspring in the CBCL-JBD subsample met criteria for BD at young adult follow-up. Rather, the value of the profile appeared to be in its capacity to predict ongoing comorbidity and impairment rather than any one specific diagnosis. There was notable stability in a pattern of concurrent mood/anxiety, attention, and behavioral problems, with accompanying functional impairment, that remained fairly consistent from middle childhood through young adulthood. Thus, at the diagnostic level of analysis, the data appear to be consistent with the concept of multifinality; that is, early on these children fit a behavioral profile believed to be associated with bipolar illness, but at longitudinal follow-up the majority no longer met diagnostic criteria for a bipolar spectrum condition and instead showed a broad array of outcomes. However, if one examines the data at the level of symptom and functional expression, there was striking continuity from childhood through young adulthood (Meyer et al., 2009).

The concept of equifinality was borne out in Duffy and colleagues' (2007) prospective follow-up study of the offspring of parents with BD. Results revealed significant variability in antecedent psychiatric diagnoses among offspring who later developed bipolar spectrum disorder (n = 26). Anxiety and sleep disorders were the most common diagnoses to precede BD in this high-risk sample. Interestingly, results suggested that parental response to lithium was an important source of heterogeneity with regard to premorbid conditions. In particular, ADHD, learning disabilities, and cluster A personality traits frequently preceded onset of BD among offspring of lithium nonresponders, whereas these phenotypes were not common among offspring of lithium responders who later developed bipolar illness. Reasons for these findings are speculative at this point but suggest that parent symptom control with lithium decreases the psychosocial impact that active illness has on offspring. In addition, parents who do not respond to lithium have more depression, mixed episodes, and a chronic course that is a more complex form of BD and that may have its own genetic subtype.

In the Stony Brook high-risk study (Carlson & Weintraub, 1993), offspring of hospitalized adults with BD, normal controls, and offspring of parents psychiatrically hospitalized for other reasons were compared. Within the sample as a whole, childhood behavior and attention problems were associated with diagnosable psychopathology in adulthood across all three groups. These problems were associated with mood disorder outcomes only in the bipolar risk group. Nevertheless, as observed by Hammen, Burge, Burney, and Adrian (1990) two decades ago, a child with a parent with BD and with attention/behavior problems was just as much at risk for developing other psychopathology and impaired social and occupational competence as the offspring of other psychiatrically ill parents.

Few studies that have observed children from childhood to adulthood have examined rates of BD. Using the Diagnostic Interview Schedule in a sample of young adults from the New Zealand Dunedin Study, Kim-Cohen and colleagues (2003) found rates of 3% for BD, although it was unclear whether this meant bipolar I or any of the bipolar spectrum disorders. More than half (58%) had had disorders before the age of 15, and it appeared that childhood depression and oppositional defiant disorder/conduct disorder occurred in rates significantly higher than in the non-"manic" sample. Rates of anxiety disorder were also high. ADHD rates were negligible.

It will be important for future studies to identify forces in development that maintain a child on a path toward adult-type bipolar illness versus other outcomes. Recent studies suggest that impaired family interaction patterns may be an important vulnerability factor for BD episodes (Du Rocher-Schudlich, Youngstrom, Calabrese, & Findling, 2008; Meyer et al., 2006; Miklowitz & Goldstein, 1997; Schenkel et al., 2008). Geller and colleagues (Geller, Craney, et al., 2002; Geller, Tillman, et al., 2004) showed that maternal warmth was highly predictive of relapse among children and adolescents diagnosed with BD, while Townsend, Demeter, Youngstrom, Drotar, and Findling (2007) found that impaired family problem-solving skills inhibited response to pharmacological treatment among youth with BD. Additional findings from the NIH high-risk study (Meyer et al., 2006) shed light on a possible mechanism through which family dysfunction may increase risk for BD in youth. In that study, exposure to extreme maternal negativity, as measured during toddlerhood through middle childhood via lab-based observational assessments, was associated with offspring executive function deficits (as measured by performance on the Wisconsin Card Sorting Test) in adolescence, which, in turn, increased risk for developing bipolar illness at young adult follow-up. Although speculative, these findings suggest that early exposure to high levels of maternal negativity may contribute to alterations in offspring neurocognitive functioning, which may interact with underlying genetic risk to increase risk for the expression of bipolar symptomatology. Alternatively, it may be that mothers become more negative and reactive in response to a child who has poor executive skills (and is more impulsive, lacks foresight, will not follow rules, and so on). Finally, another possibility is that maternal negativity and offspring executive function impairment may be reflective of a common heritable trait.

CONCLUSIONS

To further our understanding of the phenomenology of bipolar spectrum conditions, we need to adopt a theoretical framework that goes beyond symptom counts to consider transactional processes involved in the manifestation and course of illness. A developmental psychopathology approach holds much promise in this regard. Within this framework, psychopathology is conceptualized as developmental deviation rather than a categorical phenomenon (Cicchetti, 1993). As such, it becomes necessary to trace behavior and adaptation over the life course in order to detect meaningful patterns of deviancy during the periods before and after illness is manifest (Sroufe, 1989; see Table II). This entails careful study of biological and psychological factors that may be influencing the course of development. Such an approach has the potential to provide important insights with regard to phenomenology as well as early detection and the development of effective intervention strategies (Masten & Coatsworth, 1995; Sroufe, 1989). Conversely, the tendency to reify established criteria for bipolar spectrum conditions, with the underlying assumption that these are inherent characteristics, moves us away from developmental analysis (Sroufe, 2007) and, therefore, deprives us of opportunities to identify places where we might intervene before the full manifestation of manic symptomatology.

It is perhaps unpopular to suggest that most of our current assessment instruments fall short in being able to address phenomenology, but that is not what they were designed to do. The Washington University K-SADS may be an exception insofar as it asks about symptoms other than those in DSM and obtains onset and offset of specific symptoms. Although this may be a disadvantage in distinguishing DSM-IV mania from other maladaptive behavioral patterns, it may be useful in understanding the time course of phenomenology. However, insofar as all assessment instruments depend on parent memory without any effort to substantiate this information, the field is fraught with considerable bias. Documentation from past school reports, home movies, and other data gathered at different time points is needed to verify and elaborate informant recall.

Cicchetti (1993) argues that as geneticists begin to tackle more complex questions, such as "What is inherited?" and "What is the mode of genetic transmission?," psychopathology research must allow for the simultaneous assessment of multiple domains of influence within and outside each individual, "thereby minimizing fragmentation of individual functioning" (p. 495). Such a perspective encourages the study of individuals across development rather than merely focusing on a single time point.

Why must we study individuals over time? A disorder may look very different from a longitudinal versus cross-sectional perspective. In an important volume of the *Journal of Affective Disorders*, Weller, Weller, and Dogin (1998) and Carlson and Fahim (1998) each presented an individual case of a child who had been diagnosed with BD. If examined cross-sectionally, the two children resembled each other in many ways. However, it became evident in the case prepared by Carlson and Fahim that the environment was a more pathogenic force than genetic makeup. In fact, when the child was removed from his environment, his manic symptoms disappeared. Thus, a cross-sectional approach to assessing these two children led to identical diagnostic conclusions, whereas longitudinal follow-up revealed critical differences in terms of etiology and course of symptoms. We would argue that manic-like symptoms that are only expressed under certain environmental conditions most likely do not merit a bipolar diagnosis. However, this continues to be an area of controversy.

Understanding the phenomenology of BD across the life span will require acknowledgment of the fact that the spectrum of bipolar conditions seems to be conceptualized in two ways. One way is as an early-onset developmental delay in emotion regulation that may have its own trajectory, and the other is an adult-onset disorder that occasionally begins in prepubertal children. The two conditions may also co-occur and continue into adulthood. In fact, the observation that there are several different forms of BD based on age of onset fits with this notion. Efforts into understanding the similarities and differences between these populations will be needed, with collaborative research emanating from child, adolescent, and adult specialists. Efforts will also be needed to ascertain whether what is called "mania" in one research group is the same as what is called "mania" in another.

A common view is that temperament plays a major role in determining the type and intensity of developmental experiences leading to psychopathology and vice versa (Akiskal, 1996). Cicchetti and Tucker (1994) wrote, "Particularly in the temperamentally sensitive brain, less severe forms of psychological insult may create emotional sensitizations that ripple through the developmental process" (p. 546) and may lead to subsequent forms of maladaptation. Of course, not all individuals who are at risk for BD will manifest premorbid signs of vulnerability, but there is empirical evidence suggesting that a substantial subgroup of children and adolescents at risk for BD do display temperamental, neuropsychological, and behavioral differences. Thus, an important question arises: Among those individuals who are at risk for BD, what are the developmental experiences that interact with predisposition to place an individual on a pathway to disorder? Conversely, what are the protective factors in the environment that may deter individuals from proceeding along such a path?

The 2006 American Academy of Child and Adolescent Psychiatry research forum (Carlson et al., 2009) regarding risk and protective factors in the development of early-onset bipolar illness suggested that future research will need to focus on understanding the role of temperament, social cognition, language development, and reality testing on the development of BD as well as factors influencing the development of emotion regulation. Moreover, it is critical that we begin to establish normative parameters for various aspects of BD in young people, including the natural history of irritability, grandiosity, elation, emotional lability, and so-called mood swings and the age at which children understand the concepts being asked of them on interviews.

Gender is another variable that may influence pathways to BD. At this juncture, there is very little research that has looked at the ways in which gender differences influence the course of BD. This has been a more common focus in studies of unipolar depression because of the differing rates of disorder among males and females. However, it may be that gender impacts the course of BD in more subtle ways. For example, future research should attempt to understand why females experience more depressive episodes relative to manic episodes, while the opposite is true for males (Daly, 1997). Furthermore, why is it that females are more prone to rapid cycling than males (Robb, Young, Cooke, & Joffe, 1998)? Finally, little research has been done to study the effects of puberty on the development of both mania and depression in BD and why symptom expression may change between childhood and adolescence. Future investigations that address peripubertal brain changes and neurodevelopmental trajectories in girls and boys associated with the emergence of bipolar symptoms may be pivotal in our understanding of the pathophysiology of the disorder.

So, what can we say for certain at this point? From the existing literature, we know that there is a group of significantly impaired children with severe delays in emotion regulatory skills who are at heightened risk for broad-ranging and severe symptomatology as young adults. There is growing evidence that this phenotype runs in families and that environmental factors play an important role in the early manifestation of symptoms (Hudziak, Althoff, Derks, Faraone, & Boomsma, 2005), thus making it a worthwhile target for early intervention efforts. From a clinical standpoint, this group of children, who are increasingly being diagnosed with BD, require immediate attention. The appeal of calling their problems "bipolar" is that it is a familiar term that provides parents and professionals with a sense that they have identified what is wrong with the child and allows them to adopt strategies that have been developed for adults with bipolar spectrum conditions. However, given the paucity of longitudinal follow-up data, it is our view that it is premature to draw such conclusions.

An alternative conceptualization is that what is being called bipolar disorder in youth represents a developmental disorder of emotion regulation, which is less

TABLE 2.2. Summary of Conclusions

- Developmental psychopathology is a theoretical framework that has the potential to deepen our understanding of the phenomenology of bipolar illness across the life span.
- At this juncture, there is a need for longitudinal follow-up studies that assess transactional influences within and outside individuals across development, before and after manifestation of illness.
- Future research efforts will need to focus on the role of temperament, social cognition, language development, and reality testing on the development of BD as well as factors influencing the development of emotion regulation.
- It is imperative that we begin to establish normative parameters for such constructs as grandiosity, elation, and mood swings across childhood and adolescence as well as their relationship to various forms of psychopathology.
- Our current interview-based child assessment instruments are generally not designed to address the phenomenology of mania and are limited by parent and child recall. For purposes of research and clinical data collection, these instruments must be supplemented with past school reports, home movies, and other sources of information.
- Variable methods of diagnosis ascertainment across research sites have complicated our ability to draw conclusions about BD in youth.
- BD is being conceptualized in two ways: (1) an early-onset developmental delay in emotion regulation and (2) an adult-onset disorder that occasionally begins before puberty. These conditions may manifest individually or may co-occur. Both need to be better understood. Longitudinal studies are necessary to confirm that the early-onset phenotype is continuous with the adult form of illness.
- Age of onset continues to have variable definitions (putative age of symptoms defined retrospectively as mood symptoms, age of depression if a manic episode occurs subsequently, age of mania/hypomania). In addition, its significance may vary depending on whether one focuses on cognitive or biological age. If age of onset is going to be a marker, consistent definition is needed. That said, evidence exists that there are subgroups of patients based on age of onset.
- Still unaddressed are the issues of (a) whether manic symptoms in children identify a condition that is continuous with adult BD or is a developmental phenocopy and (b) methods of distinguishing which children have which.

diagnostically specific but just as important to understand. Before we conclude that these conditions are the same, we need to know whether the childhood phenotype is continuous with the adult form. From our reading of the literature, there are no data to suggest continuity with classic adult BD, but a complex, mixed, rapid cycling subtype has not been ruled out.

References

Akiskal, H. S. (1996). The temperamental foundations of affective disorders. In C. Mundt, M. J. Goldstein, K. Hahlweg, & P. Fiedler (Eds.), *Interpersonal factors in the origin and course of affective disorders* (pp. 3–30). Dorchester, UK: Dorset Press.

Akiskal, H. S., Djenderedjian, A. M., Rosenthal, R. H., & Khani, M. K. (1977). Cyclothymic disorder: Validating criteria for inclusion in the bipolar affective group. *American Journal of Psychiatry, 134*(11), 1227–1233.

Alloy, L. B., Abramson, L. Y., Walshaw, P. D., Keyser, J., & Gerstein, R. K. (2006). A cognitive-vulnerability-stress perspective on bipolar spectrum disorders in a normative adolescent brain, cognitive and emotional development context. *Development and Psychopathology*, *18*, 1055–1103.

American Psychiatric Association. (2000). *Diagnostic and statistical manual of mental disorders* (4th ed., text rev.). Washington, DC: Author.

Andreasen, N. C. (2007). DSM and the death of phenomenology in America: An example of unintended consequences. *Schizophrenia Bulletin*, *33*, 108–112.

Angermeyer, M. C., & Kühn, L. (1988). Gender differences in age at onset of schizophrenia. An overview. *European Archives of Psychiatric and Neurological Science*, *237*(6), 351–364.

Angold, A., Costello, E. J., Erkanli, A., & Worthman, C. M. (1999). Pubertal changes in hormone levels and depression in girls. *Psychological Medicine*, *29*(5), 1043–1053.

Anthony, J., & Scott, P. (1960). Manic-depressive psychosis in childhood. *Child Psychology and Psychiatry*, *1*, 53–72.

Bellivier, F., Golmard, J. L., Henry, C., Leboyer, M., & Schurhoff, F. (2001). Admixture analysis of age at onset in bipolar I affective disorder. *Archives of General Psychiatry*, *58*(5), 510–512.

Bellivier, F., Golmard, J. L., Rietschel, M., Schulze, T. G., Malafosse, A., Preisig, M., et al. (2003). Age at onset in bipolar I affective disorder: Further evidence for three subgroups. *American Journal of Psychiatry*, *160*(5), 999–1001.

Berrettini, W. (1998). Progress and pitfalls: Bipolar molecular linkage studies. *Journal of Affective Disorders*, *50*, 287–297.

Biederman, J., Faraone, S. V., Wozniak, J., Mick, E., Kwon, A., Cayton, G. A., et al. (2005). Clinical correlates of bipolar disorder in a large, referred sample of children and adolescents. *Journal of Psychiatric Research*, *39*(6), 611–622.

Biederman, J., Mick, E., Faraone, S. V., Spencer, T., Wilens, T. E., & Wozniak, J. (2000). Pediatric mania: A developmental subtype of bipolar disorder? *Biological Psychiatry*, *48*, 458–466.

Birmaher, B., Axelson, D., Strober, M., Gill, M. K., Valeri, S., Chiappetta, L., et al. (2006). Clinical course of children and adolescents with bipolar spectrum disorders. *Archives of General Psychiatry*, *63*, 175–183.

Birmaher, B., Axelson, D., Strober, M., Gill, M. K., Yang, M., Ryan, N., et al. (2009). Comparison of manic and depressive symptoms between children and adolescents with bipolar spectrum disorders. *Bipolar Disorders*, *11*(1), 52–62.

Blehar, M. C., DePaulo, J. R., Gershon, E. S., Reich, T., Simpson, S. G., & Nurnberger, J. I. (1998). Women with bipolar disorder: Findings from the NIMH genetics initiative sample. *Psychopharmacology Bulletin*, *34*(3), 239–243.

Blumberg, H. P., Kaufman, J., Martin, A., Whiteman, R., Zhang, J. H., Gore, J. C., et al. (2003). Amygdala and hippocampal volumes in adolescents and adults with bipolar disorder. *Archives of General Psychiatry*, *60*, 1201–1208.

Blumberg, H. P., Krystal, J. H., Bansal, R., Martin, A., Dziura, J., Durkin, K., et al. (2006). Age, rapid-cycling, and pharmacotherapy effects on ventral prefrontal cortex in bipolar disorder: A cross-sectional study. *Biological Psychiatry*, *59*, 611–618.

Calderoni, D., Wudarsky, M., Bhangoo, R., Dell, M. L., Nicolson, R., Hamburger, S. D., et al. (2001). Differentiating childhood-onset schizophrenia from psychotic mood disorders. *Journal of the American Academy of Child and Adolescent Psychiatry*, *40*(10), 1190–1196.

Carlson, G. A. (1979). Affective psychoses in mental retardates. *Psychiatric Clinics of North America*, *2*, 499–510.

Carlson, G. A. (1981). Manic-depressive illness and cognitive immaturity. In R. H. Belmaker & H. M. van Praag (Eds.), *Mania: An evolving concept* (pp. 281–289). Jamaica, NY: Spectrum.

Carlson, G. A., Bromet, E. J., Driessens, C., Mojtabai, R., & Schwartz, J. E. (2002). Age at onset, childhood psychopathology, and 2-year outcome in psychotic bipolar disorder. *American Journal of Psychiatry, 159*, 307–309.

Carlson, G. A., Bromet, E. J., & Jandorf, L. (1998). Conduct disorder and mania: What does it mean in adults. *Journal of Affective Disorders, 48*(2–3), 199–205.

Carlson, G. A., Bromet, E. J., & Sievers, S. (2000). Phenomenology and outcome of subjects with early- and adult-onset psychotic mania. *American Journal of Psychiatry, 157*(2), 213–219.

Carlson, G. A., & Fahim, F. (1998). George. *Journal of Affective Disorders, 51*, 195–198.

Carlson, G. A., Findling, R. L., Post, R. M., Birmaher, B., Blumberg, H. P., Correll, C., et al. (2009). AACAP 2006 Research Forum—Advancing research in early-onset bipolar disorder: Barriers and suggestions. *Journal of Child and Adolescent Psychopharmacology, 19*(1), 3–12.

Carlson, G. A., & Meyer, S. E. (2006). Phenomenology and diagnosis of bipolar disorder in children, adolescents, and adults: Complexities and developmental issues. *Development and Psychopathology, 18*, 939–969.

Carlson, G. A., & Weintraub, S. (1993). Childhood behavior problems and bipolar disorder: Relationship or coincidence? *Journal of Affective Disorders, 28*, 143–153.

Carter, T. D., Mundo, E., Parikh, S. V., & Kennedy, J. L. (2003). Early age at onset as a risk factor for poor outcome of bipolar disorder. *Journal of Psychiatric Research, 37*(4), 297–303.

Chang, K., Adleman, N. E., Dienes, K., Simeonova, D. I., Menon, V., & Reiss, A. (2004). Anomalous prefrontal-subcortical activation in familial pediatric bipolar disorder: A functional magnetic resonance imaging investigation. *Archives of General Psychiatry, 61*(8), 781–792.

Chang, K., Karchemskiy, A., Barnea-Goraly, M., Garrett, A., Simeonova, D. I., & Reiss, A. (2005). Reduced amygdalar gray matter volume in familial pediatric bipolar disorder. *Journal of the American Academy of Child and Adolescent Psychiatry, 44*(6), 565–573.

Chang, K. D., Blasey, C., Ketter, T. A., & Steiner, H. (2001). Family environment of children and adolescents with bipolar parents. *Bipolar Disorders, 3*(2), 73–78.

Chang, K. D., Blasey, C. M., Ketter, T. A., & Steiner, H. (2003). Temperament characteristics of child and adolescent bipolar offspring. *Journal of Affective Disorders, 77*(1), 11–19.

Chengappa, K. N., Kupfer, D. J., Frank, E., Houck, P. R., Grochocinski, V. J., Cluss, P. A., et al. (2003). Relationship of birth cohort and early age at onset of illness in a bipolar disorder case registry. *American Journal of Psychiatry, 160*(9), 1636–1642.

Cicchetti, D. (1993). Developmental psychopathology: Reactions, reflections, projections. *Developmental Review, 13*, 471–502.

Cicchetti, D., & Rogosch, F. A. (1996). Equifinality and multifinality in developmental psychopathology. *Development and Psychopathology, 8*(4), 597–600.

Cicchetti, D., & Toth, S. L. (1995). Developmental psychopathology and disorders of affect. In D. Cicchetti & D. J. Cohen (Eds.), *Developmental psychopathology* (Vol. 2, pp. 369–420). New York: Wiley.

Cicchetti, D., & Tucker, D. (1994). Development and self-regulatory structures of the mind. *Development and Psychopathology, 6*, 533–549.

Craddock, N., & Sklar, P. (2009). Genetics of bipolar disorder: Successful start to a long journey. *Trends in Genetics, 25*(2), 99–105.

Daly, I. (1997). Mania. *Lancet, 349*, 1157–1160.

Davenport, Y. B., Zahn-Waxler, C., Adland, M. L., & Mayfield, A. (1984). Early child-rearing practices in families with a manic-depressive parent. *American Journal of Psychiatry, 141*(2), 230–235.

Davis, R. E. (1979). Manic-depressive variant syndrome of childhood: A preliminary report. *American Journal of Psychiatry, 136*(5), 702–706.

DelBello, M. P., Zimmerman, M. E., Mills, N. P., Getz, G. E., & Strakowski, S. M. (2004). Magnetic resonance imaging analysis of amygdala and other subcortical brain regions in adolescents with bipolar disorder. *Bipolar Disorders, 6,* 43–52.

Depue, R. A., Slater, J. F., Wolfstetter-Kausch, H., Klein, D., Goplerud, E., & Farr, D. (1981). A behavioral paradigm for identifying persons at risk for bipolar depressive disorder: A conceptual framework and five validation studies. *Journal of Abnormal Psychology, 90*(5), 381–437.

Dickstein, D. P., Milham, M. P., Nugent, A. C., Drevets, W. C., Charney, D. S., Pine, D. S., et al. (2005). Frontotemporal alterations in pediatric bipolar disorder. *Archives of General Psychiatry, 62,* 734–741.

Dickstein, D. P., Nelson, E. E., McClure, E. B., Grimley, M. E., Knopf, L., Brotman, M. A., et al. (2007). Cognitive flexibility in phenotypes of pediatric bipolar disorder. *Journal of the American Academy of Child and Adolescent Psychiatry, 46*(3), 341–355.

Doyle, A. E., Wilens, T. E., Kwon, A., Seidman, L. J., Faraone, S. V., Fried, R., et al. (2005). Neuropsychological functioning in youth with bipolar disorder. *Biological Psychiatry, 58,* 540–548.

Du Rocher-Schudlich, T. D., Youngstrom, E. A., Calabrese, J. R., & Findling, R. L. (2008). The role of family functioning in bipolar disorder in families. *Journal of Abnormal Child Psychology, 36*(6), 849–863.

Duffy, A., Alda, M., Crawford, L., Milin, R., & Grof, P. (2007). The early manifestations of bipolar disorder: A longitudinal prospective study of the offspring of bipolar parents. *Bipolar Disorders, 9,* 828–838.

Duffy, A., Alda, M., Kutcher, S., Cavazzoni, P., Robertson, C., Grof, E., et al. (2002). A prospective study of the offspring of bipolar parents responsive and nonresponsive to lithium treatment. *Journal of Clinical Psychiatry, 63*(12), 1171–1178.

Faraone, S. V., Biederman, J., Wozniak, J., Mundy, E., Mennin, D., & O'Donnell, D. (1997). Is comorbidity with ADHD a marker for juvenile-onset mania? *Journal of the American Academy of Child and Adolescent Psychiatry, 36*(8), 1046–1055.

Faraone, S. V., Lasky-Su, J., Glatt, S. J., Van Eerdewegh, P., & Tsuang, M. T. (2006). Early onset bipolar disorder: Possible linkage to chromosome 9q34. *Bipolar Disorders, 8,* 144–151.

Findling, R. L., Gracious, B. L., McNamara, N. K., Youngstrom, E. A., Demeter, C. A., Branicky, L. A., et al. (2001). Rapid, continuous cycling and psychiatric co-morbidity in pediatric bipolar I disorder. *Bipolar Disorders, 3*(4), 202–210.

Forty, L., Jones, L., Jones, I., Smith, D. J., Caesar, S., Fraser, C., et al. (2009). Polarity at illness onset in bipolar I disorder and clinical course of illness. *Bipolar Disorders, 11*(1), 82–88.

Frazier, J. A., Ahn, M. S., DeJong, S., Bent, E. K., Breeze, J. L., & Giuliano, A. J. (2005). Magnetic resonance imaging studies in early-onset bipolar disorder: A critical review. *Harvard Review of Psychiatry, 13,* 125–140.

Galanter, C., Goyal, P., Jenna, L., & Fisher, P. (2008, March). *Sources of diagnostic variability in pediatric bipolar disorder diagnostic instruments.* Paper presented at the Pediatric Bipolar Disorder Conference, Cambridge, MA.

Geller, B., Badner, J. A., Tillman, R., Christian, S. L., Bolhofner, K., & Cook, E. H. (2004). Linkage disequilibrium of the brain-derived neurotrophic factor Val66Met polymorphism in children with a prepubertal and early adolescent bipolar disorder phenotype. *American Journal of Psychiatry, 161*(9), 1698–1700.

Geller, B., Craney, J. L., Bolhofner, K., Nickelsburg, M. J., Williams, M., & Zimerman, B. (2002). Two-year prospective follow-up of children with a prepubertal and early adolescent bipolar disorder phenotype. *American Journal of Psychiatry, 159*(6), 927–933.

Geller, B., Tillman, R., Craney, J. L., & Bolhofner, K. (2004). Four-year prospective outcome and natural history of mania in children with a prepubertal and early adolescent bipolar disorder phenotype. *Archives of General Psychiatry, 61,* 459–467.

Geller, B., Zimerman, B., Williams, M., Bolhofner, K., Craney, J. L., DelBello, M. P., et al. (2000). Diagnostic characteristics of 93 cases of a prepubertal and early adolescent bipolar disorder phenotype by gender, puberty and comorbid attention deficit hyperactivity disorder. *Journal of Child and Adolescent Psychopharmacology, 10*(3), 157–164.

Geller, B., Zimerman, B., Williams, M., DelBello, M. P., Bolhofner, K., Craney, J. L., et al. (2002). DSM-IV mania symptoms in a prepubertal and early adolescent bipolar disorder phenotype compared to attention-deficit hyperactive and normal controls. *Journal of Child and Adolescent Psychopharmacology, 12,* 11–25.

Geller, B., Zimerman, B., Williams, M., DelBello, M. P., Frazier, J., & Beringer, L. (2002). Phenomenology of prepubertal and early adolescent bipolar disorder: Examples of elated mood, grandiose behaviors, decreased need for sleep, racing thoughts, and hypersexuality. *Journal of Child and Adolescent Psychopharmacology, 12*(1), 3–9.

Gershon, E. S., Badner, J. A., Goldin, L. R., Sanders, A. R., Cravchik, A., & Detera-Wadleigh, S. D. (1998). Closing in on genes for manic-depressive illness and schizophrenia. *Neuropsychopharmacology, 18*(4), 233–242.

Goodwin, F. K., & Jamison, K. R. (2007). *Manic-depressive illness: Bipolar disorders and recurrent depression.* New York: Oxford University Press.

Hammen, C., Burge, D., Burney, E., & Adrian, C. (1990). Longitudinal study of diagnoses in children of women with unipolar and bipolar affective disorder. *Archives of General Psychiatry, 47*(12), 1112–1117.

Harms, E. (1952). Differential patterns of manic-depressive disease in childhood. *Nervous Child, 9,* 326–356.

Harrington, R., Fudge, H., Rutter, M., Pickles, A., & Hill, J. (1990). Adult outcomes of childhood and adolescent depression: I. Psychiatric status. *Archives of General Psychiatry, 47,* 465–473.

Hudziak, J. J., Althoff, R. R., Derks, E. M., Faraone, S. V., & Boomsma, D. I. (2005). Prevalence and genetic architecture of Child Behavior Checklist-juvenile bipolar disorder. *Biological Psychiatry, 58,* 562–568.

Jairam, R., Srinath, S., Girimaji, S. C., & Seshadri, S. P. (2004). A prospective 4–5 year follow-up of juvenile onset bipolar disorder. *Bipolar Disorders, 6,* 386–394.

Jensen, P. S., Rubio-Stipec, M., Canino, G., Bird, H. R., Dulcan, M. K., Schwab-Stone, M. E., et al. (1999). Parent and child contributions to diagnosis of mental disorder: Are both informants always necessary? *Journal of the American Academy of Child and Adolescent Psychiatry, 38,* 1569–1579.

Kaufman, J., Birmaher, B., Brent, D., Rao, U., Flynn, C., Moreci, P., et al. (1997). Schedule for Affective Disorders and Schizophrenia for School-Age Children—Present and Lifetime Version (K-SADS-PL): Initial reliability and validity data. *Journal of the American Academic of Child and Adolescent Psychiatry, 36*(7), 980–988.

Kennedy, N., Everitt, B., Boydell, J., van Os, J., Jones, P. B., & Murray, R. M. (2005). Incidence and distribution of first-episode mania by age: Results from a 35-year study. *Psychological Medicine, 35*(6), 855–863.

Kessler, R. C., Berglund, P., Demler, O., Jin, R., Merikangas, K. R., & Walters, E. E. (2005). Lifetime prevalence and age-of-onset distributions of DSM-IV disorders in the National Comorbidity Survey Replication. *Archives of General Psychiatry, 62*(6), 593–602.

Kim-Cohen, J., Caspi, A., Moffitt, T. E., Harrington, H., Milne, B. J., & Poulton, R. (2003). Prior juvenile diagnoses in adults with mental disorder: Developmental follow-back of a prospective-longitudinal cohort. *Archives of General Psychiatry, 60*(7), 709–717.

Kraepelin, E. (1921). *Manic-depressive insanity and paranoia* (R. M. Barclay, Trans.). Edinburgh, UK: Livingstone.

Kupfer, D. J., Frank, E., Grochocinski, V. J., Cluss, P. A., Houck, P. R., & Stapf, D. A. (2002). Demographic and clinical characteristics of individuals in a bipolar disorder case registry. *Journal of Clinical Psychiatry, 63*(2), 120–125.

Kutcher, S., Robertson, H. A., & Bird, D. (1998). Premorbid functioning in adolescent onset bipolar I disorder: A preliminary report from an ongoing study. *Journal of Affective Disorders, 51,* 137–144.

Leboyer, M., Bellivier, F., McKeon, P., Albus, M., Borrman, M., Perez-Diaz, F., et al. (1998). Age at onset and gender resemblance in bipolar siblings. *Psychiatry Research, 81,* 125–131.

Leibenluft, E., Charney, D. S., Towbin, K. E., Bhangoo, R. K., & Pine, D. S. (2003). Defining clinical phenotypes of juvenile mania. *American Journal of Psychiatry, 160*(3), 430–437.

Leverich, G. S., McElroy, S. L., Suppes, T., Keck, P. E., Denicoff, K. D., Nolen, W. A., et al. (2002). Early physical and sexual abuse associated with an adverse course of bipolar illness. *Biological Psychiatry, 51*(4), 288–297.

Lin, P. I., McInnis, M. G., Potash, J. B., Willour, V., MacKinnon, D. F., DePaulo, J. R., et al. (2006). Clinical correlates and familial aggregation of age at onset in bipolar disorder. *American Journal of Psychiatry, 163*(2), 240–246.

Lish, J. D., Dime-Meenan, S., Whybrow, P. C., Price, R. A., & Hirschfeld, R. M. (1994). The National Depressive and Manic-Depressive Association (DMDA) survey of bipolar members. *Journal of Affective Disorders, 31*(4), 281–294.

Loranger, A. W., & Levine, P. M. (1978). Age at onset of bipolar affective illness. *Archives of General Psychiatry, 35,* 1345–1348.

Manchia, M., Lampus, S., Chillotti, C., Sardu, C., Ardau, R., Severino, G., et al. (2008). Age at onset in Sardinian bipolar I patients: Evidence for three subgroups. *Bipolar Disorders, 10*(3), 443–446.

Masi, G., Perugi, G., Millepiedi, S., Mucci, M., Toni, C., Bertini, N., et al. (2006). Developmental differences according to age at onset in juvenile bipolar disorder. *Journal of Child and Adolescent Psychopharmacology, 16*(6), 679–685.

Masten, A. S., & Coatsworth, J. D. (1995). Competence, resilience, and psychopathology. In D. Cicchetti & D. J. Cohen (Eds.), *Developmental psychopathology* (Vol. 2, pp. 715–752). New York: Wiley.

McClellan, J., Kowatch, R. A., & Findling, R. L. (2007). Practice parameter for the assessment and treatment of children and adolescents with bipolar disorder. *Journal of the American Academy of Child and Adolescent Psychiatry, 46*(1), 107–125.

McElroy, S. L., Strakowski, S. M., West, S. A., Keck, P. E., & McConville, B. J. (1997). Phenomenology of adolescent and adult mania in hospitalized patients with bipolar disorder. *American Journal of Psychiatry, 154*(1), 44–49.

McGlashan, T. H. (1988). Adolescent versus adult onset of mania. *American Journal of Psychiatry, 145*(2), 221–223.

Mendlewicz, J. (1998). Acceptance speech for the Lieber Prize for Affective Illness Research. *NARSAD Research Newsletter, 10,* 11–12.

Meyer, S. E., Carlson, G. A., Wiggs, E. A., Martinez, P. E., Ronsaville, D. S., Klimes-Dougan, B., et al. (2004). A prospective study of the association among impaired executive functioning, childhood attentional problems, and the development of bipolar disorder. *Development and Psychopathology, 16*(2), 461–476.

Meyer, S. E., Carlson, G. A., Wiggs, E. A., Ronsaville, D. S., Martinez, P. E., Klimes-Dougan, B., et al. (2006). A prospective high-risk study of the association among maternal negativity, apparent frontal lobe dysfunction, and the development of bipolar disorder. *Development and Psychopathology, 18*(2), 573–589.

Mick, E., Biederman, J., Faraone, S. V., Murray, K., & Wozniak, J. (2003). Defining a developmental subtype of bipolar disorder in a sample of nonreferred adults by age at onset. *Journal of Child and Adolescent Psychopharmacology, 13*(4), 453–462.

Mick, E., Spencer, T., Wozniak, J., & Biederman, J. (2005). Heterogeneity of irritability in attention-deficit/hyperactivity disorder subjects with and without mood disorders. *Biological Psychiatry, 58*(7), 576–582.

Miklowitz, D. J., & Chang, K. D. (2008). Prevention of bipolar disorder in at-risk children: Theoretical assumptions and empirical foundations. *Development and Psychopathology, 20*(3), 881–897.

Miklowitz, D. J., & Goldstein, M. J. (1997). *Bipolar disorder: A family-focused treatment approach.* New York: Guilford Press.

O'Connor, M. J., Shah, B., Whaley, S., Cronin, P., Gunderson, B., & Graham, J. (2002). Psychiatric illness in a clinical sample of children with prenatal alcohol exposure. *American Journal of Drug and Alcohol Abuse, 28,* 743–754.

Olfson, M., Crystal, S., Gerhard, T., Huang, C., & Carlson, G. A. (2009). Mental health treatment received by youths in the year before and after a new diagnosis of bipolar disorder. *Psychiatric Services, 60*(8), 1098–1106.

Papadakis, A. A., Prince, R. P., Jones, N. P., & Strauman, T. J. (2006). Self-regulation, rumination, and vulnerability to depression in adolescent girls. *Development and Psychopathology, 18,* 815–829.

Pavuluri, M. N., Birmaher, B., & Naylor, M. (2005). Pediatric bipolar disorder: A review of the past 10 years. *Journal of the American Academy of Child and Adolescent Psychiatry, 44*(9), 846–871.

Pavuluri, M. N., Henry, D. B., Nadimpalli, S. S., O'Connor, M. M., & Sweeney, J. A. (2006). Biological risk factors in pediatric bipolar disorder. *Biological Psychiatry, 60,* 936–941.

Pavuluri, M. N., Schenkel, L. S., Aryal, S., Harral, E. M., Hill, S. K., Herbener, E. S., et al. (2006). Neurocognitive function in unmedicated manic and medicated euthymic pediatric bipolar patients. *American Journal of Psychiatry, 163,* 286–293.

Pellegrini, D., Kosisky, S., Nackman, D., Cytryn, L., McKnew, D. H., Gershon, E., et al. (1986). Personal and social resources in children of patients with bipolar affective disorder and children of normal control subjects. *American Journal of Psychiatry, 143*(7), 856–861.

Perlis, R. H., Miyahara, S., Marangell, L. B., Wisniewski, S. R., Ostacher, M., DelBello, M. P., et al. (2004). Long-term implications of early onset in bipolar disorder: Data from the first 1000 participants in the Systematic Treatment Enhancement Program for Bipolar Disorder (STEP-BD). *Biological Psychiatry, 55*(9), 875–881.

Perris, C., & d'Elia, G. (1966). A study of bipolar (manic-depressive) and unipolar recurrent depressive psychoses: IX. Therapy and prognosis. *Acta Psychiatrica Scandinavica Supplement, 194,* 153–171.

Perugi, G., Micheli, C., Akiskal, H. S., Madaro, D., Socci, C., Quilici, C., et al. (2000). Polarity of the first episode, clinical characteristics, and course of manic depressive illness: A systematic retrospective investigation of 320 bipolar I patients. *Comprehensive Psychiatry, 41*(1), 13–18.

Petti, T., Reich, W., Todd, R. D., Joshi, P., Galvin, M., Reich, T., et al. (2004). Psychosocial variables in children and teens of extended families identified through bipolar affective disorder probands. *Bipolar Disorders, 6*(2), 106–114.

Radke-Yarrow, M. (1998). *Children of depressed mothers: From early childhood to maturity.* New York: Cambridge University Press.

Rich, B. A., Schmajuk, M., Perez-Edgar, K. E., Fox, N. A., Pine, D. S., & Leibenluft, E. (2007). Different psychophysiological and behavioral responses elicited by frustration in pediatric bipolar disorder and severe mood dysregulation. *American Journal of Psychiatry, 164*(2), 309–317.

Robb, J. C., Young, L. T., Cooke, R. G., & Joffe, R. T. (1998). Gender differences in patients with bipolar disorder influence outcome in the Medical Outcomes Survey (SF-20) sub-scale scores. *Journal of Affective Disorders, 49*(3), 189–193.

Romero, S., DelBello, M. P., Soutullo, C. A., Stanford, K., & Strakowski, S. M. (2005). Family environment in families with versus families without parental bipolar disorder: A pre-liminary comparison study. *Bipolar Disorders, 7*(6), 617–622.

Rucklidge, J. J. (2006). Impact of ADHD on the neurocognitive functioning of adolescents with bipolar disorder. *Biological Psychiatry, 60*, 921–928.

Ruggero, C. J., Carlson, G. A., Kotov, R., & Bromet, E. J. (in press). 10-year diagnostic consis-tency of bipolar disorder in a first-admission sample. *Bipolar Disorders.*

Rutter, M., Kim-Cohen, J., & Maughan, B. (2006). Continuities and discontinuities in psycho-pathology between childhood and adult life. *Journal of Child Psychology and Psychiatry, 47*, 276–295.

Schenkel, L. S., West, A. E., Harral, E. M., Patel, N. B., & Pavuluri, M. N. (2008). Parent-child interactions in pediatric bipolar disorder. *Journal of Clinical Psychology, 64*, 422–437.

Schürhoff, F., Bellivier, F., Jouvent, R., Mouren-Siméoni, M. C., Bouvard, M., Allilaire, J. F., et al. (2000). Early and late onset bipolar disorders: Two different forms of manic-depressive illness? *Journal of Affective Disorders, 58*(3), 215–221.

Schwartz, J. E., Fennig, S., Tanenberg-Karant, M., Carlson, G., Craig, T., Galambos, N., et al. (2000). Congruence of diagnoses 2 years after a first-admission diagnosis of psychosis. *Archives of General Psychiatry, 57*(6), 593–600.

Shaw, J. A., Egeland, J. A., Endicott, J., Allen, C. R., & Hostetter, A. M. (2005). A 10-year pro-spective study of prodromal patterns for bipolar disorder among Amish youth. *Journal of the American Academy of Child and Adolescent Psychiatry, 44*(11), 1104–1111.

Shibley Hyde, J., Mezulis, A. H., & Abramson, L. Y. (2008). The ABCs of depression: Integrat-ing affective, biological, and cognitive models to explain the emergence of gender differ-ence in depression. *Psychological Review, 115*(2), 291–313.

Soares, J. C., & Mann, J. J. (1997). The anatomy of mood disorders—Review of structural neuroimaging studies. *Biological Psychiatry, 41*, 86–106.

Sroufe, L. A. (1989). Pathways to adaptation and maladaptation: Psychopathology as develop-mental deviation. In D. Cicchetti (Ed.), *Rochester Symposia on Developmental Psychopa-thology* (Vol. 1, pp. 13–40). Rochester, NY: University of Rochester Press.

Sroufe, L. A. (2007). The place of development in developmental psychopathology. In A. Mas-ten (Ed.), *Multilevel dynamics in developmental psychopathology: pathways to the future. The Minnesota symposia on child psychology* (Vol. 34, pp. 285–299). Mahwah, NJ: Erlbaum.

Staner, L., Tracy, A., Dramaix, M., Genevrois, C., Vanderelst, M., Vilane, A., et al. (1997). Clinical and psychosocial predictors of recurrence in recovered bipolar and unipolar depressives: A one-year controlled prospective study. *Psychiatry Research, 69*, 39–51.

Stefos, G., Bauwens, F., Staner, L., Pardoen, D., & Mendlewicz, J. (1996). Psychosocial predic-tors of major affective recurrences in bipolar disorder: A 4-year longitudinal study of patients on prophylactic treatment. *Acta Psychiatrica Scandinavica, 93*, 420–426.

Stephens, J. H., & McHugh, P. R. (1991). Characteristics and long-term follow-up of patients hospitalized for mood disorders in the Phipps Clinic, 1913–1940. *Journal of Nervous and Mental Disease, 179*(2), 64–73.

Strakowski, S. M., DelBello, M. P., & Adler, C. M. (2005). The functional neuroanatomy of bipolar disorder: A review of neuroimaging findings. *Molecular Psychiatry, 10*, 105–116.

Thapar, A., & Rice, F. (2006). Twin studies in pediatric depression. *Child and Adolescent Psy-chiatry Clinics of North America, 15*, 869–881.

Townsend, L. D., Demeter, C. A., Youngstrom, E., Drotar, D., & Findling, R. L. (2007). Family conflict moderates response to pharmacological intervention in pediatric bipolar disorder. *Journal of Child and Adolescent Psychopharmacology, 17*(6), 843–852.

Turvey, C. L., Coryell, W. H., Arndt, S., Solomon, D. A., Leon, A. C., Endicott, J., et al. (1999). Polarity sequence, depression, and chronicity in bipolar I disorder. *Journal of Nervous and Mental Disease, 187*(3), 181–187.

Weinberg, W. A., & Brumback, R. A. (1976). Mania in childhood. *American Journal of Diseases of Children, 130*, 380–385.

Weissman, M. M., Wolk, S., Wickramaratne, P., Goldstein, R. B., Adams, P., Greenwald, S., et al. (1999). Children with prepubertal-onset major depressive disorder and anxiety grown up. *Archives of General Psychiatry, 56*, 794–801.

Weller, E., Weller, R. A., & Dogin, J. W. (1998). A rose is a rose is a rose. *Journal of Affective Disorders, 51*, 189–193.

West, A. E., Henry, D. B., & Pavuluri, M. N. (2007). Maintenance model of integrated psychosocial treatment in pediatric bipolar disorder: A pilot feasibility study. *Journal of the American Academy of Child and Adolescent Psychiatry, 46*(2), 205–212.

Wilke, M., Kowatch, R. A., DelBello, M. P., Mills, N. P., & Holland, S. K. (2004). Voxel-based morphometry in adolescents with bipolar disorder: First results. *Psychiatry Research, 131*, 57–69.

Winokur, G., Clayton, P. J., & Reich, T. (1969). *Manic-depressive illness.* St. Louis, MO: Mosby.

Wozniak, J., Biederman, J., Kiely, K., Ablon, J. S., Faraone, S. V., Mundy, E., et al. (1995). Mania-like symptoms suggestive of childhood-onset bipolar disorder in clinically referred children. *Journal of the American Academy of Child and Adolescent Psychiatry, 34*(7), 867–876.

Wozniak, J., Biederman, J., Kwon, A., Mick, E., Faraone, S., Orlovsky, K., et al. (2005). How cardinal are cardinal symptoms in pediatric bipolar disorder?: An examination of clinical correlates. *Biological Psychiatry, 58*(7), 583–588.

Youngerman, J., & Canino, I. A. (1978). Lithium carbonate use in children and adolescents. A survey of the literature. *Archives of General Psychiatry, 35*(2), 216–224.

A Developmental Psychopathology Perspective on the Assessment and Diagnosis of Bipolar Disorder

Eric A. Youngstrom

Now is a time of great change in the way we think about bipolar disorder (BD). After decades where the prevailing belief was that BD was a highly severe, categorical illness that typically manifested in young adulthood, data are challenging each piece of the conventional wisdom. Evidence is mounting to suggest that BD falls along a spectrum (e.g., Akiskal & Pinto, 1999; Judd et al., 2003; Phelps, Angst, Katzow, & Sadler, 2008), and that there are not firm natural boundaries between positions along the continuum. Nor is there necessarily a dividing line between BD and normal emotional and motivational experience. There is growing recognition that BD can manifest in adolescence, and research findings are accumulating to support the validity of the diagnosis in childhood as well (Geller & Tillman, 2005; Youngstrom, Birmaher, & Findling, 2008). There is increasing consensus that BD is a neurodevelopmental condition, in which a genetic diathesis is present from the moment of conception and environmental experiences begin to exert harmful and protective influences from the womb through at least young adulthood and probably throughout life (Goodwin & Jamison, 2007).

This chapter is organized around five themes from developmental psychopathology, with the traditional topics of assessment (e.g., rating scales, norms, interviews, performance measures) woven around the threads of the five themes. The guiding threads are

1. *Normal developmental processes*: Which ones are implicated in BD, and what can BD teach us about normal development? How do we distinguish pathological mood states from the emotional extremes of normal development?

2. *Developmental trajectories* and emergence over time: How do the classic themes of developmental discontinuity, equifinality, and multifinality, and comorbidity illuminate our understanding of BD?

3. *Risk and protective factors*: What is the impact of adversity, and are there any self-righting tendencies associated with BD?

4. *Assessment of stage-salient developmental tasks* and their interplay with BD: How do peer functioning, academic functioning, conflict and individuation from the family, and the cascade of changes associated with puberty influence the onset and course of BD?

5. *Sex differences*: Gender differences are a focal issue in developmental psychopathology, and sex is a well-investigated moderator variable with potent effects on the course and presentation of mood disorders. What do we know about its influence on BD?

The first two sections are longer because they combine content about BD with developmental psychopathology concepts. The three later sections are briefer illustrations of other facets of the implications of a developmental psychopathology model for BD.

Developmental psychopathology offers a rich model for examining BD, with a theoretical framework and a vocabulary for describing reciprocal interactions between the developing individuals and their environment and examining the interplay among biological, intrapsychic, and social factors (e.g., Cicchetti & Cohen, 2006). However, the developmental psychopathology framework has been underutilized in the area of BD as a result of accidents of history and sociology rather than relative merit or heuristic value. When BD was considered firmly in the purview of adult biological psychiatry, there was no impetus for adult psychiatry researchers to consider psychosocial or developmental models. Conversely, BD remained "off the radar" for developmental psychopathology researchers. The condition does not map neatly onto either the externalizing or internalizing dimensions of childhood psychopathology but instead involves both major dimensions. Similarly, the most popular rating scales have not included mania items because of the conventional wisdom that these symptoms were part of a syndrome that only manifested in adulthood (e.g., Achenbach & Edelbrock, 1983). For decades the field operated as though BD sprang fully formed from the brow of young adults rather than having deep roots in constructs such as temperament and environmental experiences.

This chapter starts to integrate some concepts and constructs from developmental psychopathology with issues in the assessment and diagnosis of BD. The charge was to focus on child and adolescent assessment issues, but both the nature of developmental psychopathology and the emerging consensus about the bipolar diagnosis necessitate taking a life span perspective. This chapter will *not* provide a systematic review of the diagnostic criteria for mood states or bipolar diagnoses. These are fully articulated in the *Diagnostic and Statistical Manual of Mental Disorders* (DSM-IV-TR; American Psychiatric Association, 2000) and the *International Classification of Diseases* (ICD-10; World Health Organization, 1992).

In sharp contrast to the popular perception that there is rampant disagreement about the definition of BD in youth (Healy, 2006), the DSM and ICD frameworks are essentially identical. The consensus appears to be that when the same criteria used for adults are applied to youth, then a research diagnosis of pediatric BD has good reliability and validity (Findling et al., 2001; Youngstrom et al., 2008). Discussions about potential revisions to DSM criteria for children and adolescents appear to be converging on a conservative stance, with recommendations to make only minor changes to the current criteria (Leibenluft & Rich, 2008; Youngstrom et al., 2008) and the same changes to the adult criteria (Ghaemi et al., 2008; Vieta & Suppes, 2008). This chapter also does not provide a detailed review of the different rating scales or interview batteries available to assess pediatric BD, on which several comprehensive and recent reviews are available (Johnson, Miller, & Eisner, 2008; Quinn & Fristad, 2004; Youngstrom, 2007). *Instead, this chapter brings the arsenal of developmental psychopathology to bear on the target of BD and works to expose areas that would benefit from focused empirical investigation.*

NORMAL DEVELOPMENT AND BIPOLAR DISORDER

BD affects multiple systems of functioning, both within the affected individual and also interpersonally. Within the individual, BD influences cognitive functioning, emotion recognition and expression, energy levels, and somatic symptoms (Goodwin & Jamison, 2007; Kraepelin, 1921). Interpersonally, BD affects close personal relationships with family, friends, and partners; and it also exacts a heavy toll on academic and vocational functioning (Birmaher & Axelson, 2006; Judd & Akiskal, 2003; Judd et al., 2005; Miklowitz, Goldstein, Nuechterlein, Snyder, & Mintz, 1988). There are increasing indications that BD is associated with heart disease, increased risk of obesity, and substance misuse, each potentially contributing to the earlier mortality associated with the illness (McElroy et al., 2002; Toalson, Ahmed, Hardy, & Kabinoff, 2004). Mind, body, and relationships all can be pressed and shifted by disturbances of mood.

Emotional Development

Emotions play a fundamental role in organizing our responses to the environment. Normal human development involves learning to express emotions, recognize emotions in others, respond effectively and appropriately to affectively charged situations, and regulate emotions (Izard, Youngstrom, Fine, Mostow, & Trentacosta, 2006). BD does not appear to involve some unique emotional state that is outside the ken of the rest of human experience, nor does it seem to involve an abnormal sequencing in the developmental pattern of emergence of emotions. Although there is some evidence of emotion recognition deficits in youth affected by BD (Dickstein & Leibenluft, 2006; Rich et al., 2008), these do not appear to be a specific feature of the illness. Similar patterns are also found in youth who are peer rejected (Dodge, 1991), some of whom have mood disorder, in youth with histories of abuse, again with an unknown proportion also potentially having mood disorders (Pollak, Cicchetti, Klorman, & Brumaghim, 1997), as well as in youth and adults with Asperger syndrome and other pervasive developmental disorders (Baron-Cohen, Wheelwright, Hill, Raste, & Plumb, 2001). It is also uncertain whether these changes in emotion perception are preexisting factors that contribute to a diathesis for BD versus being state-dependent effects that occur once mood is disrupted for other reasons.

More clearly, BD involves extremes in the intensity of emotion expression and also pronounced affective instability (Lovejoy & Steuerwald, 1992). Conceptually, extreme intensity could result from changes in the threshold for emotion activation, such that it requires less stimulation to trigger a similar emotional response in persons with BD, or the intensity could reflect an exaggerated response to the same stimulus (Izard et al., 2006). A third possibility is that BD may compromise the ability to downregulate intense affect, so that it takes longer to recover from an emotion provocation. It also is possible that a combination of all three factors contributes to the disruption of the emotional systems.

BD involves disruption of at least three major dimensions of affect. In this review I use the labels "positive affect" (PA) and "negative affect" (NA) for the two dimensions describing the emotion circumplex (instead of "valence" and "activation," which are statistically interchangeable definitions of the major dimensions) because these are more commonly used in psychopathology research (Barrett & Russell, 1999; Tellegen, Watson, & Clark, 1999). The PA dimension has emotions such as elation, joy, and excitement at the high end and sadness as the polar opposite. The NA dimension has anger and fear at the high end and relaxation and tranquility (low activation, positive valence) emotions at the low end (Tellegen et al., 1999).

The tripartite model has used the two dimensions of PA and NA to describe the shared and unique features of anxiety disorders and depression (Watson, Clark, et al., 1995; Watson, Weber, et al., 1995). Both anxiety and depression involve high levels of NA, contributing to the perception that they overlap. To the extent that both measures of anxiety and depression tend to include items loaded with NA, NA becomes a nonspecific factor that elevates scores across measures. The distinguishing feature of depression, according to the tripartite model, is low levels of PA, which clinically is described as anhedonia or loss of interests (Watson, Clark, et al., 1995). The discriminating feature of anxiety disorders was hypothesized to be physiological hyperarousal. The high NA plus low PA formulation of depression has proven robust, generalizing across multiple samples, age groups, and measures (e.g., Chorpita, 2002; Joiner, Catanzaro, & Laurent, 1996). The anxiety disorders have proven more complex, with generalized anxiety disorder (GAD) appearing to be mostly congruent with high NA and physiological hyperarousal and the discrete emotion of fear aligning more with panic and some phobias (e.g., Greaves-Lord et al., 2007; Joiner & Lonigan, 2000). Obsessive–compulsive disorder, some aspects of eating disorders, and other phobias may be more specifically related to the negative emotion of disgust rather than fear or physiological hyperarousal (Davey, Buckland, Tantow, & Dallos, 1998; Davey, McDonald, et al., 1998; Ware, Jain, Burgess, & Davey, 1994).

Although it has not yet been empirically tested, the tripartite model also generates some logical predictions about BD. During the depressed phase of a bipolar illness, an individual will experience low PA and high NA, consistent with the evidence for unipolar depression. During a pure manic phase, the presentation is reversed: High PA occurs with low levels of NA. During a mixed state, the person will either display high levels of activation of both PA and NA (a "dysphoric mania"; Goodwin & Jamison, 2007) or will rapidly oscillate between high and low extremes on each dimension (high mood lability or a "conglomerate" mixed episode; Youngstrom et al., 2008). Over the long term, BD might be characterized by a greater range of emotional shifts, perhaps indexed as a larger standard deviation for repeated measures of PA and NA over time (Lovejoy & Steuerwald, 1995). It is interesting to note that depression is not the same as elevated NA in the tripartite model. Instead, pure depression would involve simultaneous elevation of NA coupled with low PA, and euphoric mania would involve the reverse. Interestingly, anger in many respects is an "approach" emotion that activates similar brain regions as PA (Demaree & Harrison, 1997). Thus, irritable manias may make sense from an affective neuroscience perspective inasmuch as anger is more similar to other positive, approach-oriented emotions than are other negative-valenced emotions.

Another aspect of emotion that could be relevant to BD pertains to a third dimension of emotion, labeled "dominance," "potency," "surgency," or "perceived controllability" (Fontaine, Scherer, Roesch, & Ellsworth, 2007; Mehrabian, 1997; Russell & Mehrabian, 1977). The third dimension discriminates between equally activating and negative valenced emotions such as fear versus anger: If the negative, activating situation is perceived as uncontrollable, then the response is fear; if perceived as controllable, then the person experiences anger. Similarly, pride versus awe can both be positive valenced and similarly activating but differ on the dominance dimension. Emotions theorists have noted that depression appears to involve low levels of dominance, and mania high levels of dominance (Mehrabian, 1997; Plutchik, 1980). Evolutionary psychologists have theorized that depression is an evolved response to situations of loss and failure that allows one to remain a member of a social group versus representing a continued challenge that might evoke responses of attack, exile, or other aggression (Gilbert, Allan, Brough, Melley, & Miles, 2002). By extension, mania may involve high-dominance emotions (pride, grandiosity, joy, as well as anger), coupled with a propensity to switch to a depression response if thwarted. This formulation accommodates findings that BD appears to be associated with rejection sensitivity (Benazzi, 2000; Chang, Steiner, & Ketter, 2000) inasmuch as rejection sensitivity involves a focus on interpersonal relationships and placement in a larger social hierarchy.

A dominance model could contribute to models of conflict and dysfunction in families (Emery, 1992), predicting that youth with BD might be prone to challenge for more autonomy and control than would be developmentally appropriate and to respond with intense emotion displays to limit setting from authority figures. Parents with mood disorder, in turn, might be more likely to react aggressively to challenges to their authority (Du Rocher Schudlich, Youngstrom, Calabrese, & Findling, 2008). Parents might also be more vulnerable to depression if they perceive their efforts at maintaining parental control as being ineffective. Given the relative paucity of recent work on the dominance dimension, this formulation is more speculative than the tripartite model, but it generates an intriguing set of hypotheses with regard to mania. An emotional dominance model would predict that mania is associated with high levels of dominance-related emotions, and the failure of efforts to attain social goals is associated with decreases in perceived dominance and corresponding increases in the subjective experience of low-dominance emotions, including depression.

In short, BD is likely to involve individual differences in the tendency to experience and express basic dimensions of emotion. A child at risk of BD may have biological predispositions that lower the threshold for eliciting a strong affective response from the child, differences in the intensity of the response, or differences in the ability to regulate the affective response. Furthermore, the high heritability of BD suggests that at-risk youth will often be exposed to an "extended phenotype" (Rende & Plomin, 1993), where their parents carry similar genes and have similar propensities toward affective lability. The family environment thus combines emotionally labile parents with highly reactive youth, creating the potential for extremely chaotic environments with intensely expressed negative emotion. Furthermore, parents often may model suboptimal emotional display rules and coping strategies (poor "meta-emotion"; Gottman, Katz, & Hooven, 1997) as a result of their own mood dysregulation and related issues (e.g., substance use). The result could potentiate gene × environment interactions, where family conflict might activate or amplify other gene effects that, in turn, feed back into heightened environmental disruption.

Motivational Systems

An alternate way of formulating mood disorders is that they involve dysregulation of basic motivational systems. One such model is Gray's behavioral inhibition system (BIS) and behavioral activation system (BAS) theory (Gray & McNaughton, 1996). BIS and BAS are thought to be basic neurophysiological systems that motivate approach and appetitive behaviors (BAS) or focus on cues of threat and punishment and inhibit behavior (BIS). BIS and BAS have behavioral correlates and established connections with temperament and personality traits: High BIS is associated with high neuroticism and high NA, and high BAS is associated with extraversion, novelty and thrill seeking, and surgency (Corr, 2001; Matthews & Gilliland, 1999). The correlation with surgency is intriguing, because it suggests that BAS may also be positively correlated with the dominance dimension of affect. Psychopathology theorists have also used BIS and BAS as an explanatory framework for several disorders, including mood, anxiety, antisocial personality, and schizophrenia in adults (Depue & Lenzenweger, 2006; Fowles, 1994) and attention-deficit/hyperactivity disorder (ADHD), anxiety disorders, conduct disorder, and depression in youth (Quay, 1993, 1997). A BIS–BAS model could account for most mood states occurring in the context of BD in similar fashion to a PA–NA model. BAS dysregulation is in some ways a better model of mania than the formulation of high PA plus low NA, because elevated BAS would be associated with both anger as well as positive emotions. This prediction is also consistent with neurocognitive findings that anger involves more left hemispheric activation (as do positive emotions), whereas fear, sadness, and depression are associated with right hemispheric activation (Demaree, Robinson, Everhart, & Youngstrom, 2005; Tomarken & Keener, 1998). Again, these findings are consistent with BAS drive showing a positive correlation with dominance.

The BAS dysregulation model of mania has accumulated substantial evidence, particularly in terms of trait BAS predicting future episodes of mania (Alloy et al., 2008; Meyer, Johnson, & Carver, 1999). The BAS dysregulation model is also gaining support in terms of laboratory findings (Gruber, Johnson, Oveis, & Keltner, 2008). A disadvantage of the BAS model is that the BAS dimension does not correlate in a straightforward manner with symptom expression (Biuckians, Miklowitz, & Kim, 2007), although BAS scores do appear to be somewhat elevated during hypomania and suppressed during depression (Meyer et al., 1999).

In summary, BD involves dysfunction of emotional and motivational systems that are intrinsic to normal development. What appears to change with BD is the propensity to experience different emotions, the intensity with which they are experienced, and changes in the duration with which moods persist (or alternately changes in the capacity to downregulate intense emotions). Further investigation needs to elaborate the relative contributions of each of these components. The next section addresses the crucial issue of understanding normal emotional development as a way of establishing benchmarks against which to chart the course of BD.

Assessing Normative versus Clinical Development of Mood and Behavior

Normal child and adolescent development provides a backdrop against which behavior must be compared in order to determine whether or not it is statistically abnormal. For parents and policymakers as well as clinicians, it is often not easy to decide what is "just being a child" or "just being a teenager" versus behaviors that constitute a social or clinical problem. Sociological critiques charge that psychiatric diagnoses often represent a reification and stigmatization of childhood behavior that used to be tolerated or fall within normal limits. This criticism has been leveled at the diagnosis of ADHD in boys and now is a component in accusations of "disease mongering" aimed at pediatric BD (Healy, 2006). Parents may be at a disadvantage when it comes to gauging the developmental appropriateness of behaviors, especially if they only have a single child, compared with teachers or clinicians, who gain the benefit of experience working with multiple youth of the same age (McDermott & Weiss, 1995).

In principle, the issue of teasing apart normal development from clinical pathology is tractable. Clinical judgment is supposed to involve a familiarity with normative behavior as well as a set of diagnostic prototypes against which profiles of behavior can be matched to recognize pathological disorders. In the context of BD, experts recommend that clinicians gauge whether a behavior is developmentally unusual in terms of the "FIND" criteria (Kowatch, Fristad, et al., 2005; Quinn & Fristad, 2004): Is it exceptional in terms of the Frequency of episodes, the Intensity with which the behavior occurs, the Number of repetitions of an act within an episode, or the Duration of the episode of behavior? Exceeding each of these comparative thresholds sets the behavior apart from what is developmentally normative, and makes it more likely that the behavior is symptomatic of an episodic mood disorder. In similar fashion, there are published descriptions of behaviors that exemplify expressions of pediatric mania versus ADHD (Geller et al., 2002; Quinn & Fristad, 2004), which are intended to help clinicians grasp the prototype and improve their performance at classifying new cases correctly. However, such training needs to overcome the tremendous range of opinion about what constitutes "normal" behavior, let alone what signifies a mood disorder. There can be wide differences in diagnostic opinions even when clinicians are presented with identical vignettes (Dubicka, Carlson, Vail, & Harrington, 2008).

Norm-referenced or "standardized" tests provide an alternate way of appraising development. Instruments such as the Achenbach System of Empirically Based Assessments (Achenbach & Rescorla, 2001) or the Behavior Assessment Scales for Children (BASC2; Reynolds & Kamphaus, 2004) gather data on large standardization samples that are meant to be representative of the general population, and then determine what constitutes average and above-average levels of behaviors compared with peers of the same sex and age. Examining the raw scores on these types of tests reveals a variety of developmental trends, including decreases in the amount of shyness and separation anxiety, attention problems, and some impulsive acting-out behaviors with age (especially in boys) and increases in depressive symptoms (especially with the onset of puberty and especially in girls), substance use, delinquent behavior, and thought disorder with age (Achenbach, Howell, McConaughy, & Stanger, 1995a).

There are three major issues in applying standardized rating scales to the investigation of BD in children and adolescents and to a lesser extent in adults. The first issue is related to the concept of establishing norms for subgroups. Age and sex differences in the typical amount of behaviors are anchored to standardized scores (usually T-scores: mean = 50, SD = 10). These standard scores provide an index of how the person's behavior compares with his or her peers. A boy and a girl with a *T*-score of 70 are both showing 2 *SD*s more of the behavior problem than their age and sex peers (putting them in the 98th percentile). However, the meaning of the raw scores could vary considerably across age and sex. Thus, the same *T*-score might correspond to a raw score of 24 for depressive symptoms in female adolescents, a raw score of 18 in preadolescent girls, and scores of 12 and 8 for similar-aged boys, respectively. In short, identical *T*-scores could refer to markedly different amounts of behavior.

Test developers debate whether it is desirable to have more fine-grained norms that take into account factors such as sex and age differences in behavior. If a consistent set of definitions is used for both sexes and across a broad swath of ages, then developmental trends and sex differences are exposed (McDermott & Weiss, 1995). For example, using a single set of norms across a wide span of ages would reveal that few preadolescents achieve clinically elevated depression scores, and more adolescent females than males would have high depression *T*-scores. The trade-off is a loss of information about whether the behavior is developmentally unusual compared with typical patterns of behavior for a specific subset of individuals. If a single, global set of norms is used, then it is not possible to compare an individual's behavior with other adolescents or other young children.

These normative trends need not influence all features of an illness in lockstep. With regard to BD, developmental issues are likely to affect the presentation and interpretation of depressive and internalizing symptoms in a different way than manic or externalizing symptoms. Hyperactivity and impulsivity are more common in boys than girls, and they decrease on average with age (Achenbach & Rescorla, 2001). Other manic symptoms, including increased energy and elated mood as well as irritability, also appear to occur more commonly in males (Duax, Youngstrom, Calabrese, & Findling, 2007) and possibly to decrease in intensity with age (Kraepelin, 1921), although this appears to contrast with aspects of typical age trends in emotion experience in adulthood and late life (Carstensen, Pasupathi, Mayr, & Nesselroade, 2000). Some anxious symptoms, such as shyness and separation anxiety, tend to decrease with age, whereas other aspects, such as trait neuroticism or generalized anxiety, show greater stability (Achenbach, Howell, McConaughy, & Stanger, 1995b; Srivastava, John, Gosling, & Potter, 2003). Sex and age norms would *reduce* the apparent changes with development and would also decrease the pronounced difference in depressive symptoms with the onset of adolescence, particularly in girls.

The second issue is that being statistically unusual is not a completely satisfactory definition of pathology. Statistical extremity, whether indexed by norms or standard scores, is neither sufficient nor necessary for pathological status. Even rare phenomena may have no clinical import if they do not result in impairment. Conversely, if the behavior is associated with impairment, then it may be interpreted as pathological regardless of statistical abnormality (Wakefield, 1992). Some recent investigations of subthreshold manic symptoms have consistently found that they are more prevalent in the general population than is full-blown mania, but even the subthreshold symptoms are associated with considerable impairment (Judd & Akiskal, 2003; Lewinsohn, Klein, & Seeley, 2000), including issues such as increased risk of substance misuse (Merikangas et al., 2008).

The third issue is the practical limitation that most norm-referenced behavior checklists do not include mania scales, nor do they include many of the symptoms that would be specific to mania. A few of the "broadband" instruments have added mania scales and items to revised versions, but these are still usually only adding the content to the adolescent versions of the instrument (e.g., Gadow & Sprafkin, 1999) or to the self-report version (e.g., BASC-2; Reynolds & Kamphaus, 2004). Both of these are significant limitations. Only by systematically gathering consistent information with younger age groups will it be possible to determine whether the behaviors cohere into similar diagnostic constellations and how they compare to normative behavior. Cross-informant data will also be crucial given the growing body of evidence that self-report may be a less valid source of information about manic symptoms (Youngstrom et al., 2004; Youngstrom, Meyers, Youngstrom, Calabrese, & Findling, 2006), particularly when the reporter is currently hypomanic or manic (Dell'Osso et al., 2002). Although there are now a variety of more specific mania-related scales available, as yet none of them have been standardized on a nationally representative sample rather than a clinical sample. Given the mounting evidence that mood symptoms can become problematic in youth, and that even subthreshold presentations may portend impairment and poor longitudinal outcomes in adulthood (Birmaher & Axelson, 2006; Birmaher et al., 2009; Geller, Tillman, Bolhofner, & Zimerman, 2008; Lewinsohn, Seeley, & Klein, 2003; Merikangas et al., 2008), the development and investigation of these types of instruments have the potential to be highly informative about the role of mood in normal and pathological developmental trajectories.

DEVELOPMENTAL TRAJECTORIES AND CHANGE IN PRESENTATION OVER TIME: EQUIFINALITY, MULTIFINALITY, AND COMORBIDITY

This section examines normal development as a baseline against which to measure pathological mood development and then discusses developmental trends in clinical mood states and correlated diagnostic entities (such as ADHD), followed by a brief examination of the ideas of equifinality (different paths converging on the same outcome) and multifinality (the same starting point leading to divergent outcomes) in the context of BD. The section concludes with mention of the ways that studying the course of mood disorders might be informative about developmental processes.

Equifinality

Equifinality refers to the possibility that several different developmental pathways could arrive at a common end point. For example, adolescent depression could be the end point for trajectories involving high levels of biological risk, early inter-personal losses, acute trauma, chronic interpersonal rejection, or any combination of these factors (Garber, Keiley, & Martin, 2002; Izard et al., 2006). Examination of the concept of BD reveals examples of equifinality at different levels of analysis, including the symptom level, the syndrome level, and the social system level.

Symptom-Level Equifinality

At the symptom level, there are multiple processes that could all lead to manifes-tations of similar-appearing behaviors. In behavioral genetics, this is sometimes described as a "phenocopy," where different genotypes, or even nongenetic pro-cesses, result in a behavioral expression that looks similar to the product of a par-ticular genotype. Poor long-term memory could be due to the expression of any of several different genes to a traumatic event or substance use, leading to cell death in the septohippocampal regions, for example (Bremner & Narayan, 1998).

Symptomatic equifinality is evident when perusing the DSM diagnostic crite-ria too. Certain symptoms are included in the criteria for multiple disorders, sug-gesting that these symptoms might be a common end point of distinct etiological pathways, if the diagnostic disorders truly represent separate entities (Angold, Costello, & Erkanli, 1999; Caron & Rutter, 1991). Figure 3.1 illustrates how irri-tability is a diagnostic feature of multiple disorders that are frequently diagnosed in childhood and adolescence as well as a common feature of BD during each of the clinical mood states: mania, hypomania, mixed, as well as pediatric depres-sion. Figure 3.1 concentrates on the disorders in which irritable mood or overt aggression is a part of the diagnostic criteria. If we consider how often irritabil-

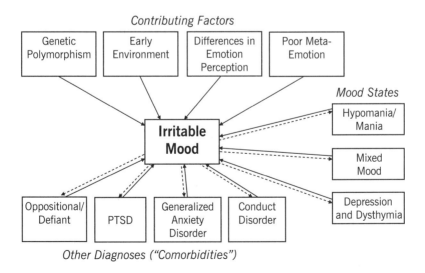

FIGURE 3.1. Interplay among contributing factors, mood states, and other diagnoses in equifinality of "irritable mood." (PTSD, posttraumatic stress disorder.)

ity presents as an associated feature of a condition, then the list would expand considerably, because most children and adolescents will respond irritably when confronted with situations that exceed their capacity for coping.

Symptomatic equifinality can also be conceptualized as the product of developmental processes. Irritable mood could be the product of genetic polymorphisms, such as the expression of single-nucleotide polymorphisms (SNPs) of genes involved in the regulation of serotonin (which have been correlated with impulsive and offensive aggression) (Burt & Mikolajewski, 2008; Haberstick, Smolen, & Hewitt, 2006; Olivier & van Oorschot, 2005). Propensity for irritable mood could also result from early environmental experiences, including prenatal exposure to testosterone (Bailey & Hurd, 2005; Benderlioglu & Nelson, 2004) or changes in maternal diet (Hibbeln et al., 2007). More developmentally downstream, the irritable mood could be due to a youth's own endocrine function or diet or to differences in emotion perception (such as the hostile attribution bias) or poor meta-emotion and impaired emotion regulation. Irritable mood can also be linked to suboptimal parenting, as well documented in the work on the coercive process in the development of antisocial behavior (Patterson, DeBaryshe, & Ramsey, 1989).

Irritable mood is a common and highly impairing symptom associated with pediatric BD (Kowatch, Youngstrom, Danielyan, & Findling, 2005). Viewed from the symptom level through the lens of equifinality, it becomes clear that there are multiple processes that could add to the risk of expressing irritable mood for an individual case and not just across different people. For example, a child might inherit an SNP associated with serotonergic impulsivity from his mother. He might also be exposed to higher levels of testosterone in utero, and his mother might have consumed almost no fish or other sources of important micronutrients during pregnancy. This constellation of factors added to the child having a more difficult temperament. Coupled with the parent's own tendency to respond impulsively and with negative affect to challenging situations, there is an increased risk of child maltreatment. As the child becomes older, there are even more opportunities for "child effects" on the parent, where the aversive behavior of the youth may feed into coercive cycles that degrade parenting efficacy and increase the chances of the parent becoming depressed. Parental depression would, in turn, further change the emotional climate and diminish the repertoire of effective parenting behaviors. The product is a feedback loop that reinforces a trajectory promoting emotional intensity and instability in the youth, eventually exceeding the thresholds for a formal diagnosis of a major mood episode. Figure 3.2 uses the tree metaphor to illustrate the idea of BD as a confluence of multiple risk factors—multiple "roots" that all feed into the "trunk" of BD.

Syndrome-Level Equifinality

At the syndrome level, equifinality reflects the fact that not all cases meeting criteria for the same diagnosis will have the same etiological processes leading to

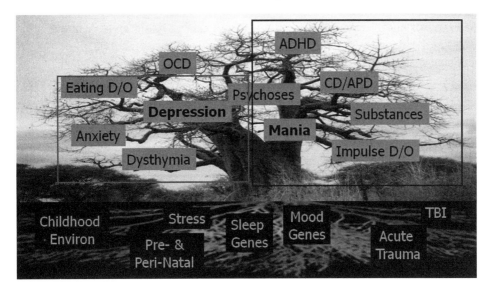

FIGURE 3.2. The tree metaphor for bipolar disorder: Equipotentiality of roots, multifinality of clinical course and presentations. (OCD, obsessive–compulsive disorder; ADHD, attention-deficit/hyperactivity disorder; D/O, disorder; CD/APD, conduct disorder/antisocial personality disorder; TBI, traumatic brain injury.)

that end point. If we identified 100 cases with pediatric BD, there is no single risk process that all 100 instances would implicate. This is a fact of using a polythetic definition of a disorder: Even if there were a single cause underlying each symptom of mania (an obvious oversimplification based on the preceding discussion), people need not have the same symptoms to meet strict criteria for a diagnosis of BD. Making a permutational expansion of the number of different combinations of mood disorder symptoms and course specifiers generates literally billions of possible configurations of symptoms (Lieberman, Peele, & Razavi, 2008).

Sleep–wake disturbance represents an interesting example. For a subset of people with BD, decreases in need for sleep are a core feature of hypomania or mania, and interruption of sleep onset may be a powerful trigger for mania (Benedetti et al., 2007; Goodwin & Jamison, 2007; Malkoff-Schwartz et al., 1998). The biological mechanisms of circadian regulation are becoming well understood, including the identification of brain structures such as the suprachiasmatic nucleus, endocrine systems involved in regulation, and even specific genes that are linked to individual differences in sleep patterns. Polymorphisms of clock genes are implicated with a fair degree of consistency as risk factors for BD (e.g., *GRK3* [Barrett et al., 2003]; *GSK3* [Benedetti et al., 2004]). However, decreased need for sleep only appears to affect approximately 60% of cases with pediatric BD (Kowatch, Youngstrom, et al., 2005) and well less than 80% of adults with BD (Goodwin & Jamison, 2007). Thus, on the one hand, the field has articulated a physiological pathway leading from gene through brain development and functioning to interactions with environmental factors, culminating in manic episodes; yet, on the other hand, this pathway is not involved in a substantial percentage of people who meet strict (albeit polythetic) criteria for BD.

Two additional factors add further complexity at the syndromal level of equifinality: diversity of definitions and diagnostic unreliability. A variety of different definitions have been included in formal nosologies as well as research programs. The DSM-IV includes bipolar II, cyclothymic disorder, and bipolar not otherwise specified (NOS) as well as bipolar I. Akiskal and colleagues have added further definitions to capture more nuanced clinical presentations (Akiskal & Pinto, 1999); others have recently revisited the Kraepelinian concept that recurrent unipolar depressions are actually a manifestation of bipolar illness (Goodwin & Jamison, 2007). Similarly, a range of definitions have been developed in the child bipolar literature, many of which are reviewed in a study by Leibenluft, Charney, Towbin, Bhangoo, and Pine (2003). These include a "narrow phenotype" that requires the presence of either elated mood or grandiosity along with an episodic presentation, an "intermediate phenotype" that encompasses the current DSM-IV definitions of bipolar I and bipolar II, and a "broad phenotype" that may not show a clear episodic presentation and can involve chronic irritability. Leibenluft has also developed more formal and narrow criteria for a syndrome called "severe mood dysregulation." Although all of these definitions may fall under a broad rubric of BD, it is unlikely that they all share identical biological, social, and developmental pathways. Indeed, evidence is emerging that there are important differences between severe mood dysregulation and bipolar I disorder (Brotman et al., 2006; Rich et al., 2007) or between chronic versus episodic presentations (Duffy, Alda, Kutchee, Fusee, & Grof, 1998; Masi et al., 2006).

A related issue is that practitioners may further expand the application of the label, using the bipolar moniker as a convenient and reimbursable diagnosis for any youth showing marked aggression. The extremely rapid recent increases in the rate of diagnosis of BD in youth (Blader & Carlson, 2007; Moreno et al., 2007) suggest a widening of usage to incorporate many cases that might otherwise seem diagnostically "homeless" (Carlson & Meyer, 2006). Recent studies using a set of vignettes indicate that there can be a wide range of diagnostic opinion and large regional differences in the rates at which ambiguous cases are labeled as falling on the bipolar spectrum (Dubicka et al., 2008). Ratings of videotapes revealed similarly large international differences in perceptions of the severity of mania in adults (Mackin, Targum, Kalali, Rom, & Young, 2006). Reliance on broader definitions increases the likelihood that many bipolar cases will reflect very different developmental processes and longitudinal trajectories.

The prior discussion has assumed that each of the different definitions is applied accurately. Unfortunately, evidence suggests that the reliability of diagnoses of mania is often lower than for other conditions (Kessler, Rubinow, Holmes, Abelson, & Zhao, 1997; Youngstrom & Youngstrom, 2008). Diagnostic unreliability, referring here to the inconsistent or inaccurate application of label, would only further compound the problems.

Social-Systems-Level Equifinality

Anyone observing a family affected by pediatric BD will be struck by the amount of tension and conflict that often characterizes interpersonal interactions (Miklowitz, Biuckians, & Richards, 2006). Such families tend to show high levels of expressed negative emotion, with much parental criticism of the youth and hostile expressions by the youth toward the parent (Coville, Miklowitz, Taylor, & Low, 2008; Du Rocher Schudlich et al., 2008; Geller et al., 2008). Youth with BD also often show deficits in the expression of social skills (although not necessarily in knowledge of social skills; Goldstein, Miklowitz, & Mullen, 2006). However, these social impairments are far from unique to BD. In that sense, dysfunctional social interactions represent a state of equifinality that bipolar disorder shares with multiple other conditions (Miklowitz, 2004).

The connection between BD and interpersonal dysfunction also creates a "chicken and egg" problem in terms of diagnosis and case formulation. Some people focus on the parent–child conflict as primary and see the youth's mood issues as being secondary to the dyadic interaction. Instead of diagnosing BD, a V-code for parent–child conflict might be preferred. Historically, family therapy approaches would tend to gravitate toward these sorts of conceptualizations, deemphasizing the formal diagnosis of an illness affecting an individual child and concentrating instead on patterns of functioning within the social system (Corsini & Wedding, 2000). The opposite extreme would be a biological psychiatric formulation that focuses on the disease, often relies on medication as a primary means of intervention, and assumes that management of the disease will result in improvements in family functioning. A developmental psychopathology framework can readily incorporate both the biological and social processes, but the clinical challenge still remains to determine which factors are more important in individual cases at different points of development or at least which constellations of factors provide more amenable points for intervention.

Multifinality and Comorbidity

A complementary idea to equifinality is multifinality: the capacity for a single risk factor or process to flow into any of several different downstream states or outcomes. Similar to equifinality, the concept of multifinality implies different things at different levels of analysis.

Modular Models of Pathology

At a fine-grained, molecular level, multifinality can refer to the shared building blocks and common mechanisms that contribute to different end points. A polymorphism of the *DRD4* gene that is associated with sensation seeking can contribute to personality traits of extraversion and openness to experience (Chen, Burton, Greenberger, & Dmitrieva, 1999), and it can also create a diathesis for

ADHD or contribute to the impulsivity seen in mania (Serretti et al., 2006). The shared-component hypothesis is consistent with the frequent findings that implicate the same genetic polymorphisms in depression, anxiety, ADHD, and schizophrenia as well as BD (Bentall, 2003; Tsuang & Faraone, 2000). In similar fashion, the common-process model accommodates the nonspecific nature of most environmental risk factors. Physical and sexual abuse are risk factors for the development of BD (Garno, Goldberg, Ramirez, & Ritzler, 2005; Romero et al., 2009), but they are also implicated in depression, posttraumatic stress disorder, borderline personality disorder, and a variety of other disorders (Fergusson, Horwood, & Lynskey, 1996).

This lack of specificity suggests a "modular model" of disorders (Youngstrom, 2009). Evolutionary and cognitive psychology are finding that brain and behavior are organized into systems that are distinct but interconnected. Specific behaviors or processes might have distinct roots and result in distinct modules of functioning, such as attachment behaviors, territorial aggression, and memory for social group membership versus memory of food locations and type (Cosmides & Tooby, 2000). Polygenic and multicausal disorders may often involve disruption of constellations of discrete modules. Psychotic mania, for example, might involve dysregulation of modules governing sleep–wake cycle, impulsivity, reward dominance, and psychosis, whereas a mixed state might require additional involvement of a threat-monitoring BIS module. Many people who meet criteria for BD do not show circadian dysregulation (Goodwin & Jamison, 2007; Kowatch, Youngstrom, et al., 2005). In a modular model of disorder, they lack the corresponding endophenotype and would not be expected to show the relevant polymorphism on circadian clock-related genes. Throughout his writings on taxometric methods, Meehl (1995) anticipated that the effects of single genes might be more focal and not directly related to all of the symptoms of a disorder.

The modular argument has evolved in parallel in the writing of Bentall (2003), who asserts that at bottom there are only symptoms, not disorders as discrete entities. The "endophenotype-as-module" position offers a more nuanced, intermediate model, where a specific biological process could be related to a constellation of symptoms and behaviors. The modular model offers a parsimonious explanation for two challenges to the existing nosology: The lack of clear diagnostic boundaries can be explained by the definitions of a disorder encompassing multiple possible endophenotype modules, and the high rates of comorbidity may be a direct result of the same endophenotype contributing to multiple syndromes. An impulsivity endophenotype may be a component of mania, ADHD, substance abuse, or all three; a "high-BIS" endophenotype may contribute to depression, generalized anxiety, panic, or mixed states.

An appropriate metaphor might be a card game, such as cribbage. Biological and environmental risk factors are each a "card." People are dealt a hand at birth and then actively modify it during development. The choices of what to discard and replace include some element of volition but also are influenced by what else is in the hand. In a game, a particular card could become part of many different "hands"—a pair, four of a kind, a straight, a flush—all depending on the rest of the hand, in much the same way that impulsivity could be a component of multiple disorders or a personality attribute without associated pathology. Cribbage is a particularly apt metaphor, because there is a "shared" environment (the "crib," a set of shared cards to which each player contributes, which counts, in turn, toward each player's score) as well as dyadic influences on the scoring (the "peg out," a round of scoring where players take turns revealing cards and competing for points as they react to other player's cards). Thus, final outcomes are the product of starting points, individual choices, shared factors, and interpersonal interactions. One of the key conceptual points illustrated by the metaphor is that there is no "gene for bipolar" and no "biological litmus test." Nor is there a single bipolar-generating environment, just as there is no single card that completes a hand or a game.

Syndrome-Level Multifinality

At a more global, molar level, BD is associated with a wide variety of clinical presentations. Even limiting discussion to the "simple" case of classic bipolar I disorder, the condition can manifest as periods of normal or even high functioning or as a major depressive episode, a manic episode, or a mixed episode with significant features of both mania and depression. When persons are monitored prospectively, their moods and behaviors reveal even greater complexity. "Subthreshold" mood presentations, with low-grade depressions or hypomanias or mixed hypomanic states, are often even more frequent than the extreme, pronounced mood states associated with syndromal episodes. Kraepelin (1921) described eight different mood states that resulted from being high or low on each of three aspects of functioning: intellective (cognitive), vegetative (somatic, or energy level), and affective (mood). There is no simple answer to the question of what BD looks like or what the typical end point of a bipolar developmental trajectory might be.

This plethora of presentations applies even to the rare cases without significant psychiatric comorbidity. However, comorbidity appears to be the rule and not the exception with BD, both in pediatric (Axelson et al., 2006; Kowatch, Youngstrom, et al., 2005) and adult (Kessler, Merikangas, & Wang, 2007) cases. The rates of comorbidity for many conditions are too high for them to be independent. It is possible to have a comorbid BD and a broken arm, for example, but the probability of having both should be a product of the base rates of each condition separately, because breaking a bone does not increase risk for BD (and for the sake of argument we assume that the effects of mania or depression on risk for bone fractures are also negligible). BD shows high rates of association with many other disorders, including panic attacks, anxiety disorders, ADHD, conduct disorder, substance misuse, oppositional defiant disorder (ODD), pervasive developmental disorders, physical and sexual abuse, and posttraumatic stress disorder. In many samples, the rate of co-occurrence is significantly higher than would be expected if the two conditions were statistically independent, although this is not always the case (cf. Youngstrom, 2009).

Elevated rates of comorbidity have prompted critical discussions of the concept and potential implications of comorbidity in mental health in general (e.g., Angold et al., 1999; Caron & Rutter, 1991; Youngstrom, Findling, & Calabrese, 2003) as well as heated debate in the area of pediatric BD in particular (Klein, Pine, & Klein, 1998). Caron and Rutter (1991) delineated several different mechanisms that could result in "artifactual" and "true" comorbidity, all of which are potentially contributing to some degree to the apparent multifinality observed across BD. Possible sources of artifactual comorbidity include the following.

1. *Using categorical labels where dimensions might be more appropriate.* As discussed in the Emotional Development section, there is no sharp dividing line between normal experience and the pathological mood states of BD; nor are there clear quantitative or qualitative boundaries between disorders within the bipolar spectrum or between bipolar versus unipolar depression (Youngstrom, 2009). Formal statistical evaluations indicate that there is no distinct category underlying GAD (Ruscio, Borkovec, & Ruscio, 2001), nor has one been found for ADHD (Frazier, Youngstrom, & Naugle, 2007). If these findings are robust, then there is no firm boundary between the distress or inattention associated with BD versus the symptoms being the product of other syndromes. The comorbidity appearing between bipolar, GAD, and ADHD could be a by-product of superimposing a categorical map of boundaries on what actually is a seamless flow of symptoms growing out of a developmental pathological process (see Figure 3.2, at the branch level of the metaphoric tree). Similarly, anxiety and depressive disorders may be labels that describe places along a continuum of trait NA and physiological hyperarousal (Bradley, 2000; Clark & Watson, 1991).

2. *Overlap in diagnostic criteria.* The potential for overlap between ADHD and BD has generated much discussion (e.g., Biederman, Klein, Pine, & Klein, 1998; Klein et al., 1998). It appears that BD is a distinct phenomenon, even when eliminating the overlapping items (Kim & Miklowitz, 2002). The nonspecificity of irritable mood also can contribute to the "overlap" phenomenon, as discussed in the context of equifinality: Not only are irritable mood and aggression common features of mania, but they are also diagnostic symptoms of unipolar depression, GAD, posttraumatic stress disorder, ODD, and intermittent explosive disorder (American Psychiatric Association, 2000) and are common associated features of a welter of other childhood conditions. Similarly, motor agitation and poor concentration are highly nonspecific symptoms. If a symptom is counted toward multiple diagnoses, it lowers the number of additional symptoms required to pass threshold for the additional diagnosis. Invoking the card game analogy again, nonspecific symptoms are like wild cards that can be used to construct multiple hands.

3. *Artificial subdivision of syndromes.* In the classic debate between "lumpers," who favor parsimony, versus "splitters," who prefer carefully nuanced description,

oversplitting would create a falsely inflated rate of comorbidity by treating multiple components of the same larger diagnostic entity as separate conditions that frequently co-occur. High rates of comorbidity thus raise questions of whether the nosological system is oversplitting. Within the bipolar spectrum, cyclothymic disorder and dysthymia can be coded separately from mania or major depressive episodes if they occur for at least a year before the onset of the major mood episode (2 years before in adults), resulting in the coding of two "comorbid" mood disorders (e.g., a cyclothymic disorder and bipolar I, or a "double depression").

A more pernicious issue is that one pathological condition can affect multiple aspects of functioning, creating apparent comorbidities that at root are really part of a single problem. A bipolar illness might involve high levels of anxiety, manifesting as high NA during a depressive episode or as high energy and fear during a dysphoric mania when the person feels that he or she is losing control or becoming preoccupied with a specific goal and then tense and irritable when thwarted from pursuing it. In each case, the anxiety is due to a bipolar illness, and Caron and Rutter (1991) would argue that it creates artifactual comorbidity to diagnose two conditions (a BD and a comorbid anxiety or obsessive–compulsive disorder) even though the person might show sufficient symptoms and impairment to meet criteria for the second diagnosis. The idea of a core phenotype of pediatric BD embraces this argument and posits that features commonly diagnosed as comorbid disorders may actually be an expression of a single core pathological phenotype in pediatric BD (Papolos, 2003). DSM currently also recognizes the possibility of overlap and instructs that anxiety disorders should not be diagnosed as comorbid with mood disorders unless the anxious symptoms also manifest outside the context of the mood episode. However, DSM does not include similar guidance about excluding diagnoses of ADHD, oppositional defiant disorder, conduct disorder, or other family conflicts or disruptive behavior problems if they appear to be secondary to a mood disorder. Figure 3.2 illustrates how BD can branch in multiple directions, growing into a variety of different multifinality "leaves" that could be diagnosed as comorbid conditions but may, in a fundamental sense, be either secondary to the BD or an expression of the illness itself, not second disorders in their own right.

4. *Developmental sequencing.* Another potential source of spurious comorbidity can be that one disorder is an early manifestation of another. In developmental psychopathology terms, this can be an example of "heterotypic continuity," where one process shows different presentations at different ages or in different developmental contexts. This possibility is relevant to BD in multiple ways. Some conditions may represent prodromes for BDs. Cyclothymic disorder and bipolar NOS both are logical potential prodromes for bipolar II and bipolar I disorders. In both cases, the evidence indicates multifinality: Some persons with cyclothymic disorder or bipolar NOS do "progress" to bipolar I or II when followed prospectively (Angst et al., 2003; Birmaher et al., 2009; Lewinsohn et al., 2000), roughly one-third of cases over a 3-year period. Another third continue to show a presentation similar to their baseline assessment, and another third appear to change to a dif-

ferent, nonbipolar diagnosis (Birmaher et al., 2009). Conversely, cases that show affective dysregulation that fits even less clearly on the bipolar spectrum, such as elevated scores on multiple scales of the Child Behavior Checklist or meeting the criteria for severe mood dysregulation, tend to continue to be highly impaired at follow-up but unlikely to develop BD (Brotman et al., 2006; Meyer et al., 2009). More controversially, some have speculated that ADHD might be a prodrome for BD (Tillman & Geller, 2006), but longitudinal studies of cohorts with ADHD have found that few cases actually develop it (Galanter et al., 2003; Hazell, Carr, Lewin, & Sly, 2003). A more tenable description appears to be that ADHD might increase risk for later mania but not necessarily be a prodrome for it (because most cases with ADHD will not develop mania and many adults with BD never had ADHD). There is evidence that anxiety disorders, and GAD in particular, may often be developmental precursors to depression (Mineka, Watson, & Clark, 1998). It is plausible that anxiety disorders might also precede bipolar depression (Birmaher et al., 2002), although this remains to be demonstrated with prospective longitudinal data.

5. *Referral or surveillance biases.* Both of these design concerns represent a last major source of artifactual comorbidity (Caron & Rutter, 1991). They have had substantial impact on some published findings with regard to pediatric BD. One pioneering research group ascertained almost all of its cases with BD from an ADHD clinic, with the result that almost 100% of cases with BD also met criteria for ADHD (Wozniak et al., 1995). This rate of comorbidity was a consequence of the referral and ascertainment pattern, not a product of BD itself, as has become clear in subsequent publications that have consistently found lower rates of ADHD (although still quite high) (Kowatch, Youngstrom, et al., 2005). Interestingly, there is not strong evidence that the rates of comorbid ADHD in bipolar cases exceeds the rates of ADHD in nonbipolar cases at the same clinical settings. Similar problems could apply to other clinical samples where local reputation, expertise, or patterns of service provision influence referral patterns.

Reliance on clinical samples also introduces other potential confounds that could distort our understanding of risk factors (e.g., Berkson's, 1946, fallacy of ascertainment bias) and longitudinal course as well as comorbidity. Clinical samples often underestimate the rate of hypomania, for example, because hypomania does not lead to sufficient impairment to motivate treatment seeking. Research in college student samples has demonstrated the existence of a group of people with recurrent hypomanias but no lifetime history of depression or mania (Alloy et al., 2008; Depue, Krauss, Spoont, & Arbisi, 1989), a group that is essentially invisible in clinical samples because of the lack of motivation (and often lack of need) to seek treatment.

Surveillance biases are a major issue in studying pediatric BD. Older research systematically underestimated the rates of hypomania, mania, and mixed episodes in youth, especially when it was theoretically rare for these to manifest in adolescence and impossible in childhood, much as was the pattern with unipolar depression in previous decades (Kovacs, 1989). Conversely, studies with adults affected by BD systematically underestimated rates of ADHD, often failing to formally assess for it because it was assumed to be a pediatric illness (Kessler, Berglund, Demler, Jin, & Walters, 2005; Nierenberg et al., 2005). Unfortunately, semistructured and structured interviews provide no guarantee of protection from surveillance effects. Meta-analyses find significant inconsistencies in the rates of comorbid anxiety disorders, ODD, and other conditions across studies (Kowatch, Youngstrom, et al., 2005). Although referral biases undoubtedly contribute to this variance across sites, there is mounting evidence of sizable differences in rates of mania identified even when clinicians are presented with identical vignettes (Dubicka et al., 2008) or in ratings of the severity of mania even when using rating tools such as the Young Mania Rating Scale (Young, Biggs, Ziegler, & Meyer, 1978) to code videotaped interviews (Mackin et al., 2006).

Surveillance bias need not always result in a bias toward underestimating risk factors or comorbidity rates, however. If certain factors cue clinicians to do a better job of assessment for particular features, then this will often induce an apparent correlation. Better monitoring may contribute to the perception of an association between BD and physical or sexual abuse, inflate the degree of association between familial risk and rates of BD in offspring, or exaggerate the degree of association between exposure to medications and subsequent rates of mania (Carlson, 2003). The literature about antidepressant-congruent pediatric mania may provide the strongest example of this, where elevated rates of mania are found in open studies (the observer and family know that they are receiving active medication) and fail to achieve statistical significance in double-blind studies (Joseph, Youngstrom, & Soares, 2009; Licht, Gijsman, Nolen, & Angst, 2008).

It also is possible to encounter syndrome-level multifinality as a result of "true comorbidity." Possible explanations of true comorbidity include (1) overlapping risk factors or common underlying dimensions of cognitive, behavioral, or affective dysfunction; (2) comorbidity creating a distinct, meaningful syndrome; and (3) one disorder creating an increased risk for the other. Again, all three probably apply to pediatric BD. First, the risk factors identified for BD are all nonspecific (Tsuchiya, Byrne, & Mortensen, 2003). The genes of risk for BD also have been implicated in unipolar depression, schizophrenia, and ADHD, among other conditions (Faraone, Glatt, & Tsuang, 2003); and low birthweight, pre- and perinatal insult, abuse and trauma, high trait NA/BIS/neuroticism, and BAS dysregulation all are associated with multiple other forms of psychopathology (Fowles, 1994; Hack et al., 2004). Even a family history of BD is not a specific risk factor for its development: Offspring of a parent with BD are at elevated risk for a variety of different poor outcomes (Hodgins, Faucher, Zarac, & Ellenbogen, 2002). The overlapping risk factor explanation is an example of the classic "third variable" problem in research design: The correlation between two variables may be the product of each being independently associated with the same underlying third variable, in this case the shared risk factor or underlying affective dimension.

The second possibility, of comorbidity resulting in a distinct, meaningful syndrome, also may apply to BD. Comorbid anxiety disorders appear to augur a more refractory course of illness, for example (Perlis et al., 2004; Wagner, 2006). The symptoms of comorbid ADHD often persist even after mood symptoms have responded to intervention and then respond well to adjunctive treatment with stimulants (Findling et al., 2006; Scheffer, Kowatch, Carmody, & Rush, 2005), suggesting that the ADHD either is a true comorbidity or is reflective of a subtype of BD (Faraone, Biederman, Mennin, Wozniak, & Spencer, 1997). The comorbid ADHD and bipolar subtype might be a version that has more chronic course and impairment. The presence or absence of ODD may be a marker or proxy for dysfunctional family interactions and high expressed emotion, which have large effects on the trajectory of illness and development (Hooley & Hiller, 2001; Miklowitz, 2004).

The third possibility, that BD might itself create an increased risk of other conditions, is also highly likely. The evidence clearly indicates a greater hazard of substance misuse associated with BD, and although bidirectional influences are likely, mood disorder is well established as a risk factor for later substance problems (Geller et al., 2008; Grant et al., 2005; Merikangas et al., 2008). BD may also create additional anxiety as the person feels embarrassed and afraid of the consequences of manic episodes. Although the literature on stress generation is more developed with unipolar depression (Rudolph et al., 2000), bipolar depressions would be associated with at least similar levels of interpersonal conflict and stress generation (Geller et al., 2008; Tillman et al., 2003). Manic and mixed states probably entail even greater relational stress. These processes will result in increased risk of trauma and posttraumatic stress disorder and probably also put children at greater risk of abuse (Garno et al., 2005). Pediatric BD is also likely to be mechanism for child effects models (Lytton, 1990), where the dysregulated behavior of the youth contributes to increased stress and depression in the parent and heightened dysfunction in the family (Du Rocher Schudlich et al., 2008).

Yet another possibility is that BD may result in the disruption of multiple systems and the expression of enough behavior problems to technically satisfy criteria for a second disorder, but in this instance the behaviors are a bipolar-induced phenocopy of the other condition. Referring to Figure 3.2 again, this model would posit that the comorbidity suggested at the branch level actually is a direct result of the BD, creating a set of behaviors that would satisfy the criteria for an additional diagnosis but reflecting a different set of risk factors and processes than those that would lead to the disorder in the absence of a bipolar process. Papolos's (2003) idea of a core phenotype of pediatric BD describes how a set of symptoms and features in addition to those captured in the current DSM criteria may be an intrinsic part of the bipolar phenotype and should be considered part of a single syndrome instead of comorbid conditions.

A final possibility derives from the kindling model (Post, Leverich, Xing, & Weiss, 2001), suggesting that comorbidities arise from the cumulative effects of mood episodes on reorganizing brain structures and social interactions. In this view, attention problems could result from the scarring effects of severe mood episodes, and recurrent depressions might establish trait-like changes in emotion perception and mood-congruent recall that increase later levels of anxiety. There are various plausible neural mechanisms for such developmental changes, including inhibition of neurogenesis as well as changes in synaptic connectivity.

Developmental Changes in Mood and Emotion Regulation: What Do They Teach Us about Normal Development?

In light of the meager amount of research to date on the developmental psychopathology of BD, there is not a large set of "lessons learned" from BD about normal development. However, there are several ways in which research on BD could be highly informative about developmental processes. One example would be by investigating the increasing ratio of depressive to manic episodes with age, which appears to increase to more than 3:1 by adulthood (Judd et al., 2002; Kraepelin, 1921). The elucidation of what factors contribute to this change is likely to be highly informative, not just about BD but about normal developmental processes in mood and emotion regulation. Is the shift due to acute treatments being more effective for mania? That possibility cannot account for the secular trend being observed before the advent of lithium therapy (Kraepelin, 1921), nor does it address the sharp increase in depression at puberty, especially among girls (Cyranowski, Frank, Young, & Shear, 2000). Is it an artifact of relying on clinical samples, where people are unlikely to seek treatment for hypomania or, conversely, where people suffering from predominantly depressive courses of illness might be overrepresented? Certainly, the age differences in mood episode polarity are much more pronounced than secular trends in emotion experience that have been documented in the general population, such as a general increase in positive affectivity achieved by preferential selection of interactions with fulfilling persons (Carstensen et al., 2000). A third possibility is that psychosocial factors have strong depressogenic effects, such that expressed emotion, peer rejection, abuse, and other environmental factors may cumulate over time to produce more depressive episodes. A fourth possibility is that at least some aspects of mania may reflect developmental delays in the maturation of executive functioning or emotion-regulation circuitry, with the result that impulsive and emotionally labile behaviors are common in youth and become less frequent or intense with age. Similar models of developmental delay are being applied productively to antisocial behavior (Tremblay et al., 1997) and ADHD (Barkley, 2001).

RISK AND PROTECTIVE FACTORS

The prior discussions of equifinality and multifinality have emphasized that the risk factors contributing to BD are not specific to it but can also contribute to the development of other conditions as well. The developmental trajectory of each individual is going to be shaped by the constellation of risk and protective factors with which they start as well as the experiences and factors that accrue as they navigate their life course. Some risk factors deserve additional comment because they may moderate or change the risk conveyed by other factors. Sexual abuse and neglect are an interesting illustration: Not only are they bad in their own right, with a main effect increasing the risk of psychopathology, but they may moderate the course of bipolar illness, possibly contributing to the higher rate of depression and bipolar II disorder in women (Garno et al., 2005) and to suicidality (Leverich & Post, 2006) and decreasing the threshold for relapse in response to stressful life events (Dienes, Hammen, Henry, Cohen, & Daley, 2006).

One risk factor that is conspicuous in its absence from the bipolar literature is low socioeconomic status (SES). The relationship between SES and BD is likely to be complex: The association between BD and creativity and productivity could induce a positive correlation with SES in some cases, whereas the burden of illness and poor functioning with recurrent episodes may result in downward SES drift in other cases (Goodwin & Jamison, 2007; Kessler et al., 2006; Lopez, Mathers, Ezzati, Jamison, & Murray, 2006). Another consideration is that BD has often been underrecognized in minority populations (DelBello, Lopez-Larson, Soutullo, & Strakowski, 2001; Strakowski et al., 1996), potentially further distorting the relationship with SES in samples within the United States. It seems likely that many of the advantages that pertain to higher SES, including better educational support and access to more and superior health care services, are likely to moderate the effect of other risk factors on the trajectories of persons at risk of developing or relapsing into bipolar episodes. Cultural beliefs and norms are also likely to influence the expression of risk factors in ways that will further moderate relationships with SES, including the effects of attitudes toward mental illness, stigma, and help seeking, as well as varying degrees of familism and reliance on the extended family as a source of social support (Coelho, Strauss, & Jenkins, 1998; Loue & Sajatovic, 2008; Yeh et al., 2005).

Less is known about protective factors that buffer against or modify the course of BD. Knowledge in this regard is poised to advance rapidly, as gains are consolidated in terms of establishing genetic and environmental risk factors. With the risk factors clearly demarcated, it becomes easier to define high-risk groups and then investigate the factors associated with resiliency and positive trajectories. There are some obvious candidates for study as protective factors based on their widespread importance in developmental psychopathology. These include higher general cognitive ability (Gottfredson, 1997), positive family functioning (more positive emotion expression, warmth, good communication, authoritative parenting), good early environment (including good pre- and postnatal diet, good access to general preventive health care, and secure attachment), good meta-emotion skills (emotion recognition, regulation, and family or cultural rules or mores around emotion expression; Gottman, Katz, & Hooven, 1996), and the formation of constructive peer relationships. Each of these are likely to exert a beneficial influence, but research needs to isolate whether the benefits are due to positive main effects, interactions that blunt the negative effects of risk factors, or even changes in the variability of outcomes. Spectacular successes and failures may otherwise be lost in the description of "average" or "typical" trajectories.

From a developmental perspective, there are likely to be critical periods where the effects of risk and protective factors are much more important. Nutrients involved in brain development will probably have greater impact during periods of rapid growth or neural reorganization, including prenatal, infancy, and peripubertal epochs. It is possible that the timing of exposure to risk factors will also have major consequences for the degree of effect they have on development, as has been found in the case of lead poisoning and marijuana exposure. The neurotoxic effects of lead are greatest when the brain is actively growing but can also recur years later as bone loss releases bioactive lead back into the body in late life (Agency for Toxic Substances & Disease Registry, 2007). Similarly, if toxins accrete in adipose tissue, then obesity could heighten risk of accumulation, and weight loss might actually result in at least brief reexposure of other biological systems to the toxin. Marijuana may be a major potentiator of psychotic symptoms, but only for a subset of the population with a particular genetic diathesis and only if sufficient exposure occurs before a threshold is passed in brain development (Henquet, Di Forti, Morrison, Kuepper, & Murray, 2008; van Winkel et al., 2008). Lead, obesity, and marijuana each provide an example of how environmental factors can interact with genes, with each other, with timing of exposure during development, and with yet other factors to produce a diversity of outcomes.

ASSESSMENT OF STAGE-SALIENT TASKS

Even before birth, some risk factors and moderators of development relevant to BD may be present. Thus, it is valuable to assess stage-salient tasks throughout development and examine their association with bipolar trajectories. The recent neurodevelopmental imaging/mapping project provides normative benchmarking data against which patterns of development in cases affected by BD can be compared (Gogtay et al., 2007). There is evidence for particular regions being implicated in BD, such as the amygdala, which appears to be smaller in pediatric BD, and average or slightly enlarged in adults with BD (Miklowitz & Chang, 2008). Similarly, assessment of body mass index will help clarify whether obesity is a risk factor for BD versus being a consequence of medication-induced weight gain or mood-induced changes in activity and appetite (Correll, 2008); and prospective longitudinal neurocognitive assessment will clarify whether differences in cognitive functioning represent a diathesis for illness, a state-dependent change in processing, a scarring effect of mood episodes that can endure even after recovery from episode, or a side effect of pharmacological treatments (Joseph, Frazier, Youngstrom, & Soares, 2008).

At a psychosocial level of analysis, stage-salient tasks that are decidedly relevant for BD include the formation of early attachment and corresponding internal working models, the development of social competence and the formation of healthy peer relationships, and the adolescent transition to greater autonomy. Youth with BD may not have deficits in knowledge about social skills but instead have difficulty enacting the skills (Goldstein et al., 2006), possibly because of mood-dependent changes in emotion perception (Rich et al., 2008), or mood-dependent changes in motivation to engage socially (Fowles, 1994; Frank et al., 2005). The adolescent goals of individuation and autonomy already create conflict as a part of normal development (Emery, 1992). Mood disorder amplifies the conflict, as the affected teenager challenges for more authority when manic and reacts more hopelessly and helplessly (yet also irritably) when depressed. Both responses potentially provoke more extreme reactions from the rest of the family system.

It also is crucial to assess academic achievement vis-à-vis BD. Academic success may moderate other risk factors, and without longitudinal data, it cannot be certain whether academic decline is mediated by state effects of mood on cognition, disruptive behaviors associated with mood states, or the side effects of pharmacological treatments. As youth mature, the emphasis will shift from evaluating academic achievement to vocational success; however, in a global sense, both reflect developmentally appropriate aspects of role functioning. BD has the potential to disrupt educational attainment, job success, and the successful formation of long-term relationships, including marriage and a new family. The formal examination of the relationship between BD and quality of life is only beginning (Freeman et al., 2009; Michalak, Yatham, Wan, & Lam, 2005). Research already makes clear that BD on average exacts a steep toll on quality of life, yet there also is a wide range of functioning and the possibility of exceptionally good outcomes.

SEX DIFFERENCES: INTERACTIONS IN DEVELOPMENT OF MOOD PROBLEMS

Sex differences offer an intriguing lens through which to view BD from a developmental psychopathology vantage. Sex is a construct that involves biological differences, including genetic factors, endocrinological differences, and differences in socialization that are driven in part by environment selection as well as expectations and responses from parents, teachers, and peers. The field is gaining a deeper appreciation of how these factors may be influenced by macrosystem factors such as culture and how these factors can moderate each other from the level of gene × environment interactions on up. Sex also is related to exposure to different environmental risk factors, the willingness to seek treatment, and adherence and outcome for some treatments as well. In short, sex has the potential to interact with BD at many, if not all, levels and facets.

At an epidemiological level, studies have not found sex differences in the rate of bipolar I disorder, and data are scant about bipolar NOS or cyclothymic disorder (Goodwin & Jamison, 2007). Bipolar II disorder appears more common in women than men (Goodwin & Jamison, 2007), but there is no evidence that it is a genetically sex-linked condition. There are at least two plausible explanations for the higher rate found in women: (1) ascertainment bias and (2) differences in exposure to risk factors. The potential for ascertainment bias arises because bipolar II disorder involves a combination of depression and hypomanic episodes. Neither men nor women are likely to self-refer for treatment for hypomania. However, women are more likely to seek treatment for depression (cf. Marcus et al., 2005; e.g., Morey, Thacher, & Craighead, 2007; Sen, 2004). Consequently, clinical samples will find higher rates of women presenting with bipolar II disorder. It is also possible that women will admit depressive symptoms at a higher rate in research contexts as well, leading to a higher rate of identification, even in epidemiological samples (Kessler et al., 1997). The second hypothesis, differential exposure to risk factors, is also plausible given the association between sexual abuse and bipolar II disorder. Bipolar II disorder appears more linked to sexual, and not physical, abuse (Garno et al., 2005); and girls are much more likely to be exposed to sexual abuse than are boys (Fergusson, Lynskey, & Horwood, 1996). Abuse appears to be associated with an earlier age of onset of mood disorder, greater mood instability and reactivity, greater suicidality, and more frequent relapse (Post & Leverich, 2006). Abuse might be an environmental potentiator that mediates the effect of biological risk factors (Miklowitz & Chang, 2008), and it also might have some of its effects on affective lability and episode recurrence by reducing the threshold for later life events to trigger relapse through "stress sensitization" (Dienes et al., 2006).

There appear to be larger sex differences in the tendency to present with specific mood states versus specific lifetime bipolar diagnoses. Clinic-referred young males appear to have higher rates of mania and comorbid ADHD, whereas adolescent and older females have higher rates of depression (Duax et al., 2007). There also may be sex differences in the pattern of family interactions associated with BD, with expressed negative emotions and criticism being more severe for adolescent-onset females (Coville et al., 2008). Other trends in sex differences in attention problems, anxiety, and aggressive behavior have been described previously and are incorporated into the age and sex norms of many standardized behavior checklists. It remains an open question whether these differences represent a shifting background against which behaviors need to be evaluated to measure extremity versus indicating real differences in risk and rate of illness. An informative framework for examining these issues would be to use the "differential item functioning" measurement techniques to examine whether the relationship of symptoms and behaviors to the core constructs of mania and depression are the same for males versus females and also whether they show similar levels of the behavior after controlling for the mood factors (Embretson, 1996). Detailed psychometric investigation of sex differences could speak directly to whether depression and mania should be measured using the same scales and benchmarks for both sexes, as is currently the practice, versus having separate sex norms for the same scales or developing sex-specific content to the scales. Documenting the measurement properties in such detail would establish a fulcrum against which to leverage studies of treatment seeking and outcomes: If there are major sex differences in the items associated with mania or depression, then this will obscure differences in rates of service utilization as well as the size of treatment responses.

SUMMARY: A DEVELOPMENTAL PSYCHOPATHOLOGY AGENDA FOR RESEARCH AND PRACTICE IN ASSESSMENT OF BIPOLAR DISORDER

BD is not an affliction that strikes spontaneously in adulthood. Even instances in which the first major mood episode occurs in later life will have roots in earlier biological risk factors and environmental experiences. Recent increases in the rate of diagnosis of BD in youth have provoked controversy that has challenged researchers to examine rigorously the validity of applying mood disorder labels to adolescents and prepubertal children. One consequence has been a surge in research addressing criterion validity, including comparisons with the standards established by Robins and Guze (Cantwell, 1996; Robins & Guze, 1970). Longitudinal prospective investigations are beginning to chart the developmental continuity of pediatric presentations with adult functioning (Birmaher et al., 2006; Geller et al., 2008). The accumulating evidence is also revealing examples of developmental discontinuities and opening new areas for investigation that will rapidly inform both developmental theories and clinical practice.

Examination of normal development with regard to BD raises issues of growth and change in the systems related to emotion expression and regulation. The major dimensions of PA, NA, and dominance/surgency have strong relationships to basic systems of motivation, such as the BAS and BIS, as well as temperament and personality. These dimensional models have already informed work with unipolar depression and ADHD, and they generate a provocative set of hypotheses with regard to manic and mixed states. Assimilation of BIS/BAS or emotion models also helps connect symptoms to biological substrates and to social processes. A developmental psychopathology framework also brings new tools, such as norm-referenced assessments that explicitly benchmark mood and behavior against what is age appropriate. The concepts of equifinality and multifinality also will add much value to discussions of BD: Equifinality reminds us that the same phenotypic expression could derive from many different processes; and multifinality challenges observers to remember the diversity of end points that can grow from a bipolar diathesis, including resilient and positive outcomes.

Both equifinality and multifinality are concepts likely to advance understanding of the mechanisms generating the appearance of psychiatric comorbidity in the majority of persons affected by BD. The high rate of co-occurrence of BD and diagnoses such as anxiety disorders, ADHD, substance use, trauma, and conduct problems could be due to a variety of methodological artifacts, including the imposition of categorical boundaries where the underlying conditions are dimensional or developmentally sequenced in a way that cross-sectional evaluations fail to capture. There also are likely to be developmental mechanisms that result in multiple constellations of symptoms over time, generating the appearance of comorbidity when diagnostic criteria are applied to a snapshot of behaviors without mapping the trajectories or processes involved.

The examination of risk factors has established that the causes and contributing factors to the development of BD are both many and nonspecific. Even the genetic and biological processes conferring risk for BD also appear to be implicated in a variety of other conditions. The good news, from a clinical and policy perspective, is that BD may benefit from nonspecific interventions too: Improvements in nutrition, early attachment experiences, or refined communication skills and meta-emotion strategies have the potential to prevent or ameliorate the mood dysregulation associated with BD much as they influence externalizing and internalizing problems more generally. Protective factors with regard to BD are less well studied, but the lack of specificity in risk factors suggests that many of the general protective factors, such as secure attachment, supportive family environment, higher SES, and better general cognitive ability, are good candidates for having beneficial effects on BD as well.

Shifting to a developmental psychopathology framework also exposes the need for more research and clinical assessment around accomplishment of stage-salient developmental tasks. Relatively little is known about the developmental associations between BD and the successful navigation of educational and vocational goals or the formation of significant peer and intimate relationships. Epidemiological studies of the impact of the disorder on adults are demonstrating that the long-term consequences of BD are severe in terms of lost years of productivity and increased morbidity.

In short, a developmental psychopathology perspective on BD both challenges and guides research and practice. Developmental models compel us to look at risk and protective factors that have effects long before symptoms evolve into a clinically diagnosable disorder. Developmental psychopathology models also direct our attention to focus on change over time, and they expand the scope of our view to include consideration of age- and stage-appropriate tasks rather than concentrating solely on symptoms.

ACKNOWLEDGMENT

This work was supported in part by Grant No. NIMH R01 MH066647 from the National Institute of Mental Health.

REFERENCES

Achenbach, T. M., & Edelbrock, C. (1983). *Manual for the Child Behavior Checklist and Revised Child Behavior Profile*. Burlington: University of Vermont, Department of Psychiatry.

Achenbach, T. M., Howell, C. T., McConaughy, S. H., & Stanger, C. (1995a). Six-year predictors of problems in a national sample of children and youth: I. Cross-informant syndromes. *Journal of the American Academy of Child and Adolescent Psychiatry, 34*(3), 336–347.

Achenbach, T. M., Howell, C. T., McConaughy, S. H., & Stanger, C. (1995b). Six-year predictors of problems in a national sample: III. Transitions to young adult syndromes. *Journal of the American Academy of Child and Adolescent Psychiatry, 34*(5), 658–669.

Achenbach, T. M., & Rescorla, L. A. (2001). *Manual for the ASEBA School-Age Forms & Profiles.* Burlington: University of Vermont.

Agency for Toxic Substances & Disease Registry. (2007). *Case studies in environmental medicine (SEM): Who is at risk of lead exposure?* Retrieved October 12, 2008, from *www.atsdr. cdc.gov/csem/lead/pbwhoisat_risk2.html*

Akiskal, H. S., & Pinto, O. (1999). The evolving bipolar spectrum. Prototypes I, II, III, and IV. *Psychiatric Clinics of North America, 22*(3), 517–534.

Alloy, L. B., Abramson, L. Y., Walshaw, P. D., Cogswell, A., Grandin, L. D., Hughes, M. E., et al. (2008). Behavioral approach system and behavioral inhibition system sensitivities and bipolar spectrum disorders: Prospective prediction of bipolar mood episodes. *Bipolar Disorders, 10*(2), 310–322.

American Psychiatric Association. (2000). *Diagnostic and statistical manual of mental disorders* (4th ed., text rev.). Washington, DC: Author.

Angold, A., Costello, E. J., & Erkanli, A. (1999). Comorbidity. *Journal of Child Psychology and Psychiatry, 40*(1), 57–87.

Angst, J., Gamma, A., Benazzi, F., Ajdacic, V., Eich, D., & Rossler, W. (2003). Toward a redefinition of subthreshold bipolarity: Epidemiology and proposed criteria for bipolar-II, minor bipolar disorders and hypomania. *Journal of Affective Disorders, 73*(1–2), 133–146.

Axelson, D. A., Birmaher, B., Strober, M., Gill, M. K., Valeri, S., Chiappetta, L., et al. (2006). Phenomenology of children and adolescents with bipolar spectrum disorders. *Archives of General Psychiatry, 63*(10), 1139–1148.

Bailey, A. A., & Hurd, P. L. (2005). Finger length ratio (2D:4D) correlates with physical aggression in men but not in women. *Biological Psychology, 68*(3), 215–222.

Barkley, R. A. (2001). The executive functions and self-regulation: An evolutionary neuropsychological perspective. *Neuropsychology Review, 11*(1), 1–29.

Baron-Cohen, S., Wheelwright, S., Hill, J., Raste, Y., & Plumb, I. (2001). The "Reading the Mind in the Eyes" Test revised version: A study with normal adults, and adults with Asperger syndrome or high-functioning autism. *Journal of Child Psychology and Psychiatry, 42*(2), 241–251.

Barrett, L. F., & Russell, J. A. (1999). The structure of current affect: Controversies and emerging consensus. *Current Directions in Psychological Science, 8*(1), 10–14.

Barrett, T. B., Hauger, R. L., Kennedy, J. L., Sadovnick, A. D., Remick, R. A., Keck, P. E., et al. (2003). Evidence that a single nucleotide polymorphism in the promoter of the G protein receptor kinase 3 gene is associated with bipolar disorder. *Molecular Psychiatry, 8*(5), 546–557.

Benazzi, F. (2000). Exploring aspects of DSM-IV interpersonal sensitivity in bipolar II. *Journal of Affective Disorders, 60*(1), 43–46.

Benderlioglu, Z., & Nelson, R. J. (2004). Digit length ratios predict reactive aggression in women, but not in men. *Hormones and Behavior, 46*(5), 558–564.

Benedetti, F., Bernasconi, A., Blasi, V., Cadioli, M., Colombo, C., Falini, A., et al. (2007). Neural and genetic correlates of antidepressant response to sleep deprivation: A functional magnetic resonance imaging study of moral valence decision in bipolar depression. *Archives of General Psychiatry, 64*(2), 179–187.

Benedetti, F., Bernasconi, A., Lorenzi, C., Pontiggia, A., Serretti, A., Colombo, C., et al. (2004). A single nucleotide polymorphism in glycogen synthase kinase 3-beta promoter gene influences onset of illness in patients affected by bipolar disorder. *Neuroscience Letters, 355*(1–2), 37–40.

Bentall, R. (2003). *Madness explained: Psychosis and human nature.* New York: Penguin Group.

Berkson, J. (1946). Limitations of the application of fourfold tables to hospital data. *Biometrics Bulletin, 2*(3), 47–53.

Biederman, J., Klein, R. G., Pine, D. S., & Klein, D. F. (1998). Resolved: Mania is mistaken for ADHD in prepubertal children. *Journal of the American Academy of Child and Adolescent Psychiatry, 37,* 1091–1093.

Birmaher, B., & Axelson, D. (2006). Course and outcome of bipolar spectrum disorder in children and adolescents: A review of the existing literature. *Development and Psychopathology, 18*(4), 1023–1035.

Birmaher, B., Axelson, D., Goldstein, B., Strober, M., Gill, M. K., Hunt, J., et al. (2009). Four-year longitudinal course of children and adolescents with bipolar spectrum disorders: The Course and Outcome of Bipolar Youth (COBY) Study. *American Journal of Psychiatry, 166*(7), 795–804.

Birmaher, B., Axelson, D., Strober, M., Gill, M. K., Valeri, S., Chiappetta, L., et al. (2006). Clinical course of children and adolescents with bipolar spectrum disorders. *Archives of General Psychiatry, 63*(2), 175–183.

Birmaher, B., Kennah, A., Brent, D., Ehmann, M., Bridge, J., & Axelson, D. (2002). Is bipolar disorder specifically associated with panic disorder in youths? *Journal of Clinical Psychiatry, 63*(5), 414–419.

Biuckians, A., Miklowitz, D. J., & Kim, E. Y. (2007). Behavioral activation, inhibition and mood symptoms in early-onset bipolar disorder. *Journal of Affective Disorders, 97*(1–3), 71–76.

Blader, J. C., & Carlson, G. A. (2007). Increased rates of bipolar disorder diagnoses among U.S. child, adolescent, and adult inpatients, 1996–2004. *Biological Psychiatry, 62*(2), 107–114.

Bradley, S. J. (2000). *Affect regulation and the development of psychopathology.* New York: Guilford Press.

Bremner, J. D., & Narayan, M. (1998). The effects of stress on memory and the hippocampus throughout the life cycle: Implications for childhood development and aging. *Development and Psychopathology, 10*(4), 871–885.

Brotman, M. A., Schmajuk, M., Rich, B. A., Dickstein, D. P., Guyer, A. E., Costello, E. J., et al. (2006). Prevalence, clinical correlates, and longitudinal course of severe mood dysregulation in children. *Biological Psychiatry, 60*(9), 991–997.

Burt, S. A., & Mikolajewski, A. J. (2008). Preliminary evidence that specific candidate genes are associated with adolescent-onset antisocial behavior. *Aggressive Behavior, 34*(4), 437–445.

Cantwell, D. P. (1996). Classification of child and adolescent psychopathology. *Journal of Child Psychology and Psychiatry, 37,* 3–12.

Carlson, G. A. (2003). The bottom line. *Journal of Child and Adolescent Psychopharmacology, 13*(2), 115–118.

Carlson, G. A., & Meyer, S. E. (2006). Phenomenology and diagnosis of bipolar disorder in children, adolescents, and adults: Complexities and developmental issues. *Development and Psychopathology, 18*(4), 939–969.

Caron, C., & Rutter, M. (1991). Comorbidity in child psychopathology: Concepts, issues and research strategies. *Journal of Child Psychology and Psychiatry, 32*(7), 1063–1080.

Carstensen, L. L., Pasupathi, M., Mayr, U., & Nesselroade, J. R. (2000). Emotional experience in everyday life across the adult life span. *Journal of Personality and Social Psychology, 79*(4), 644–655.

Chang, K. D., Steiner, H., & Ketter, T. A. (2000). Psychiatric phenomenology of child and adolescent bipolar offspring. *Journal of the American Academy of Child and Adolescent Psychiatry, 39*(4), 453–460.

Chen, C., Burton, M., Greenberger, E., & Dmitrieva, J. (1999). Population migration and the variation of dopamine D4 receptor (DRD4) allele frequencies around the globe. *Evolution and Human Behavior, 20*(5), 309–324.

Chorpita, B. F. (2002). The tripartite model and dimensions of anxiety and depression: An examination of structure in a large school sample. *Journal of Abnormal Child Psychology, 30*(2), 177–190.

Cicchetti, D., & Cohen, D. J. (Eds.). (2006). *Developmental psychopathology: Developmental neuroscience* (2nd ed., Vol. 2). Hoboken, NJ: Wiley.

Clark, L. A., & Watson, D. (1991). Tripartite model of anxiety and depression: Psychometric evidence and taxonomic implications. *Journal of Abnormal Psychology, 100*(3), 316–336.

Coelho, V. L. D., Strauss, M. E., & Jenkins, J. H. (1998). Expression of symptomatic distress by Puerto Rican and Euro-American patients with depression and schizophrenia. *Journal of Nervous and Mental Disease, 186*(8), 477–483.

Corr, P. J. (2001). Testing problems in J. A. Gray's personality theory: A commentary on Matthews and Gilliland (1999). *Personality and Individual Differences, 30,* 333–352.

Correll, C. U. (2008). Antipsychotic use in children and adolescents: Minimizing adverse effects to maximize outcomes. *Journal of the American Academy of Child and Adolescent Psychiatry, 47*(1), 9–20.

Corsini, R., & Wedding, D. (Eds.). (2000). *Current psychotherapies* (6th ed.). Itasca, IL: Peacock.

Cosmides, L., & Tooby, J. (2000). Evolutionary psychology and the emotions. In M. Lewis & J. M. Haviland-Jones (Eds.), *Handbook of emotions* (2nd ed., pp. 91–115). New York: Guilford Press.

Coville, A. L., Miklowitz, D. J., Taylor, D. O., & Low, K. G. (2008). Correlates of high expressed emotion attitudes among parents of bipolar adolescents. *Journal of Clinical Psychology, 64*(4), 438–449.

Cyranowski, J. M., Frank, E., Young, E., & Shear, K. (2000). Adolescent onset of the gender difference in lifetime rates of major depression. *Archives of General Psychiatry, 57*(1), 21–27.

Davey, G. C. L., Buckland, G., Tantow, B., & Dallos, R. (1998). Disgust and eating disorders. *European Eating Disorders Review, 6*(3), 201–211.

Davey, G. C. L., McDonald, A. S., Hirisave, U., Prabhu, G. G., Iwawaki, S., Jim, C. I., et al. (1998). A cross-cultural study of animal fears. *Behaviour Research and Therapy, 36*(7–8), 735–750.

DelBello, M. P., Lopez-Larson, M. P., Soutullo, C. A., & Strakowski, S. M. (2001). Effects of race on psychiatric diagnosis of hospitalized adolescents: A retrospective chart review. *Journal of Child and Adolescent Psychopharmacology, 11*(1), 95–103.

Dell'Osso, L., Pini, S., Cassano, G. B., Mastrocinque, C., Seckinger, R. A., Saettoni, M., et al. (2002). Insight into illness in patients with mania, mixed mania, bipolar depression and major depression with psychotic features. *Bipolar Disorders, 4,* 315–322.

Demaree, H. A., & Harrison, D. W. (1997). Physiological and neuropsychological correlates of hostility. *Neuropsychologia, 35*(10), 1405–1411.

Demaree, H. A., Robinson, J. L., Everhart, D. E., & Youngstrom, E. A. (2005). Behavioral inhibition system (BIS) strength and trait dominance are associated with affective response and perspective taking when viewing dyadic interactions. *International Journal of Neuroscience, 115*(11), 1579–1593.

Depue, R., & Lenzenweger, M. (2006). Toward a developmental psychopathology of personality disturbance: A neurobehavioral dimensional model. In D. Cicchetti & D. J. Cohen (Eds.), *Developmental psychopathology: Developmental neuroscience* (2nd ed., Vol. 2, pp. 762–796). Hoboken, NJ: Wiley.

Depue, R. A., Krauss, S., Spoont, M. R., & Arbisi, P. (1989). General Behavior Inventory identification of unipolar and bipolar affective conditions in a nonclinical university population. *Journal of Abnormal Psychology, 98*(2), 117–126.

Dickstein, D. P., & Leibenluft, E. (2006). Emotion regulation in children and adolescents: Boundaries between normalcy and bipolar disorder. *Development and Psychopathology, 18*(4), 1105–1131.

Dienes, K. A., Hammen, C., Henry, R. M., Cohen, A. N., & Daley, S. E. (2006). The stress sensitization hypothesis: Understanding the course of bipolar disorder. *Journal of Affective Disorders, 95*(1–3), 43–49.

Dodge, K. A. (1991). Emotion and social information processing. In J. Garber & K. A. Dodge (Eds.), *The development of emotion regulation and dysregulation* (pp. 159–181). New York: Cambridge University Press.

Du Rocher Schudlich, T. D., Youngstrom, E. A., Calabrese, J. R., & Findling, R. L. (2008). The role of family functioning in bipolar disorder in families. *Journal of Abnormal Child Psychology, 36*(6), 849–863.

Duax, J. M., Youngstrom, E. A., Calabrese, J. R., & Findling, R. L. (2007). Sex differences in pediatric bipolar disorder. *Journal of Clinical Psychiatry, 68*(10), 1565–1573.

Dubicka, B., Carlson, G. A., Vail, A., & Harrington, R. (2008). Prepubertal mania: Diagnostic differences between US and UK clinicians. *European Child and Adolescent Psychiatry, 17*(3), 153–161.

Duffy, A., Alda, M., Kutchee, S., Fusee, C., & Grof, P. (1998). Psychiatric symptoms and syndromes among adolescent children of parents with lithium-responsive or lithium-nonresponsive bipolar disorder. *American Journal of Psychiatry, 155*, 431–433.

Embretson, S. E. (1996). The new rules of measurement. *Psychological Assessment, 8*(4), 341–349.

Emery, R. (1992). Family conflicts and their developmental implications: A conceptual analysis of meanings for the structure of relationships. In W. Hartup & C. Shantz (Eds.), *Family conflicts* (pp. 270–298). New York: Cambridge University Press.

Faraone, S. V., Biederman, J., Mennin, D., Wozniak, J., & Spencer, T. (1997). Attention-deficit hyperactivity disorder with bipolar disorder: A familial subtype? *Journal of the American Academy of Child and Adolescent Psychiatry, 36*(10), 1378–1387.

Faraone, S. V., Glatt, S. J., & Tsuang, M. T. (2003). The genetics of pediatric-onset bipolar disorder. *Biological Psychiatry, 53*(11), 970–977.

Fergusson, D. M., Horwood, L. J., & Lynskey, M. T. (1996). Childhood sexual abuse and psychiatric disorder in young adulthood: II. Psychiatric outcomes of childhood sexual abuse. *Journal of the American Academy of Child and Adolescent Psychiatry, 35*, 1365–1374.

Fergusson, D. M., Lynskey, M. T., & Horwood, L. J. (1996). Childhood sexual abuse and psychiatric disorder in young adulthood: I. Prevalence of sexual abuse and factors associated with sexual abuse. *Journal of the American Academy of Child and Adolescent Psychiatry, 35*, 1355–1364.

Findling, R. L., Gracious, B. L., McNamara, N. K., Youngstrom, E. A., Demeter, C., & Calabrese, J. R. (2001). Rapid, continuous cycling and psychiatric co-morbidity in pediatric bipolar I disorder. *Bipolar Disorders, 3*, 202–210.

Findling, R. L., McNamara, N. K., Stansbrey, R. J., Gracious, B. L., Whipkey, R. E., Demeter, C. A., et al. (2006). Combination lithium and divalproex sodium in pediatric bipolar symptom re-stabilization. *Journal of the American Academy of Child and Adolescent Psychiatry, 45*, 142–148.

Fontaine, J. R., Scherer, K. R., Roesch, E. B., & Ellsworth, P. C. (2007). The world of emotions is not two-dimensional. *Psychological Science, 18*(12), 1050–1057.

Fowles, D. C. (1994). A motivational theory of psychopathology. In W. D. Spaulding (Ed.),

Integrative views of motivation, cognition, and emotion (Vol. 41, pp. 181–238). Lincoln: University of Nebraska Press.

Frank, E., Kupfer, D. J., Thase, M. E., Mallinger, A. G., Swartz, H. A., Fagiolini, A. M., et al. (2005). Two-year outcomes for interpersonal and social rhythm therapy in individuals with bipolar I disorder. *Archives of General Psychiatry, 62*(9), 996–1004.

Frazier, T. W., Youngstrom, E. A., & Naugle, R. I. (2007). The latent structure of attention-deficit/hyperactivity disorder in a clinic-referred sample. *Neuropsychology, 21*(1), 45–64.

Freeman, A. J., Youngstrom, E. A., Michalak, E., Siegel, R., Meyers, O. I., & Findling, R. L. (2009). Quality of life in pediatric bipolar disorder. *Pediatrics, 123*(3), e446–e452.

Gadow, K. D., & Sprafkin, J. (1999). *Youth's Inventory–4 manual.* Stony Brook, NY: Checkmate Plus.

Galanter, C., Carlson, G., Jensen, P., Greenhill, L., Davies, M., Li, W., et al. (2003). Response to methylphenidate in children with attention deficit hyperactivity disorder and manic symptoms in the multimodal treatment study of children with attention deficit hyperactivity disorder titration trial. *Journal of Child and Adolescent Psychopharmacology, 13*(2), 123–136.

Garber, J., Keiley, M. K., & Martin, C. (2002). Developmental trajectories of adolescents' depressive symptoms: Predictors of change. *Journal of Consulting and Clinical Psychology, 70*(1), 79–95.

Garno, J. L., Goldberg, J. F., Ramirez, P. M., & Ritzler, B. A. (2005). Impact of childhood abuse on the clinical course of bipolar disorder. *British Journal of Psychiatry, 186*, 121–125.

Geller, B., & Tillman, R. (2005). Prepubertal and early adolescent bipolar I disorder: Review of diagnostic validation by Robins and Guze criteria. *Journal of Clinical Psychiatry, 66*(Suppl. 7), 21–28.

Geller, B., Tillman, R., Bolhofner, K., & Zimerman, B. (2008). Child bipolar I disorder: Prospective continuity with adult bipolar I disorder; characteristics of second and third episodes; predictors of 8-year outcome. *Archives of General Psychiatry, 65*(10), 1125–1133.

Geller, B., Zimerman, B., Williams, M., DelBello, M. P., Frazier, J., & Beringer, L. (2002). Phenomenology of prepubertal and early adolescent bipolar disorder: Examples of elated mood, grandiose behaviors, decreased need for sleep, racing thoughts and hypersexuality. *Journal of Child and Adolescent Psychopharmacology, 12*(1), 3–9.

Ghaemi, S. N., Bauer, M., Cassidy, F., Malhi, G. S., Mitchell, P., Phelps, J., et al. (2008). Diagnostic guidelines for bipolar disorder: A summary of the International Society for Bipolar Disorders Diagnostic Guidelines Task Force Report. *Bipolar Disorders, 10*(1, Pt. 2), 117–128.

Gilbert, P., Allan, S., Brough, S., Melley, S., & Miles, J. N. (2002). Relationship of anhedonia and anxiety to social rank, defeat and entrapment. *Journal of Affective Disorders, 71*(1–3), 141–151.

Gogtay, N., Ordonez, A., Herman, D. H., Hayashi, K. M., Greenstein, D., Vaituzis, C., et al. (2007). Dynamic mapping of cortical development before and after the onset of pediatric bipolar illness. *Journal of Child Psychology and Psychiatry, 48*(9), 852–862.

Goldstein, T. R., Miklowitz, D. J., & Mullen, K. L. (2006). Social skills knowledge and performance among adolescents with bipolar disorder. *Bipolar Disorders, 8*(4), 350–361.

Goodwin, F. K., & Jamison, K. R. (2007). *Manic-depressive illness* (2nd ed.). New York: Oxford University Press.

Gottfredson, L. S. (1997). Why g matters: The complexity of everyday life. *Intelligence, 24*(1), 79–132.

Gottman, J. M., Katz, L. F., & Hooven, C. (1996). Parental meta-emotion philosophy and the emotional life of families: Theoretical models and preliminary data. *Journal of Family Psychology, 10*(3), 243–268.

Gottman, J. M., Katz, L. F., & Hooven, C. (1997). *Meta-emotion: How families communicate emotionally*. Mahwah, NJ: Erlbaum.

Grant, B. F., Stinson, F. S., Hasin, D. S., Dawson, D. A., Chou, S. P., Ruan, W. J., et al. (2005). Prevalence, correlates, and comorbidity of bipolar I disorder and axis I and II disorders: Results from the National Epidemiologic Survey on Alcohol and Related Conditions. *Journal of Clinical Psychiatry, 66*(10), 1205–1215.

Gray, J. A., & McNaughton, N. (1996). The neuropsychology of anxiety: Reprise. In D. A. Hope (Ed.), *Perspectives in anxiety, panic and fear* (Vol. 43, pp. 61–134). Lincoln: University of Nebraska Press.

Greaves-Lord, K., Ferdinand, R. F., Sondeijker, F. E., Dietrich, A., Oldehinkel, A. J., Rosmalen, J. G., et al. (2007). Testing the tripartite model in young adolescents: Is hyperarousal specific for anxiety and not depression? *Journal of Affective Disorders, 102*(1–3), 55–63.

Gruber, J., Johnson, S. L., Oveis, C., & Keltner, D. (2008). Risk for mania and positive emotional responding: Too much of a good thing? *Emotion, 8*(1), 23–33.

Haberstick, B. C., Smolen, A., & Hewitt, J. K. (2006). Family-based association test of the 5HTTLPR and aggressive behavior in a general population sample of children. *Biological Psychiatry, 59*(9), 836–843.

Hack, M., Youngstrom, E. A., Cartar, L., Schluchter, M., Gerry, T. H., Flannery, D., et al. (2004). Behavioral outcomes and evidence of psychopathology among very low birth weight infants at age 20 years. *Pediatrics, 114*, 932–940.

Hazell, P. L., Carr, V., Lewin, T. J., & Sly, K. (2003). Manic symptoms in young males with ADHD predict functioning but not diagnosis after 6 years. *Journal of the American Academy of Child and Adolescent Psychiatry, 42*(5), 552–560.

Healy, D. (2006). The latest mania: Selling bipolar disorder. *PLoS Medicine, 3*(4), e185.

Henquet, C., Di Forti, M., Morrison, P., Kuepper, R., & Murray, R. M. (2008). Gene–environment interplay between cannabis and psychosis. *Schizophrenia Bulletin, 34*(6), 1111–21.

Hibbeln, J. R., Davis, J. M., Steer, C., Emmett, P., Rogers, I., Williams, C., et al. (2007). Maternal seafood consumption in pregnancy and neurodevelopmental outcomes in childhood (ALSPAC study): An observational cohort study. *Lancet, 369*, 578–585.

Hodgins, S., Faucher, B., Zarac, A., & Ellenbogen, M. (2002). Children of parents with bipolar disorder. A population at high risk for major affective disorders. *Child and Adolescent Psychiatric Clinics of North America, 11*(3), 533–553.

Hooley, J. M., & Hiller, J. B. (2001). Family relationships and major mental disorder: Risk factors and preventive strategies. In B. R. Sarason & S. Duck (Eds.), *Personal relationships: Implications for clinical and community psychology* (pp. 61–87). New York: Wiley.

Izard, C. E., Youngstrom, E. A., Fine, S. E., Mostow, A. J., & Trentacosta, C. J. (2006). Emotions and developmental psychopathology. In D. Cicchetti & D. J. Cohen (Eds.), *Developmental psychopathology: Vol. 1. Theory and method* (2nd ed., pp. 244–292). New York: Wiley.

Johnson, S. L., Miller, C. J., & Eisner, L. (2008). Bipolar disorder. In J. Hunsley & E. J. Mash (Eds.), *A guide to assessments that work* (pp. 121–137). New York: Oxford University Press.

Joiner, T. E., Jr., Catanzaro, S. J., & Laurent, J. (1996). Tripartite structure of positive and negative affect, depression, and anxiety in child and adolescent psychiatric inpatients. *Journal of Abnormal Psychology, 105*(3), 401–409.

Joiner, T. E. J., & Lonigan, C. J. (2000). Tripartite model of depression and anxiety in youth psychiatric inpatients: Relations with diagnostic status and future symptoms. *Journal of Clinical Child Psychology, 29*(3), 372–382.

Joseph, M., Frazier, T. W., Youngstrom, E. A., & Soares, J. C. (2008). A quantitative and qualitative review of neurocognitive performance in pediatric bipolar disorder. *Journal of Child and Adolescent Psychopharmacology, 18*, 595–605.

Joseph, M., Youngstrom, E. A., & Soares, J. C. (2009). Antidepressant-coincident mania in children and adolescents treated with selective serotonin reuptake inhibitors. *Future Neurology, 4*(1), 87–102.

Judd, L. L., & Akiskal, H. S. (2003). The prevalence and disability of bipolar spectrum disorders in the US population: Re-analysis of the ECA database taking into account subthreshold cases. *Journal of Affective Disorders, 73*(1–2), 123–131.

Judd, L. L., Akiskal, H. S., Schettler, P. J., Coryell, W., Maser, J., Rice, J. A., et al. (2003). The comparative clinical phenotype and long term longitudinal episode course of bipolar I and II: A clinical spectrum or distinct disorders? *Journal of Affective Disorders, 73*(1–2), 19–32.

Judd, L. L., Akiskal, H. S., Schettler, P. J., Endicott, J., Leon, A. C., Solomon, D., et al. (2005). Psychosocial disability in the course of bipolar I and II disorders: A prospective, comparative, longitudinal study. *Archives of General Psychiatry, 62*, 1322–1330.

Judd, L. L., Akiskal, H. S., Schettler, P. J., Endicott, J., Maser, J., Solomon, D. A., et al. (2002). The long-term natural history of the weekly symptomatic status of bipolar I disorder. *Archives of General Psychiatry, 59*, 530–537.

Kessler, R. C., Akiskal, H. S., Ames, M., Birnbaum, H., Greenberg, P., Hirschfeld, R. M. A., et al. (2006). Prevalence and effects of mood disorders on work performance in a nationally representative sample of U.S. workers. *American Journal of Psychiatry, 163*(9), 1561–1568.

Kessler, R. C., Berglund, P., Demler, O., Jin, R., & Walters, E. E. (2005). Lifetime prevalence and age-of-onset distributions of DSM-IV disorders in the National Comorbidity Survey replication. *Archives of General Psychiatry, 62*(6), 593–602.

Kessler, R. C., Merikangas, K. R., & Wang, P. S. (2007). Prevalence, comorbidity, and service utilization for mood disorders in the United States at the beginning of the twenty-first century. *Annual Review of Clinical Psychology, 3*, 137–158.

Kessler, R. C., Rubinow, D. R., Holmes, C., Abelson, J. M., & Zhao, S. (1997). The epidemiology of DSM-III-R bipolar I disorder in a general population survey. *Psychological Medicine, 27*(5), 1079–1089.

Kim, E. Y., & Miklowitz, D. J. (2002). Childhood mania, attention deficit hyperactivity disorder and conduct disorder: A critical review of diagnostic dilemmas. *Bipolar Disorders, 4*(4), 215–225.

Klein, R. G., Pine, D. S., & Klein, D. F. (1998). Resolved: Mania is mistaken for ADHD in prepubertal children. *Journal of the American Academy of Child and Adolescent Psychiatry, 37*(10), 1093–1096.

Kovacs, M. (1989). Affective disorders in children and adolescents. *American Psychologist, 44*(2), 209–215.

Kowatch, R. A., Fristad, M. A., Birmaher, B., Wagner, K. D., Findling, R. L., & Hellander, M. (2005). Treatment guidelines for children and adolescents with bipolar disorder. *Journal of the American Academy of Child and Adolescent Psychiatry, 44*(3), 213–235.

Kowatch, R. A., Youngstrom, E. A., Danielyan, A., & Findling, R. L. (2005). Review and meta-analysis of the phenomenology and clinical characteristics of mania in children and adolescents. *Bipolar Disorders, 7*(6), 483–496.

Kraepelin, E. (1921). *Manic-depressive insanity and paranoia.* Edinburgh, UK: Livingstone.

Leibenluft, E., Charney, D. S., Towbin, K. E., Bhangoo, R. K., & Pine, D. S. (2003). Defining clinical phenotypes of juvenile mania. *American Journal of Psychiatry, 160*, 430–437.

Leibenluft, E., & Rich, B. A. (2008). Pediatric bipolar disorder. *Annual Review of Clinical Psychology, 4*, 163–187.

Leverich, G., & Post, R. M. (2006). Course of bipolar illness after history of childhood trauma. *Lancet, 367,* 1040–1042.

Lewinsohn, P. M., Klein, D. N., & Seeley, J. (2000). Bipolar disorder during adolescence and young adulthood in a community sample. *Bipolar Disorders, 2,* 281–293.

Lewinsohn, P. M., Seeley, J. R., & Klein, D. N. (2003). Bipolar disorders during adolescence. *Acta Psychiatrica Scandinavica, 108,* 47–50.

Licht, R. W., Gijsman, H., Nolen, W. A., & Angst, J. (2008). Are antidepressants safe in the treatment of bipolar depression?: A critical evaluation of their potential risk to induce switch into mania or cycle acceleration. *Acta Psychiatrica Scandinavica, 118*(5), 337–346.

Lieberman, D. Z., Peele, R., & Razavi, M. (2008). Combinations of DSM-IV-TR criteria sets for bipolar disorders. *Psychopathology, 41*(1), 35–38.

Lopez, A. D., Mathers, C. D., Ezzati, M., Jamison, D. T., & Murray, C. J. (2006). Global and regional burden of disease and risk factors, 2001: Systematic analysis of population health data. *Lancet, 367,* 1747–1757.

Loue, S., & Sajatovic, M. (2008). Research with severely mentally ill Latinas: Successful recruitment and retention strategies. *Journal of Immigrant and Minority Health, 10*(2), 145–153.

Lovejoy, M. C., & Steuerwald, B. L. (1992). Psychological characteristics associated with sub-syndromal affective disorder. *Personality and Individual Differences, 13*(3), 303–308.

Lovejoy, M. C., & Steuerwald, B. L. (1995). Subsyndromal unipolar and bipolar disorders: Comparisons on positive and negative affect. *Journal of Abnormal Psychology, 104*(2), 381–384.

Lytton, H. (1990). Child and parent effects in boys' conduct disorder: A reinterpretation. *Developmental Psychology, 26*(5), 683–697.

Mackin, P., Targum, S. D., Kalali, A., Rom, D., & Young, A. H. (2006). Culture and assessment of manic symptoms. *British Journal of Psychiatry, 189,* 379–380.

Malkoff-Schwartz, S., Frank, E., Anderson, B., Sherrill, J. T., Siegel, L., Patterson, D., et al. (1998). Stressful life events and social rhythm disruption in the onset of manic and depressive bipolar episodes. *Archives of General Psychiatry, 55*(8), 702–707.

Marcus, S. M., Young, E. A., Kerber, K. B., Kornstein, S., Farabaugh, A. H., Mitchell, J., et al. (2005). Gender differences in depression: Findings from the STAR*D study. *Journal of Affective Disorders, 87*(2–3), 141–150.

Masi, G., Perugi, G., Toni, C., Millepiedi, S., Mucci, M., Bertini, N., et al. (2006). The clinical phenotypes of juvenile bipolar disorder: Toward a validation of the episodic–chronic distinction. *Biological Psychiatry, 59*(7), 603–610.

Matthews, G., & Gilliland, K. (1999). The personality theories of H. J. Eysenck and J. A. Gray: A comparative review. *Personality and Individual Differences, 26*(4), 583–626.

McDermott, P. A., & Weiss, R. V. (1995). A normative typology of healthy, subclinical, and clinical behavior styles among American children and adolescents. *Psychological Assessment, 7*(2), 162–170.

McElroy, S. L., Frye, M. A., Suppes, T., Dhavale, D., Keck, P. E., Jr., Leverich, G. S., et al. (2002). Correlates of overweight and obesity in 644 patients with bipolar disorder. *Journal of Clinical Psychiatry, 63*(3), 207–213.

Meehl, P. E. (1995). Bootstraps taxometrics: Solving the classification problem in psychopathology. *American Psychologist, 50,* 266–275.

Mehrabian, A. (1997). Comparison of the PAD and PANAS as models for describing emotions and for differentiating anxiety from depression. *Journal of Psychopathology and Behavioral Assessment, 19*(4), 331–357.

Merikangas, K. R., Herrell, R., Swendsen, J., Rossler, W., Ajdacic-Gross, V., & Angst, J. (2008). Specificity of bipolar spectrum conditions in the comorbidity of mood and substance use disorders: Results from the Zurich cohort study. *Archives of General Psychiatry, 65*(1), 47–52.

Meyer, B., Johnson, S. L., & Carver, C. S. (1999). Exploring behavioral activation and inhibition sensitivities among college students at risk for bipolar spectrum symptomatology. *Journal of Psychopathology and Behavioral Assessment, 21*(4), 275–292.

Meyer, S. E., Carlson, G. A., Youngstrom, E., Ronsaville, D. S., Martinez, P. E., Gold, P. W., et al. (2009). Long-term outcomes of youth who manifested the CBCL-Pediatric Bipolar Disorder phenotype during childhood and/or adolescence. *Journal of Affective Disorders, 113,* 227–235.

Michalak, E. E., Yatham, L. N., Wan, D. D., & Lam, R. W. (2005). Perceived quality of life in patients with bipolar disorder. Does group psychoeducation have an impact? *Canadian Journal of Psychiatry, 50,* 95–100.

Miklowitz, D. J. (2004). The role of family systems in severe and recurrent psychiatric disorders: A developmental psychopathology view. *Development and Psychopathology, 16*(3), 667–688.

Miklowitz, D. J., Biuckians, A., & Richards, J. A. (2006). Early-onset bipolar disorder: A family treatment perspective. *Development and Psychopathology, 18*(4), 1247–1265.

Miklowitz, D. J., & Chang, K. D. (2008). Prevention of bipolar disorder in at-risk children: Theoretical assumptions and empirical foundations. *Development and Psychopathology, 20*(3), 881–897.

Miklowitz, D. J., Goldstein, M. J., Nuechterlein, K. H., Snyder, K. S., & Mintz, J. (1988). Family factors and the course of bipolar affective disorder. *Archives of General Psychiatry, 45*(3), 225–231.

Mineka, S., Watson, D., & Clark, L. A. (1998). Comorbidity of anxiety and unipolar mood disorders. *Annual Review of Psychology, 49,* 377–412.

Moreno, C., Laje, G., Blanco, C., Jiang, H., Schmidt, A. B., & Olfson, M. (2007). National trends in the outpatient diagnosis and treatment of bipolar disorder in youth. *Archives of General Psychiatry, 64*(9), 1032–1039.

Morey, E., Thacher, J. A., & Craighead, W. E. (2007). Patient preferences for depression treatment programs and willingness to pay for treatment. *Journal of Mental Health Policy and Economics, 10*(2), 73–85.

Nierenberg, A. A., Miyahara, S., Spencer, T., Wisniewski, S. R., Otto, M. W., Simon, N., et al. (2005). Clinical and diagnostic implications of lifetime attention-deficit/hyperactivity disorder comorbidity in adults with bipolar disorder: Data from the first 1000 STEP-BD participants. *Biological Psychiatry, 57*(11), 1467–1473.

Olivier, B., & van Oorschot, R. (2005). 5-HT1B receptors and aggression: A review. *European Journal of Pharmacology, 526*(1–3), 207–217.

Papolos, D. F. (2003). Bipolar disorder and comorbid disorders: The case for a dimensional nosology. In B. Geller & M. P. DelBello (Eds.), *Bipolar disorder in childhood and early adolescence* (pp. 76–106). New York: Guilford Press.

Patterson, G. R., DeBaryshe, B. D., & Ramsey, E. (1989). A developmental perspective on antisocial behavior. *American Psychologist, 44*(2), 329–335.

Perlis, R., Miyahara, S., Marangell, L. B., Wisniewski, S. R., Ostacher, M., DelBello, M. P., et al. (2004). Long-term implications of early onset in bipolar disorder: Data from the first 1000 participants in the systematic treatment enhancement program for bipolar disorder (STEP-BD). *Biological Psychiatry, 55,* 875–881.

Phelps, J., Angst, J., Katzow, J., & Sadler, J. (2008). Validity and utility of bipolar spectrum models. *Bipolar Disorders, 10*(1, Pt. 2), 179–193.

Plutchik, R. (1980). *Emotion: A psychoevolutionary synthesis.* New York: Harper & Row.

Pollak, S. D., Cicchetti, D., Klorman, R., & Brumaghim, J. T. (1997). Cognitive brain event-related potentials and emotion processing in maltreated children. *Child Development, 68,* 773–787.

Post, R. M., & Leverich, G. S. (2006). The role of psychosocial stress in the onset and progression of bipolar disorder and its comorbidities: The need for earlier and alternative modes of therapeutic intervention. *Development and Psychopathology, 18*(4), 1181–1211.

Post, R. M., Leverich, G. S., Xing, G., & Weiss, S. R. B. (2001). Developmental vulnerabilities to the onset and course of bipolar disorder. *Development and Psychopathology, 13,* 581–598.

Quay, H. C. (1993). The psychobiology of undersocialized aggressive conduct disorder: A theoretical perspective. *Development and Psychopathology, 5*(1–2), 165–180.

Quay, H. C. (1997). Inhibition and attention deficit hyperactivity disorder. *Journal of Abnormal Child Psychology, 25*(1), 7–13.

Quinn, C. A., & Fristad, M. A. (2004). Defining and identifying early onset bipolar spectrum disorder. *Current Psychiatry Reports, 6*(2), 101–107.

Rende, R., & Plomin, R. (1993). Families at risk for psychopathology: Who becomes affected and why? *Development and Psychopathology, 5*(4), 529–540.

Reynolds, C. R., & Kamphaus, R. (2004). *BASC-2 Behavior Assessment System for Children.* Circle Pines, MN: AGS.

Rich, B. A., Fromm, S. J., Berghorst, L. H., Dickstein, D. P., Brotman, M. A., Pine, D. S., et al. (2008). Neural connectivity in children with bipolar disorder: Impairment in the face emotion processing circuit. *Journal of Child Psychology and Psychiatry, 49*(1), 88–96.

Rich, B. A., Schmajuk, M., Perez-Edgar, K. E., Fox, N. A., Pine, D. S., & Leibenluft, E. (2007). Different psychophysiological and behavioral responses elicited by frustration in pediatric bipolar disorder and severe mood dysregulation. *American Journal of Psychiatry, 164,* 309–317.

Robins, E., & Guze, S. B. (1970). Establishment of diagnostic validity in psychiatric illness: Its application to schizophrenia. *American Journal of Psychiatry, 126*(7), 983–986.

Romero, S., Birmaher, B., Axelson, D., Goldstein, T., Goldstein, B. I., Gill, M. K., et al. (2009). Prevalence and correlates of physical and sexual abuse in children and adolescents with bipolar disorder. *Journal of Affective Disorders, 112*(1–3), 144–150.

Rudolph, K. D., Hammen, C., Burge, D., Lindberg, N., Herzberg, D., & Daley, S. E. (2000). Toward an interpersonal life-stress model of depression: The developmental context of stress generation. *Development and Psychopathology, 12*(2), 215–234.

Ruscio, A. M., Borkovec, T. D., & Ruscio, J. (2001). A taxometric investigation of the latent structure of worry. *Journal of Abnormal Psychology, 110*(3), 413–422.

Russell, J. A., & Mehrabian, A. (1977). Evidence for a three-factor theory of emotions. *Journal of Research in Personality, 11,* 273–294.

Scheffer, R. E., Kowatch, R. A., Carmody, T., & Rush, A. J. (2005). Randomized, placebo-controlled trial of mixed amphetamine salts for symptoms of comorbid ADHD in pediatric bipolar disorder after mood stabilization with divalproex sodium. *American Journal of Psychiatry, 162*(1), 58–64.

Sen, B. (2004). Adolescent propensity for depressed mood and help seeking: Race and gender differences. *Journal of Mental Health Policy and Economics, 7*(3), 133–145.

Serretti, A., Mandelli, L., Lorenzi, C., Landoni, S., Calati, R., Insacco, C., et al. (2006). Temperament and character in mood disorders: Influence of DRD4, SERTPR, TPH and MAO-A polymorphisms. *Neuropsychobiology, 53*(1), 9–16.

Srivastava, S., John, O. P., Gosling, S. D., & Potter, J. (2003). Development of personality in early and middle adulthood: Set like plaster or persistent change? *Journal of Personality and Social Psychology, 84*(5), 1041–1053.

Strakowski, S. M., Flaum, M., Amador, X., Bracha, H. S., Strakowski, S. M., Pandurangi, A.

K., et al. (1996). Racial differences in the diagnosis of psychosis. *Schizophrenia Research*, *21*(2), 117–124.

Tellegen, A., Watson, D., & Clark, L. A. (1999). On the dimensional and hierarchical structure of affect. *Psychological Science*, *10*(4), 297–303.

Tillman, R., & Geller, B. (2006). Controlled study of switching from attention-deficit/hyperactivity disorder to a prepubertal and early adolescent bipolar I disorder phenotype during 6-year prospective follow-up: Rate, risk, and predictors. *Development and Psychopathology*, *18*(4), 1037–1053.

Tillman, R., Geller, B., Nickelsburg, M. J., Bolhofner, K., Craney, J. L., DelBello, M. P., et al. (2003). Life events in a prepubertal and early adolescent bipolar disorder phenotype compared to attention-deficit hyperactive and normal controls. *Journal of Child and Adolescent Psychopharmacology*, *13*(3), 243–251.

Toalson, P., Ahmed, S., Hardy, T., & Kabinoff, G. (2004). The metabolic syndrome in patients with severe mental illnesses. *Journal of Clinical Psychiatry*, *6*(4), 152–158.

Tomarken, A. J., & Keener, A. D. (1998). Frontal brain asymmetry and depression: A self-regulatory perspective. *Cognition and Emotion*, *12*(3), 387–420.

Tremblay, R. E., Schaal, B., Boulerice, B., Arseneault, L., Soussignan, R., & Perusse, D. (1997). Male physical aggression, social dominance, and testosterone levels at puberty: A developmental perspective. In A. Raine, P. Brennan, D. P. Farrington, & S. A. Mednick (Eds.), *Biosocial bases of violence* (pp. 271–291). New York: Plenum Press.

Tsuang, M. T., & Faraone, S. (2000). The genetic epidemiology of bipolar disorder. In A. Marneros & J. Angst (Eds.), *Bipolar disorders: 100 years after manic depressive insanity* (pp. 231–241). Norwell, MA: Kluwer Academic.

Tsuchiya, K. J., Byrne, M., & Mortensen, P. B. (2003). Risk factors in relation to an emergence of bipolar disorder: A systematic review. *Bipolar Disorders*, *5*(4), 231–242.

van Winkel, R., Henquet, C., Rosa, A., Papiol, S., Fananas, L., De Hert, M., et al. (2008). Evidence that the COMT(Val158Met) polymorphism moderates sensitivity to stress in psychosis: An experience-sampling study. *American Journal of Medical Genetics*, *147B*(1), 10–17.

Vieta, E., & Suppes, T. (2008). Bipolar II disorder: Arguments for and against a distinct diagnostic entity. *Bipolar Disorders*, *10*(1, Pt. 2), 163–178.

Wagner, K. D. (2006). Bipolar disorder and comorbid anxiety disorders in children and adolescents. *Journal of Clinical Psychiatry*, *67*(Suppl. 1), 16–20.

Wakefield, J. C. (1992). The concept of mental disorder: On the boundary between biological facts and social values. *American Psychologist*, *47*(3), 373–388.

Ware, J., Jain, K., Burgess, I., & Davey, G. C. (1994). Disease-avoidance model: Factor analysis of common animal fears. *Behaviour Research and Therapy*, *32*(1), 57–63.

Watson, D., Clark, L. A., Weber, K., Assenheimer, J. S., Strauss, M. E., & McCormick, R. A. (1995). Testing a tripartite model: II. Exploring the symptom structure of anxiety and depression in student, adult, and patient samples. *Journal of Abnormal Psychology*, *104*(1), 15–25.

Watson, D., Weber, K., Assenheimer, J. S., Clark, L. A., Strauss, M. E., & McCormick, R. A. (1995). Testing a tripartite model: I. Evaluating the convergent and discriminant validity of anxiety and depression symptom scales. *Journal of Abnormal Psychology*, *104*(1), 3–14.

World Health Organization. (1992). *The ICD-10 Classification of Mental and Behavioural Disorders: Clinical Descriptions and Diagnostic Guidelines*. London: Author.

Wozniak, J., Biederman, J., Kiely, K., Ablon, J. S., Faraone, S., Mundy, E., et al. (1995). Mania-like symptoms suggestive of childhood-onset bipolar disorder in clinically referred children. *Journal of the American Academy of Child and Adolescent Psychiatry*, *34*(7), 867–876.

Yeh, M., Hough, R. L., Fakhry, F., McCabe, K. M., Lau, A. S., & Garland, A. F. (2005). Why bother with beliefs? Examining relationships between race/ethnicity, parental beliefs about causes of child problems, and mental health service use. *Journal of Consulting and Clinical Psychology, 73*(5), 800–807.

Young, R. C., Biggs, J. T., Ziegler, V. E., & Meyer, D. A. (1978). A rating scale for mania: Reliability, validity, and sensitivity. *British Journal of Psychiatry, 133,* 429–435.

Youngstrom, E. A. (2007). Pediatric bipolar disorder. In E. J. Mash & R. A. Barkley (Eds.), *Assessment of childhood disorders* (4th ed., pp. 253–304). New York: Guilford Press.

Youngstrom, E. A. (2009). Definitional issues in bipolar disorder across the life cycle. *Clinical Psychology: Science and Practice, 16,* 140–160.

Youngstrom, E. A., Birmaher, B., & Findling, R. L. (2008). Pediatric bipolar disorder: Validity, phenomenology, and recommendations for diagnosis. *Bipolar Disorders, 10*(Suppl. 1), 194–214.

Youngstrom, E. A., Findling, R. L., & Calabrese, J. R. (2003). Who are the comorbid adolescents? Agreement between psychiatric diagnosis, parent, teacher, and youth report. *Journal of Abnormal Child Psychology, 31,* 231–245.

Youngstrom, E. A., Findling, R. L., Calabrese, J. R., Gracious, B. L., Demeter, C., DelPorto Bedoya, D., et al. (2004). Comparing the diagnostic accuracy of six potential screening instruments for bipolar disorder in youths aged 5 to 17 years. *Journal of the American Academy of Child and Adolescent Psychiatry, 43,* 847–858.

Youngstrom, E. A., Meyers, O., Youngstrom, J. K., Calabrese, J. R., & Findling, R. L. (2006). Diagnostic and measurement issues in the assessment of pediatric bipolar disorder: Implications for understanding mood disorder across the life cycle. *Development and Psychopathology, 18,* 989–1021.

Youngstrom, J. K., & Youngstrom, E. A. (2008, February). *Pediatric bipolar disorder underdiagnosed in community mental health.* Paper presented at the biennial meeting of the International Society of Bipolar Disorders, Delhi, India.

CHAPTER 4

Bipolar Disorder in the Preschool Period
Development and Differential Diagnosis

Joan L. Luby, Andy C. Belden, and Mini Tandon

There has been a tremendous increase in public health attention and concern related to the diagnosis of childhood bipolar disorder (BD) over the past 2 decades. In keeping with this trend, there has also been a surge of empirical research investigating the application of the bipolar diagnosis to childhood populations (for a review, see Kowatch & DelBello, 2006). Despite a growing scientific database, diagnosing children with BD remains highly controversial and hotly debated in both scientific and public forums (Carey, 2007; Ghaemi & Martin, 2007; Groopman, 2007). At the center of the BD controversy is whether the disorder is currently being overdiagnosed in child and adolescent populations. Recent data demonstrating a 40-fold increase in the diagnosis of childhood BD within clinical settings over a 10-year period (1994–2004) has escalated controversy and heightened public concerns (Moreno et al., 2007).

In addition to escalating concerns about stigma and inappropriate labeling often associated with childhood mental disorders, there is growing alarm about the frequent use of psychotropic agents as a first-line treatment for presumptive childhood BD. The psychotropic agents used for the treatment of BD include mood-stabilizing medications that have an array of potentially serious side effects. Most of these remain insufficiently tested in child and adolescent populations in general and more specifically in the treatment of BD (see Kowatch, Strawn, & DelBello, Chapter 13, and Thase, Chapter 14, this volume).

Currently, the salient controversies among researchers and clinicians specializing in child BD include distinguishing clinical symptoms from developmental extremes, defining diagnostic criteria, and defining temporal features. Furthermore, most would agree that when these same issues are discussed within the preschool period, the debate/controversy becomes more intense, ambiguous, and alarming to the general public. The purpose of this chapter is to discuss these issues in the context of preschool development. In addition, we provide new longitudinal findings from the Preschool Depression Study (PDS), which included a subsample who met DSM-IV bipolar I symptom criteria that has been previously described (Luby & Belden, 2006).

CONTROVERSIES IN THE NOSOLOGY OF CHILDHOOD BIPOLAR DISORDER: IMPLICATIONS FOR STUDY OF THE PRESCHOOL DISORDER

A current debate in the nosology of childhood BD is how to define the disorder with regard to the adult-based DSM-IV (American Psychiatric Association, 1994) criteria. Three different viewpoints have received the most attention in the scientific literature to date. A central question is whether children must manifest discrete episodes of mania as seen in adults to meet formal criteria for the diagnosis or whether developmental modifications to the temporal features of some DSM diagnoses in children are needed. Geller and colleagues propose one view in which adherence to all DSM-IV criteria, with the exception of standard duration criteria, are required (Geller, Zimerman, Williams, DelBello, Frazier, et al., 2002). Geller and other research groups have suggested that developmental modifications to the duration criteria for childhood BD are necessary (Biederman et al., 2000; Geller & Luby, 1997; Geller, Tillman, Craney, & Bolhofner, 2004). The need to modify duration criteria has been supported by several independent investigations, which have described a very rapid, continuous or so-called ultradian cycling combined with mixed mania as the most common manifestation of BD in children and adolescents (Findling et al., 2001; Geller & Cook, 2000; Geller & Luby, 1997; Geller et al., 1995; Geller & Tillman, 2005; Tillman & Geller, 2003).

Biederman and colleagues have proposed alternative criteria for the BD diagnosis, emphasizing the importance of severe irritability and mood lability and not requiring the adherence to all other DSM-IV symptom or duration criteria (Biederman, 1995; Biederman, Faraone, Chu, & Wozniak, 1999; Wozniak, Biederman, & Richards, 2001). Their broader definition of the disorder does not require that all DSM-IV "cardinal symptoms" (e.g., elation, grandiosity) are met. Leibenluft, Charney, Towbin, Bhangoo, and Pine (2003) have proposed an alternate, more conservative view in which all adult-based DSM-IV criteria, including duration criteria, must be met to make the diagnosis of BD. Related to this view, this group has proposed a distinction between "narrow" and "broad" definitions of childhood BD and suggested that children who fall into either of the developmentally modified groups (i.e., those with chronic irritability, mood lability, oppositionality, and hyperarousal without elation or grandiosity) should be labeled as "severely emotionally dysregulated" rather than bipolar (Leibenluft et al., 2003). According to this proposed schema, the narrow definition of the disorder requires full adherence to DSM-IV criteria, for which discrete episodes of mania must be evident (Leibenluft et al., 2003; see Youngstrom, Chapter 3, this volume, for further details).

Contributing to the skepticism and controversy about the definition of childhood BDs are the high rates of comorbidity with attention-deficit/hyperactivity disorder (ADHD) reported by several groups in the empirical literature (e.g., Faraone, Biederman, & Monuteaux, 2001; Findling et al., 2001; Geller et al., 2000; Tillman & Geller, 2003). At the core of this phenomenon is the high degree of symptom overlap between ADHD and BD, making differential diagnosis especially challenging. Children with severe ADHD sometimes erroneously receive a bipolar diagnosis, and the reverse may be true as well (Carlson, 1998; Kim & Miklowitz, 2002). In addition to overlap with ADHD, children with BD are also known to have high rates of other comorbid disruptive disorders such as oppositional defiant disorder (ODD) and conduct disorder (CD) (e.g., Biederman et al., 1999; Geller et al., 2000; Kim & Miklowitz, 2002; Kovacs & Pollock, 1995; Kutcher, Marton, & Korenblum, 1989; Spencer et al., 2001; Wozniak, Biederman, Faraone, Blier, & Monuteaux, 2001). Rates of comorbidity among children with BD, which are notably higher than those found in other childhood psychiatric disorders, have raised doubts about the specificity and subsequently the validity of the bipolar diagnosis.

Results from several studies investigating school-age children typically find that approximately 80% of children diagnosed with BD also met criteria for ADHD (Faraone et al., 2001; Findling et al., 2001; Geller et al., 2000; Tillman & Geller, 2003). Although the two disorders may coexist in many children and share similar features, several symptoms may be specific markers, which are especially useful in differentiating BD from ADHD (Geller, Zimerman, Williams, DelBello, Bolhofner, et al., 2002). Geller and colleagues found that grandiosity and elation are symptoms common in BD but rare in prepubertal and early-adolescent children with ADHD. Similarly, the symptoms of sharpened thinking and increased goal-directed behavior, two descriptions from the broad symptom of increased energy, were both more prevalent in those with BD versus ADHD (Geller et al., 2000). Importantly, symptoms of decreased need for sleep, hypersexuality, racing thoughts, elation, and grandiosity were found to best differentiate BD from ADHD in prepubertal and early-adolescent children (Geller et al., 1998; Geller, Zimerman, Williams, DelBello, Bolhofner, et al., 2002; Geller, Zimerman, Williams, DelBello, Frazier, et al., 2002).

As controversial as this area of research has been when focusing on children and adolescents, the ambiguity and debate surrounding BD diagnoses are even greater when applied to children younger than 6 years. There has been a great deal of public health concern about the application and accurate diagnosis of mental disorders in general, and serious Axis I mood disorders in particular, among young children (Carey, 2007; Moreno et al., 2007; Weller, Weller, & Fristad, 1995; Williams, Klinepeter, Palmes, Pulley, & Foy, 2004). The controversy surrounds the risks of inappropriate labeling and stigmatization versus the benefits of proper identification and early intervention. Adding to the complexity of diagnosing preschool-age children with BD is the very real challenge that researchers and clinicians face when attempting to disentangle and differentiate normative aberrations in emotional, social, and cognitive functioning from those that are clinically significant. Episodes of emotional or behavioral dysregulation that remain within a normative range must be distinguished from variations in the same behaviors that cross the normative threshold into "clinically relevant" domains and that may ultimately be early manifestations of an Axis I mood disorder. Along this line, the distinction between normative but intense emotional experiences well known during the preschool period, such as high levels of joy and elevated self-concept, with clinically significant alterations in mood and self-concept (e.g., elation, grandiosity), are examples of this difficult distinction. These concerns are underscored further by the potential use and dangers of inadequately tested psychotropic medications in this very young population.

GAPS IN UNDERSTANDING PRESCHOOL BIPOLAR DISORDER

Over the last decade, there has been significant progress in our understanding of the nosology of several psychiatric disorders in the preschool period (Luby & Belden, 2006; Pine et al., 2002; Scheeringa, Peebles, Cook, & Zeanah, 2001; Scheeringa, Zeanah, Myers, & Putnam, 2003; Task Force on Research Diagnostic Criteria: Infancy and Preschool, 2003). The availability of developmentally appropriate measures of psychopathology and impairments designed for young children has catalyzed work in this area (Carter, Briggs-Gowan, & Davis, 2004; Egger et al., 2006; Hodges, 1994). A basic principle in the design of these measures has been the need to capture developmentally adjusted manifestations of symptom states as they arise in preschool-age children. Earlier studies that assessed the presence of symptoms as detailed in the DSM system and that described adult-based behaviors and emotions often failed to find preschool children who met diagnostic criteria for any mental disorder. The problems with nondevelopmentally informed approaches to diagnosing childhood-onset mental disorders are akin to using a large net when attempting to capture small fish: One could erroneously conclude they don't exist if they are not captured by the net. Through increased attention to age-adjusted and developmentally appropriate methods used to assess DSM symptom states in very young children, our understanding of psychiatric nosology for several preschool-onset mental disorders has improved significantly.

There continues to be a dearth of empirical investigations examining mania or BD in children younger than 6 years. The lagging progress in this area is likely related to the skepticism and controversy about the disorder in older children, which provides an uncertain framework for downward extension of studies to young children. In the absence of large-scale controlled investigations, numerous case reports and chart reviews have described mania symptoms and syndromes in preschool children (Luby, Tandon, & Nicol, 2007; Mota-Castillo et al., 2001; Pavuluri, Janicak, & Carbray, 2002; Tumuluru, Weller, Fristad, & Weller, 2003; Tuzun, Zoroglu, & Savas, 2002; Wilens et al., 2002). Furthermore, and related in part to the numerous controversial issues cited previously, the lack of an age-appropriate psychiatric interview to assess mania symptoms has thwarted empirical investigations in this area.

In collaboration with the authors of the Preschool Age Psychiatric Assessment (PAPA; Egger, Ascher, & Angold, 1999), Luby and colleagues developed a mania module for the PAPA based on DSM-IV bipolar I criteria. Results examining the test–retest reliability have been previously reported with an intraclass correlation coefficient of $r = .71$ (Luby & Belden, 2006). Although validity testing of this module is still needed, initial results (described next) suggest that a specific bipolar I symptom constellation can be identified in the preschool period. Specifically, a constellation of mania symptoms in preschoolers between the ages of 3 and 6 that showed discriminant validity from DSM-IV major depressive disorder (MDD) and disruptive (ADHD/ODD/CD) psychiatric disorders has been identified (Luby & Belden, 2006).

Several findings emerged from this exploratory investigation of the validity of preschool-onset BD. Findings provided support for a specific symptom constellation that distinguished BD from other early-onset disruptive disorders. Especially noteworthy was that children diagnosed with preschool BD were 74 times as likely as children in the disruptive group to have exhibited hypersexuality and 23 times as likely as those in the disruptive group to have exhibited grandiosity. Some examples of grandiosity include a preschooler who tries to make executive decisions for family, is brazenly directive with authority figures outside the home, or holds fixed false beliefs about his sports skills. Second, results indicated that, even when controlling for the impulsive and inattentive ADHD symptoms of preschoolers with BD, these children continued to be rated as significantly more impaired on all six subscales of a well-validated measure of functional impairment (Preschool and Early Childhood Functional Assessment Scale; Hodges, 1994) compared with healthy children and same-age peers with MDD, ADHD, ODD, or CD. Similarly, children in the BD group scored significantly lower (i.e., poor developmental adaptive abilities) on the Communication, Daily Living, Social, and Motor subscales of the Vineland (Sparrow, Carter, & Cicchetti, 1987) compared with same-age peers in the healthy, MDD, and disruptive comparison groups (Luby & Belden, 2006).

SPECIFIC MARKERS OF PRESCHOOL BIPOLAR DISORDER

Finally, Luby and Belden (2006) reported that when using only five (i.e., hypersexuality, elation, grandiosity, hypertalkative, and flight of ideas) of the 13 BD symptoms, preschoolers with a BD diagnosis could be differentiated from those who had ADHD, ODD, or CD (without BD) 92% of the time. The symptom of hypersexuality, although less common in this early age compared with prepubertal and early-adolescent BD samples, was more prevalent in those with BD compared with preschoolers with disruptive disorders (Luby & Belden, 2006). Although these findings are limited by small sample size, they are very similar to those reported in older bipolar children by Geller, Zimerman, Williams, DelBello, Bolhofner, and colleagues (2002). It is important to note that hypersexuality is, and in the current sample was, statistically rare in preschoolers. However, the clinical manifestations of hypersexuality in preschoolers have been previously observed and described. Preschoolers who (1) are flirtatious and romantic with adults, making them uncomfortable, or (2) have no history of suspected sexual abuse but disrobe among peers or touch them inappropriately are some examples cited in published case reports (Danielyan, Pathak, Kowatch, Arszman, & Johns, 2007; Luby et al., 2007; Maia, Boaratima, Kleinman, & Fu-l, 2007; Mota-Castillo et al., 2001; Scheffer & Niskala Apps, 2004; Tumuluru et al., 2003; Tuzun et al., 2002). Importantly, in at least some of these case reports, sexual abuse was ruled out.

In addition to clinical symptom descriptions of hypersexuality, there have been a growing number of case reports detailing symptoms generally thought to be consistent with preschool BD (Danielyan et al., 2007; Dilsaver & Akiskal, 2004; Luby et al., 2007; Maia et al., 2007). Symptom manifestations in many of the cited case reports appear to overlap, including descriptions of euphoria, elation, irritability, decreased need for sleep, and pressured speech or elevations in motor activity. Common to several studies cited previously was the consistent finding of family history of affective disorders (including mood and anxiety disorders) among first-degree relatives. Also noteworthy was the impairment that such children faced as a result of their symptomatology, including expulsion from preschool or day care settings and increased risk of injury, sometimes resulting in hospitalization at such early age. High recovery and relapse rates, defined by meeting criteria for hypomania or mania with moderate symptoms requiring intervention (Clinical Global Impression-Severity ≥ 5) and minimally improved for at least 2 weeks, have been reported (Danielyan et al., 2007). High rates of comorbidity with ADHD are also described in these case series, with some comorbid cases having shown increased sensitivities and side effects to stimulants such as worsening motor hyperactivity.

DIFFERENTIATING BIPOLAR DISORDER FROM ATTENTION-DEFICIT/ HYPERACTIVITY DISORDER IN PRESCHOOL CHILDREN

Few investigations have examined preschoolers with BD comorbid with ADHD. Luby and Belden (2006) reported that, similar to comorbidity rates reported in several samples of older BD children, 81% of preschoolers who met all DSM-IV symptom criteria for BD (based on an age-appropriate structured diagnostic interview) also had ADHD. In contrast, another study aimed to examine comorbidity in a sample of clinically referred preschoolers and school-age children ages 4 to

9. In this investigation, diagnoses were made by structured interview with parent informants using DSM III-R criteria (American Psychiatric Association, 1987) and confirmed by clinical consensus of a panel of mental health professionals (Wilens et al., 2002). Using these methods, 26% of preschoolers with ADHD had comorbid BD and were functionally impaired socially, behaviorally, and academically to a similar level as their school-age peers who also had ADHD and BD (Wilens et al., 2002).

The differential diagnosis between BD and ADHD is made even more challenging in preschoolers based on normative high activity levels in this age group, some ongoing ambiguity about the diagnostic characteristics of preschool ADHD, and the previously mentioned lack of well-validated age-appropriate measures to assess mania in this age group. The use of age-appropriate measures to assist in diagnosis has proven to be helpful, and a few empirical investigations have informed which measures differentiate the two disorders in school-age children.

Measurement Tools

Prior literature has reviewed the risks of missing pertinent psychopathology in young children when measures designed for older children are applied (Task Force on Research Diagnostic Criteria: Infancy and Preschool, 2003). That is, when questions about symptoms as manifested in older children and adults are used to assess symptoms in young children, one can erroneously conclude that the symptoms are not present because age-appropriate manifestations will not be captured. Given the lack of available measures for mania in preschoolers, a new mania module for the PAPA (Egger et al., 1999) was developed incorporating developmental manifestations of bipolar symptoms as observed and previously described in preschoolers (e.g., Findling et al., 2001; Luby et al., 2007; Pavuluri et al., 2002; Tumuluru et al., 2003). Items address the symptoms of elation, grandiosity, hypersexuality, flight of ideas/racing thoughts, decreased need for sleep, and increased energy/motor pressure/hyperactivity. Following the PAPA format, each symptom is detailed for intensity, duration, frequency, context, and onset and resulting impairment when present. When rating intensity, consideration is given to normative levels of these phenomena appropriate to some symptom dimensions in this age group (e.g., normative elation in response to a special event).

The Central Importance of Play in Assessing Symptoms

Emphasis is given to manifestations of symptoms in play, given its central role in the preschool period (Piaget, 1951). Fantasy play is normative, and children may pretend they have special powers similar to their favorite action heroes or abilities like famous athletes; however, the PAPA elicits information to ascertain whether such grandiosity is outside the realm of normative play and is held as a fixed and false belief rather than a fanciful construction. Furthermore, the interviewer gathers history about whether any resulting functional impairment or injury related to such beliefs has occurred. For instance, it is important to ascertain whether the child truly believes he or she has the authority to make executive decisions for the family and begins acting on this, demonstrated, for example, by packing for a desired trip or moving into a master bedroom suite, two specific grandiose behaviors that have been observed in BD preschoolers in our clinic.

As noted previously, context specificity is a key consideration in distinguishing between normative versus fantasy play characteristic of the preschool period and pathological symptoms of elation and/or grandiosity. Along this line, Geller, Zimerman, Williams, DelBello, Frazier, and colleagues (2002) provided useful clinical examples of the distinction between normative behaviors and clinical mania in prepubertal children. For instance, the child who pretends he is a teacher and directs peers playfully after school is not displaying psychopathology, given appropriate context and lack of impairment. In contrast, the child who teaches class because he actually believes he is the teacher and gets suspended demonstrates both inappropriate context and impairment, described as pathological grandiosity (Geller, Zimerman, Williams, DelBello, Frazier, et al., 2002). Similarly, it would be normative for a child to pretend she is a princess and to dress up as such and behave in an imperial fashion in play but can let go of this persona when playtime is over. In contrast, a grandiose child may believe he or she has age-inappropriate powers and may display inappropriate expectations of control over outside authority figures (e.g., doctors, preschool directors) by giving them instructions, teasing them, or advising them on life plans.

DEPRESSION IN PRESCHOOL BIPOLAR DISORDER

In an attempt to further elucidate the nosology of preschool BD, Luby and Belden (2008) examined whether manifestations of distinct depressive episodes were identifiable in children with preschool bipolar I. We compared a subsample of preschool participants in a larger ongoing longitudinal PDS who were identified as having preschool bipolar or unipolar depression. We reported several notable findings regarding the clinical characteristics of MDD in children with preschool-onset BD. First, children in the preschool bipolar group experienced significantly more symptoms of unipolar MDD than those in the preschool unipolar depressed group. That is, on average BD preschoolers manifested 3.2 (mean $SD = 3.5$) more unipolar depressive symptoms than unipolar depressed preschoolers without BD. When testing for differences in specific unipolar symptom manifestations, results indicated that 100% of BD preschoolers ($n = 22$) versus 76% of unipolar preschoolers ($n = 54$) exhibited irritability, $\chi^2 (1) = 6.12$, $p < .01$. Furthermore, preschoolers with BD were significantly more likely than those with unipolar MDD to have displayed the following symptoms of depression: being easily annoyed, sleep problems, self-hatred, death themes in play, and suicidal/intentional self-injurious behaviors. Although death themes in play may be normative, preoccupation with death themes is seen in the play of preschoolers with mood disorders to the exclusion of other themes. Self-injurious behaviors such as head banging or hitting self may also arise during tantrums or expressions of anger in both preschoolers with depression and those with BD.

Results indicated two significant differences in unipolar depression symptom frequencies for children with preschool bipolar versus unipolar MDD. That is, in addition to irritability (described previously) children with preschool BD more frequently had the symptom of anhedonia at clinical levels than same-age peers diagnosed with unipolar MDD. Anhedonia in a preschooler is evidenced by a lack of ability to enjoy activities and play, a highly clinically significant symptom during this developmental period. Luby and Belden (2008) also reported that bipolar and unipolar preschoolers' expressions of clinical-level sadness were very similar. However, when sadness was expressed at a clinically relevant level by preschoolers with BD, the average total duration (obtained using the PAPA) of the expression was 4 hours versus an average duration of 26 minutes in unipolar depressed preschoolers. On the basis of their findings, Luby and Belden concluded that, similar to BD in adults, preschoolers with a BD syndrome suffer from clinically significant and severe episodes of depression. Findings underscored the marked depression that characterizes preschool BD and suggested that further investigation of this domain may clarify the nosology of preschool BD.

A 4-Year-Old with Aggression, Guilt, and Sadness

A 4.2-year-old boy was referred to the clinic because of concerns about extreme irritability associated with aggression interrupted by periods of extreme sadness, guilt, and remorse. His mother was unable to manage the child's intense tantrums arising with little or no apparent provocation multiple times daily, but the greatest concern was aggression toward his younger sibling. The child was hospitalized after pushing his younger sister down a flight of stairs and subsequently becoming inconsolably sad and crying for several hours.

FAMILIAL TRANSMISSION OF BIPOLAR DISORDER IN CHILDREN AND ADOLESCENTS

Previous studies provide extensive support for familial transmission, including strong genetic contributions to childhood BD. Estimates of heritability of BD have been reported between 85 and 89% (McGuffin et al., 2003). Unprecedented scientific efforts have been underway to identify candidate genes or components of genetic anticipation associated with BD. However, to date there is no widely accepted or replicated association between any one gene and BD. Taken together, the existing literature suggests that single-gene effects in BD disorder are rare, if not nonexistent (Baum et al., 2008). The most recent findings indicate that BD is most likely a polygenetic disease influenced by several genes, each having a small effect (Perlis et al., 2008).

Luby and Mrakotsky (2003) examined whether depressed preschoolers had a significantly greater proportion of family members diagnosed with BD compared with preschoolers in healthy and psychiatric comparison groups. Results indicated that preschoolers with MDD had significantly more family members with BD than those in the healthy and psychiatric comparison groups. Findings also indicated that, among preschoolers with depression, those with a family history of BD had a significantly higher rate of "restlessness" than those without this family history. The authors suggested this may be evidence of a more agitated depressive subtype in preschoolers with a family history of BD and speculated that this depressive subgroup may be at a heighted risk for switching to mania later in their development.

Equally important as obtaining a better understanding of the heritability of BD at the molecular genetic level are studies examining familial and environmental factors that may function as risk or protective factors for children genetically at risk for BD. To date, no studies have examined environmental risk/protective factors in preschool BD. However, Curtis and Cicchetti (2003) review factors involved in the study of biological contributors to resilience as might be applied to affective disorders in general. For example, they review the theory set forth by Post, Leverich, Weiss, Zhang, and Xing (2003) that adaptive changes in gene expression may impact how individuals cope with adversity in both positive and negative ways, thereby changing the propensity for recurrence of affective illness. In addition to these biological risk/protective factors, there is also a body of literature implicating several familial factors as having moderate to large effects on the etiology, course, psychosocial outcomes, and treatment response in adolescents with BD spectrum disorders (for a review, see DelBello & Geller, 2001). Findings from older children and adolescents with BD, as well as from samples of depressed preschoolers, provide a useful empirical foundation for hypothesis generation regarding familial factors that may be associated with age of onset, course, and developmental outcomes in children with preschool BD.

FAMILIAL ENVIRONMENT AND BIPOLAR DISORDER COURSE IN CHILDREN AND ADOLESCENTS

Findings from developmental psychopathology research have suggested that caregiving strategies, emotional expressivity, and parenting attributions play a critical role in the development of more broadly defined internalizing and externalizing disorders in children younger than 6 years (Denham et al., 2000; Dix, 1991; Eisenberg et al., 2001). Given the doubts surrounding the existence and validity of BD in young children, it is not surprising that no research has examined associations between preschool BD and these risk/protective factors. Prospective longitudinal studies of young children at risk for BD (by virtue of having an affected parent) or who have been diagnosed with very early-onset BD are well poised to inform key questions related to risk, timing, course, severity, and outcomes of BD throughout childhood.

A growing body of evidence suggests that biological, psychological, and social variables interact to affect the onset and course of many forms of psychopathology (Caspi et al., 2003; Fish et al., 2004; Kandel, 1998; Weaver, Meaney, & Szyf, 2006). Adolescents with BD who experience high levels of caregiver hostility, criticism, and emotional overinvolvement (i.e., high expressed emotion [EE]) are at a significantly higher risk for severe BD symptoms during family treatment (Miklowitz, Biuckians, & Richards, 2006). Similarly, Craney and Geller (2003) found that among children with BD, those whose mothers were rated as being low in expressed warmth were four times as likely to have a BD recurrence within a 4-year period following a recovery compared with those whose mothers expressed high warmth. Miklowitz (2007) proposed that, through bidirectional processes, chronic parent–child interactions that include high amounts of criticism, hostility, and conflict hinder children's developing capacities to self-regulate their emotion states, a core deficit in BDs. When children are unable to regulate their emotions in socially appropriate ways, their subsequent misbehaviors may elicit and reinforce parents' high EE propensity as well as parents' subsequent use of maladaptive caregiving behaviors. This bidirectionality may create a vicious cycle of perpetuation of psychopathology.

Unipolar depression severity in a preschool sample was found to be negatively associated with mothers' observed use of supportive caregiving strategies during a mildly stressful parent–child problem-solving task (Belden & Luby, 2006). Results also indicated that preschoolers with more severe unipolar depression were significantly less compliant (e.g., did not follow caregiver directions), persistent (e.g., gave up on the task), and enthusiastic during the dyadic task. Interestingly, the association between preschool unipolar depression severity and children's observed compliance and persistence during the task was no longer significant when mothers' observed use of emotionally supportive caregiving strategies was included as a mediator within the model. Therefore, the link between preschool unipolar depression severity and observed negative behavioral outcomes was at least partially a result of caregivers' lack of supportive strategies during the task. Using the same task, results from Luby and colleagues (2006) indicated that raters blind to preschool diagnosis and using a standardized coding scheme were able to detect differences between melancholic and nonmelancholic unipolar depressed preschoolers based on preschoolers' expressions of enthusiasm, avoidance, and compliance during the task.

Preschoolers' internal representations of parenting using the MacArthur Story Stem Battery (a narrative task) were investigated in another larger sample of depressed preschoolers (Belden, Sullivan, & Luby, 2007). Findings from this investigation indicated that even as early as the preschool period unipolar depression severity was significantly associated with preschool children's internal representations of the mothers' caregiving strategies. That is, when asked to act out the end of an emotionally evocative story stem (e.g., complete a story stem in which a child is at the store with his or her mother and loses a favorite stuffed animal), preschoolers with higher unipolar depression severity scores were observed and coded as representing their mothers as being significantly more controlling, hostile, critical, and punitive. These same internal representations predicted the observed use of negative and nonsupportive caregiving strategies by mothers 1 year later during a mildly stressful parent–child interaction task.

Conceptually, findings from unipolar depressed preschoolers are consistent with the hypothetical model developed by Miklowitz (2007) describing the reciprocal and dysfunctional processes that occur within caregiver–child dyads, which function to increase the occurrence of relapse in older children. That is, in two independent samples, we found that the higher MDD severity scores of preschoolers were associated with more frequent use of high emotional expressivity among mothers, including hostility, coercion, and emotional overinvolvement. Mothers' more frequent use of negative parenting was also associated with preschoolers' use of behaviors often associated with poor emotion self-regulation strategies in early childhood, such as noncompliance, poor persistence, and tantrums (Belden, 2007; Belden & Luby, 2006; Luby et al., 2006). Furthermore, preschoolers with higher MDD scores represented their mothers' caregiving strategies as more hostile, coercive, and negative on the MacArthur Story Stem Battery. Presumably these representations were based on the children's caregiving experiences, suggesting that even as early as the preschool period children have begun to internalize and develop expectations and attributions about the types of caregiving strategies they will receive from their mothers. This is especially interesting considering that preschoolers' internal representations of their mothers as expressing negative emotionality and related behaviors predicted mothers' actual observed use of the same behaviors while interacting with their children 1 year later.

Integrating these findings with the Miklowitz model suggests that preschoolers who experience greater depressive symptoms early on may intensify and increase their negative reactions to caregiving strategies and behaviors. Preschoolers' frequent negative reactions, partially a result of residual mood symptoms, within the caregiver–child relationship may result in the caregivers' misattribution of the cause of the children's behaviors (i.e., "My child is behaving maliciously" vs. "This behavior is out of my child's control and due to a biologically based illness"). Increasing negative caregiving cognitions and schemata for the caregiver–child relationship on the part of the caregiver is then proposed to result in caregivers reacting to their children's misbehavior with high EE or related negative strategies. Hence, the vicious cycle associated with increased relapse of mood disorders in children is perpetuated. Based on our findings in unipolar depressed children, the dysfunctional dyadic processes proposed by Miklowitz (2007) may emerge as early as the preschool period of development. Such a negative interactive process may be particularly salient in the context of the early symptoms of BD such as extreme irritability, resulting in severe tantrums and intense negative emotional expressions (e.g., a preschooler stating "I hate you" to a parent in response to minor frustrations). These expressions may be particularly provocative for parents and difficult to keep in perspective, setting off the vicious cycle outlined previously.

PRESCHOOL BIPOLAR DISORDER AS A DISORDER OF EMOTION REGULATION

An interesting area relevant to developmental psychopathology models is the question of whether preschool BD can be conceptualized as a fundamental disorder of emotion regulation. At face value, highly emotionally labile children with BD who manifest intense periods of extreme negative and positive mood states would seem to have a fundamental impairment in their ability to regulate emotions. In this way, the mood lability inherent in BD is an obvious form of poor emotion regulation. However, developmental models of emotion regulation, focusing on the child's developmental capacity for emotional control and its antecedents and consequences, have not been applied to conceptualizations of BD. Furthermore, such a conceptualization, if proven valid, may help to guide early intervention strategies and suggest that greater focus on enhancing the child's emotional regulatory skills in early development would be useful. Such models have been previously described for mood disorders and are currently being tested in depressed preschool populations (Luby, Stalets, Blankenship, Pautsch, & McGrath, 2008).

Despite its potential utility, there are several ways in which the symptom manifestations of early childhood BD may not be well described by a simple developmental emotion dysregulation model. The phenomena of a new onset of symptoms arising after a period of normal development, as well as episodicity, fail to fit this developmental model. That is, in some young children with BD, emotion dysregulation characterized by intense and labile mood onsets after a period of adequate capacity for emotion regulation has already been demonstrated. This trajectory of symptom onset suggests that the disorder is not just a developmental delay or failure to achieve a developmental capacity. Those children who manifest episodes of mood dysregulation separated by periods of normal emotional functioning (a common pattern in at least 50% of adults with BD) do not appear to have impairments in the underlying capacity for emotion regulation. In these cases, the capacity for adequate or appropriate emotion regulation remains intact for periods of time. Neither of these circumstances are consistent with a typical emotion dysregulation model, raising questions about the application of this model to understanding the phenomenology of early-onset BD. This issue is further complicated by the ongoing debate about episodicity in childhood BD, with some groups reporting a lack of discrete episodes. To date, there have been no investigations of emotion regulation (using state-of-the-art developmental and diagnostic measures together) in preschool- or school-age BD.

LONGITUDINAL COURSE OF PRESCHOOL-ONSET BIPOLAR DISORDER

A question that is central to the validation of a psychiatric disorder is whether a specific symptom constellation can be identified and remains relatively stable over time (Robins & Guze, 1970). Although there are clinically significant disorders that are not longitudinally stable (e.g., some anxiety disorders), in general the issue of stability is of importance because symptoms or problems that spontaneously remit are unlikely to require treatment and may not be clinically significant. To date there have been very few longitudinal data on preschoolers with mania symptoms. Recent findings from Luby, Si, Belden, Tandon, and Spitznagel (2009) using data from a longitudinal study of preschool depression funded by the National Institute of Mental Health (PDS) indicated that preschool-onset MDD has a chronic and recurrent course similar to the course known in older children and adolescents. The hypothesis that preschool bipolar symptoms would also manifest a similar stable longitudinal course as established in at least two studies of older children with BD seems well founded (DelBello, 2007; Geller, Tillman, Bolhofner, & Zimerman, 2008; Geller et al., 2004). To test this hypothesis, data related to the diagnosis, course, and potential environmental correlates of preschool-onset BD have been obtained as a part of the PDS described previously. The sample of 306 children (ages 3–6 years) was recruited from community preschools, day care centers, and primary care sites using a screening checklist to oversample for preschoolers with mood symptoms (see Luby, Belden, Pautsch, Si, & Spitznagel, 2009, for details of sample ascertainment). As outlined previously, preschoolers were assessed using the PAPA, which included an age-appropriate mania module conducted at three annual study waves. The stability of preschool BD was investigated by analyzing the risk of the diagnosis of BD at 12 (wave 2) and 24 months (wave 3) after baseline compared with preschoolers without BD at baseline (Figure 4.1). In addition, analyses were conducted to test whether children with preschool BD were more likely to be diagnosed with BD at later waves (using raters blind to children's diagnostic history) compared with same-age peers without BD but diagnosed with preschool disruptive disorders.

Results indicated that preschoolers diagnosed with BD at wave 1 were 13 times as likely as preschoolers without BD to be diagnosed with BD 12 and 24 months later. Results also indicated that preschoolers diagnosed with BD at wave 1 were at almost eight times greater risk than preschoolers diagnosed with a disruptive disorder to be diagnosed with BD 12 and 24 months later, suggesting that preschool-onset BD is not a transient disorder.

These preliminary findings suggest that preschool BD demonstrates longitudinal stability over time, consistent with the longitudinal course known in older children and adolescents (DelBello, 2007; Geller et al., 2004, 2008). These findings lend additional support to the idea that a valid preschool BD can be identified.

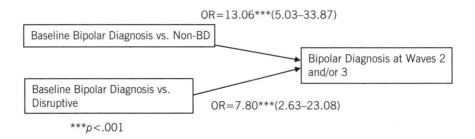

FIGURE 4.1. Odds ratios (OR) for bipolar disorder at waves 2 and/or 3 for children with bipolar disorder at baseline versus healthy or disruptive children at baseline.

TREATMENT OF PRESCHOOL BIPOLAR DISORDER

As might be expected based on the lack of clarity about the nosology of the disorder, there has been very little investigation of treatments for preschoolers with BD. Unfortunately, only a few published psychopharmacological treatment studies exist. Most of these studies are limited by small sample size, open-label or retrospective chart review designs, or lack of an appropriate control group; some are simply individual case reports (e.g., Scheffer & Niskala Apps, 2004). Another problem is that many studies are conducted primarily in older children but include only a small number of preschoolers. The majority of these reports address the use of mood stabilizers or second-generation antipsychotics. For example, lithium monotherapy successfully improved symptoms in five hospitalized preschoolers in one case report series (Tumuluru et al., 2003). Other case series and reports have reviewed the effectiveness of valproic acid or carbamazepine as monotherapy to improve symptoms in outpatient clinic samples of preschoolers with a clinical diagnosis of BD (Mota-Castillo et al., 2001; Tuzun et al., 2002). For preschoolers who did not improve with lithium treatment alone, augmentation with risperidone was shown to improve response in an open-label trial that included older children (Pavuluri et al., 2006). Conversely, in a single case report of a 4½-year-old preschooler described as manic, risperidone monotherapy response was augmented successfully by the addition of the mood stabilizer topiramate when side effects of lithium augmentation were intolerable (Pavuluri et al., 2002). Furthermore, the second-generation antipsychotics risperidone and olanzapine showed efficacy in a prospective, open-label trial of preschoolers (*n* = 31) with a form of BD based on a broader definition of the disorder (Biederman et al., 2005).

Given the dearth of psychopharmacological treatment studies that use double-blind designs, continued caution in the use and monitoring of any psychotropic in a preschool child is warranted. Currently, the empirical literature suggests that risperidone has the most available published evidence for efficacy in the amelioration of irritability or aggression in the treatment of young children with pervasive developmental disorders/autism spectrum disorders (Luby et al., 2006; Masi, Cosenza, Mucci, & De Vito, 2001; Nagaraj, Singhi, & Malhi, 2006; Pandina,

Bossie, Youssef, Zhu, & Dunbar, 2007; Shea et al., 2004; Williams et al., 2006). Open-label studies that have tested the medication in preschoolers with presumed BD support dosage ranges between 0.25 to 2.0 mg/day, with the need for ongoing risk–benefit analysis in preschool-age children (Gleason et al., 2007).

Lack of data and related concerns about the potential dangers and side effects of pharmacological treatments with preschool-age children underscore the importance of psychotherapeutic strategies in preschool BD. A number of early psychotherapeutic interventions have been used and have proven effective for the treatment of disruptive behavioral problems in preschool-age children, including parent–child interaction therapy (PCIT; Eyberg, 1988; Eyberg, Boggs, & Algina, 1995) and the Incredible Years Series (Webster-Stratton & Hammond, 1997) among others (Burke, Loeber, & Birmaher, 2002; Farmer, Compton, Bums, & Robertson, 2002; Webster-Stratton, Reid, & Hammond, 2004). Although not yet tested in preschoolers with a diagnosis of BD, an adaptation of PCIT has been developed for preschool mood disorders (Luby et al., 2008). PCIT is a manualized treatment designed to enhance the parent–child relationship and teach the parent effective and nurturing strategies for setting limits with disruptive and noncompliant behavior (Eyberg et al., 1995). PCIT has been empirically tested and shown to be effective for the treatment of disruptive behavior among preschoolers (Hood & Eyberg, 2003). Highly unusual in psychotherapy research was the finding that gains made in response to this early intervention were sustained after 6 years without booster sessions (Hood & Eyberg, 2003). These promising findings suggest that early intervention during the preschool period of development may be a window of opportunity for more sustained gains.

Based on these impressive outcomes, PCIT was adapted for application to the treatment of mood disorders by Luby and colleagues. This adaptation, so-called PCIT emotion development (ED), includes a new and additional module focused on enhancing emotional competence. Among the goals of this emotion development module are to enhance the preschoolers' capacity to regulate intense emotions, an area of obvious application to BD. In addition, enhancing the preschoolers' capacity to identify, label, and understand a broad range of emotions in themselves and others is emphasized as a major treatment goal. The preschooler and primary caregiver attend 1-hour weekly sessions over the course of 14 weeks during which the emotional and dynamic relationship of the parent and child is optimized and facilitated by a trained therapist. This trained therapist guides the dyad's interaction and application of skills directly but unobtrusively using a "bug-in-the-ear" device. A series of progressively more challenging homework assignments consolidates skills learned in treatment sessions, allows monitoring of progress, and enhances the generalizability of these skills outside of the clinical setting.

More specifically, the PCIT-ED therapy is divided into three main modules. The first of this series, child-directed interaction (CDI), targets the development of a nurturing relationship of the dyad. In general, the caregiver is taught to allow the child to direct the play and follow along, fostering an accepting and approving relationship. Such a secure relationship is then thought to promote skills needed to start the more challenging parent-directed interaction (PDI) module. This second component aims to decrease socially inappropriate and disruptive behaviors and to facilitate the child's ability to comply with parental directives. Unlike CDI, PDI emphasizes specific and direct instructions given to children by caregivers, to be followed by positive attention. When these explicit directions are not followed, a series of predictable, sequential consequences follow each incident; for instance, a specific verbal warning is followed by a time-out chair and subsequently use of a time-out room as indicated. Consistency is emphasized. Caregivers are supported in their challenges through ongoing coaching of PDI throughout the therapy sessions. Such consistency and predictability of consequences set the stage for the final and key component of ED. In this last module, as stated previously, the focus is on the central importance of the emotional experience through teaching an understanding of, and the ability to generate, vocabulary to articulate feeling states. This ability to describe feelings in self and others and training in age-appropriate relaxation techniques provide alternatives to the socially inappropriate or displaced and maladaptive (or dysregulated) manifestations of feeling states. For example, the child is encouraged to use a relaxation technique such as squeezing imaginary lemons to calm him-or herself as rehearsed in therapy instead of hitting a sibling for taking away a favorite toy. This psychotherapeutic treatment is currently being tested in a randomized controlled trial with depressed preschoolers (see the following case example). Randomized controlled studies in preschoolers with BD are now needed.

To date, PCIT-ED has been successfully applied to preschoolers in a National Institute of Mental Health phase I trial at the Washington University School of Medicine Early Emotion Development Program. One of several cases is now presented in de-identified form.

A 3-Year-Old with Temper Tantrums

A 3-year-old preschool girl with a notable family history of MDD presented with screaming tantrums, including undressing and kicking others accompanied by crying spells with mood lability. These tantrums were often triggered by incidents like not being able to buy a toy at the store or fighting for a toy with an older sibling. Her mother was overwhelmed and felt helpless in her ability to help her child to calm in such instances.

After detailing incidents as described, mother and child engaged in therapy and completed related homework for each of the three therapy components, the first of which was CDI. The mother and child engaged each other in child-selected play. The mother applied PRIDE skills (**P**raise, **R**eflection, **I**mitation, **D**escription of behavior, and use of **E**nthusiam) to help convey approval of the child and her emotional tones; simultaneously, she fostered vocabulary to convey emotional expression. The young child was readily engaged and displayed increasingly noteworthy expression of her feeling states during observed therapy sessions.

This "special time" was part of daily homework and was reviewed at weekly therapy sessions with the therapist. The avoidance of any commands, questions, or criticism during this uninterrupted special time was reviewed during each session. Any challenges throughout the week were addressed as they arose.

During the second phase of treatment, PDI, the child's tantrums became more apparent in sessions. She was noted to cry in response to directions to clean up, for example. She would then kick her feet and scream for several minutes. The sequential use of a simple verbal command repeated only once often required escalation to the use of a time-out chair and then the time-out room in the clinic. This sequence then generalized to the home. After several weeks, when consistently applied at home, these principles helped the mother to feel more able to intervene in such emotionally provocative displays of anger or sadness.

The child eventually decreased the behaviors by learning the skills involved in all phases, most notably the final component: ED. This phase promoted recognition of emotional expression states on homework sheets, describing how such feeling states occurred within and outside of the child, using personally applied examples (e.g., her brother taking her toy) and practicing her response with the use of relaxation techniques such as squeezing lemons when angry. This 3-year-old child's ability to describe provoking triggers at home and to apply the skills in therapy were noted to increase throughout the 14 sessions. Furthermore, an increase in self-awareness of emotional states allowed the child to recall when to use the techniques learned in therapy. The child was noted to have a rich use of emotionally expressive words and was more apt to listen to her mother, with more socially acceptable displays of anger by the end of treatment. She was able to utilize the relaxation techniques and her relaxation spot in her room when needed as alternatives to kicking and screaming, as had been the norm at the start of the treatment.

At the same time as the child showed greater emotional competence, increases in parental effectiveness and positive experience were also reported. Her mother reported an increasingly positive relationship because she was able to feel more connected with the child through the use of daily special time. Her mother also reported feeling more in control and engaged with the child when she learned to tolerate emotion from the child more effectively and to help cue the child to use verbal and other techniques to self-soothe after routine distressing events, such as when problems sharing among the siblings occurred at home. Mom felt supported in her challenges with her child and felt less distressed as the treatment progressed.

CONCLUSION

Despite the empirical and theoretical work reviewed in this chapter, preschool BD remains a highly ambiguous diagnostic area. Whereas there is a small but growing body of empirical literature suggesting that the disorder can be identified during the preschool period (as early as age 3), large-scale empirical investigations that include appropriate disruptive control groups are needed. The public health urgency for these data is underscored by the high and rising rates of prescriptions for mood-stabilizing agents for preschool children with a presumptive bipolar diagnosis. Clarifying the nosology of very early-onset BD is an important endeavor in the interests of preschoolers themselves. However, it may also have important implications for our understanding of the developmental psychopathology of the disorder during childhood and, therefore, for earlier and potentially more preventive interventions that may have implications for the disorder across the life span. One early intervention strategy, reviewed in this chapter, may be applicable to preschoolers with BD or BD subsyndromes. Further controlled testing of the efficacy of this intervention is warranted. The question of whether improvements arising from these early interventions are sustained over time (e.g., several years later) is of interest to address the question of whether earlier intervention has more enduring effects than standard treatments applied later in childhood.

REFERENCES

American Psychiatric Association. (1987). *Diagnostic and statistical manual of mental disorders* (3rd ed., rev.). Washington, DC: Author.

American Psychiatric Association. (1994). *Diagnostic and statistical manual of mental disorders* (4th ed.). Washington, DC: Author.

Baum, A. E., Hamshere, M., Green, E., Cichon, S., Rietschel, M., Noethen, M. M., et al. (2008). Meta-analysis of two genome-wide association studies of bipolar disorder reveals important points of agreement. *Molecular Psychiatry, 13*(5), 466–467.

Belden, A. C. (2007). Preschoolers' emotion regulation: The role of mothers' caregiving strategies and emotional expressivity. *Dissertation Abstracts International: Section B: The Sciences and Engineering, 67*(10-B), 6093.

Belden, A. C., & Luby, J. L. (2006). Preschoolers' depression severity and behaviors during dyadic interactions: The mediating role of parental support. *Journal of the American Academy of Child and Adolescent Psychiatry, 45*(2), 213–222.

Belden, A. C., Sullivan, J. P., & Luby, J. L. (2007). Depressed and healthy preschoolers' internal representations of their mothers' caregiving: associations with observed caregiving behaviors one year later. *Attachment and Human Development, 9*(3), 239–254.

Biederman, J. (1995). Developmental subtypes of juvenile bipolar disorder. *Harvard Review of Psychiatry, 3*(4), 227–230.

Biederman, J., Faraone, S. V., Chu, M. P., & Wozniak, J. (1999). Further evidence of a bidirectional overlap between juvenile mania and conduct disorder in children. *Journal of the American Academy of Child and Adolescent Psychiatry, 38*(4), 468–476.

Biederman, J., Mick, E., Faraone, S., Spencer, T., Wilens, T., & Wozniak, J. (2000). Pediatric mania: A developmental subtype of bipolar disorder? *Biological Psychiatry, 48*, 458–466.

Biederman, J., Mick, E., Hammerness, P., Harpold, T., Aleardi, M., Dougherty, M., et al. (2005). Open-label, 8-week trial of olanzapine and risperidone for the treatment of bipolar disorder in preschool-age children. *Biological Psychiatry, 58*(7), 589–594.

Burke, J. D., Loeber, R., & Birmaher, B. (2002). Oppositional defiant disorder and conduct disorder: A review of the past 10 years, part II. *Journal of the American Academy of Child and Adolescent Psychiatry, 41*(11), 1275–1293.

Carey, B. (2007, September 4). Bipolar illness soars as a diagnosis for the young. *New York Times*. Retrieved from *http://www.nytimes.com/2007/09/04/health/04psych.html*

Carlson, G. A. (1998). Mania and ADHD: Comorbidity or confusion. *Journal of Affective Disorders, 51*(2), 177–187.

Carter, A. S., Briggs-Gowan, M. J., & Davis, N. O. (2004). Assessment of young children's social-emotional development and psychopathology: Recent advances and recommendations for practice. *Journal of Child Psychology and Psychiatry, 45*(1), 109–134.

Caspi, A., Sugden, K., Moffitt, T. E., Taylor, A., Craig, I. W., Harrington, H., et al. (2003). Influence of life stress on depression: Moderation by a polymorphism in the 5-HTT gene. *Science, 301*, 386–389.

Craney, J. L., & Geller, B. (2003). A prepubertal and early adolescent bipolar disorder-I phenotype: Review of phenomenology and longitudinal course. *Bipolar Disorder, 5*(4), 243–256.

Curtis, W. J., & Cicchetti, D. (2003). Moving research on resilience into the 21st century: Theoretical and methodological considerations in examining the biological contributors to resilience. *Development and Psychopathology, 15*(3), 773–810.

Danielyan, A., Pathak, S., Kowatch, R. A., Arszman, S., & Johns, E. (2007). Clinical characteristics of bipolar disorder in very young children. *Journal of Affective Disorders, 97*(1–3), 51–59.

DelBello, M. P. (2007). The phenomenology and assessment of childhood and adolescent mental health: Progress in research. *Journal of Clinical Psychiatry, 68*(9), 1418.

DelBello, M. P., & Geller, B. (2001). Review of studies of child and adolescent offspring of bipolar parents. *Bipolar Disorder, 3*(6), 325–334.

Denham, S., Workman, E., Cole, P., Weissbrod, C., Kendziora, K., & Zahn-Waxler, C. (2000). Prediction of externalizing behavior problems from early to middle childhood: The role of parental socialization and emotion expression. *Development and Psychopathology, 12*, 23–45.

Dilsaver, S. C., & Akiskal, H. S. (2004). Preschool-onset mania: Incidence, phenomenology and family history. *Journal of Affective Disorders, 82*(Suppl. 1), S35–S43.

Dix, T. (1991). The affective organization of parenting: Adaptive and maladaptive processes. *Psychological Bulletin, 110*(1), 3–25.

Egger, H. L., Ascher, B., & Angold, A. (1999). *Preschool Age Psychiatric Assessment (PAPA): Version 1.1.* Durham, NC: Center for Developmental Epidemiology, Department of Psychiatry and Behavioral Sciences, Duke University Medical Center.

Egger, H. L., Erkanli, A., Keeler, G., Potts, E., Walter, B., & Angold, A. (2006). Test–Retest reliability of the Preschool Age Psychiatric Assessment (PAPA). *Journal of the American Academy of Child and Adolescent Psychiatry, 45*(5), 538–549.

Eisenberg, N., Cumberland, A., Spinrad, T. L., Fabes, R. A., Shepard, S. A., Reiser, M., et al. (2001). The relations of regulation and emotionality to children's externalizing and internalizing problem behavior. *Child Development, 72*, 1112–1134.

Eyberg, S. M. (1988). Parent–child interaction therapy: Integration of traditional and behavioral concerns. *Child and Family Behavior Therapy, 10*(1), 33–46.

Eyberg, S. M., Boggs, S. R., & Algina, J. (1995). Parent–child interaction therapy: A psychosocial model for the treatment of young children with conduct problem behavior and their families. *Psychopharmacology Bulletin, 31*(1), 83–91.

Faraone, S. V., Biederman, J., & Monuteaux, M. C. (2001). Attention deficit hyperactivity disorder with bipolar disorder in girls: Further evidence for a familial subtype? *Journal of Affective Disorders, 64*(1), 19–26.

Farmer, E. M., Compton, S. N., Bums, B. J., & Robertson, E. (2002). Review of the evidence base for treatment of childhood psychopathology: Externalizing disorders. *Journal of Consulting and Clinical Psychology, 70*(6), 1267–1302.

Findling, R. L., Gracious, B. L., McNamara, N. K., Youngstrom, E. A., Demeter, C. A., Branicky, L. A., et al. (2001). Rapid, continuous cycling and psychiatric co-morbidity in pediatric bipolar I disorder. *Bipolar Disorders, 3,* 202–210.

Fish, E. W., Shahrokh, D., Bagot, R., Caldji, C., Bredy, T., Szyf, M., et al. (2004). Epigenetic programming of stress responses through variations in maternal care. *Annals of the New York Academy of Sciences, 1036,* 167–180.

Geller, B., & Cook, E. H., Jr. (2000). Ultradian rapid cycling in prepubertal and early adolescent bipolarity is not in transmission disequilibrium with val/met COMT alleles. *Biological Psychiatry, 47*(7), 605–609.

Geller, B., & Luby, J. (1997). Child and adolescent bipolar disorder: A review of the past 10 years. *Journal of the American Academy of Child and Adolescent Psychiatry, 36*(9), 1168–1176.

Geller, B., Sun, K., Zimerman, B., Luby, J., Frazier, J., & Williams, M. (1995). Complex and rapid-cycling in bipolar children and adolescents: A preliminary study. *Journal of Affective Disorders, 34*(4), 259–268.

Geller, B., & Tillman, R. (2005). Prepubertal and early adolescent bipolar I disorder: Review of diagnostic validation by Robins and Guze criteria. *Journal of Clinical Psychiatry, 66*(Suppl. 7), 21–28.

Geller, B., Tillman, R., Bolhofner, K., & Zimerman, B. (2008). Child bipolar I disorder: Prospective continuity with adult BP-I; characteristics of second and third episodes; predictors of 8-year outcome. *Archives of General Psychiatry, 65,* 1125–1236.

Geller, B., Tillman, R., Craney, J. L., & Bolhofner, K. (2004). Four-year prospective outcome and natural history of mania in children with a prepubertal and early adolescent bipolar disorder phenotype. *Archives of General Psychiatry, 61*(5), 459–467.

Geller, B., Williams, M., Zimerman, B., Frazier, J., Beringer, L., & Warner, K. (1998). Prepubertal and early adolescent bipolarity differentiate from ADHD by manic symptoms, grandiose delusions, ultra-rapid or ultradian cycling. *Journal of Affective Disorders, 51*(2), 81–91.

Geller, B., Zimerman, B., Williams, M., Bolhofner, K., Craney, J. L., DelBello, M. P., et al. (2000). Diagnostic characteristics of 93 cases of a prepubertal and early adolescent bipolar disorder phenotype by gender, puberty and comorbid attention deficit hyperactivity disorder. *Journal of Child and Adolescent Psychopharmacology, 10*(3), 157–164.

Geller, B., Zimerman, B., Williams, M., DelBello, M. P., Bolhofner, K., Craney, J. L., et al. (2002). DSM-IV mania symptoms in a prepubertal and early adolescent bipolar disorder phenotype compared to attention-deficit hyperactive and normal controls. *Journal of Child and Adolescent Psychopharmacology, 12*(1), 11–25.

Geller, B., Zimerman, B., Williams, M., DelBello, M. P., Frazier, J., & Beringer, L. (2002). Phenomenology of prepubertal and early adolescent bipolar disorder: Examples of elated mood, grandiose behaviors, decreased need for sleep, racing thoughts and hypersexuality. *Journal of Child and Adolescent Psychopharmacology, 12*(1), 3–9.

Ghaemi, S., & Martin, A. (2007). Defining the boundaries of childhood bipolar disorder. *American Journal of Psychiatry, 164*(2), 185–188.

Gleason, M. M., Egger, H. L., Emslie, G. J., Greenhill, L. L., Kowatch, R. A., Lieberman, A. F., et al. (2007). Psychopharmacological treatment for very young children: Contexts and guidelines. *Journal of the American Academy of Child and Adolescent Psychiatry, 46,* 1532–1572.

Groopman, J. (2007, April 9). What's normal?: Diagnosing bipolar disorder in children. *The New Yorker*, pp. 28–33.

Hodges, K. (1994). *The Preschool and Early Childhood Functional Assessment Scale (PECFAS).* Ypsilanti: Eastern Michigan University.

Hood, K., & Eyberg, S. (2003). Outcomes of parent–child interaction therapy: Mothers' reports of maintenance three to six year after treatment. *Journal of Clinical Child and Adolescent Psychology, 32*(3), 419–429.

Kandel, E. R. (1998). A new intellectual framework for psychiatry. *American Journal of Psychiatry, 155*, 457–469.

Kim, E. Y., & Miklowitz, D. J. (2002). Childhood mania, attention deficit hyperactivity disorder and conduct disorder: A critical review of diagnostic dilemmas. *Bipolar Disorder, 4*(4), 215–225.

Kovacs, M., & Pollock, M. (1995). Bipolar disorder and comorbid conduct disorder in childhood and adolescence. *Journal of the American Academy of Child and Adolescent Psychiatry, 34*(6), 715–723.

Kowatch, R., & DelBello, M. P. (2006). Pediatric bipolar disorder: Emerging diagnostic and treatment approaches. *Child and Adolescent Psychiatric Clinics of North America, 15*(1), 73–108.

Kutcher, S. P., Marton, P., & Korenblum, M. (1989). Relationship between psychiatric illness and conduct disorder in adolescents. *Canadian Journal of Psychiatry, 34*(6), 526–529.

Leibenluft, E., Charney, D. S., Towbin, K. E., Bhangoo, R. K., & Pine, D. S. (2003). Defining clinical phenotypes of juvenile mania. *American Journal of Psychiatry, 160*(3), 430–437.

Luby, J., & Belden, A. (2006). Defining and validating bipolar disorder in the preschool period. *Development and Psychopathology, 18*(4), 971–988.

Luby, J. L., & Belden, A. C. (2008). Clinical characteristics of bipolar vs. unipolar depression in preschool children: An empirical investigation. *Journal of Clinical Psychiatry, 69*(12), 1960–1969.

Luby, J. L., Belden, A., Pautsch, J., Si, X., & Spitznagel, E. (2009). The clinical significance of preschool depression: Impairment in functioning and clinical markers of the disorder. *Journal of Affective Disorders, 112*(1–3), 111–119

Luby, J. L., & Mrakotsky, C. (2003). Depressed preschoolers with bipolar family history: A group at high risk for later switching to mania? *Journal of Child and Adolescent Psychopharmacology, 13*(2), 187–197.

Luby, J. L., Si, X., Belden, A., Tandon, M., & Spitznagel, E. (2009). Preschool depression: Homotypic continuity and course over two years. *Archives of General Psychiatry, 66*, 897–905.

Luby, J. L., Stalets, M. M., Blankenship, S., Pautsch, J., & McGrath, M. (2008). Treatment of preschool bipolar disorder: A novel parent–child interaction therapy and review of data on psychopharmacology. In B. Geller & M. P. DelBello (Eds.), *Treatment of bipolar disorder in children and adolescents* (pp. 270–286). New York: Guilford Press.

Luby, J. L., Sullivan, J., Belden, A., Stalets, M., Blankenship, S., & Spitznagel, E. (2006). An observational analysis of behavior in depressed preschoolers: Further validation of early-onset depression. *Journal of the American Academy of Child and Adolescent Psychiatry, 45*(2), 203–212.

Luby, J. L., Tandon, M., & Nicol, G. (2007). Three clinical cases of DSM-IV mania symptoms in preschoolers. *Journal of Child and Adolescent Psychopharmacology, 17*(2), 237–243.

Maia, F., Boaratima, K. A., Kleinman, A., & Fu-l, L. (2007). Preschool bipolar disorder: Brazilian children case reports. *Journal of Affective Disorders, 104*(1–3), 237–243.

Masi, G., Cosenza, A., Mucci, M., & De Vito, G. (2001). Risperidone monotherapy in preschool children with pervasive developmental disorders. *Journal of Child Neurology, 16*(6), 395–400.

McGuffin, P., Rijsdijk, F., Andrew, M., Sham, P., Katz, R., & Cardno, A. (2003). The heritability of bipolar affective disorder and the genetic relationship to unipolar depression. *Archives of General Psychiatry, 60*(5), 497–502.

Miklowitz, D. J. (2007). The role of the family in the course and treatment of bipolar disorder. *Current Directions in Psychological Science, 16*(4), 192–196.

Miklowitz, D. J., Biuckians, A., & Richards, J. A. (2006). Early-onset bipolar disorder: A family treatment perspective. *Development and Psychopathology, 18*(4), 1247–1265.

Moreno, C., Laje, G., Blanco, C., Jiang, H., Schmidt, A. B., & Olfson, M. (2007). National trends in the outpatient diagnosis and treatment of bipolar disorder in youth. *Archives of General Psychiatry, 64*(9), 1032–1039.

Mota-Castillo, M., Torruella, A., Engels, B., Perez, J., Dedrick, C., & Gluckman, M. (2001). Valproate in very young children: An open case series with a brief follow-up. *Journal of Affective Disorders, 67*, 193–197.

Nagaraj, R., Singhi, P., & Malhi, P. (2006). Risperidone in children with autism: Randomized, placebo-controlled, double-blind study. *Journal of Child Neurology, 21*(6), 450–455.

Pandina, G. J., Bossie, C. A., Youssef, E., Zhu, Y., & Dunbar, F. (2007). Risperidone improves behavioral symptoms in children with autism in a randomized, double-blind, placebo-controlled trial. *Journal of Autism and Developmental Disorders, 37*(2), 367–373.

Pavuluri, M. N., Henry, D. B., Carbray, J. A., Sampson, G. A., Naylor, M. W., & Janicak, P. G. (2006). A one-year open-label trial of risperidone augmentation in lithium nonresponder youth with preschool-onset bipolar disorder. *Journal of Child and Adolescent Psychopharmacology, 16*(3), 336–350.

Pavuluri, M. N., Janicak, P. G., & Carbray, J. (2002). Topiramate plus risperidone for controlling weight gain and symptoms in preschool mania. *Journal of Child and Adolescent Psychopharmacology, 12*(3), 271–273.

Perlis, R. H., Purcell, S., Fagerness, J., Kirby, A., Petryshen, T. L., Fan, J., et al. (2008). Family-based association study of lithium-related and other candidate genes in bipolar disorder. *Archives of General Psychiatry, 65*(1), 53–61.

Piaget, J. (1951). *Play, dreams, and imitation in childhood.* New York: Norton.

Pine, D. S., Alegria, M., Cook, E. H., Jr., Costello, E. J., Dahl, R. E., Merikangas, K. R., et al. (2002). Advances in developmental science and DSM-V. In V. D. Kupfer, M. R. First, & D. A. Reiger (Eds.), *A research agenda for DSM* (pp. 85–122). Washington, DC: American Psychiatric Publishing.

Post, R. M., Leverich, G. S., Weiss, S. R., Zhang, L., & Xing, G. (2003). Psychosocial stressors as predisposing factors to affective illness and PTSD: Potential neurobiological mechanisms and theoretical implications. In D. Cicchetti & E. F. Walker (Eds.), *Neurodevelopmental mechanisms in psychopathology* (pp. 491–525). New York: Cambridge University Press.

Robins, E., & Guze, S. B. (1970). Establishment of diagnostic validity in psychiatric illness: Its application to schizophrenia. *American Journal of Psychiatry, 126*(7), 983–987.

Scheeringa, M., Peebles, C., Cook, C., & Zeanah, C. (2001). Toward establishing procedural, criterion and discriminant validity for PTSD in early childhood. *Journal of the American Academy of Child and Adolescent Psychiatry, 40*(1), 52–60.

Scheeringa, M., Zeanah, C., Myers, L., & Putnam, F. (2003). New findings on alternative criteria for PTSD in preschool children. *Journal of the American Academy of Child and Adolescent Psychiatry, 42*, 561–570.

Scheffer, R. E., & Niskala Apps, J. A. (2004). The diagnosis of preschool bipolar disorder presenting with mania: Open pharmacological treatment. *Journal of Affective Disorders*, 82(Suppl. 1), S25–S34.

Shea, S., Turgay, A., Carroll, A., Schulz, M., Orlik, H., Smith, I., et al. (2004). Risperidone in the treatment of disruptive behavioral symptoms in children with autistic and other pervasive developmental disorders. *Pediatrics, 114*(5), 634–641.

Sparrow, S., Carter, A. S., & Cicchetti, D. (1987). *Vineland Screener: Overview, reliability, validity, administration and scoring.* New Haven, CT: Yale University.

Spencer, T. J., Biederman, J., Wozniak, J., Faraone, S. V., Wilens, T. E., & Mick, E. (2001). Parsing pediatric bipolar disorder from its associated comorbidity with the disruptive behavior disorders. *Biological Psychiatry, 49*(12), 1062–1070.

Task Force on Research Diagnostic Criteria: Infancy and Preschool. (2003). Research diagnostic criteria for infants and preschool children: The process and empirical support. *Journal of the American Academy of Child and Adolescent Psychiatry, 42*(12), 1504–1512.

Tillman, R., & Geller, B. (2003). Definitions of rapid, ultrarapid, and ultradian cycling and of episode duration in pediatric and adult bipolar disorders: A proposal to distinguish episodes from cycles. *Journal of Child and Adolescent Psychopharmacology, 13*(3), 267–271.

Tumuluru, R. V., Weller, E. B., Fristad, M. A., & Weller, R. A. (2003). Mania in six preschool children. *Journal of Child and Adolescent Psychopharmacology, 13*(4), 489–494.

Tuzun, U., Zoroglu, S. S., & Savas, H. A. (2002). A 5-year-old boy with recurrent mania successfully treated with carbamazepine. *Psychiatry and Clinical Neuroscience, 56*(5), 589–591.

Weaver, I. C., Meaney, M. J., & Szyf, M. (2006). Maternal care effects on the hippocampal transcriptome and anxiety-mediated behaviors in the offspring that are reversible in adulthood. *Proceedings of the National Academy of Sciences USA, 103*, 343480–343485.

Webster-Stratton, C., & Hammond, M. (1997). Treating children with early-onset conduct problems: A comparison of child and parent training interventions. *Journal of Consulting and Clinical Psychology, 65*(1), 93–109.

Webster-Stratton, C., Reid, M. J., & Hammond, M. (2004). Treating children with early-onset conduct problems: Intervention outcomes for parent, child, and teacher training. *Journal of Clinical Child and Adolescent Psychology, 33*(1), 105–124.

Weller, E. B., Weller, R. A., & Fristad, M. A. (1995). Bipolar disorder in children: Misdiagnosis, underdiagnosis, and future directions. *Journal of the American Academy of Child and Adolescent Psychiatry, 34*(6), 709–714.

Wilens, T. E., Biederman, J., Brown, S., Tanguay, S., Monuteaux, M. C., Blake, C., et al. (2002). Psychiatric comorbidity and functioning in clinically referred preschool children and school-age youths with ADHD. *Journal of the American Academy of Child and Adolescent Psychiatry, 41*(3), 262–268.

Williams, J., Klinepeter, K., Palmes, G., Pulley, A., & Foy, J. M. (2004). Diagnosis and treatment of behavioral health disorders in pediatric practice. *Pediatrics, 114*(3), 601–606.

Williams, S. K., Scahill, L., Vitiello, B., Aman, M. G., Arnold, L. E., McDougle, C. J., et al. (2006). Risperidone and adaptive behavior in children with autism. *Journal of the American Academy of Child and Adolescent Psychiatry, 45*(4), 431–439.

Wozniak, J., Biederman, J., Faraone, S. V., Blier, H., & Monuteaux, M. C. (2001). Heterogeneity of childhood conduct disorder: Further evidence of a subtype of conduct disorder linked to bipolar disorder. *Journal of Affective Disorders, 64*(2–3), 121–131.

Wozniak, J., Biederman, J., & Richards, J. A. (2001). Diagnostic and therapeutic dilemmas in the management of pediatric-onset bipolar disorder. *Journal of Clinical Psychiatry, 62*(Suppl. 14), 10–15.

PART II

ONSET, PROGNOSIS, AND COURSE

Clinical Presentation and Longitudinal Course of Bipolar Spectrum Disorders in Children and Adolescents

Rasim Somer Diler, Boris Birmaher, and David J. Miklowitz

The view that pediatric bipolar disorder (BD) is nonexistent has been increasingly challenged by systematic research. Historically, several factors have made the accurate diagnosis of BD in childhood difficult, including lack of awareness, diagnostic confusion, clinical bias against the diagnosis of mania in children, low base rate of the disorder, symptom overlap between BD and other more prevalent childhood-onset psychiatric disorders such as attention-deficit/hyperactivity disorder (ADHD), and developmental issues and variability in clinical presentation (Pavuluri, Birmaher, & Naylor, 2005; Soutullo et al., 2005). Consistent with Kraepelin's early descriptions (1921), it is now well established that BD occurs in children and adolescents (Kowatch, Fristad, et al., 2005; Pavuluri et al., 2005) and is associated with high rates of mixed- and rapid-cycling presentations, substance abuse, suicidal risk, and social, family, vocational, and academic impairment (Birmaher & Axelson, 2006; Pavuluri et al., 2005). A community study reported that approximately 1% of adolescents had BD (mainly bipolar II and cyclothymia) and 5.6% had "soft" BD subthreshold symptoms (Lewinsohn, Klein, & Seeley, 1995). Retrospective studies in adults with BD have reported that up to 60% had the onset of their mood symptoms before the age of 20 (Chengappa et al., 2003; Egeland et al., 2003); however, the real prevalence of BD in children and adolescents is still unknown.

Despite the growing evidence that the consequences of BD arising during childhood can be devastating, the clinical characteristics of pediatric BD are still debated, and the onset, course, and outcome of BD in youth have been insufficiently studied (Birmaher & Axelson, 2006; Pavuluri et al., 2005). In this chapter, we describe the clinical presentation and longitudinal course of BD spectrum in children and adolescents. In addition, we discuss differential diagnosis, sub-threshold manifestations, dimensional presentation of BD, differences and similarities of the clinical presentation of BD in children and adolescents, and the limitations of current studies.

CATEGORICAL ASSESSMENT OF BIPOLAR DISORDER

Three approaches have dominated research for BD diagnosis in children and adolescents, including applying the existent DSM-IV-TR (*Diagnostic and Statistical Manual of Mental Disorders*, 4th ed., text rev.; American Psychiatry Association, 2000) criteria to children and adolescents, emphasizing cardinal symptoms (e.g., euphoria and grandiosity) as required for the diagnosis and emphasizing irritability as a key symptom (Geller et al., 2003; Leibenluft & Rich, 2008; Wozniak et al., 2005). There is consensus in the field that children and adolescents sometimes fulfill the DSM-IV criteria for bipolar I and II disorder (McClellan, Kowatch, Findling, & Work Group on Quality Issues, 2007), but it appears that this presentation occurs in a minority of youth (Birmaher & Axelson, 2006). Some of these youth meet the mania or hypomania criteria but do not meet the time requirement to be diagnosed as bipolar I or II (Leibenluft, Charney, Towbin, Bhangoo, & Pine, 2003). These children usually received the diagnosis of BD not otherwise specified (NOS).

In this chapter, we refer to Course and Outcome of Bipolar Youth (COBY) study at several points, and we report the methodology of this study to familiarize the readers to the study design and sample characteristics. The COBY study is the first report on the systematic assessment and comparison of children and adolescents with bipolar spectrum disorders (bipolar I, II, and NOS) (Axelson et al., 2006; Birmaher et al., 2006). Subjects were enrolled at three academic medical centers: Brown University (n = 144), University of California, Los Angeles (n = 90), and University of Pittsburgh Medical Center (n = 204). Four hundred and thirty-eight children and adolescents (12.7 ± 3.2 years old) with bipolar I (n = 255), bipolar II (n = 30), and BD NOS (n = 153) were included in the study. Study inclusion criteria were (1) current age of 7 years 0 months to 17 years 11 months and (2) fulfilling DSM-IV criteria for bipolar I or bipolar II disorder, or the COBY established criteria for bipolar disorder NOS (Axelson et al., 2006). The COBY study used DSM-IV criteria for bipolar I and II. However, because the DSM-IV criteria for BD NOS are vague, the COBY investigators (Axelson et al., 2006; Birmaher et al., 2006) set the minimum inclusion threshold for the BD NOS group (one DSM-IV symptom criterion less than full criteria for a manic or hypomanic episode, clear change in functioning, mood and symptom duration of a minimum of 4 hours within a day and a minimum of four episodes). Mood symptoms were assessed by the mood disorder sections of the Kiddie Schedule for Affective

Disorders and Schizophrenia for School-Age Children (Present Episode; K-SADS-P, fourth revision; Puig-Antich, Chambers, & Ryan, 1986) plus additional items from the K-SADS—Mania Rating Scale (Axelson et al., 2003). A total of 263 subjects were interviewed an average of every 35 weeks for 94.8 ± 51.5 weeks using the Longitudinal Interval Follow-up Evaluation (LIFE; Keller et al., 1987).

As discussed later, youth with bipolar I/II and BD NOS usually have elation or grandiosity above and beyond what is considered normal for their developmental stage (Axelson et al., 2006). However, other children and adolescents do not have these key symptoms but have severe irritability and rages that are very difficult to control. These children presumably show chronic symptoms and not the mood periodicity typically described in BD (Biederman et al., 2005; Wozniak et al., 2005). The question is whether these children actually have BD. Some investigators claim so (Biederman et al., 2005; Wozniak et al., 1995), especially if the outbursts are very severe and accompanied by other manic symptoms such as decreased need of sleep and hypersexuality. Others have claimed that these children have other psychiatric disorders such as oppositional defiant disorder (ODD) or ADHD with severe mood dysregulation (Leibenluft & Rich, 2008).

Concepts from developmental psychopathology help to bring these discrepant viewpoints into focus. Similar genetic predispositions may result in a multifinality of outcomes, some of which may fit the diagnostic boundaries of BD and some of which may not. Thus, the underlying biological or psychological organization may be the same, but behaviors reflecting these vulnerabilities may change at different phases of development ("heterotypic continuity") (Cicchetti & Dawson, 2002). A child with classic bipolar symptoms and a child with ADHD and ODD may have similar "molar organizations" but may express it differently depending on developmental differences shaped by environmental forces.

Recently, the American Academy of Child and Adolescent Psychiatry (AACAP) released the practice parameters for BD and recommended that clinicians should adhere to the DSM-IV, including the duration criteria (requirement of an episodic change in mood lasting at least 4 days for hypomania and 7 days for mania) (McClellan et al., 2007). The AACAP also defined BD NOS as manic symptoms that are not present for a sufficient time to meet the DSM-IV duration criteria for a manic, hypomanic, or mixed episode. Despite the evidence discussed next, the practice parameters included manic symptoms that do not occur in distinct episodes in BD NOS.

CLINICAL CHARACTERISTICS

An increased interest in youth with BD during the past decade has fueled research elucidating clinical features of the diagnosis. However, consensus is lacking on key issues such as the requirement of clearly identified mood episodes, the role of cardinal symptoms and irritable mood, the temporal relation between manic and depressive symptoms, the validity and significance of manic symptoms that do not meet the DSM-IV criteria (e.g., symptoms or duration thresholds), and differentiation of manic symptoms (e.g., distractibility, irritability) from other pediatric psychiatric disorders (Birmaher & Axelson, 2005). We discuss these key issues next.

Episodic versus Chronic Mania

The DSM-IV criteria for a manic, mixed, or hypomanic episode require a distinct period of abnormal mood and accompanying symptoms. Considering possible developmental differences in the presentation of mania in youth (e.g., chronic symptoms and rapid mood cycles rather than discreet mood episodes; characterization of mania by severe irritability or grandiosity), some authors (Geller et al., 2003; Wozniak et al., 1995) adapted diagnostic guidelines for youth that differed from those for adults. Biederman and colleagues reported that more than 75% of their patients with BD had a chronic course and presented with rapid cycling (four or more episodes per year) or episodes longer than a year, but none had daily cycling (Biederman et al., 2004). In contrast, Geller, Tillman, and Bolhofner (2007) emphasized the significance of daily cycles (daily switching of mood states) when diagnosing BD in youth. They also argued that youth with BD present with chronic manic symptoms, with mean durations of 3 to 4 years for manic or mixed episodes (Geller, Tillman, Craney, & Bolhofner, 2004). It is not clear why there are differences among the investigators, but perhaps the problems reside in the requirements for illness duration versus episode duration.

Although the discussion continues about how to conceptualize chronic mood symptoms in youth with BD, other authors have agreed that these youth may have chronic symptomatology with short symptom-free periods but emphasize that it is an episodic illness and that the duration of full threshold manic and mixed episodes are shorter than 3 or 4 years in most cases (Birmaher et al., 2006; Leibenluft & Rich, 2008). Consistent with AACAP recommendations (McClellan et al., 2007), Leibenluft and Rich (2008) suggested focusing first on determining the presence of mood episodes and ascertaining the extent to which symptoms occurred during an identifiable time frame rather than viewing the disorder as having a persistent and unremitting presentation. Similarly, available follow-up studies have emphasized that high recovery accompanied by high recurrence is a very common course of BD in youth (Birmaher et al., 2006; DelBello, Hanseman, Adler, Fleck, & Strakowski, 2007; Geller, Tillman, Bolhofner, & Zimerman, 2008).

Future longitudinal studies will help us better understand whether children with different descriptions of BD (e.g., chronic manic symptoms vs. episodic course) will have similar final outcomes as BD when they reach adulthood (equifinality). However, as detailed next, the few available longitudinal studies report low risk for developing BD when bipolar spectrum was softly defined and episodicity was not required (Brotman et al., 2006; Leibenluft, Charney, Towbin, Bhangoo, & Pine, 2006).

Cardinal Symptoms

The overlap of manic symptoms with features of other psychiatric disorders suggests giving more weight to symptoms that are more specific to mania (Birmaher & Axelson, 2005). Elated mood and grandiosity are advocated by some authors as "cardinal," or hallmark, symptoms (Geller et al., 2002; Leibenluft, Charney, & Pine, 2003). Although the presence of elated/elevated mood and/or grandiosity were not required for inclusion in the COBY study, there were nonetheless high rates of elated/elevated mood (91.8%) and grandiosity (75.5%) in children and adolescents with bipolar I (Axelson et al., 2006). On the other hand, about 10% of children and adolescents with BD in the same study did not have either elation or grandiosity. Similar to the cross-sectional phenomenology studies of adolescents with bipolar I disorder that used semistructured interviews (Table 5.1) (Biederman, Faraone, Chu, & Wozniak, 1999; Findling et al., 2001; Geller et al., 2000), a meta-analysis of pediatric BD suggested that grandiosity and irritability symptoms are present in most manic youth, although there was considerable heterogeneity among studies in the rates of euphoria/elation (Kowatch, Fristad, et al., 2005).

Emotion dysregulation, an inability to sustain positive emotions and minimize negative emotions, can be a key characteristic of BD in children. Persistent and inappropriate elated mood or uncontrollable feelings of joy could represent an inability to regulate mood (Luby & Belden, 2006). An important question in young children is whether they have sufficient emotional, cognitive, and social development for experiencing manic symptoms such as elation and grandiosity. Birmaher, Axelson, Strober, and colleagues (2009) compared children with BD (<12 years old) with adolescents with childhood-onset BD and adolescents with adolescent-onset BD (Figure 5.1). Both adolescent groups showed more severe grandiosity than children with BD; adolescents with adolescent-onset BD had more severe elation than both children and adolescents with childhood-onset BD, suggesting the significance of maturation in the presentation of elation and grandiosity.

Some authors have suggested that elated mood is not common in young children and that children may be unable to accurately self-evaluate and distinguish between fantasy and reality or may misinterpret questions about their moods (Carlson & Meyer, 2006). According to the AACAP guidelines, clinicians should be cautious when making BD diagnoses in children younger than 6 (McClellan et al., 2007). On the other hand, two recent studies and a case series in children with BD reported that preschool children (ages 3–7) can manifest elation and grandiosity (Luby, Tandon, & Nicol, 2009); children as young as 3 to 4 years may have enough cognitive and emotional development and self-conception to experience manic symptoms. Luby and Belden (2006) demonstrated that clinically elevated mood is not a normative phenomenon in preschool children and can be helpful when differentiating BD from other disorders such as major depressive disorder (MDD) and disruptive behavior disorder (DBD). In summary, available studies

TABLE 5.1. Phenomenology of Bipolar I Disorder: Comparison across Four Samples

	Mass General (n = 110/186)	Wash-U (n = 93)	Case Western (n = 90)	COBY BD-I (age adjusted)[a] (n = 133/150)
Age (years)	10.9 ± 4.1	10.9 ± 2.6	10.8 ± 3.5	11.1 ± 2.7
% male	74%	61%	71%	57%
Age at mania onset (years)	6.4 ± 0.5	6.8 ± 3.4	6.7 ± 4.0	8.8 ± 3.4
Presence of manic symptoms				
Elated/elevated mood	25%	89%	86%	90%
Irritability	84%	98%	92%	84%
Increased energy	79%	100%	81%	90%
Grandiosity	57%	86%	83%	72%
Decreased need for sleep	53%	40%	72%	81%
Pressured speech	68%	97%	81%	93%
Racing thoughts	71%	50%	88%	74%
Distractibility	93%	94%	84%	89%
Motor hyperactivity	90%	99%	81%	95%
Poor judgment	90%	90%	86%	84%
Hypersexuality	25%	43%	32%	47%
Comorbid disorders				
ADHD	87%	87%	70%	69 %
ODD	86%	79%	47%	46%
CD	41%	12%	17%	12%
AD	54%	23%	14%	37%
SUD	7%	0%	7%	5%
Other features of illness				
Mixed episode	83%	55%	20%	34%[b]/ 43%[c]
Psychosis	20%	60%	17%	38%
Prior psychiatric hospitalization	23%	—	31%	60%
Global functioning	42 ± 7[d]	43 ± 8[e]	—	53 ± 12[f,g]

Note. The table compares findings from the COBY bipolar I sample (bipolar I disorder and a random subsample of bipolar I subjects) at the University of Pittsburgh (Axelson et al., 2006) with those from Massachusetts General Hospital (Mass General; Biederman et al., 1999), Washington University in St. Louis (Wash-U; Geller et al., 2000; Tillman et al., 2003), and Case Western Reserve University (Findling et al., 2001). ADHD, attention-deficit/hyperactivity disorder; ODD, oppositional defiant disorder; CD, conduct disorder; AD, anxiety disorder; SUD, substance use disorder. From Axelson et al. (2006). Copyright 2006 by the American Medical Association. Reprinted by permission.
[a]For comparison, only COBY bipolar I disorder subjects ages younger than 13 plus a random subsample of COBY bipolar I adolescents were included.
[b]Current or most recent episode.
[c]Lifetime.
[d]Global Assessment of Functioning.
[e]Child Global Assessment Scale.
[f]At intake.
[g]Most severe lifetime.

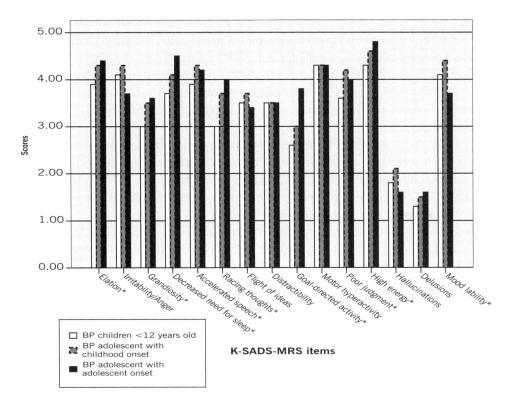

FIGURE 5.1. Symptoms of mania in children versus adolescents with bipolar disorder. BD, bipolar disorder; K-SADS-MRS, Schedule for Affective Disorders and Schizophrenia for School-Age Children—Mania Rating Scale (Axelson et al., 2003); group 1, children with BD (*n* = 173); group 2, adolescents with childhood-onset BD (*n* = 101); group 3, adolescents with adolescent-onset BD (*n* = 90); *p < .05 between three groups after adjusting for sex, socioeconomic status, duration of illness, and significantly different comorbid disorders. The scale anchors are as follows: 1 = *none*, 2 = *slight*, 3 = *mild*, 4 = *moderate*, 5 = *severe*, 6 = *extreme*.

suggest that both elation and grandiosity can be present in young children with BD; however, these symptoms become more prominent during adolescence.

Irritability

Irritability has been defined as "an emotional state characterized by having a low threshold for experiencing anger in response to negative emotional events" (Birmaher & Axelson, 2005; Leibenluft, Charney, et al., 2003). The DSM-IV criteria for a manic episode explicitly allows for the presence of irritable mood alone to satisfy the "A" criterion, although it qualifies this by requiring an additional "B" symptom criterion beyond what is required for elated mood (American Psychiatric Association, 2000). Some investigators stress that the irritability seen in BD can be considered an equally meaningful mood criterion for pediatric mania (Mick, Spencer, Wozniak, & Biederman, 2005; Wozniak et al., 2005). Wozniak and colleagues (2005) reported that irritability was more common than euphoria (94% vs. 51%) in children with BD, and that the presence or the absence of euphoria had no effects on the symptom profile, patterns of comorbidity, and measures of functioning.

In the meta-analysis of the phenomenology and clinical characteristics of mania in children and adolescents, irritability was frequently present in children and adolescents with BD (Kowatch, Youngstrom, Danielyan, & Findling, 2005) and could be considered as a sensitive marker for pediatric BD (Table 5.1). However, irritability is also part of the DSM-IV diagnostic criteria for other disorders such as ODD, MDD, generalized anxiety, posttraumatic stress disorder, ADHD, and pervasive developmental disorders; therefore, irritability has low specificity for BD (Birmaher & Axelson, 2005; Geller et al., 2003; Leibenluft & Rich, 2008). Accordingly, Kowatch and colleagues pointed out that irritability must be considered as analogous to fever or pain; it can be regarded as a sensitive indicator that "something is wrong" (Kowatch, Fristad, et al., 2005). In the same vein, Youngstrom, Birmaher, and Findling (2008) suggested that the absence of any episodes of irritability and aggressive behavior may help in ruling out BD.

Impairment and symptoms that accompany irritability are particularly important considerations when differentiating BD from normal development. The severity and duration of irritability are also important clinical factors when assessing individuals for BD. Mick and colleagues (2005) suggested that irritability that is extreme and explosive can distinguish BD from other disorders. Notably, the "super-angry/grouchy/cranky-type" of irritability, but not the "mad/cranky" or ODD-type irritability, was correlated with BD. However, others suggested that this classification can be misleading in different environments (Youngstrom et al., 2008).

Leibenluft and colleagues (2006) reported that both episodic and chronic irritability in adolescents appear to show the same characteristics (episodic vs. chronic) over time, but only episodic irritability was associated with manic outcomes. The same authors reported that chronic irritability was associated with future ADHD, ODD, and MDD rather than BD. Episodic irritability was also associated with future anxiety (Leibenluft et al., 2006), suggesting that different initial presentations of irritability in children may result in different psychiatric diagnoses unfolding over the course of development.

Studies have also focused on the significance of irritability from the developmental perspective and whether irritability is the prominent mood symptom in subsyndromal BD or in younger children with BD (Birmaher & Axelson, 2006; Carlson & Meyer, 2006; Geller et al., 2003; Leibenluft & Rich, 2008). The few available studies in preschool children reported that irritability was the predominant mood symptom in individuals with BD (Danielyan, Pathak, Kowatch, Arszman, & Johns, 2007; Luby & Belden, 2006; Scheffer & Niskala Apps, 2004). Preschoolers with both BD and MDD were more likely to exhibit irritability compared with healthy controls and preschoolers with DBD, respectively (Luby & Belden, 2006), suggesting that severe irritability may be a precursor to mood symptoms in young children and that it can be considered as a changing behavioral manifestation of the same underlying process at different periods of development (e.g., heterotypic continuity).

Because children and adolescents have not passed through the major risk period for BD, elucidation of prodromal organizations that may subsequently evolve into adult BD is very important (Cicchetti & Rogosch, 2002). When a soft definition of bipolar spectrum disorders was used to define subthreshold presentations of BD, chronic and irritable mood were reported as more common in BD NOS compared with the other subtypes (Masi et al., 2007). However, in the COBY study, in which BD NOS was strictly defined, irritability did not differentiate between bipolar I and BD NOS (Axelson et al., 2006) and was uncorrelated with age at onset (Birmaher, Axelson, Strober, et al., 2009), supporting its high sensitivity for BD across different ages and BD subtypes. Attention to developmental pathways emerging earlier in development that eventuate in BD is critical for understanding variation in trajectories operating for different individuals (Cicchetti & Dawson, 2002). We need longitudinal studies that evaluate irritability from the developmental perspective and follow its course and significance in syndromal and subsyndromal BD children.

Other Manic Symptoms in Children and Adolescents

A meta-analysis of seven published phenomenology studies of pediatric mania determined weighted rates and confidence intervals for 11 symptoms of mania that were measured across most of the studies (Kowatch, Youngstrom, et al., 2005). Increased energy and distractibility were the most common manic symptoms, whereas hypersexuality was the least frequent. There was also significant heterogeneity in the rates of individual manic symptoms, including decreased need for sleep, racing thoughts, poor judgment, pressured speech, distractibility, elated/euphoric mood, and irritability. Sampling issues and methodological differences among the studies, such as the mood state (mixed vs. manic) (see Table 5.1), average subject age, and the use of the child in addition to the parent as informants, may have accounted for much of the variability in symptom rates (Kowatch, Youngstrom, et al., 2005).

To date, few studies have compared the symptoms of mania between children and adolescents with BD. Faraone and colleagues (1997) compared manic symptoms among a group of children with bipolar I ($n = 68$) and adolescents with early-onset ($n = 25$) and late-onset ($n = 17$) mania. Increased energy was twice as common in children and adolescents with early-onset mania compared with the late-onset manic group. Geller and colleagues (2000) and Findling and colleagues (2001) did not find any differences in the rates of manic symptoms between children and adolescents with bipolar I ($n = 93$ and 90, respectively).

Birmaher, Axelson, Monk, and colleagues (2009) evaluated 173 children with BD (< 12 years), 101 adolescents with childhood-onset BD, and 90 adolescents with adolescent-onset BD (Figure 5.1). Adjusting for confounding factors (socioeconomic status, duration of illness, and rates of comorbid disorders), both adolescent BD groups showed significantly higher total manic scores, racing thoughts, poor judgment, and increased productivity compared with children with BD. Adolescents with adolescent-onset BD had more severe goal-directed activity, racing thoughts, and high energy than both children and adolescents with childhood-onset BD. They also had more decreased need for sleep, accelerated speech, delusions, and sharpened thinking compared with children with BD (Birmaher, Axelson, Strober, et al., 2009).

Typically, childhood-onset BD has a different clinical presentation, a higher familial loading for mood disorders, and a different pattern of comorbid disorders than adolescent-onset BD. Furthermore, older age is associated with more severe and more classic typical mood symptomatology. Birmaher, Axelson, Strober, and colleagues (2009) suggest that childhood-onset BD may have a different trajectory than adolescent-onset BD, which appears to be more similar to adult BD. We need extensive longitudinal studies to understand the degree of convergence or divergence in the organization of biological, psychological, and social systems as they relate to symptom manifestation of BD in youth (Cicchetti & Dawson, 2002). Longitudinal studies will help determine the conditions under which youth who begin with a variety of symptom constellations have similar outcomes in adulthood (equifinality) and, in turn, why youth who appear to be phenotypically similar in childhood show a wide dispersion of outcomes in adulthood (multifinality) (Geller et al., 2008).

Depression

Depressive episodes are reported to be the most common manifestation of BD in children and adults alike, but depression is underdiagnosed in adults and commonly undiagnosed in children (Karippot, 2006). Children with bipolar depression were more likely to have severe depression with suicidality, anhedonia, and hopelessness and had higher rates of comorbid disruptive behavior, anxiety, and substance use disorders compared with children with unipolar depression (Wozniak et al., 2004). They also had lower Global Assessment of Functioning scores and higher rates of hospitalization and psychiatric disorders in first-degree relatives (Wozniak et al., 2004).

The majority of youth at risk for developing BD disorder (e.g., offspring of BD parents) had depression and other nonspecific psychopathology before they developed BD (Birmaher, Axelson, Monk, et al., 2009; Duffy, Alda, Crawford, Milin, & Grof, 2007). Although the specificity of depression as a risk factor for BD in the absence of other risk factors (e.g., family history, mood cycles) is not high (Miklowitz & Chang, 2008), major depressive episode (MDE) may precede the onset of mania, so that some children and adolescents who appear to have unipolar depression may actually have BD with depression as their initial presentation (Birmaher, Axelson, Monk, et al., 2009).

Both adolescents with childhood-onset and adolescent-onset BD showed more severe depressive symptoms and higher rates of melancholic, atypical depressive symptoms, and suicide attempts than children with BD (Birmaher, Axelson, Strober, et al., 2009). Birmaher, Axelson, Strober, and colleagues (2009) also reported that the expression of major depression in BD seemed to be related to developmental pubertal changes and age of onset (e.g., heterotypic continuity). As we reported earlier, irritability was the only symptom that was moderately higher in depressed children when compared with adolescents with adolescent-onset BD.

A history of an MDE is needed when making bipolar II diagnosis (MDE plus at least one hypomanic episode), but the presentation of full DSM-IV criteria for bipolar II disorder does not appear to be common in youth with bipolar spectrum illness (Axelson et al., 2006; Birmaher, Axelson, Monk, et al., 2009). In the COBY study, subjects with bipolar II disorder were older, generally late or postpubertal, and more likely to be female. Functional impairment was less severe in the subjects with bipolar II compared with those with bipolar I, but overall there were few detectable differences between the subjects with bipolar II and those with either bipolar I or BD NOS (Axelson et al., 2006).

Subthreshold Presentations

Some children and adolescents present in clinical and research settings with what appears to be significant manic symptomatology but do not meet full DSM-IV criteria for BD disorders. In the COBY study, 263 children with BD spent more time in subsyndromal pure depression and subsyndromal mixed states during the 2-year follow-up compared with syndromal pure major depression and mixed states (Birmaher et al., 2006). The assessment, diagnosis, and management of subthreshold presentations of BD in children and adolescents are controversial, although many children present for mental health treatment with significant impairment and are frequently assigned a diagnosis of BD NOS (Birmaher & Axelson, 2005). Clinicians must pay particular attention to subsyndromal presentations during the assessment and treatment of BD given their association with significant morbidity (e.g., functional impairment, high rates of comorbidities and suicidal ideation) and increased risk for relapse (Birmaher et al., 2006; Pavuluri et al., 2005; Pavuluri, Graczyk, et al., 2004).

In the COBY study, the main difference between children with BD NOS and the other two BD subgroups was the lack of sufficient duration to fulfill criteria for bipolar I or II. Axelson and colleagues (2006) reported that children and adolescents with bipolar spectrum disorders presented with a history of substantial impairment and high rates of prior hospitalization, medication treatment, major depression, suicidal ideation, comorbid disruptive behavior disorders, and anxiety disorders. Children and adolescents with BD-NOS were similar to those with bipolar I on many factors, including age of onset, duration of illness, rates of comorbid diagnoses and prior MDEs, family history, and the types of manic symptoms that were present during the most serious lifetime episode.

A recent study from Italy reported that BD NOS and bipolar I disorder were equally severe in terms of clinical symptomatology, functional impairment, and need for hospitalization (Masi et al., 2007). However, this study used a soft definition of BD NOS (e.g., no specific minimal duration of manic episodes were required) and reported that children and adolescents with BD NOS presented with an earlier onset, a chronic course, an irritable mood, and higher comorbidity with DBD compared with the other BD subtypes (Masi et al., 2007). In summary, available studies suggest a bipolar NOS phenotype that exists on a continuum with youth with bipolar I (Axelson et al., 2006).

Of particular importance, children of parents with BD are reported to have an elevated risk for developing BD and other psychiatric disorders (Singh et al., 2007); thus, the presence of syndromal and subthreshold presentations of BD should be carefully evaluated in such children. Studies that prospectively followed offspring of BD parents have reported that the initial presentation in at-risk youth was usually non-BD mood symptoms or subthreshold BD, with rates of BD NOS between 33 and 66% (Birmaher, Axelson, Monk, et al., 2009; Duffy et al., 2007).

Applying knowledge of normative adolescent development to the study of psychopathology will be critical for identifying abnormal developmental processes in children at risk for BD. Certain pathways that signify adaptational compromises or failures will almost certainly predict subsequent BD in some genetically predisposed children, but it is likely that there will be a significant proportion of false positives as well (Cicchetti & Rogosch, 2002). For example, BD NOS probably reflects an adaptational compromise, but not all children with BD NOS will go on to develop bipolar I or II disorder. Knowledge of the intervening risk and protective factors—in the genetic, social, biological, psychological, or cultural vein—will do much to sharpen our ability to predict conversion to fully syndromal BD.

DIMENSIONAL ASSESSMENT OF BIPOLAR DISORDER

The categorical approach, like DSM, views psychopathological states as distinct syndromes requiring a predetermined number of symptoms, an age of onset, and a certain duration of symptoms for diagnosis. In contrast, the dimensional approach views psychopathology as a quantitative deviation from normal, with no clear threshold demarcating individuals with and without a disorder (Biederman, Faraone, Mick, Moore, & Lelon, 1996). Because of their ease of administration, good psychometric properties, and cross-cultural validation, the Achenbach Rating Scales (mainly parent-rated Child Behavior Checklist [CBCL]; Achenbach & Rescorla, 2001) have been in widespread use, most recently in studies of pediatric

BD (Mick, Biederman, Pandina, & Faraone, 2003). Cutoff scores of 70 (2 *SD* above normal level) have been recommended as clinically meaningful thresholds for a deviation from age- and sex-matched healthy children. It has been suggested that both categorical and dimensional methods are complementary and preferable in making clinical decisions (Eiraldi, Power, Karustis, & Goldstein, 2000), and that the CBCL is suitable as a method of providing dimensional findings based on categorical diagnoses in pediatric BD (Biederman et al., 1996). However, others suggest that high scores on the CBCL might be due to symptom severity, comorbidity, or functional impairment among youth with BD (Kahana, Youngstrom, Findling, & Calabrese, 2003, Youngstrom, Youngstrom, & Starr, 2005).

A recent study reported that CBCL and its subscales should not be used as a proxy for DSM-IV BD diagnosis (Diler et al., 2009). In the COBY sample, after controlling for significant demographic and clinical variables, parent-rated CBCL scores were similar between bipolar I, II, and NOS in children with BD younger than 12 years, but adolescents diagnosed with BD NOS and bipolar II had higher CBCL Withdrawn/Depressed scores compared with those with bipolar I disorder. When all subjects were analyzed, those with BD NOS had higher Internalizing, Externalizing, and total CBCL scores compared with bipolar I and II subgroups, even though global functioning was worse in the bipolar I subgroup. Except for the Somatic Problems subscale, children with BD (<12 years old) had significantly higher psychopathology on all CBCL scores compared with adolescents with BD (≥12 years old). Our findings from the CBCL analysis confirm our results from categorical assessments that childhood BD may have a different presentation than adolescent BD.

COMORBIDITY

Children and adolescents with bipolar spectrum disorders present with a history of substantial impairment, high rates of prior hospitalization, medication treatment, major depression, suicidal ideation, and comorbid disruptive and anxiety disorders (Axelson et al., 2006). Comorbid disorders in subjects with bipolar disorder in different studies are reported in Table 5.1. They frequently have histories of psychotic symptoms and suicide attempts. Depending on the population studied, approximately 50–80% have ADHD, 20–60% DBD, and 30–70% anxiety disorders (Birmaher & Axelson, 2005). Other psychiatric disorders, such as obsessive–compulsive disorder, as well as medical conditions can also accompany BD. The COBY sample was similar to that of the other studies in regard to the high rates of comorbid ADHD and ODD (Table 5.1) and showed that children and adolescents with BD NOS were similar to those with bipolar I regarding the comorbid diagnoses (Axelson et al., 2006; Goldstein et al., 2008). A few studies compared comorbidity in BD children and adolescents. Masi and colleagues (2006) reported more comorbid ADHD and ODD in children (*n* = 80) compared with adolescents (*n* = 56) with bipolar spectrum disorders. Birmaher, Axelson, Strober, and colleagues (2009) reported that both adolescents with adolescent-onset and childhood-onset BD had higher prevalence of lifetime conduct and substance use disorders than children with BD in the COBY sample.

The prevalence of substance abuse in child studies has been low compared with adult BD studies (Geller et al., 2008; Goodwin & Jamison, 1990; Post et al., 2003), and beginning in adolescence the rate of comorbid substance abuse progressively increases (Pavuluri et al., 2005). A better understanding of how comorbid conditions develop and evolve during childhood and adolescent BD is very crucial. The presence of these disorders affects children's and adolescents' response to treatment and prognosis, indicating the need to identify and treat them effectively (Kowatch, Fristad, et al., 2005). For example, there usually is a window between first mood episode and substance abuse: During an 8-year naturalistic follow-up study, 35.2% of youth with bipolar I developed substance use disorders when they were 18 years or older (Geller et al., 2008). In the COBY study, adolescents with adolescent-onset BD had more substance abuse than adolescents with childhood-onset BD (Birmaher, Axelson, Strober, et al., 2009). Available findings emphasize the importance of prompt treatment of youth with BD before they begin to use substances that could complicate the management of their mood disorder and worsen their long-term prognosis (Birmaher & Axelson, 2006, Geller et al., 2008).

Of particular importance, adults patients with BD die prematurely not only from suicide but also from cardiovascular and other metabolic disorders. These concurrent medical conditions can be related to BD or its treatments (Scheffer & Linden, 2007). We need to learn more about the development of concurrent medical conditions in youth with BD and their associations with demographic variables (e.g., age, sex), phenomenology of BD, other comorbid conditions, and treatments given so that preventive interventions can be implemented.

DIFFERENTIAL DIAGNOSIS

It may be difficult to diagnose pediatric BD given the variability in the clinical presentation (e.g., severity, subtype of BD disorder, phase of the illness), high comorbidity and overlap in symptom presentation with other psychiatric disorders, effects of development on symptom expression (e.g., grandiosity and adult-like mania presentation in adolescence), children's difficulties in verbalizing their symptoms, and the potential effects of medications on children's mood (Birmaher & Axelson, 2005). A few studies have reported that preschool children with BD can be distinguished from healthy children and children with DBDs (Danielyan et al., 2007; Luby & Belden, 2006). It is critical that clinicians have a working knowledge of normative cognitive, behavioral, and affective development so that it can be determined whether a certain behavior is expected or pathological during the children's present stage of development (Carlson & Meyer, 2006). As noted, elated mood and grandiosity can help differentiate children with BD from healthy children and children with other psychopathology. BD should be a part of the differential diagnosis for a wide range of clinical presentations of Axis I diagnoses such as anxiety, pervasive developmental, eating, impulse control, disruptive behavior (including ADHD, conduct disorder [CD], and ODD), psychotic, and substance abuse disorders; Axis II diagnoses (Pavuluri et al., 2005); and physical and sexual abuse (Romero et al., 2008). It is very important to observe whether the symptoms of the comorbid disorder disappear or persist while the child with BD is euthymic.

The presence of psychosis in youth with BD has varied (see Table 5.1) from 17 to 87.5% across studies (Pavuluri, Herbener, & Sweeney, 2004; Tillman et al., 2008). When patients present with psychotic symptoms, the onset of schizophrenia is usually insidious and the patients lack the engaging quality associated with mania (Yazgan, Fis, & Scahill, 2007). In BD, affective contact is fairly good; incoherence and poverty of content are transitory rather than persistent; treatment response to mood stabilizers is dramatic; and a family history of affective disorders, namely BD, is found at a considerable rate (Yazgan et al., 2007).

ADHD and BD can be confused with each other, they may co-occur, or BD can be superimposed on ADHD (Carlson & Meyer, 2006). Leibenluft and colleagues suggested that manic symptoms should represent a distinct change from the usual level of functioning (e.g., change or worsening of distractibility during a mood episode in children with ADHD) (Leibenluft & Rich, 2008). There are some symptoms that mainly occur in youth with BD compared with other disorders (e.g., ADHD) and may help to differentiate between BD and these disorders, such as clinically relevant euphoria, grandiosity, decreased need for sleep, hypersexuality (without history of sexual abuse or exposure to sex) and hallucinations (Diler, Uguz, Seydaoglu, Erol, & Avci, 2007; Geller et al., 2002). Similarly, hypersexuality, elated mood, grandiosity, talkativeness, and flight of ideas were the most prevalent symptoms to distinguish preschool children with BD from those with DBDs.

Although irritability is posited as a clinical feature of pediatric BD, the specificity of this symptom remains uncertain (see prior discussion). If chronic irritability is part of severe ADHD, it would not be a useful symptom for the differential diagnosis of BD and ADHD in children. However, data from the Multimodal Treatment Study of Children with ADHD is suggestive of irritability as a marker for BD and not ADHD (Galanter et al., 2003). Irritability associated with BD is more severe and persistent than the frustration commonly found with ADHD and is often associated with violent outbursts (Yazgan et al., 2007). Leibenluft and colleagues (2006) reported that episodic irritability was associated with future BD and chronic irritability was associated with ADHD and ODD and future MDD. Children with ADHD alone do not manifest significant disturbances in mood. Therefore, the presence of mood instability is more consistent with a diagnosis of BD than ADHD.

FAMILY HISTORY

A meta-analysis of the high-risk child BD ("top-down") literature reported that offspring of parents with BD had an average of 4–15% lifetime prevalence of BD compared with 0–2% in offspring of healthy parents (Lapalme, Hodgins, & LaRoche, 1997). Similarly, the Pittsburgh Bipolar Offspring Study showed that children (ages 6–18 years) of parents with BD had a 13.4-fold higher risk for developing BD compared with children of community controls. Moreover, the risk was 3.6-fold higher when both parents had BD compared with only one parent (Birmaher, Axelson, Monk, et al., 2009). "Bottom-up" studies of childhood-onset BD also provide further evidence of the familial nature of BD. Studies have shown increased risk for BD and depression in first-degree relatives of children and adolescents with BD compared with relatives of adolescents with other disorders (Lewinsohn et al., 1995; Strober et al., 1988).

COURSE AND OUTCOME OF BIPOLAR DISORDER

Retrospective Studies

Retrospective studies of adults with BD report that between 10–20% of patients have onset before 10 years of age (Pavuluri et al., 2005). Up to 60% reported onset of their mood symptoms before the age of 20 (Chengappa et al., 2003; Egeland et al., 2003). BD in adults is frequently preceded by childhood disruptive behavior and anxiety disorders (Henin et al., 2007). A retrospective study of 983 patients with BD found that early-onset BD was associated with a severe course of illness and poor outcome (Perlis et al., 2004).

Prospective Studies

There are few prospective studies available regarding youth with BD. Prospective follow-up studies of children with BD may help validate the presence of this condition in youth and help us better understand natural course and factors associated with its onset and recurrences, which may also be useful for preventive strategies and to improve current acute and maintenance treatments (Birmaher, 2007).

Community Prospective Studies

One community study evaluated 1,709 adolescents ages 14 to 18 and found that 1.0% had BD (mainly bipolar II and cyclothymia) (Lewinsohn et al., 1995). Over a 14-month follow-up, adolescents who reported symptoms in the bipolar spectrum had more functional impairment, psychosis, suicidality, comorbid anxiety, disruptive disorders, and mental health utilization than adolescents with a history of MDD and healthy adolescents (Lewinsohn et al., 1995). The authors reassessed the subjects at age 24 and, on the basis of youth reports only, found that

BD in adolescence showed significant continuity across developmental periods and was associated with adverse outcomes during young adulthood (Lewinsohn, Klein, & Seeley, 2000). Lewinsohn and colleagues (1995, 2000) found that 5.7% of the adolescents had soft "subsyndromal BD" symptoms (a distinct period of abnormally and persistently elevated, expansive, or irritable mood), and these adolescents had high levels of impairment, comorbidity, and family history of BD and depression that were comparable to the BD group; however, they only showed increased risk for depression, not BD, as young adults. These findings raise questions about the continuity of bipolar spectrum disorders across the life span when the spectrum is softly defined (e.g., multifinality), at least in community samples.

Clinical Prospective Studies

There have been few prospective naturalistic studies of the course of BD in children and adolescents in clinical samples. We report these studies in Table 5.2 and detail them next.

Strober and colleagues (1995) followed 52 adolescents for 5 years and reported that 98% of bipolar I adolescents fully recovered from their index episode during the follow-up. Adolescents with pure depression at intake had longer time to recovery compared with those adolescents with pure mania, mixed states, and cycling at intake. About 70% had at least one syndromal or subsyndromal recurrence. Adolescents with cycling or mixed episodes at intake had the highest probability of multiple recurrences. Approximately 20% of the sample made a suicide attempt requiring medical attention (Strober et al., 1995).

In a study conducted in India, Srinath, Janardhan, Reddy, Girimaji, Seshadri, and Subbakrishna (1998) reevaluated 30 children and adolescents (age range = 11–16 years) 4 to 5 years after they were diagnosed with BD using the DSM-III. At intake, subjects were drug-naive. They were intensively treated for index episodes with antimanic (mainly lithium) and antipsychotic drugs and all eventually recovered from their index episode; however, 67% had at least one recurrence. Polarity of the index episodes was mainly mania (63%) followed by depression (10%), cycling (10%), and mixed (7%). One subject had committed suicide (3%) and one had attempted (3%). No risk factor was identified to predict recovery or relapse (Srinath et al., 1998).

A multicenter study followed 73 outpatient adolescents (mean age = 17.1 ± 1.8) with bipolar I for a mean of 76 ± 62 weeks (Birmaher, 2004). Longitudinal changes in psychiatric symptomatology, functioning, and treatment exposure since the previous evaluation were assessed using the LIFE (Keller et al., 1987). During follow-up, almost all patients were on psychotropic medications and 70% had at least one hospitalization. In this study, approximately 68% of the adolescents with BD recovered in 20 to 40 weeks. Adolescents with mixed index episodes had longer time to recovery (mean = 58 weeks) than those with manic (mean = 42 weeks) or depressive (mean = 20 weeks) index episodes. Although the recovery rate was

TABLE 5.2. Prospective Naturalistic Studies of Youth with Bipolar Disorder

Study	BD diagnoses/ origin of most of the sample	Mean age (years)	Sample size	Frequency and duration of follow-up (months)	% Remission/ recovery[a]	% Relapse/ recurrence[a]	Predictors of outcome
Strober et al. (1995)	BD-I, inpatients	16	54	Every 6 months for 5 years	98%	44%	Pure depression (longer time to recovery); cycling and mixed episodes (higher recurrences)
Srinath et al. (1998)	BD-I, outpatient	14	30	Once after 4–5 years	100%	67%	None identified
Birmaher (2004)	BD-I outpatients	17	73	Every 6 months for 19 months	68%	59%	Mixed episodes (longer time to recovery and higher recurrences)
Jairam et al. (2004)	BD-I outpatients	14	25	Every 6 months for 52 months	100%	64%	Lifetime depressive episode, longer duration of index episode, poorer CGAS scores at follow-up, noncompliance with treatment (more relapse)

Study	Diagnosis/sample		N	Assessment interval	Recovery	Relapse/recurrence	Predictors
Birmaher et al. (2006)	BD-I, II, NOS outpatients	13	263	Every 6 months for 24 months	70%	50%	BD-I (more recurrence); BD NOS (longer time to recovery and greater number of changes in polarity); low SES, prepubertal BD onset, lifetime psychosis (greater number of changes in polarity); mixed episodes, psychosis, low SES, comorbid ADHD, conduct, anxiety, substance abuse, and family psychopathology (more time with syndromal and subsyndromal symptoms)
DelBello et al. (2007)	BD-I, mania, inpatients	15	71	1, 4, 8, 12 months after hospitalization	85% (40% functional recovery)	52%	Comorbid ADHD and anxiety disorders, low SES, and poor adherence to pharmacological treatment (longer time to recovery); alcohol use disorder, lack of psychotherapy, and use of antidepressants (shorter time to recurrence).
Geller et al. (2008)	BD-I, mania outpatients	11	115	Every 6 months for 3 years and then once a year for 8 years	87.8%	73.3%	Low maternal warmth (relapse to mania, longer time in mania), younger baseline age (longer time in mania), older age at follow-up (higher risk for substance use disorders)

Note. BD, bipolar disorder; NOS, not otherwise specified; SES, socioeconomic status; ADHD, attention-deficit/hyperactivity disorder; C-GAS, Global Assessment Score for Children (Shaffer et al., 1983).
[a]Some investigators did not differentiate between the terms remission/recovery or relapse/recurrences.

high, 59% of the patients had at least one recurrence; patients with mixed BD had more recurrences and shorter intervals before recurrence (Birmaher, 2004).

Jairam, Srinath, Girimaji, and Seshadri (2004) followed 25 youth (9–16 years old) with DSM-IV mania (with elation and/or grandiosity) for 4 to 5 years. Youth were diagnosed using the Diagnostic Interview for Children and Adolescents—Revised (Herjanic & Reich, 1982). This study was conducted in India and, similar to Srinath and colleagues' (1998) report, the rates of mixed episode, rapid cycling, and comorbidities were low (e.g., 4% with ADHD). All 25 adolescents showed recovery (mean = 44 ± 46 days), but 64% of the subjects had at least one relapse (36% had multiple relapses) in about 18 months. Manic relapses were the most common (58%), followed by depressive (23%), mixed affective (16%), and hypomanic relapses (3%). Subsyndromal relapse were seen in nine (36%) subjects. The rate of relapse was 53% for the treatment-compliant group and 100% for the noncompliant group, but a majority of the relapses (72.4%) were breakthrough episodes that occurred during intense pharmacological treatment. One completed suicide and two had suicide attempts. A lifetime history of depressive episodes, a longer duration of the index episode, and poorer Children's Global Assessment Scale (Shaffer et al., 1983) scores at follow-up predicted relapse.

The COBY is the first study that systematically followed children and adolescents with bipolar spectrum disorders (Birmaher et al., 2006). As detailed previously, subjects with BD NOS were diagnosed with COBY established criteria and showed similar clinical characteristics and psychiatric family history to the subjects with bipolar I and II at intake (Axelson et al., 2006). About 70% of the subjects with BD showed recovery during follow-up, and about 50% of them had at least one full syndromal recurrence in a mean period of 15 months after recovery. Subjects were mostly (95%) in pharmacological treatment at baseline, but they were symptomatic approximately 60% of the follow-up time (22% with full syndromal episodes and 38% with subsyndromal symptoms) (Birmaher et al., 2006). In the COBY study (Birmaher et al., 2006), preliminary analyses showed that subjects with prepubertal-onset BD were approximately two times less likely than those with postpubertal-onset BD to recover. In addition, subjects with prepubertal-onset BD had more chronic symptoms, spent more follow-up time with subsyndromal mood symptoms, and had more polarity changes per year than those with postpubertal-onset BD. Preliminary analyses showed that mixed episodes, psychosis, low socioeconomic status (SES), comorbid ADHD, conduct, anxiety, substance abuse, and family psychopathology were associated with significantly more time with syndromal and subsyndromal symptoms. Older adolescents had more functional impairment than younger children both in episode and in remission/recovery. Given that psychosocial demands generally increase throughout development, it is possible that older youth may find it more difficult to meet these increased demands.

On average, the COBY subjects had 1.5 syndromal recurrences per year, particularly depressive episodes (Birmaher et al., 2006). Subjects with bipolar I had more manic/hypomanic and mixed episodes than those with BD NOS, subjects with bipolar II had more depression that those with bipolar I and NOS, and subjects with BD NOS showed more subsyndromal mania and mixed symptomatology (Figure 5.2). Subjects with BD NOS had a more protracted illness, but they showed a longer time to recurrence than those with bipolar I and II once they recovered from their index episode. On the other hand, subjects with bipolar I recovered and recurred from their index episode more frequently than those with BD NOS (Birmaher et al., 2006). In the COBY study, approximately 20% of subjects with bipolar II converted to bipolar I during 2-year follow-up and 25% of the BD NOS subjects converted to either bipolar I or II.

These findings from the longitudinal assessment (Birmaher et al., 2006) support the report from the intake assessment (Axelson et al., 2006) of the COBY study that the bipolar NOS phenotype exists on a continuum with bipolar I disorder. In contrast to the high switch rates of BD NOS in the COBY study, two previous studies (Brotman et al., 2006; Lewinsohn et al., 2000) did not find high switch rates in subjects with subsyndromal bipolar symptomatology. In comparison to the COBY's definition of BD NOS, these studies, as detailed previously, defined subsyndromal BD less stringently, suggesting less liability for full BD than captured by the COBY's more restrictive definition (Birmaher & Axelson, 2006). In addition, the Lewinsohn and colleagues (2000) study based their intake diagnoses only on the adolescents' report without parental input.

A post hoc analysis of the Great Smoky Mountain Study indicated subjects who were softly defined as BD NOS (severe mood dysregulation with chronic,

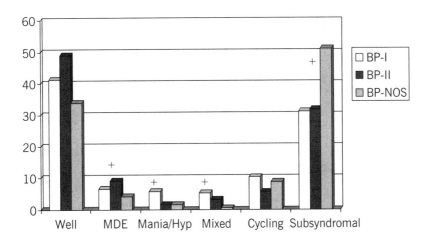

FIGURE 5.2. Comparison of weekly symptom status between youth with bipolar I disorder (BD-I), bipolar II disorder (BD-II), and bipolar disorder not otherwise specified (BD NOS). Weekly symptom status is the percentage of follow-up weeks spent asymptomatic or symptomatic in different mood categories; +p < .05 between three groups; MDE, major depressive episode. From Birmaher and Axelson (2006). Copyright 2006 by Cambridge University Press. Reprinted by permission.

nonepisodic, and explosive irritability) were prone to developing more recurrent MDD than BD over the 8-year follow-up (Brotman et al., 2006). This suggests the possibility of multifinality (similar initial conditions lead to different end stages) of the BD NOS diagnosis when it is not strictly defined.

DelBello and colleagues (2007) evaluated the 1-year outcome of 71 bipolar I adolescents admitted for their first manic or mixed episode. Adolescents were followed for 12 months after hospitalization, and 81% showed syndromic recovery in about 27 weeks after the onset of their index episode; however, only 40% of adolescents achieved functional recovery. Furthermore, about 52% of the subjects showed at least one syndromal recurrence. BD adolescents spent about 40% of their time with syndromic symptomatology (mainly mixed symptoms), 46% of their time with subsyndromal symptoms, and 16% of their time asymptomatic. ADHD, anxiety disorders, low SES, and poor adherence to pharmacological treatment predicted longer time to recovery, and alcohol use disorder, lack of psychotherapy treatment, and use of antidepressants predicted shorter time to recurrence. However, we need to be cautious when interpreting the effects on course and outcome of medications in the longitudinal naturalistic course of BD. It is not completely clear whether some of these medications were prescribed because subjects had a more severe illness and were already depressed and, as a consequence, were at high risk to manifest suicide ideation or behaviors (Birmaher, 2007).

Geller and colleagues (2008) followed a cohort of 115 children with bipolar I disorder (age 7–16 years) for 8 years. Subjects were required to have their first manic or mixed episode at intake, with elation or grandiosity as a criterion symptom for study inclusion. Psychiatric symptomatology was ascertained using the Washington University K-SADS. Approximately 88% of the subjects recovered in a mean time of 55.6 ± 51.9 weeks. However, 73.3% of these subjects had at least one recurrence in an average time of 99 ± 81 weeks. Subjects spent 60.2% of weeks with any mood episodes and 39.6% of weeks with mania episodes. There were 24 (44.4%) subjects who had mania after they reached age 18 years, but the percentage of weeks with mood episodes were not different across ages. When baseline characteristics of youth were compared with the subjects who were 18 years or older, CGAS (Shaffer et al., 1983), mixed mania, ADHD, CD, and ODD were higher and substance dependency was lower in younger children. Lower maternal warmth, which was correlated with lower baseline age, predicted more weeks with mania or mixed mania and relapse to mania (Geller et al., 2008). Similarly, Miklowitz, Biuckians, and Richards (2006) reported that highly critical expressed emotion among parents of adolescents with BD was associated with poorer course of BD over 2 years.

The results and comparisons among the studies (see Table 5.2) should be interpreted with caution given the different methodologies used in these studies (e.g., differences in inclusion and exclusionary criteria, definition of BD, demographics, instruments, and definitions of recovery, remission, relapse, and recurrence). Furthermore, most of the pediatric samples were small and were followed infrequently or for a relatively brief period. The studies focused primarily on bipolar I, most did not identify syndromal and subsyndromal course, and some did not interview the youth (or the parents) directly. Although they have methodological differences, available studies consistently show high rates of hospitalizations and health service utilization, psychosis, suicide attempts and completion, high rates of switching from BD NOS to bipolar I or II and from bipolar II to I, substance abuse, unemployment, legal problems, and poor academic and psychosocial functioning (Birmaher, 2007). Studies have indicated that 70–100% of children and adolescents with BD will eventually recover (e.g., no significant symptoms for 2 months) from their index episode; however, up to 75% will experience one or more recurrences in a period of 2 to 8 years (Table 5.2).

Comparison of Studies in Adults versus Children

Considerable debate exists about the distinction of early-onset (pediatric) BD from late-onset (adult) BD (Chang, 2007) and whether different initial stages (early onset vs. late onset) can lead to the same condition (e.g., equifinality). Given that longitudinal studies are limited in youth with BD as detailed previously, comparison of BD in adults versus children may help us answer some of these questions. A recent 8-year naturalistic study of youth with bipolar I (Geller et al., 2008) reported that the percentage of weeks youth were ill with mood symptoms was similar to the findings of a 12.8-year follow-up of bipolar I adults (Judd et al., 2002). Similar to the few available studies in youth (Birmaher & Axelson, 2006), poor prognosis among adults is associated with early onset, mixed, rapid cycling, and depressive presentations, longer duration, recurrent episodes, persistence of subsyndromal affective symptoms, psychosis, comorbid substance abuse, exposure to negative events, poor adherence to treatment, family discord, and low SES (Coryell, Keller, Lavori, & Endicott, 1990; Coryell et al., 1997; Cruz et al., 2008; Himmelhoch & Garfinkel, 1986; Judd et al., 2002, 2003; Miklowitz, Goldstein, Nuechterlein, Snyder, & Mintz, 1988; O'Connell, Mayo, Flatow, Cuthbertson, & O'Brien, 1991; Post et al., 1989; Schneck et al., 2008; Tohen, Waternaux, & Tsuang, 1990; Valtonen et al., 2006).

Studies also suggest developmental differences in the course of BD between children and adults (Birmaher & Axelson, 2006). The COBY study (Birmaher et al., 2006) showed that youth with bipolar I had significantly more polarity switches, spent significantly more time symptomatic, and had more mixed/cycling and subsyndromal episodes than adults with bipolar I (Judd et al., 2003) (Figure 5.3). These results are consistent with what other investigators, including Kraepelin, have reported (Angst, Gerber-Werder, Zuberbühler, & Gamma, 2004; Coryell et al., 1998; Kraepelin, 1921). These results showed that bipolar II and perhaps BD NOS are less developmentally stable in the pediatric age group (e.g., heterotypic continuity). Thus, BD in youth follows a changeable and sinuous course with patients developing a wide spectrum of mood symptoms ranging from mild to severe depression, mania, and hypomania (Birmaher & Axelson, 2006).

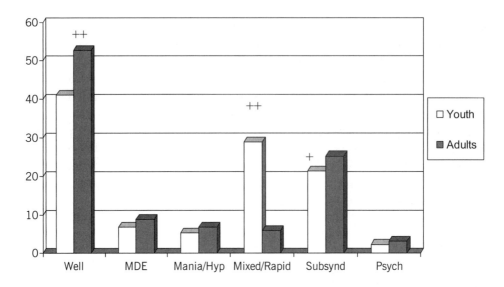

FIGURE 5.3. Comparison of weekly symptom status between youth with bipolar I disorder (BD-I) and adults with BD-I. Weekly symptom status is the percentage of follow-up weeks spent asymptomatic or symptomatic in different mood categories; $+p = .05$; $++p < .001$; MDE, major depressive episode. From Birmaher and Axelson (2006). Copyright 2006 by Cambridge University Press. Reprinted by permission.

CONCLUSION

Many children and adolescents with BD have very short and frequent periods of syndromal or subsyndromal mania, hypomania, or depression, making their diagnosis especially difficult (Birmaher & Axelson, 2005). A large multicenter study of children and adolescents with BD spectrum disorders (COBY study) demonstrated that youth with bipolar II disorder and BD NOS (*especially when strictly defined*) have a phenotype that *exists on a continuum* with youth with bipolar I (Axelson et al., 2006; Birmaher et al., 2006). Family studies confirmed this dimensional continuum by providing further evidence that the initial presentation of mania in the offspring of BD parents was usually BD NOS (Birmaher, Axelson, Monk, et al., 2009; Duffy et al., 2007).

Studies that used categorical and dimensional assessments have reported that early-onset BD has a somewhat different phenotype, suggesting that the early onset of mania and depression is associated with maturation and developmental changes. The fluctuating course of BD in children and adolescents (high rates of recovery and recurrences) shows a dimensional continuum of BD symptom severity from subsyndromal to mood syndromes meeting full DSM-IV criteria and appears to be more accentuated than in adults with BD (Birmaher & Axelson, 2006). Children and adolescents with early onset, low SES, long duration, rapid mood fluctuation, mixed episodes, psychosis, comorbid disorders, and family psychopathology have worse longitudinal outcomes.

It is essential to view youth in a life span perspective and to examine both past and current risk as well as protective processes and how they have influenced the evolving individual's vulnerability and resilience over the course of development. The cross-disciplinary investigations that utilize multiple levels of analysis methodologies (Cicchetti & Dawson, 2002; Miklowitz, 2004) promise to strengthen our capacity to facilitate developmentally sensitive assessments and interventions. Similar to the studies of other psychopathologies in youth (Cicchetti & Blender, 2006; Cicchetti & Cannon, 1999), longitudinal studies using developmental psychopathology concepts (e.g., equifinality and multifinality, homotypic and heterotypic continuity, and risk, protective and resilience factors) are needed in youth with and at risk for BD.

BD affects children very early in life and deprives them of the opportunity for normal psychosocial development at crucial stages of their lives (Birmaher & Axelson, 2006). Early recognition and acute pharmacological and psychotherapeutic interventions, as well as maintenance treatments to avoid recurrences, are vital in youth with BD to ameliorate syndromal and subsyndromal symptoms and to reduce or prevent the morbidity that frequently accompanies this illness (Birmaher & Axelson, 2006).

REFERENCES

Achenbach, T. M., & Rescorla, L. A. (2001). *Manual for the ASEBA School-Age Forms and Profiles.* Burlington: Department of Psychiatry, University of Vermont.

American Psychiatric Association. (2000). *Diagnostic and statistical manual of mental disorders* (4th ed., text rev.). Washington, DC: Author.

Angst, J., Gerber-Werder, R., Zuberbühler, H. U., & Gamma, A. (2004). Is bipolar I disorder heterogeneous? *European Archives of Psychiatry and Clinical Neuroscience, 254,* 82–91.

Axelson, D., Birmaher, B., Strober, M., Gill, M. K., Valeri, S., Chiappetta, L., et al. (2006). Phenomenology of children and adolescents with bipolar spectrum disorders. *Archives of General Psychiatry, 63*(10), 1139–1148.

Axelson, D., Birmaher, B. J., Brent, D., Wassick, S., Hoover, C., Bridge, J., et al. (2003). A preliminary study of the Kiddie Schedule for Affective Disorders and Schizophrenia for School-Age Children mania rating scale for children and adolescents. *Journal of Child and Adolescent Psychopharmacology, 13*(4), 463–470.

Biederman, J., Faraone, S., Mick, E., Moore, P., & Lelon, E. (1996). Child Behavior Checklist findings further support comorbidity between ADHD and major depression in a referred sample. *Journal of the American Academy of Child and Adolescent Psychiatry, 35*(6), 734–742.

Biederman, J., Faraone, S. V., Chu, M. P., & Wozniak, J. (1999). Further evidence of a bidirectional overlap between juvenile mania and conduct disorder in children. *Journal of the American Academy of Child and Adolescent Psychiatry, 38*(4), 468–476.

Biederman, J., Faraone, S. V., Wozniak, J., Mick, E., Kwon, A., & Aleardi, M. (2004). Further evidence of unique developmental phenotypic correlates of pediatric bipolar disorder:

Findings from a large sample of clinically referred preadolescent children assessed over the last 7 years. *Journal of Affective Disorders, 82*(Suppl. 1), S45–S58.

Biederman, J., Faraone, S. V., Wozniak, J., Mick, E., Kwon, A., Cayton, G. A., et al. (2005). Clinical correlates of bipolar disorder in a large, referred sample of children and adolescents. *Journal of Psychiatric Research, 39*(6), 611–622.

Birmaher, B. (2004). Bipolare und Depressive Storungen im Kindes—und Jugendalter [Bipolar and depressive disturbances in children and youths]. In A. Maneros (Ed.), *Das Neue Handbuch der Bipolaren und Depressiven Erkrankungen* [The new manual of bipolar and depressive disorders] (pp. 573–590). Stuttgart, Germany: George Thieme Verlag.

Birmaher, B. (2007). Longitudinal course of pediatric bipolar disorder. *American Journal of Psychiatry, 164*(4), 537–539.

Birmaher, B., & Axelson, D. (2005). Pediatric psychopharmacology. In B. J. Sadock & V. A. Sadock (Eds.), *Kaplan and Sadock's comprehensive textbook of psychiatry* (8th ed., Vol. II, pp. 3363–3375). Philadelphia: Lippincott Williams & Wilkins.

Birmaher, B., & Axelson, D. (2006). Course and outcome of bipolar spectrum disorder in children and adolescents: A review of the existing literature. *Development and Psychopathology, 18*(4), 1023–1035.

Birmaher, B., Axelson, D., Monk, K., Kalas, C., Goldstein, B., Hickey, M. B., et al. (2009). Lifetime psychiatric disorders in school-aged offspring of parents with bipolar disorder: The Pittsburgh Bipolar Offspring study. *Archives of General Psychiatry, 66*(3), 287–296.

Birmaher, B., Axelson, D., Strober, M., Gill, M. K., Valeri, S., Chiappetta, L., et al. (2006). Clinical course of children and adolescents with bipolar spectrum disorders. *Archives of General Psychiatry, 63*(2), 175–183.

Birmaher, B., Axelson, D., Strober, M., Gill, M. K., Yang, M., Ryan, N., et al. (2009). Comparison of manic and depressive symptoms between children and adolescents with bipolar spectrum disorders. *Journal of Bipolar Disorders, 11*(1), 52–62.

Brotman, M. A., Schmajuk, M., Rich, B. A., Dickstein, D. P., Guyer, A. E., Costello, E. J., et al. (2006). Prevalence, clinical correlates, and longitudinal course of severe mood dysregulation in children. *Biological Psychiatry, 60*(9), 991–997.

Carlson, G. A., & Meyer, S. E. (2006). Phenomenology and diagnosis of bipolar disorder in children, adolescents, and adults: Complexities and developmental issues. *Development and Psychopathology, 18*(4), 939–969.

Chang, K. (2007). Adult bipolar disorder is continuous with pediatric bipolar disorder. *Canadian Journal of Psychiatry, 52*(7), 418–425.

Chengappa, K. N., Kupfer, D. J., Frank, E., Houck, P. R., Grochocinski, V. J., Cluss, P. A., et al. (2003). Relationship of birth cohort and early age at onset of illness in a bipolar disorder case registry. *American Journal of Psychiatry, 160*(9), 1636–1642.

Cicchetti, D., & Blender, J. A. (2006). A multiple-levels-of-analysis perspective on resilience: Implications for the developing brain, neural plasticity, and preventive interventions. *Annals of the New York Academy of Sciences, 1094*, 248–258.

Cicchetti, D., & Cannon, T. D. (1999). Neurodevelopmental processes in the ontogenesis and epigenesis of psychopathology. *Development and Psychopathology, 11*(3), 375–393.

Cicchetti, D., & Dawson, G. (2002). Multiple levels of analysis. *Development and Psychopathology, 14*(3), 417–420.

Cicchetti, D., & Rogosch, F. A. (2002). A developmental psychopathology perspective on adolescence. *Journal of Consulting and Clinical Psychology, 70*(1), 6–20.

Coryell, W., Keller, M., Lavori, P., & Endicott, J. (1990). Affective syndromes, psychotic features, and prognosis: II. Mania. *Archives of General Psychiatry, 47*(7), 658–662.

Coryell, W., Turvey, C., Endicott, J., Leon, A. C., Mueller, T., Solomon, D., et al. (1998). Bipolar

I affective disorder: Predictors of outcome after 15 years. *Journal of Affective Disorders*, *50*(2–3), 109–116.

Coryell, W., Winokur, G., Solomon, D., Shea, T., Leon, A., & Keller, M. (1997). Lithium and recurrence in a long-term follow-up of bipolar affective disorder. *Psychological Medicine*, *27*(2), 281–289.

Cruz, N., Vieta, E., Comes, M., Haro, J. M., Reed, C., & Bertsch, J. (2008). Rapid-cycling bipolar I disorder: Course and treatment outcome of a large sample across Europe. *Journal of Psychiatric Research*, *42*(13), 1068–1075.

Danielyan, A., Pathak, S., Kowatch, R. A., Arszman, S. P., & Johns, E. S. (2007). Clinical characteristics of bipolar disorder in very young children. *Journal of Affective Disorders*, *97*(1–3), 51–59.

DelBello, M. P., Hanseman, D., Adler, C. M., Fleck, D. E., & Strakowski, S. M. (2007). Twelve-month outcome of adolescents with bipolar disorder following first hospitalization for a manic or mixed episode. *American Journal of Psychiatry*, *164*(4), 582–590.

Diler, R. S., Birmaher, B., Axelson, D., Goldstein, B., Gill, M., Strober, M., et al. (2009). The Child Behavior Checklist (CBCL) and the CBCL-Bipolar Phenotype are not useful in diagnosing pediatric bipolar disorder. *Journal of Child and Adolescent Psychopharmacology*, *19*, 23–30.

Diler, R. S., Uguz, S., Seydaoglu, G., Erol, N., & Avci, A. (2007). Differentiating bipolar disorder in Turkish prepubertal children with attention-deficit hyperactivity disorder. *Bipolar Disorders*, *9*(3), 243–251.

Duffy, A., Alda, M., Crawford, L., Milin, R., & Grof, P. (2007). The early manifestations of bipolar disorder: A longitudinal prospective study of the offspring of bipolar parents. *Bipolar Disorders*, *9*(8), 828–838.

Egeland, J. A., Shaw, J. A., Endicott, J., Pauls, D. L., Allen, C. R., Hostetter, A. M., et al. (2003). Prospective study of prodromal features for bipolarity in well Amish children. *Journal of the American Academy of Child and Adolescent Psychiatry*, *42*(7), 786–796.

Eiraldi, R. B., Power, T. J., Karustis, J. L., & Goldstein, S. G. (2000). Assessing ADHD and comorbid disorders in children: The Child Behavior Checklist and the Devereux Scales of Mental Disorders. *Journal of Clinical Child Psychology*, *29*(1), 3–16.

Faraone, S. V., Biederman, J., Wozniak, J., Mundy, E., Mennin, D., & O'Donnell, D. (1997). Is comorbidity with ADHD a marker for juvenile-onset mania? *Journal of the American Academy of Child and Adolescent Psychiatry*, *36*, 1046–1055.

Findling, R. L., Gracious, B. L., McNamara, N. K., Youngstrom, E. A., Demeter, C. A., Branicky, L. A., et al. (2001). Rapid, continuous cycling and psychiatric co-morbidity in pediatric bipolar I disorder. *Bipolar Disorders*, *3*(4), 202–210.

Galanter, C. A., Carlson, G. A., Jensen, P. S., Greenhill, L. L., Davies, M., Li, W., et al. (2003). Response to methylphenidate in children with attention deficit hyperactivity disorder and manic symptoms in the multimodal treatment study of children with attention deficit hyperactivity disorder titration trial. *Journal of Child and Adolescent Psychopharmacology*, *13*(2), 123–136.

Geller, B., Craney, J. L., Bolhofner, K., DelBello, M. P., Axelson, D., Luby, J., et al. (2003). Phenomenology and longitudinal course of children with a prepubertal and early adolescent bipolar disorder phenotype. In B. Geller & M. P. DelBello (Eds.), *Bipolar disorder in childhood and early adolescence* (pp. 25–50). New York: Guilford Press.

Geller, B., Tillman, R., & Bolhofner, K. (2007). Proposed definitions of bipolar I disorder episodes and daily rapid cycling phenomena in preschoolers, school-aged children, adolescents, and adults. *Journal of Child and Adolescent Psychopharmacology*, *17*(2), 217–222.

Geller, B., Tillman, R., Bolhofner, K., & Zimerman, B. (2008). Child bipolar I disorder: Prospective continuity with adult bipolar I disorder; characteristics of second and third episodes; predictors of 8-year outcome. *Archives of General Psychiatry, 65*(10), 1125–1133.

Geller, B., Tillman, R., Craney, J. L., & Bolhofner, K. (2004). Four-year prospective outcome and natural history of mania in children with a prepubertal and early adolescent bipolar disorder phenotype. *Archives of General Psychiatry, 61*(5), 459–467.

Geller, B., Zimerman, B., Williams, M., Bolhofner, K., Craney, J. L., DelBello, M. P., et al. (2000). Diagnostic characteristics of 93 cases of a prepubertal and early adolescent bipolar disorder phenotype by gender, puberty and comorbid attention deficit hyperactivity disorder. *Journal of Child and Adolescent Psychopharmacology, 10*(3), 157–164.

Geller, B., Zimerman, B., Williams, M., DelBello, M. P., Bolhofner, K., Craney, J. L., et al. (2002). DSM-IV mania symptoms in a prepubertal and early adolescent bipolar disorder phenotype compared to attention-deficit hyperactive and normal controls. *Journal of Child and Adolescent Psychopharmacology, 12*(1), 11–25.

Goldstein, B. I., Strober, M. A., Birmaher, B., Axelson, D. A., Esposito-Smythers, C., Goldstein, T. R., et al. (2008). Substance use disorders among adolescents with bipolar spectrum disorders. *Bipolar Disorders, 10*(4), 469–478.

Goodwin, F. K., & Jamison, K. R. (1990). *Manic-depressive illness.* New York: Oxford University Press.

Henin, A., Biederman, J., Mick, E., Hirshfeld-Becker, D. R., Sachs, G. S., Wu, Y., et al. (2007). Childhood antecedent disorders to bipolar disorder in adults: A controlled study. *Journal of Affective Disorders, 99*(1–3), 51–57.

Herjanic, B., & Reich, W. (1982). Development of a structured psychiatric interview for children: Agreement between children and parents on individual symptoms. *Journal of Abnormal Child Psychology, 10*, 307–324.

Himmelhoch, J. M., & Garfinkel, M. E. (1986). Sources of lithium resistance in mixed mania. *Psychopharmacology Bulletin, 22*(3), 613–620.

Jairam, R., Srinath, S., Girimaji, S. C., & Seshadri, S. P. (2004). A prospective 4–5 year follow-up of juvenile onset bipolar disorder. *Bipolar Disorders, 6*(5), 386–394.

Judd, L. L., Akiskal, H. S., Schettler, P. J., Coryell, W., Endicott, J., Maser, J. D., et al. (2003). A prospective investigation of the natural history of the long-term weekly symptomatic status of bipolar II disorder. *Archives of General Psychiatry, 60*(3), 261–269.

Judd, L. L., Akiskal, H. S., Schettler, P. J., Endicott, J., Maser, J., Solomon, D. A., et al. (2002). The long-term natural history of the weekly symptomatic status of bipolar I disorder. *Archives of General Psychiatry, 59*(6), 530–537.

Kahana, S. Y., Youngstrom, E. A., Findling, R. L., & Calabrese, J. R. (2003). Employing parent, teacher, and youth self-report checklists in identifying pediatric bipolar spectrum disorders: An examination of diagnostic accuracy and clinical utility. *Journal of Child and Adolescent Psychopharmacology, 13*(4), 471–488.

Karippot, A. (2006). Pediatric bipolar depression. In R. S. El-Mallakh & S. N. Ghaemi (Eds.), *Bipolar depression: A comprehensive guide* (pp. 101–115.). Washington, DC: American Psychiatric Publishing.

Keller, M. B., Lavori, P. W., Friedman, B., Nielsen, E., Endicott, J., McDonald-Scott, P., et al. (1987). The Longitudinal Interval Follow-up Evaluation. A comprehensive method for assessing outcome in prospective longitudinal studies. *Archives of General Psychiatry, 44*(6), 540–548.

Kowatch, R. A., Fristad, M., Birmaher, B., Wagner, K. D., Findling, R. L., Hellander, M., et al. (2005). Treatment guidelines for children and adolescents with bipolar disorder. *Journal of the American Academy of Child and Adolescent Psychiatry, 44*(3), 213–235.

Kowatch, R. A., Youngstrom, E. A., Danielyan, A., & Findling, R. L. (2005). Review and meta-analysis of the phenomenology and clinical characteristics of mania in children and adolescents. *Bipolar Disorders, 7*(6), 483–496.

Kraepelin, E. (1921). *Manic depressive insanity and paranoia.* London: Livingstone.

Lapalme, M., Hodgins, S., & LaRoche, C. (1997). Children of parents with bipolar disorder: A metaanalysis of risk for mental disorders. *Canadian Journal of Psychiatry, 42*, 623–631.

Leibenluft, E., Charney, D. S., & Pine, D. S. (2003). Researching the pathophysiology of pediatric bipolar disorder. *Biological Psychiatry, 53*(11), 1009–1020.

Leibenluft, E., Charney, D. S., Towbin, K. E., Bhangoo, R. K., & Pine, D. S. (2003). Defining clinical phenotypes of juvenile mania. *American Journal of Psychiatry, 160*(3), 430–437.

Leibenluft, E., Charney, D. S., Towbin, K. E., Bhangoo, R. K., & Pine, D. S. (2006). Chronic versus episodic irritability in youth: A community-based, longitudinal study of clinical and diagnostic associations. *Journal of Child and Adolescent Psychopharmacology, 16*, 456–466.

Leibenluft, E., & Rich, B. A. (2008). Pediatric bipolar disorder. *Annual Review of Clinical Psychology, 4*, 163–187.

Lewinsohn, P. M., Klein, D. N., & Seeley, J. R. (1995). Bipolar disorders in a community sample of older adolescents: Prevalence, phenomenology, comorbidity, and course. *Journal of the American Academy of Child and Adolescent Psychiatry, 34*(4), 454–463.

Lewinsohn, P. M., Klein, D. N., & Seeley, J. R. (2000). Bipolar disorder during adolescence and young adulthood in a community sample. *Bipolar Disorders, 2*(3, Pt. 2), 281–293.

Luby, J., & Belden, A. (2006). Defining and validating bipolar disorder in the preschool period. *Development and Psychopathology, 18*(4), 971–988.

Luby, J. L., Tandon, M., & Nicol, G. (2009). Three clinical cases of DSM-IV mania symptoms in preschoolers. In J. L. Luby & M. A. Riddle (Eds.), *Advances in preschool psychopharmacology* (pp. 79–85). New Rochelle, NY: Mary Ann Liebert.

Masi, G., Perugi, G., Millepiedi, S., Mucci, M., Pari, C., Pfanner, C., et al. (2007). Clinical implications of DSM-IV subtyping of bipolar disorders in referred children and adolescents. *Journal of the American Academy of Child and Adolescent Psychiatry, 46*(10), 1299–1306.

Masi, G., Perugi, G., Millepiedi, S., Mucci, M., Toni, C., Bertini, N., et al. (2006). Developmental differences according to age at onset in juvenile bipolar disorder. *Journal of Child and Adolescent Psychopharmacology, 16*(6), 679–685.

McClellan, J., Kowatch, R., Findling, R. L., & Work Group on Quality Issues. (2007). Practice parameter for the assessment and treatment of children and adolescents with bipolar disorder. *Journal of the American Academy of Child and Adolescent Psychiatry, 46*(1), 107–125.

Mick, E., Biederman, J., Pandina, G., & Faraone, S. V. (2003). A preliminary meta-analysis of the Child Behavior Checklist in pediatric bipolar disorder. *Biological Psychiatry, 53*(11), 1021–1027.

Mick, E., Spencer, T., Wozniak, J., & Biederman, J. (2005). Heterogeneity of irritability in attention-deficit/hyperactivity disorder subjects with and without mood disorders. *Biological Psychiatry, 58*(7), 576–582.

Miklowitz, D. J. (2004). The role of family systems in severe and recurrent psychiatric disorders: A developmental psychopathology view. *Development and Psychopathology, 16*(3), 667–688.

Miklowitz, D. J., Biuckians, A., & Richards, J. A. (2006). Early-onset bipolar disorder: A family treatment perspective. *Development and Psychopathology, 18*, 1247–1265.

Miklowitz, D. J., & Chang, K. D. (2008). Prevention of bipolar disorder in at-risk children: Theoretical assumptions and empirical foundations. *Development and Psychopathology, 20*, 881–897.

Miklowitz, D. J., Goldstein, M. J., Nuechterlein, K. H., Snyder, K. S., & Mintz, J. (1988). Family factors and the course of bipolar affective disorder. *Archives of General Psychiatry, 45*(3), 225–231.

O'Connell, R. A., Mayo, J. A., Flatow, L., Cuthbertson, B., & O'Brien, B. E. (1991). Outcome of bipolar disorder on long-term treatment with lithium. *British Journal of Psychiatry, 159*, 123–129.

Pavuluri, M. N., Birmaher, B., & Naylor, M. W. (2005). Pediatric bipolar disorder: A review of the past 10 years. *Journal of the American Academy of Child and Adolescent Psychiatry, 44*(9), 846–871.

Pavuluri, M. N., Graczyk, P. A., Henry, D. B., Carbray, J. A., Heidenreich, J., & Miklowitz, D. J. (2004). Child- and family-focused cognitive-behavioral therapy for pediatric bipolar disorder: Development and preliminary results. *Journal of the American Academy of Child and Adolescent Psychiatry, 43*(5), 528–537.

Pavuluri, M. N., Herbener, E. S., & Sweeney, J. A. (2004). Psychotic symptoms in pediatric bipolar disorder. *Journal of Affective Disorders, 80*(1), 19–28.

Perlis, R. H., Miyahara, S., Marangell, L. B., Wisniewski, S. R., Ostacher, M., DelBello, M. P., et al. (2004). Long-term implications of early onset in bipolar disorder: Data from the first 1000 participants in the systematic treatment enhancement program for bipolar disorder (STEP-BD). *Biological Psychiatry, 55*(9), 875–881.

Post, R. M., Leverich, G. S., Altshuler, L. L., Frye, M. A., Suppes, T. M., Keck, P. E., Jr., et al. (2003). An overview of recent findings of the Stanley Foundation Bipolar Network (Part I). *Bipolar Disorders, 5*(5), 310–319.

Post, R. M., Rubinow, D. R., Uhde, T. W., Roy-Byrne, P. P., Linnoila, M., Rosoff, A., et al. (1989). Dysphoric mania. Clinical and biological correlates. *Archives of General Psychiatry, 46*(4), 353–358.

Puig-Antich, J., Chambers, W. J., & Ryan, N. D. (1986). *Schedule for Affective Disorders and Schizophrenia for School-Age Children (6–18 years) Kiddie-SADS—Present Episode (K-SADS-P), fourth working draft.* Pittsburgh, PA: Western Psychiatric Institute and Clinic, University of Pittsburgh School of Medicine.

Romero, S., Birmaher, B., Axelson, D., Goldstein, T., Goldstein, B. I., Gill, M. K., et al. (2008). Prevalence and correlates of physical and sexual abuse in children and adolescents with bipolar disorder. *Journal of Affective Disorders, 112*(1–3), 144–150.

Scheffer, R. E., & Linden, S. (2007). Concurrent medical conditions with pediatric bipolar disorder. *Current Opinion in Psychiatry, 20*(4), 398–401.

Scheffer, R. E., & Niskala Apps, J. A. (2004). The diagnosis of preschool bipolar disorder presenting with mania: Open pharmacological treatment. *Journal of Affective Disorders, 82*(Suppl. 1), S25–S34.

Schneck, C. D., Miklowitz, D. J., Miyahara, S., Araga, M., Wisniewski, S., Gyulai, L., et al. (2008). The prospective course of rapid-cycling bipolar disorder: Findings from the STEP-BD. *American Journal of Psychiatry, 165*(3), 370–377.

Shaffer, D., Gould, M., Brasic, J., Ambrosini, P., Fischer, P., Bird, H., et al. (1983). A Children's Global Assessment Scale (CGAS). *Archives of General Psychiatry, 40*, 1228–1231.

Singh, M. K., DelBello, M. P., Stanford, K. E., Soutullo, C., McDonough-Ryan, P., McElroy, S. L., et al. (2007). Psychopathology in children of bipolar parents. *Journal of Affective Disorders, 102*(1–3), 131–136.

Soutullo, C. A., Chang, K. D., Diez-Suarez, A., Figueroa-Quintana, A., Escamilla-Canales, I., Rapado-Castro, M., et al. (2005). Bipolar disorder in children and adolescents: International perspective on epidemiology and phenomenology. *Bipolar Disorders, 7*(6), 497–506.

Srinath, S., Janardhan Reddy, Y. C., Girimaji, S. R., Seshadri, S. P., & Subbakrishna, D. K.

(1998). A prospective study of bipolar disorder in children and adolescents from India. *Acta Psychiatrica Scandinavica, 98*(6), 437–442.

Strober, M., Morrell, W., Burroughs, J., Lampert, C., Danforth, H., & Freeman, R. (1988). A family study of bipolar I disorder in adolescence. Early onset of symptoms linked to increased familial loading and lithium resistance. *Journal of Affective Disorders, 15*, 255–268.

Strober, M., Schmidt-Lackner, S., Freeman, R., Bower, S., Lampert, C., & DeAntonio, M. (1995). Recovery and relapse in adolescents with bipolar affective illness: A five-year naturalistic, prospective follow-up. *Journal of the American Academy of Child and Adolescent Psychiatry, 34*, 724–731.

Tillman, R., Geller, B., Bolhofner, K., Craney, J. L., Williams, M., & Zimerman, B. (2003). Ages of onset and rates of syndromal and subsyndromal comorbid DSM-IV diagnoses in a prepubertal and early adolescent bipolar disorder phenotype. *Journal of the American Academy of Child and Adolescent Psychiatry, 42*(12), 1486–1493.

Tillman, R., Geller, B., Klages, T., Corrigan, M., Bolhofner, K., & Zimerman, B. (2008). Psychotic phenomena in 257 young children and adolescents with bipolar I disorder: Delusions and hallucinations (benign and pathological). *Bipolar Disorders, 10*(1), 45–55.

Tohen, M., Waternaux, C. M., & Tsuang, M. T. (1990). Outcome in mania. A 4-year prospective follow-up of 75 patients utilizing survival analysis. *Archives of General Psychiatry, 47*(12), 1106–1111.

Valtonen, H. M., Suominen, K., Mantere, O., Leppamaki, S., Arvilommi, P., & Isometsa, E. T. (2006). Prospective study of risk factors for attempted suicide among patients with bipolar disorder. *Bipolar Disorders, 8*(5, Pt. 2), 576–585.

Wozniak, J., Biederman, J., Kiely, K., Ablon, J. S., Faraone, S. V., Mundy, E., et al. (1995). Mania-like symptoms suggestive of childhood-onset bipolar disorder in clinically referred children. *Journal of the American Academy of Child and Adolescent Psychiatry, 34*(7), 867–876.

Wozniak, J., Biederman, J., Kwon, A., Mick, E., Faraone, S., Orlovsky, K., et al. (2005). How cardinal are cardinal symptoms in pediatric bipolar disorder?: An examination of clinical correlates. *Biological Psychiatry, 58*(7), 583–588.

Wozniak, J., Spencer, T., Biederman, J., Kwon, A., Monuteaux, M., Rettew, J., et al. (2004). The clinical characteristics of unipolar vs. bipolar major depression in ADHD youth. *Journal of Affective Disorders, 82*(Suppl. 1), S59–S69.

Yazgan, Y., Fis, N. P., & Scahill, L. K. (2007). Pediatric bipolar disorder: From the perspective of North America. In R. S. Diler (Ed.), *Pediatric bipolar disorder: A global perspective* (pp. 1–32). New York: Nova Science.

Youngstrom, E., Youngstrom, J. K., & Starr, M. (2005). Bipolar diagnoses in community mental health: Achenbach Child Behavior Checklist profiles and patterns of comorbidity. *Biological Psychiatry, 58*(7), 569–575.

Youngstrom, E. A., Birmaher, B., & Findling, R. L. (2008). Pediatric bipolar disorder: Validity, phenomenology, and recommendations for diagnosis. *Bipolar Disorders, 10*(1, pt. 2), 194–214.

CHAPTER 6

Course of Early-Onset Bipolar Spectrum Disorders during the College Years

A Behavioral Approach System Dysregulation Perspective

Lauren B. Alloy, Lyn Y. Abramson, Snezana Urosevic,
Robin Nusslock, and Shari Jager-Hyman

Although bipolar disorder (BD) has a strong genetic predisposition (McGuffin et al., 2003; Merikangas et al., 2002), there is increasing recognition that genetic vulnerability does not fully account for the timing, expression, and polarity of symptoms. Thus, in the past two decades, there has been greater interest in the role of psychosocial, developmental, and neurobiological risk factors that influence the onset, course, and expression of BD (see Alloy et al., 2005; Alloy, Abramson, Walshaw, Keyser, & Gerstein, 2006; Alloy, Abramson, Urosevic, Bender, & Wagner, 2009, for general reviews).

BDs are manifested along a continuum or spectrum (cyclothymia, bipolar II, bipolar I), with some disorders in the spectrum less severe and associated with less impairment than others (Akiskal, Djenderedjian, Rosenthal, & Khani, 1977; Akiskal, Khani, & Scott-Strauss, 1979; Cassano et al., 1999; Depue et al., 1981; Goodwin & Jamison, 2007; see Baldessarini, 2000, for criticism of the bipolar spectrum concept). In addition, milder forms of BD sometimes progress to more severe forms (e.g., Akiskal et al., 1977, 1979; Birmaher et al., 2006; Shen, Alloy, Abramson, & Sylvia, 2008) and sometimes exhibit a stable course and do not progress. Moreover, whereas some individuals with a bipolar spectrum disorder exhibit a very negative course with significant impairment in academic, work, and social functioning (e.g., Angst, Stassen, Clayton, & Angst, 2002; Goodwin & Jamison, 2007; Lagace & Kutcher, 2005; Nusslock, Alloy, Abramson, Harmon-Jones,

& Hogan, 2008; Strakowski, DelBello, Fleck, & Arndt, 2000), others experience a more benign course, including high achievement (Andreasen, 1987; Coryell et al., 1989; Kutcher, Robertson, & Bird, 1998; Nusslock et al., 2008).

In this chapter, we consider the course of bipolar spectrum disorders during the late adolescent/early adult years among individuals who had an earlier onset of the disorder. Specifically, in the sections that follow, we discuss a behavioral approach system (BAS) dysregulation perspective for understanding the course of BDs. We then describe and present findings to date from the Longitudinal Investigation of Bipolar Spectrum Disorders (LIBS) Project, a longitudinal study designed to investigate the course of bipolar spectrum disorders from a BAS perspective in college students with earlier onset (mean age of onset for first hypomanic or depressive episode or beginning of cyclothymic pattern, 13 years; median age, 14). However, whether our findings on the course of bipolar spectrum disorders in college students with earlier onset generalize to a sample with bipolar I must be examined directly.

We present descriptive findings on the course of bipolar spectrum disorders in our sample, findings regarding BAS-related risk factors affecting the course of these disorders, potential mediators of those risk factors, transactional processes affecting the course of these disorders, factors that influence differential outcomes and whether or not there is progression to a more severe disorder (multifinality) among individuals with bipolar spectrum disorders, and the role of developmental variables and early adversity in influencing the course of these disorders. We begin with a brief review of some of the literature regarding the course of BD in individuals with adolescent onset.

COURSE OF ADOLESCENT-ONSET BIPOLAR SPECTRUM DISORDERS

Bellivier and colleagues (Bellivier, Golmard, Henry, Leboyer, & Schurhoff, 2001; Bellivier et al., 2003) found that there are three high-risk periods for the onset of BD, with the earliest occurring in midadolescence. Other studies have also found that the first peak in rates of BD is between the ages of 15 and 19 (Burke, Burke, Regier, & Rae, 1990; Kennedy et al., 2005; Kessler, Rubinow, Holmes, Abelson, & Zhao, 1997; Kupfer et al., 2002; Weissman et al., 1996). Recent research indicates that BD may also exhibit prepubertal onset (see Meyer & Carlson, Chapter 2 and Youngstrom, Chapter 3, this volume); however, work on adolescent onset and exacerbation of BD is more relevant to the present chapter.

Evidence suggests that childhood- or adolescent-onset BD is associated with a worse course than adult-onset BD, including more irritability, higher lifetime suicidal ideation, increased comorbidity, and greater familial loading (e.g., Carter, Mundo, Parikh, & Kennedy, 2003; Ernst & Goldberg, 2004; Mick, Biederman, Faraone, Murray, & Wozniak, 2003; Suominen et al., 2007). Childhood- or adolescent-onset BD is also characterized by greater rapid cycling, greater chronicity, and more mixed states than adult-onset BD (Biederman et al., 2005; Geller et al.,

1995; Leibenluft, Charney, & Pine, 2003; Mick et al., 2003; Strober et al., 1988; Suominen et al., 2007). Moreover, adolescent- (and childhood-) onset BD increases risk for academic, social, and interpersonal problems (see Birmaher & Axelson, 2006, for a review and Birmaher et al., 2006, for contradictory results). These findings provide a context for the results reported later from the LIBS Project.

A BEHAVIORAL APPROACH SYSTEM DYSREGULATION MODEL OF BIPOLAR SPECTRUM DISORDERS

A BAS dysregulation model of bipolar spectrum disorders may provide an overarching, explanatory model for integrating risk factors, etiological, and transactional processes that influence the course of BDs. The BAS dysregulation model integrates specific psychosocial factors and specific neurobiological systems that may combine to affect the onset and course of BD. Moreover, the BAS model provides a single theme—level of approach motivation—to organize a diverse array of symptoms (e.g., motor, affective, cognitive, vegetative) and account for both poles of BD. According to the BAS dysregulation model, individuals with a bipolar spectrum disorder have a single vulnerability—a dysregulated BAS—but polarity-specific triggers for depressive and hypomanic/manic episodes (Urosevic, Abramson, Harmon-Jones, & Alloy, 2008).

The BAS is triggered by incentive cues in reward situations and functions to put an organism in contact with a reward or goal (e.g., Depue & Collins, 1992; Depue & Iacono, 1989; Fowles, 1987; Gray, 1991). At the behavioral level, central components of an activated BAS include locomotor initiation, incentive-reward motivation, positive affect, anger, and complex cognitions (e.g., Depue & Collins, 1999; Harmon-Jones & Allen, 1998; Harmon-Jones & Sigelman, 2001; see also Carver, 2004). Fowles's (1988) hypothesis that obstructed reward is a trigger for BAS-related irritability suggests that environmental cues likely influence whether a high BAS activation state is euphoric or irritable. On the other hand, an individual in a state of low BAS activation should experience anhedonia and decreased energy and exhibit few, if any, approach behaviors. In addition, Fowles (e.g., 1988, 1993) related a high outcome expectancy of success to BAS activation and hopelessness to BAS deactivation or shutdown.

With regard to neurobiology, Depue and colleagues (e.g., Depue & Collins, 1999; Depue & Iacono, 1989) hypothesized that the BAS involves the dopaminergic (DA) system, particularly the DA activity in the central nucleus accumbens and several frontal cortex regions. Much research in humans has focused on left frontal cortical activity as a neurobiological index of the BAS (for a review, see Davidson, 1994; Urosevic et al., 2008). Studies have found a significant positive relationship between increased relative left frontal cortical activity as measured by electroencephalogram (EEG) and higher self-report measures of BAS sensitivity (Harmon-Jones & Allen, 1997; Sutton & Davidson, 1997), experimentally manipulated reward motivational states (Miller & Tomarken, 2001; Sobotka, Davidson,

& Senulis, 1992), and a positive dispositional affective style (see Davidson, Jackson, & Kalin, 2000, for a review).

From a BAS dysregulation perspective, normal developmental changes that occur in the DA system at puberty (Chambers, Taylor, & Potenza, 2003; Spear, 2000) may be relevant to why BDs often develop or worsen during adolescence. In early adolescence, there is a significant increase in functional DA activity in the prefrontal cortex (PFC) (Rosenberg & Lewis, 1995; Sisk & Foster, 2004; Sisk & Zehr, 2005). This increase in circulating PFC dopamine levels may lead to greater sensitivity and efficiency of the brain's reward circuitry and thus to greater behavioral reward seeking and responsiveness (Steinberg, 2008). Indeed, behavioral sensation seeking and reward sensitivity were found to increase in youth from age 10 to midadolescence, peaking somewhere between ages 13 and 16 (Steinberg et al., 2009). Thus, some of the neurobiological circuitry implementing BAS functioning is enhanced beginning in early adolescence and may lead to increased BAS sensitivity.

According to the BAS dysregulation model of BD (Depue & Iacono, 1989; Depue, Krauss & Spoont, 1987; Johnson, 2005; Urosevic et al., 2008), individuals vulnerable to bipolar spectrum disorders exhibit an overly sensitive BAS that is hyperreactive to relevant cues and thus becomes dysregulated easily. Such BAS hypersensitivity should lead to great variability in state levels of BAS activation over time and across situations in response to BAS activating and deactivating stimuli. Thus, in response to BAS activation-relevant events involving goal striving and attainment, reward incentive, and anger evocation, a hypersensitive BAS can lead to excessive BAS activity. In vulnerable individuals, this excessive BAS activation, in turn, is hypothesized to lead to hypomanic/manic symptoms. In contrast, in response to BAS deactivation-relevant events involving definite failure and nonattainment of goals, excessive BAS deactivation or shutdown of behavioral approach should occur, leading to depressive symptoms. Such BAS vulnerability to dysregulation may be an endophenotype that mediates the effects of the genetic predisposition to BD. Moreover, according to Depue and colleagues (1987), individuals with bipolar spectrum disorders have genetically predetermined mean trait levels of BAS that predict which type of episode (depressive vs. hypomanic/manic) will predominate in the course of their BD.

In their expansion of the BAS dysregulation model of BDs, Urosevic and colleagues (2008) added a transactional component. In general, models including transactional processes allow bidirectional influences between various causal factors in the model. In Urosevic and colleagues' expanded BAS model, an individual's level of BAS activation before the occurrence of relevant environmental cues (i.e., pre-event BAS state) can result in selection or creation of environmental events (i.e., dependent BAS-relevant events) through a process of "stress generation" (Hammen, 1991) that affects subsequent changes in BAS activation. Thus, individuals with a highly sensitive BAS may be more likely to actually generate BAS activation and deactivation events in addition to being more emotionally and behaviorally responsive to such events when they occur.

THE LONGITUDINAL INVESTIGATION
OF BIPOLAR SPECTRUM DISORDERS PROJECT

The LIBS Project is a two-site (University of Wisconsin [UW], Temple University [TU]) longitudinal study that investigates the psychosocial, cognitive, and neu-robiological predictors of the course of bipolar spectrum disorders among 18- to 24-year-olds with earlier onset of their disorder. It primarily examines predictors of bipolar spectrum course from a BAS dysregulation model perspective. In the following sections, we describe the LIBS Project and many of its findings to date.

Participant Selection

Participants in the LIBS Project were selected via a two-phase screening pro-cess. In Phase I, approximately 20,500 18- to 24-year-old students at UW and TU were administered the revised General Behavior Inventory (GBI; Depue, Krauss, Spoont, & Arbisi, 1989), a first-stage case identification procedure for bipolar spectrum disorders, to identify potential bipolar spectrum and healthy compari-son participants. Using the GBI case-scoring method and cutoffs recommended by Depue and colleagues (1989), which were also validated against diagnostic interviews in a pilot study, participants who scored 11 or higher on the Depres-sion (D) scale and 13 or higher on the Hypomanic–Biphasic (HB) scale of the GBI were identified as potential bipolar spectrum individuals (high GBI), whereas those who scored below these cutoffs on the D and HB scales were identified as potential healthy controls (low GBI). Individuals who met these GBI criteria were invited for Phase II of screening, involving an expanded Schedule for Affective Disorders and Schizophrenia—Lifetime (exp-SADS-L; Endicott & Spitzer, 1978) diagnostic interview. High-GBI participants who met DSM-IV (American Psychi-atric Association, 1994) or Research Diagnostic Criteria (RDC; Spitzer, Endicott & Robins, 1978) for bipolar II, cyclothymia, or BD not otherwise specified (BD NOS; see Axelson et al., 2006, for validation of the bipolar NOS diagnosis in chil-dren and adolescents), but having no lifetime history of mania or mixed episode, were invited to participate in the main longitudinal study. Control participants invited into the longitudinal study exhibited low GBI scores and, based on the exp-SADS-L interview, had no lifetime history of any mood disorder or any other Axis I disorder (except that they could have a specific phobia) and no family his-tory of BD. The comparison participants were matched to the participants with BD on age, sex, and ethnicity.

The final LIBS Project sample included 200 participants with bipolar spec-trum disorder (78 men, 122 women; 157 with bipolar II and 43 with cyclothy-mic or BD NOS; age range = 18–24 years [M = 19.6 ± 1.6]). The bipolar sample was 68.9% Caucasian, 13.1% African American, 5.1% Hispanic, 3.6% Asian, 0.5% Native American, and 8.2% other. The final healthy comparison sample included 86 men and 122 women ages 18 to 24 years (mean 19.7 + 1.5 years); 72.8% were

Caucasian, 12.1% African American, 3.4% Hispanic, 4.4% Asian, 0.5% Native American, and 6.8% other.

Project Assessments and Design

After agreeing to participate in the longitudinal study, all participants completed a time 1 assessment that included self-report measures of depressive and hypomanic/manic symptoms; BAS sensitivity, impulsivity, and trait aggressiveness; cognitive and coping styles; and social rhythm regularity. At time 1, participants also completed a set of tasks designed to assess self-referent information processing and Axis II personality dysfunction. In addition, at time 1, participants completed a number of measures assessing developmental factors, including their parents' inferential feedback and parenting styles, their own childhood stressful life events, and childhood emotional, physical, and sexual maltreatment.

A subset of participants also completed two EEG sessions. In one session, EEG was recorded both in the resting state and in response to monetary reward and punishment trials on an anagram task (Harmon-Jones et al., 2008). The anagrams were divided into easy, medium, and hard difficulty blocks, with half of the anagrams in each difficulty block assigned to the reward condition and half to the punishment avoidance condition. After each anagram block, participants completed a questionnaire to assess current affective state. EEG was recorded from 14 (12 homologous and two midline) electrodes, placed on the midfrontal, lateral frontal, central, anterior temporal, posterior temporal, and parietal regions of the scalp. As in previous research (e.g., Harmon-Jones & Allen, 1998), a frontal asymmetry index was computed (for each anticipatory period [7 seconds prior to each anagram]), using midfrontal and lateral frontal sites. For comparison purposes, asymmetry indexes for the other sites were also computed. In the other session, EEG was recorded in the resting state and in response to an anger-induction scenario (a radio editorial proposed a tuition increase and the participants paid at least 33% of their own tuition).

Following time 1, participants were followed longitudinally for up to 7 years (average 4.54 years, $SD = 2.74$ years), with assessments occurring approximately every 4 months. At time 1 and each 4-month follow-up, interviewers were blind to participants' diagnostic group (bipolar spectrum vs. healthy control). During each 4-month assessment, participants were assessed for depressive and hypomanic/manic symptoms and diagnosable episodes, symptoms and diagnoses of other disorders, life events, inferences about those events, and social rhythms (patterns of daily activity and sleep–wake cycles). Symptoms and diagnosable episodes of depression, hypomania/mania, and other disorders were assessed at each 4-month follow-up with self-report measures and an expanded SADS-Change diagnostic interview (exp-SADS-C; Spitzer & Endicott, 1978; see Alloy et al., 2008, for expansion). The exp-SADS-C assessed onset, offset, duration, and severity of symptoms and episodes of Axis I disorders throughout the longitudinal phase.

To assess the occurrence of positive and negative life events over the past 4 months, participants were administered a combination of a self-report questionnaire (expanded Life Events Scale [LES]; Francis-Raniere, Alloy, & Abramson, 2006) and a semistructured interview (Life Events Interview [LEI]; Francis-Raniere et al., 2006). The LEI served as a reliability and validity check on the LES (Francis-Raniere et al., 2006) by providing explicit definitional criteria for what experiences counted as each event and a priori probes to determine whether the event definition criteria were met. If the event did not meet the definitional criteria, the event was designated as "does not qualify" and was not counted in final event totals. The interviewer also dated the occurrence of each event that did qualify and rated the objective impact of the event and the degree to which it disrupted social rhythms (social rhythm disruption [SRD] events).

DESCRIPTIVE FINDINGS ON THE COURSE OF BIPOLAR DISORDER IN THE LONGITUDINAL INVESTIGATION OF BIPOLAR SPECTRUM DISORDERS PROJECT

In this section, we present some general descriptive information about the course of bipolar spectrum disorders in the LIBS Project bipolar spectrum sample. The mean age of first onset of bipolar spectrum disorder (i.e., either bipolar II, cyclothymia, or BD NOS) for the entire bipolar sample was 13.12 (SD = 4.51) and the median age was 13.82. Of 43 participants with a cyclothymia or BD NOS diagnosis at the outset of the project (who already had exhibited at least one DSM-IV or RDC hypomanic episode), 32 (74.4%) converted to either a DSM-IV or an RDC bipolar II diagnosis (had a first onset of major depressive episode) over the longitudinal follow-up, whereas 5 (11.6%) converted to a bipolar I diagnosis (had a first onset of manic episode). Note that conversion to a bipolar II and bipolar I diagnosis among individuals with cyclothymia or BD NOS at the outset was not mutually exclusive. Of 157 participants with a DSM-IV or RDC bipolar II diagnosis at the outset of the project, 26 (16.6%) converted to a bipolar I diagnosis (had a first onset of manic episode) over the follow-up period. Combining the participants with a cyclothymia/BD NOS and a bipolar II diagnosis, 31 of 200 (15.4%) converted to a bipolar I diagnosis. The participants who progressed to bipolar I disorder had a significantly younger age at onset (M = 11.11, SD = 4.91) than those who did not progress to bipolar I (M = 13.48, SD = 4.35), whereas participants diagnosed with cyclothymia and BD NOS who progressed to bipolar II did not differ on age at onset (M = 13.87, SD = 4.89) with those who did not (M = 13.91, SD = 5.95). There were no differences in the likelihood of seeking treatment for mood-related issues between participants who did and did not progress to a more severe diagnosis; 70% of the bipolar spectrum group sought treatment for mood-related problems.

Overall, the rates of lifetime comorbid diagnoses among participants with bipolar spectrum disorder were as follows: 11% generalized anxiety disorder, 11%

TABLE 6.1. Predictors of Progression to a More Severe Bipolar Disorder among LIBS Project Participants During Prospective Follow-Up

Conversion to bipolar II diagnosis	Conversion to bipolar I diagnosis
Clinical predictors	Clinical predictors
No age-of-onset differences Comorbid alcohol abuse	Earlier age of onset Comorbid alcohol abuse Comorbid substance abuse Comorbid eating disorder not otherwise specified
Temperament/personality predictors	Temperament/personality predictors
Higher BAS sensitivity	Higher BAS sensitivity Higher impulsiveness Higher physical aggression

Note. This table summarizes predictors discovered to date. Further predictors of progression to more severe bipolar disorders may yet be found in further analyses of the LIBS Project data. BAS, behavioral approach system.

panic disorder, 28% specific and social phobia, 9% obsessive–compulsive disorder, 19% posttraumatic stress disorder, 10% anxiety disorder NOS, 24% alcohol abuse, 9% alcohol dependence, 29% substance abuse, 6% anorexia, 2% bulimia, and 6% eating disorder NOS. Participants with bipolar spectrum disorder who progressed to bipolar I had significantly higher rates of comorbid alcohol abuse (39% vs. 21%), substance abuse (45% vs. 26%), and eating disorder NOS (16% vs. 5%) than those who did not convert to bipolar I. Similarly, participants diagnosed with cyclothymia and BD NOS who progressed to bipolar II had marginally significantly higher rates of comorbid alcohol abuse (25% vs. 0%) than those who did not progress to bipolar II (the SADS-Change interviewers ruled out mood episodes that were specifically substance induced). Table 6.1 summarizes the predictors of progression to more severe BDs discovered in the LIBS Project sample to date.

RISK FACTORS INFLUENCING THE COURSE OF BIPOLAR SPECTRUM DISORDERS

In this section, we review findings from the LIBS Project regarding risk factors and transactional processes in the course of bipolar spectrum disorders (see Table 6.2 for a summary of these findings). Our review focuses on risk factors primarily from a BAS dysregulation model perspective.

Behavioral Approach System–Related Risk Factors

Directly relevant to the BAS dysregulation model, as part of the LIBS Project, Alloy and colleagues (2008) found that at time 1, controlling for depressive and hypomanic/manic symptoms, the bipolar spectrum group exhibited higher levels of

TABLE 6.2. Risk Factors, Mediators, and Moderators of Outcomes in the Course of Bipolar Spectrum Disorders in the LIBS Project

Risk factors	Outcomes
BAS-related risk factors	
High BAS sensitivity	Higher likelihood of lifetime BD diagnosis
	Higher likelihood and shorter time to onset of Hyp/Ma episodes (and of MD episodes for BAS-RR)
	Progression to BD II among participants with Cyc or BD NOS
	Progression to BD I among participants with BD II or Cyc
	Higher rates of BAS activation and deactivation life events
	Greater substance abuse problems
BAS-relevant cognitive styles	Higher likelihood of lifetime BD diagnosis
	Higher likelihood of Hyp/Ma episode onset (autonomy, self-criticism) and lower likelihood of MD episode onset (autonomy)
BAS-relevant life events	
BAS-activation life events	Higher likelihood of Hyp/Ma episode onset
	Increased relative left frontal cortical activation on EEG
BAS-deactivation life events	Higher likelihood of MD episodes
	Decreased relative left frontal cortical activation on EEG
Relative left frontal cortical activity (EEG)	Higher likelihood of lifetime BD diagnosis
	Higher likelihood of Hyp/Ma and MD episode onset
Social rhythm-related risk factors	
Low social rhythm regularity	Higher likelihood of lifetime BD diagnosis
	Shorter time to onset of Hyp/Ma and MD episodes
Social rhythm disruption events	Higher likelihood of MD episode onsets and symptoms
Developmental risk factors	
Childhood stressful life events	Higher likelihood of lifetime BD diagnosis
	Earlier age of first onset of BD
"Affectionless control" or critical parenting	Higher likelihood of lifetime BD diagnosis
	BAS-relevant cognitive styles
Childhood maltreatment	Higher likelihood of lifetime BD diagnosis
Moderators	
BAS-relevant life events	
BAS-activation life events	Higher likelihood of Hyp/Ma episode onsets (in interaction with high BAS sensitivity or BAS-relevant cognitive styles)
BAS-deactivation life events	Higher likelihood of MD episode onsets (in interaction with high BAS sensitivity or BAS-relevant cognitive styles)

(cont.)

TABLE 6.2. *(cont.)*

Risk factors	Outcomes
Low impulsivity	Higher academic achievement (in interaction with high BAS-Drive) Lower likelihood of progression to BD I (in interaction with high BAS sensitivity)
Mediators	
High impulsivity	Higher substance abuse problems (impulsivity mediates BD diagnosis and high BAS sensitivity)

Note. This table summarizes findings discovered to date. Further risk factors, moderators, and mediators may yet be found in further analyses of the LIBS Project data. Please see the text for more detailed description of these findings. BAS, behavioral approach system; RR, Reward Responsiveness subscale; BD, bipolar disorder; Cyc, cyclothymia; NOS, not otherwise specified; MD, major depressive; Hyp/Ma, hypomanic/manic; EEG, electroencephalogram.

self-reported BAS sensitivity on the BAS total and BAS Drive and Fun-Seeking subscales than the matched healthy comparison group. Other cross-sectional studies have also obtained higher self-reported BAS sensitivity as well as greater reward responsiveness on behavioral tasks, in both symptomatic and euthymic bipolar spectrum individuals compared with controls (for a review, see Alloy et al., 2008; Alloy, Abramson, Urosevic, et al., 2009). Using a behavioral high-risk design in an adjunctive part of the LIBS Project, Alloy, Abramson, Walshaw, and colleagues (2006) selected 18- to 24-year-old participants with high versus moderate levels of BAS sensitivity based on two self-report measures (behavioral inhibition system [BIS]/BAS Scales [Carver & White, 1994] and Sensitivity to Punishment Sensitivity to Reward Questionnaire [Torrubia, Avila, Molto, & Caseras, 2001]), blind to their symptom levels. These high- and moderate-BAS sensitivity individuals were administered the exp-SADS-L diagnostic interview used in the LIBS Project (Endicott & Spitzer, 1978) and measures of bipolar symptoms, hypomania proneness, and impulsivity. Alloy, Abramson, Walshaw, and colleagues found that the high-BAS sensitivity group was six times more likely to meet diagnostic criteria for a lifetime bipolar spectrum disorder than the moderate-BAS sensitivity group (50% vs. 8%), but the groups did not differ in their likelihood of a lifetime unipolar depression diagnosis (14% vs. 29%). The high-BAS group also had higher impulsivity and marginally higher GBI Hypomanic/Biphasic scores than the moderate BAS group. Higher BAS Reward Responsiveness subscale scores were also associated with higher hypomania proneness. The two groups did not differ on concurrent depressive or hypomanic symptoms. Finally, in the main LIBS Project, controlling for time 1 depressive and hypomanic symptoms, Alloy and colleagues (2008) reported that higher time 1 BAS total scores significantly predicted a greater likelihood and a shorter time to onset of hypomanic/manic episodes, but not depressive episodes, among the bipolar spectrum group over an average of 3 years of follow-up. Both time 1 BAS Reward Responsiveness and BIS scores marginally predicted ($p < .10$) shorter time to onset of major depressive episodes over the follow-up. Similarly, two other longitudinal studies (Meyer, Johnson, & Winters, 2001; Salavert et al., 2007) also found that initial higher BAS sensitivity predicted manic episode/symptom relapse over time.

Similar to other studies of individuals diagnosed as euthymic bipolar and individuals at risk for BD based on exhibiting hypomanic personality (for a review, see Alloy, Abramson, Urosevic, et al., 2009; Urosevic et al., 2008), Alloy, Abramson, Walshaw, and colleagues (2009) found that, controlling for time 1 depressive and hypomanic symptoms, the bipolar group in the LIBS Project exhibited a unique profile of BAS-relevant maladaptive cognitive styles (measured by the Dysfunctional Attitudes Scale [Weissman & Beck, 1978]; Sociotropy Autonomy Scales [Beck, Epstein, Harrison, & Emery, 1983]; and Depressive Experiences Questionnaire [Blatt, D'Afflitti, & Quinlan, 1976]) characterized by perfectionism, autonomy, and self-criticism relative to the healthy controls. However, the bipolar group did not show maladaptive dependency, sociotropy, or approval-seeking attitudes typically observed among unipolar depressed individuals. Moreover, time 1 BAS-relevant autonomous and self-critical cognitive styles, but not styles involving approval seeking, dependency, and sociotropy, predicted prospective onsets of hypomanic/manic and depressive episodes during an average of 3 years of follow-up among the bipolar spectrum group (Alloy, Abramson, Walshaw, et al., 2009). Lozano and Johnson (2001) also reported that the BAS-relevant trait of achievement-striving predicted increases in manic symptoms over 6 months in a sample with bipolar I disorder.

In line with the BAS dysregulation model, longitudinal studies found that life events involving goal striving or goal attainment that are hypothesized to activate the BAS specifically trigger hypomanic/manic symptoms and episodes among individuals with BD. In two studies, Johnson and colleagues (2000, 2008) found that events involving goal attainment predicted increases in manic, but not depressive, symptoms among patients with bipolar I disorder over follow-up, whereas general positive life events did not. In the LIBS Project, Nusslock, Abramson, Harmon-Jones, Alloy, and Hogan (2007) examined the effects of a goal-striving event (studying for and taking final exams) on the course of bipolar spectrum disorders. Bipolar symptoms were assessed during the final exam period and a control period in the bipolar spectrum and control groups, with each group further subdivided into those currently taking or not taking final exams. Individuals with BD taking exams, unlike those not taking exams and the whole control group, exhibited more onsets of new hypomanic episodes in the final exam period compared with the control period. Indeed, a full 42% of the bipolar spectrum individuals experienced onset of a new hypomanic episode during the final exam period. This pattern of results was not found for depressive episodes. In addition, consistent with the BAS model, over the first year of follow-up, we found that among the participants with bipolar spectrum disorder, controlling for initial depressive and hypomanic symptoms, BAS activation-relevant events (e.g., goal striving and attainment events) prospectively predicted increases in hypomanic symptoms, whereas BAS deactivation-relevant events (e.g., definite failures and losses) prospectively predicted increases in depressive symptoms.

In the LIBS Project, we found that BAS-relevant events also combined with BAS sensitivity and BAS-related maladaptive cognitive styles to predict prospective bipolar mood symptoms. In preliminary analyses, controlling for initial depressive and hypomanic symptoms, higher time 1 BAS sensitivity interacted with BAS activation-relevant events to prospectively predict increases in hypomanic symptoms, whereas it interacted with BAS deactivation-relevant events to prospectively predict increases in depressive symptoms over the first year of follow-up. Similarly, Francis-Raniere and colleagues (2006) reported that, controlling for initial symptom levels, time 1 BAS-relevant, self-critical, perfectionistic cognitive styles interacted with BAS-relevant negative events to predict prospective increases in depressive symptoms and with BAS-relevant positive events to predict prospective increases in hypomanic symptoms at the next 4-month assessment among participants with bipolar spectrum disorder.

In sum, BAS sensitivity, BAS-related cognitive styles, and the occurrence of BAS-relevant life events each predict prospectively a greater likelihood of mood symptoms or episodes or a shorter time to onset of mood episodes and thus a worse course among individuals with bipolar spectrum disorder. Moreover, BAS-activating and deactivating life events combined with BAS sensitivity and BAS-relevant cognitive styles to predict mood symptoms and episodes, suggesting that the BAS dysregulation model may be very promising for understanding processes that contribute to the course of BD.

Behavioral Approach System–Related Transactional Processes

An important component of the expanded BAS model of BDs discussed by Urosevic and colleagues (2008) is the transactional, bidirectional influences between BAS-related life events and bipolar symptoms. In the LIBS Project, Urosevic and colleagues (2009) found that individuals with bipolar spectrum disorder reported both BAS-activating and deactivating events at significantly greater rates than controls over the follow-up. Among the bipolar spectrum group, rates of BAS activation-relevant and deactivation-relevant events were significantly positively related to each other, suggesting that the same individuals with BD were experiencing high rates of both types of events. Thus, our participants with early-onset bipolar spectrum disorders may actually experience more BAS-activating and -deactivating life events through processes of stress generation (Hammen, 1991), which, in turn, trigger onsets of additional hypomanic/manic and depressive symptoms and episodes, respectively, as our findings described previously show.

In addition, Bender, Alloy, Sylvia, Urosevic, and Abramson (2009) further examined stress-generation processes using data from the first year of follow-up in the LIBS Project. Bender and colleagues found that higher time 1 hypomanic symptoms predicted greater subsequent occurrence of BAS-related positive and negative achievement events among males, whereas higher time 1 depressive symptoms predicted greater occurrence of positive and negative interpersonal events among females. These gender differences in stress-generation processes among individuals with bipolar spectrum disorder may contribute to the gender differences typically seen in the course of BD, in which men typically show a predominance of hypomania/mania, whereas women typically show a predominance of depression (e.g., Leibenluft, 1996; Rasgon et al., 2005).

Biopsychosocial Behavioral Approach System–Related Risk Factors

Findings from the LIBS Project also suggest that a neurobiological index of BAS activation may be a risk factor that could interact with psychosocial stressors to influence the course of BD. In the LIBS Project, our main neurobiological measure of BAS activation was obtained from assessment of participants' EEG in the resting state and in response to reward and punishment trials on an anagrams task and in response to an anger-induction manipulation. Prior work has shown that increased relative left frontal cortical EEG activity is a neurobiological index of BAS activation, whereas decreased relative left frontal EEG activity indicates BAS deactivation (Harmon-Jones & Allen, 1997; Sutton & Davidson, 1997).

According to the BAS dysregulation model, individuals with BD show an excessive increase in BAS activity in response to reward incentives, goal striving, and anger evocation. If an event is perceived as a "challenge" and elicits approach-motivated perceptions of successful coping, the BAS should be activated and hypomanic/manic symptoms may follow. Consistent with this hypothesis, in the LIBS Project, Harmon-Jones and colleagues (2008) obtained a significant three-way interaction between diagnostic group, anagram difficulty level, and type of trial (reward vs. punishment) in the anagram EEG session. Specifically, individuals with bipolar spectrum disorder exhibited greater relative left frontal cortical activation on EEG to a challenging goal-striving task (the difficult anagram trials) compared with healthy controls when they confronted a potential reward but not when they faced a potential punishment. That is, whereas controls disengaged from goal pursuit in response to the most difficult reward trials (and showed decreased relative left frontal cortical activation), individuals with BD maintained a heightened motivational state (and relative increased left frontal cortical activation) in this condition. This effect was specific to frontal EEG sites. These findings may indicate that individuals with BD get "stuck" in a state of goal pursuit and cannot regulate out of this state.

In the anger-induction EEG session, Harmon-Jones and colleagues (2002) reported that individuals with higher proneness to hypomania (on the GBI) exhibited greater relative left frontal cortical EEG activation in response to the anger manipulation, whereas those with higher proneness to depression (on the GBI) showed lower relative left frontal cortical activation in response to this anger-provoking manipulation. Thus, the same event triggered either increased or decreased BAS activation on EEG, depending on whether the individual was relatively more vulnerable to hypomania/mania or to depression.

Finally, there is preliminary evidence from the LIBS Project that relative left frontal EEG activation predicts prospective onsets of both hypomanic/manic and depressive episodes over the first 3 years of follow-up over and above the self-report BAS sensitivity measure. Future analyses from the LIBS Project could examine whether the EEG indices of BAS activation interact with naturally occurring BAS-activating and -deactivating events to affect onset and other characteristics of prospectively occurring mood episodes among individuals with BD.

Potential Mediators of Behavioral Approach System–Relevant Events: Social Rhythm Disruption

Events that disrupt daily social rhythms (e.g., meal times, sleep–wake times) have been found to trigger bipolar mood episodes in several studies (for a review, see Alloy et al., 2005; Alloy, Abramson, Urosevic, et al., 2009). For example, Malkoff-Schwartz and colleagues (1998, 2000) observed that manic episodes were significantly more likely to be preceded by SRD events than depressive episodes. SRD events are hypothesized to trigger bipolar mood episodes through destabilizing circadian rhythms (see Ehlers, Frank, & Kupfer, 1988; Grandin, Alloy, & Abramson, 2006, for reviews). In the LIBS Project, Sylvia and colleagues (2009) reported that during the first year of follow-up SRD events at each 4-month assessment predicted increased depressive symptoms at the next assessment. In addition, participants with bipolar spectrum disorder were more likely to experience an SRD event before a depressive episode than during a control period without a depressive episode, and they experienced more depressive symptoms after than before an SRD event. Thus, SRD events may increase the likelihood of depressive as well as hypomanic/manic episodes. Moreover, Shen and colleagues (2008) found that individuals with BD in the LIBS Project had less regular social rhythms than healthy controls at time 1 (as measured by the Social Rhythm Metric; Monk, Flaherty, Frank, Hoskinson, & Kupfer, 1990) and lower time 1 social rhythm regularity predicted a shorter time to onset of both hypomanic/manic and depressive episodes during an average of 33 months of prospective follow-up.

It is possible that social rhythm disruption may be one of the processes that mediate the effects of BAS dysregulation on BD course. For example, events involving a loss of a goal may trigger a dysregulated BAS response with SRD as one component of this dysregulated response (e.g., a person loses his or her job, responds with BAS deactivation, helplessness, and rumination, and as a result loses hours of sleep, thus disrupting social and circadian rhythms, leading to depressive symptoms). Future work with data from the LIBS Project will need to explicitly assess whether SRD is related to and mediates dysregulated BAS response in predicting bipolar mood symptoms.

DIFFERENTIAL OUTCOMES AMONG INDIVIDUALS
WITH BIPOLAR SPECTRUM DISORDERS

It is well known that BD is associated with functional impairment, including erratic work history, divorce, substance abuse, lower academic achievement, and increased suicide (e.g., Angst et al., 2002; Conway, Compton, Stinson, & Grant, 2006; Lagace & Kutcher, 2005; Strakowski et al., 2000). However, paradoxically, BD has also been associated with high levels of accomplishment (e.g., Coryell et al., 1989; Johnson, 2005; Petterson, 1977; Tsuchiya, 2004). There are also reports of high levels of creativity among individuals with bipolar spectrum disorders (Andreasen, 1987; Jamison, 1996; Richards et al., 1988; Simeonova, Chang, Strong, & Ketter, 2005). In addition, as described previously, some individuals in the LIBS Project with an initial cyclothymia or bipolar II diagnosis went on to develop a more severe disorder in the bipolar spectrum (i.e., converted to bipolar II or bipolar I diagnosis), whereas others did not and had a more stable course. These findings demonstrate the developmental concept of multifinality in that an initial diagnosis of a bipolar spectrum disorder can lead to either a stable or a worsening course and high levels of either impairment or achievement.

In the LIBS Project, we have begun to examine predictors of progression to a more severe bipolar diagnosis over the longitudinal follow-up period among participants with BD who initially had a milder diagnosis in the bipolar spectrum at the outset of the project (see Table 6.1 for a summary of these findings). To date, among participants with an initial cyclothymia (based on DSM-IV or RDC) or BD NOS diagnosis (at least one DSM-IV or RDC hypomanic episode), controlling for length of follow-up time, higher BAS total and Fun-Seeking and Reward Responsiveness subscale scores significantly predicted conversion to a bipolar II diagnosis (first onset of a major depressive episode) on follow-up (odds ratios: 1.75–2.10). Among individuals with a bipolar II, cyclothymia, or BD NOS diagnosis at the outset of the project, controlling for length of follow-up time, higher BAS total, impulsiveness (on the Impulsive Nonconformity Scale [Chapman et al., 1984]) and physical aggression (on the Buss Aggression Questionnaire [Buss & Perry, 1992]) all significantly predicted conversion to a bipolar I diagnosis (first onset of a manic episode) over the follow-up (odds ratio = 1.08). Thus, higher BAS sensitivity, impulsiveness, and physical aggressiveness predicted a worsening of course during early adulthood among individuals with a milder adolescent-onset bipolar spectrum disorder.

What factors may contribute to a course of bipolar spectrum disorder marked by greater impairment versus greater accomplishment? We have begun to address this question in the LIBS Project with respect to substance use problems and academic achievement. Given prior theorizing and research linking heightened reward sensitivity/drive (i.e., BAS sensitivity) to substance use and addiction (see Alloy, Bender, et al., 2009, for a review), and the fact that alcohol and drugs of abuse have rewarding properties, Alloy, Bender, and colleagues (2009) hypothesized that high BAS sensitivity may predict a course marked by greater substance use problems among individuals with bipolar spectrum disorders as well as partially mediate BD–substance use comorbidity. Also, Alloy, Bender, and colleagues predicted that higher impulsiveness, referring to a tendency toward behavior that is rash, lacks planning and foresight, and occurs without reflection or deliberation (Dawe & Loxton, 2004), might predict worse substance use problems among individuals with BD. Indeed, prior research found that high trait impulsivity has been associated with increased substance abuse, suicidal behavior, and higher rates of arrest among individuals with BD (Kwapil, Miller, Zinser, Chapman, & Eckblad, 2000; Swann et al., 2005, 2007). In the LIBS Project, BAS sensitivity and impulsiveness correlated at $r = .41$ with each other, indicating that, although related, they are distinct constructs. Consistent with the hypotheses, Alloy, Bender, and colleagues (2009) found that higher BAS total scores, BAS Fun-Seeking scores, and Impulsiveness scores each significantly predicted increased substance use problems over the first year of follow-up, controlling for lifetime history of substance use. Moreover, BAS total and Fun-Seeking scores partially mediated and Impulsiveness scores fully mediated the association between bipolar spectrum diagnosis and prospective substance use problems (bipolar spectrum diagnosis did not predict substance abuse once impulsiveness was covaried). Thus, lower impulsivity protected against substance use problems among individuals with BD. BAS sensitivity and impulsiveness did not interact to predict prospective substance use problems among the bipolar spectrum group.

Nusslock and colleagues (2008) further examined the role of BAS sensitivity and impulsiveness in predicting academic achievement. Academic transcripts were gathered for a subset of the LIBS Project sample (54 with bipolar spectrum disorder and 66 control participants). Individuals with bipolar spectrum disorder obtained a significantly lower cumulative grade point average (GPA), dropped more classes, and were more likely to withdraw from college either for a semester or permanently than healthy controls, controlling for number of semesters enrolled. In addition, among individuals with bipolar spectrum disorder, there was a significant interaction between BAS Drive subscale scores and impulsivity scores in predicting cumulative GPA. Individuals with BD exhibiting a combination of high BAS Drive and low impulsivity earned higher cumulative GPAs than the remaining participants with BD. Thus, high BAS sensitivity (specifically, BAS Drive), when paired with low impulsivity, may not be impairing and may contribute to the high achievement sometimes observed among individuals with BD.

Taken together, the studies described in this section suggest that differential outcomes (multifinality) for individuals with bipolar spectrum disorders may be at least partially due to their levels of trait BAS sensitivity, impulsivity, and physical aggression. High BAS sensitivity, impulsiveness, and physical aggressiveness may be predictive of a more negative course of BD in the form of greater likelihood of mood episodes (see Alloy et al., 2008), conversion to more severe bipolar diagnoses, and substance use problems (see Alloy, Bender, et al., 2009). However, when high BAS sensitivity is accompanied by the protective factor of low impulsivity, such high BAS sensitivity may actually contribute to higher achievement (Nusslock et al., 2008) and is associated with a lower likelihood of progression to bipolar I disorder. It makes sense that a tendency to be high in goal striving and approach motivation would be associated with relatively high achievement when combined with low impulsivity, which might prevent goal striving from getting out of control.

DEVELOPMENTAL FACTORS AND EARLY ADVERSITY IN BIPOLAR SPECTRUM DISORDERS

Research and theory suggest that exposure to certain parenting practices, childhood stressors, or maltreatment experiences may increase individuals' risk for onset and a more severe course of BD (see Alloy, Abramson, Smith, Gibb, & Neeren, 2006, for a review). Early adverse experiences and parenting practices may affect a person's development of emotion regulation strategies, which, in turn, may influence the course and expression of BD, given that emotion dysregulation is a central feature of the disorder. In the LIBS Project, we have begun to examine the role of such developmental factors in the onset and course of bipolar spectrum disorders.

Grandin, Alloy, and Abramson (2007) examined the association between childhood stressors that were independent or dependent on an individual's behavior and eventual bipolar spectrum diagnosis. Grandin et al. reasoned that if childhood adversity contributes to the emergence of bipolar symptoms, then independent childhood stressful events occurring before the age of onset of participants' bipolar spectrum disorder would be associated with bipolar versus healthy control status, and a greater number of independent childhood stressors would be associated with an earlier age of onset of BD. Grandin and colleagues found that, controlling for family history of BD, age at BD onset, and depressive and hypomanic symptoms at the time participants reported their childhood stressors (at time 1), a higher number of pre-onset, independent stressful events was associated with a bipolar versus control diagnosis. Moreover, controlling for family history of BD and time 1 depressive and hypomanic symptoms, the more total childhood stressors, as well as independent, dependent, negative emotional, and achievement failure events participants with BD experienced, the younger they were when they had their first bipolar mood episode. Whereas independent events might help to directly bring about an earlier onset of a bipolar mood episode, dependent events may do so through indirect stress-generation processes. Prodromal or early-occurring symptoms of bipolarity or a highly sensitive BAS temperament may lead to the occurrence of the dependent events via stress generation, and then these events, in turn, may have increased the likelihood of an earlier onset of a full-blown affective episode.

Neeren, Alloy, and Abramson (2008) examined reported histories of negative parenting and parental maltreatment in the bipolar spectrum and healthy comparison groups. Controlling for family history of mood disorder and concurrent (time 1) depressive and hypomanic/manic symptoms, low levels of maternal warmth/acceptance and high levels of maternal and paternal negative psychological control (the "affectionless control" pattern identified by Parker [1983]) were associated with a bipolar spectrum diagnosis. In addition, controlling for family history of mood disorder and concurrent symptoms, and counting only experiences of maltreatment that occurred before the age of onset of BD, higher levels of emotional maltreatment by mothers and fathers and higher levels of physical maltreatment by mothers were associated with a bipolar spectrum diagnosis.

Wagner, Alloy, and Abramson (2009) followed up on the Neeren and colleagues findings by examining the association of critical parenting with bipolar status, course of illness, and BAS-relevant cognitive styles. Wagner and colleagues reasoned that parenting that is overtly critical may be especially likely to exacerbate BAS sensitivity and contribute to the development of a self-critical, perfectionistic cognitive style in offspring, the type of style that several studies, including our own (Alloy, Abramson, Walshaw, et al., 2009), suggest characterizes individuals with BD. Controlling for family history of mood disorders and time 1 depressive and hypomanic/manic symptoms, higher reported critical parenting by both mothers and fathers was associated with a bipolar versus control diagnosis and with BAS-relevant cognitive styles of higher perfectionism and autonomy but not with the BAS-irrelevant cognitive styles of approval seeking or sociotropy. However, critical parenting did not predict prospective occurrence (yes–no) of major depressive or hypomanic/manic episodes. It may be that parenting is related to vulnerability to BD but not episode recurrence. Alternatively, analyses that examine whether parenting predicts other aspects of BD course such as fluctuations in symptoms, time to onset of episodes, or episode number, severity, or duration might yield different results. It is also possible that critical parenting did not predict episode recurrence during the college years because the college students were no longer exposed to their parents as regularly. In addition, future studies would benefit by assessing parenting styles using behavioral observation rather than relying solely on self-reports of individuals with BD (see Alloy, Abramson, Smith, et al., 2006).

In sum, to date, the LIBS Project findings regarding developmental experiences in BD suggest that early childhood stressors, childhood emotional and physical maltreatment, and parenting characterized by low affection, high psychological control, and high criticism are associated with a bipolar spectrum diagnosis. In addition, critical parenting is specifically associated with greater BAS-relevant cognitive styles. Moreover, higher numbers of childhood stressors predict an earlier age of onset of bipolar spectrum disorder. Further analyses with LIBS Project data will examine whether aspects of parenting or early adversity (childhood stressors or maltreatment experiences) predict characteristics of the course of BD.

CONCLUSION

Much research remains to be conducted regarding the course of adolescent bipolar spectrum disorders. However, work to date from the LIBS Project has yielded much valuable information on risk factors, possible mechanisms, transactional processes, and differential outcomes in BDs from a BAS dysregulation perspective. It should be noted, though, that the findings from the LIBS Project may or may not generalize to clinical samples or to individuals with bipolar I disorder. First, our descriptive findings regarding age at onset (mean = 13.12 years) and rates of progression to more severe disorders (74.4% individuals diagnosed as cyclothymic or BD NOS progressed to bipolar II, and 15.4% of individuals diagnosed as bipolar II, cyclothymic, and BD NOS progressed to bipolar I disorder) in the bipolar spectrum are generally consistent with other findings in the literature (e.g., Akiskal et al., 1977, 1979; Birmaher et al., 2006). Second, as predicted by a BAS dysregulation model of BD, high BAS sensitivity and activation, as assessed by self-report and EEG, greater BAS-relevant cognitive styles, and BAS-relevant life events, each predicts a greater likelihood or shorter time to occurrence of bipolar mood episodes and symptoms, alone and in combination (BAS sensitivity or BAS-relevant cognitive styles in interaction with BAS-relevant life events). High BAS sensitivity also predicts progression to bipolar II disorder among individuals with cyclothymia or BD NOS and progression to bipolar I disorder among individuals with bipolar II or cyclothymia. Third, consistent with the transactional part of the BAS dysregulation model, our findings suggest that individuals with bipolar spectrum disorders may be more likely to actually generate the kinds of BAS activation and deactivation events that, in turn, worsen the course of their disorder. Thus, individuals with BD may be both more likely to experience and more reactive than other individuals to the sorts of environmental triggers that contribute to their symptoms.

Fourth, our developmental findings to date suggest that early BAS-relevant critical parenting along with low affection and early childhood stressors and maltreatment may also contribute to the risk for bipolar spectrum disorder and earlier onset of BD, as well as maladaptive BAS-relevant cognitive styles in offspring. Finally, high BAS sensitivity in combination with high versus low impulsiveness and aggressiveness may help explain which individuals with a bipolar spectrum disorder have a more negative course (progression to bipolar I, greater substance use problems, poor achievement) and which have more positive outcomes (less likelihood of progression to a more severe disorder, fewer substance use problems, high achievement).

In conclusion, the findings reviewed here suggest that the BAS dysregulation model is very promising for integrating psychosocial and neurobiological vulnerability factors and mechanisms involved in the onset and course of bipolar spectrum disorders. Moreover, the BAS dysregulation model suggests strategies for improving the effectiveness of various psychosocial interventions for BD (see Nusslock, Abramson, Harmon-Jones, Alloy, & Coan, 2009), as well as potential novel interventions that manipulate BAS activation by manipulating left versus right frontal cortical activation (Harmon-Jones, 2006; Peterson, Shackman, & Harmon-Jones, 2008). It is hoped the evidence reviewed here sets the foundation for further research on the onset and course of BDs from a BAS dysregulation perspective.

ACKNOWLEDGMENTS

Preparation of this chapter was supported by National Institute of Mental Health Grant Nos. MH 52617 and MH 077908 to Lauren B. Alloy and 52662 to Lyn Y. Abramson.

REFERENCES

Akiskal, H. S., Djenderedjian, A. H., Rosenthal, R. H., & Khani, M. K. (1977). Cyclothymic disorder: Validating criteria for inclusion in the bipolar affective group. *American Journal of Psychiatry, 134,* 1227–1233.

Akiskal, H. S., Khani, M. K., & Scott-Strauss, A. (1979). Cyclothymic temperamental disorders. *Psychiatric Clinics of North America, 2,* 527–554.

Alloy, L. B., Abramson, L. Y., Smith, J. B., Gibb, B. E., & Neeren, A. M. (2006). Role of parenting and maltreatment histories in unipolar and bipolar mood disorders: Mediation by cognitive vulnerability to depression. *Clinical Child and Family Psychology Review, 9,* 23–64.

Alloy, L. B., Abramson, L. Y., Urosevic, S., Bender, R. E., & Wagner, C. A. (2009). Longitudinal predictors of bipolar spectrum disorders: A behavioral approach system (BAS) perspective. *Clinical Psychology: Science and Practice, 16,* 206–226.

Alloy, L. B., Abramson, L. Y., Urosevic, S., Walshaw, P. D., Nusslock, R., & Neeren, A. M. (2005). The psychosocial context of bipolar disorder: Environmental, cognitive, and developmental risk factors. *Clinical Psychology Review, 25,* 1043–1075.

Alloy, L. B., Abramson, L. Y., Walshaw, P. D., Cogswell, A., Smith, J. M., Neeren, A. M., et al. (2006). Behavioral approach system (BAS) sensitivity and bipolar spectrum disorders: A retrospective and concurrent behavioral high-risk design. *Motivation and Emotion, 30,* 143–155.

Alloy, L. B., Abramson, L. Y., Walshaw, P. D., Cogswell, A., Sylvia, L. G., Hughes, M. E., et al. (2008). Behavioral approach system (BAS) and behavioral inhibition system (BIS) sensitivities and bipolar spectrum disorders: Prospective prediction of bipolar mood episodes. *Bipolar Disorders, 10,* 310–322.

Alloy, L. B., Abramson, L. Y., Walshaw, P. D., Gerstein, R. K., Keyser, J. D., Whitehouse, W. G., et al. (2009). Behavioral approach system (BAS)—relevant cognitive styles and bipolar spectrum disorders: Concurrent and prospective associations. *Journal of Abnormal Psychology, 118,* 459–471.

Alloy, L. B., Abramson, L. Y., Walshaw, P. D., Keyser, J., & Gerstein, R. K. (2006). A cognitive vulnerability-stress perspective on bipolar spectrum disorders in a normative adolescent brain, cognitive, and emotional development context. *Development and Psychopathology, 18,* 1055–1103.

Alloy, L. B., Bender, R. E., Wagner, C. A., Whitehouse, W. G., Abramson, L. Y., Hogan, M. E., et al. (2009). Bipolar spectrum–substance use comorbidity: Behavioral approach system (BAS) sensitivity and impulsiveness as shared personality vulnerabilities. *Journal of Personality and Social Psychology, 97,* 549–565.

American Psychiatric Association. (1994). *Diagnostic and statistical manual of mental disorders* (4th ed.). Washington, DC: Author.

Andreasen, N. C. (1987). Creativity and mental illness: Prevalence rates in writers and their first-degree relatives. *American Journal of Psychiatry, 144,* 1288–1292.

Angst, F., Stassen, H. H., Clayton, P. J., & Angst, J. (2002). Mortality of patients with mood disorders: Follow-up over 34–38 years. *Journal of Affective Disorders, 68,* 167–181.

Axelson, D., Birmaher, B., Strober, M., Gill, M. K., Valeri, S., Chiappetta, L., et al. (2006). Phenomenology of children and adolescents with bipolar spectrum disorders. *Archives of General Psychiatry, 63,* 1139–1148.

Baldessarini, R. J. (2000). A plea for integrity of the bipolar disorder concept. *Bipolar Disorders, 2,* 3–7.

Beck, A. T., Epstein, N., Harrison, R. P., & Emery, G. (1983). *Development of the Sociotropy-Autonomy Scale: A measure of personality factors in depression.* Unpublished manuscript, University of Pennsylvania Center for Cognitive Therapy.

Bellivier, F., Golmard, J. L., Henry, C., Leboyer, M., & Schurhoff, F. (2001). Admixture analysis of age at onset in bipolar I affective disorder. *Archives of General Psychiatry, 58,* 510–512.

Bellivier, F., Golmard, J. L., Rietschel, M., Schulze, T. G., Malafosse, A., Preisig, M., et al. (2003). Age at onset in bipolar I affective disorder: Further evidence for three subgroups. *American Journal of Psychiatry, 160,* 999–1001.

Bender, R. E., Alloy, L. B., Sylvia, L. G., Urosevic, S., & Abramson, L. Y. (2009). *Generation of life events in bipolar disorder: A replication and extension of the stress generation theory.* Manuscript submitted for publication.

Biederman, J., Faraone, S. V., Wozniak, J., Mick, E., Kwon, A., Cayton, G., et al. (2005). Clinical correlates of bipolar disorder in a large, referred sample of children and adolescents. *Journal of Psychiatric Research, 39,* 611–622.

Birmaher, B., & Axelson, D. (2006). Course and outcome of bipolar spectrum disorder in children and adolescents: A review of the existing literature. *Development and Psychopathology, S18,* 1023–1035.

Birmaher, B., Axelson, D., Strober, M., Gill, M. K., Valeri, S., Chiappetta, L., et al. (2006). Clinical course of children and adolescents with bipolar spectrum disorders. *Archives of General Psychiatry, 63,* 175–183.

Blatt, S. J., D'Afflitti, J. P., & Quinlan, D. M. (1976). Experiences of depression in normal young adults. *Journal of Abnormal Psychology, 85,* 383–389.

Burke, K. C., Burke, J. D., Regier, D. A., & Rae, D. S. (1990). Age at onset of selected mental disorders in five community populations. *Archives of General Psychiatry, 47,* 511–518.

Buss, A. H., & Perry, M. (1992). The Aggression Questionnaire. *Journal of Personality and Social Psychology, 63,* 452–459.

Carter, T. D., Mundo, E., Parikh, S. V., & Kennedy, J. L. (2003). Early age at onset as a risk factor for poor outcome of bipolar disorder. *Journal of Psychiatric Research, 37,* 297–303.

Carver, C. S. (2004). Negative affect deriving from the behavioral approach system. *Emotion, 4,* 3–22.

Carver, C. S., & White, T. L. (1994). Behavioral inhibition, behavioral activation, and affective responses to impending reward and punishment: The BIS/BAS scales. *Journal of Personality and Social Psychology, 67,* 319–333.

Cassano, G. B., Dell'Osso, L., Frank, E., Miniati, M., Fagiolini, A., Shear, K., et al. (1999). The bipolar spectrum: A clinical reality in search of diagnostic criteria and an assessment methodology. *Journal of Affective Disorders, 54,* 319–328.

Chambers, R., Taylor, J., & Potenza, M. (2003). Developmental neurocircuitry of motivation in adolescence: A critical period of addiction vulnerability. *American Journal of Psychiatry, 160,* 1041–1052.

Chapman, L. J., Chapman, J. P., Numbers, J. S., Edell, W. S., Carpenter, B. N., & Beckfield, D. (1984). Impulsive nonconformity as a trait contributing to the prediction of psychotic-like and schizotypal symptoms. *Journal of Nervous and Mental Disease, 172,* 681–691.

Conway, K. P., Compton, W., Stinson, F. S., & Grant, B. F. (2006). Lifetime comorbidity of DSM-IV mood and anxiety disorders and specific drug use disorders: Results from the National Epidemiologic Survey on Alcohol and Related Conditions. *Journal of Clinical Psychiatry, 67,* 247–257.

Coryell, W., Endicott, J., Keller, M., Andreasen, N., Grove, W., Hirschfeld, R. M. A., et al. (1989). Bipolar affective disorder and high achievement: A familial association. *American Journal of Psychiatry, 146,* 983–988.

Davidson, R. J. (1994). Cerebral asymmetry, emotion, and affective style. In P. Ekman & R. J. Davidson (Eds.), *The nature of emotion: Fundamental questions* (pp. 329–331). New York: Oxford University Press.

Davidson, R. J., Jackson, D. C., & Kalin, N. H. (2000). Emotion, plasticity, context, and regulation: Perspectives from affective neuroscience. *Psychological Bulletin, 126,* 890–909.

Dawe, S., & Loxton, N. J. (2004). The role of impulsivity in the development of substance use and eating disorders. *Neuroscience and Biobehavioral Reviews, 28,* 343–351.

Depue, R. A., & Collins, P. F. (1992). A neurobehavioral system approach to developmental psychopathology: Implications for disorders of affect. In D. Cicchetti & S. L. Toth (Eds.), *Rochester Symposium on Developmental Psychopathology: Vol. 4. Developmental perspectives on depression* (pp. 29–101). Rochester, NY: University of Rochester Press.

Depue, R. A., & Collins, P. F. (1999). Neurobiology of the structure of personality: Dopamine, facilitation of incentive motivation, and extraversion. *Behavioral and Brain Sciences, 22,* 491–569.

Depue, R. A., & Iacono, W. G. (1989). Neurobehavioral aspects of affective disorders. *Annual Review of Psychology, 40,* 457–492.

Depue, R. A., Krauss, S., & Spoont, M. (1987). A two-dimensional threshold model of seasonal bipolar affective disorder. In D. Magnusson & A. Ohman (Eds.), *Psychopathology: An interactional perspective* (pp. 95–123). New York: Academic Press.

Depue, R. A., Krauss, S. P., Spoont, M. R., & Arbisi, P. (1989). General Behavior Inventory identification of unipolar and bipolar affective conditions in a nonclinical population. *Journal of Abnormal Psychology, 98,* 117–126.

Depue, R. A., Slater, J., Wolfstetter-Kausch, H., Klein, D., Goplerud, E., & Farr, D. (1981). A behavioral paradigm for identifying persons at risk for bipolar depressive disorder: A conceptual framework and five validation studies (monograph). *Journal of Abnormal Psychology, 90,* 381–437.

Ehlers, C. L., Frank, E., & Kupfer, D. J. (1988). Social zeitgebers and biological rhythms: A unified approach to understanding the etiology of depression. *Archives of General Psychiatry, 45,* 948–952.

Endicott, J., & Spitzer, R. L. (1978). A diagnostic interview: The Schedule of Affective Disorders and Schizophrenia. *Archives of General Psychiatry, 35,* 837–844.

Ernst, C. L., & Goldberg, J. F. (2004). Clinical features related to age at onset in bipolar disorder. *Journal of Affective Disorders, 82,* 21–27.

Fowles, D. C. (1987). Application of a behavioral theory of motivation to the concepts of anxiety and impulsivity. *Journal of Research in Personality, 21,* 417–435.

Fowles, D. C. (1988). Presidential Address, 1987. Psychophysiology and psychopathology: A motivational approach. *Psychophysiology, 25,* 373–391.

Fowles, D. C. (1993). Biological variables in psychopathology: A psychobiological perspective. In P. B. Sutker & H. E. Adams (Eds.), *Comprehensive handbook of psychopathology* (2nd ed., pp. 57–82). New York: Plenum Press.

Francis-Raniere, E., Alloy, L. B., & Abramson, L. Y. (2006). Depressive personality styles and bipolar spectrum disorders: Prospective tests of the event congruency hypothesis. *Bipolar Disorders, 8*, 382–399.

Geller, B., Sun, K., Zimerman, B., Luby, J., Frazier, J., & Williams, M. (1995). Complex and rapid-cycling in bipolar children and adolescents: A preliminary study. *Journal of Affective Disorders, 18*, 259–268.

Goodwin, F. K., & Jamison, K. R. (2007). *Manic-depressive illness* (2nd ed.). New York: Oxford University Press.

Grandin, L. D., Alloy, L. B., & Abramson, L. Y. (2006). The social zeitgeber theory, circadian rhythms, and mood disorders: Review and evaluation. *Clinical Psychology Review, 26*, 679–694.

Grandin, L. D., Alloy, L. B., & Abramson, L. Y. (2007). Childhood stressful life events and bipolar spectrum disorders. *Journal of Social and Clinical Psychology, 26*, 460–478.

Gray, J. A. (1991). Neural systems, emotion and personality. In J. Madden IV (Ed.), *Neurobiology of learning, emotion and affect* (pp. 273–306). New York: Raven Press.

Hammen, C. (1991). Generation of stress in the course of unipolar depression. *Journal of Abnormal Psychology, 100*, 555–561.

Harmon-Jones, E. (2006). Unilateral right-hand contractions cause contralateral alpha power suppression and approach motivational affective experience. *Psychophysiology, 43*, 598–603.

Harmon-Jones, E., Abramson, L. Y., Nusslock, R., Sigelman, J. D., Urosevic, S., Turonie, L. D., et al. (2008). Effect of bipolar disorder on left frontal cortical responses to goals differing in valence and task difficulty. *Biological Psychiatry, 63*, 693–698.

Harmon-Jones, E., Abramson, L. Y., Sigelman, J. D., Bohlig, A., Hogan, M. E., & Harmon-Jones, C. (2002). Proneness to hypomania/mania symptoms or depression symptoms and asymmetrical frontal cortical responses to an anger-evoking event. *Journal of Personality and Social Psychology, 82*, 610–618.

Harmon-Jones, E., & Allen, J. J. B. (1997). Behavioral activation sensitivity and resting frontal EEG asymmetry: Covariation of putative indicators related to risk for mood disorders. *Journal of Abnormal Psychology, 106*, 159–163.

Harmon-Jones, E., & Allen, J. J. B. (1998). Anger and prefrontal brain activity: EEG asymmetry consistent with approach motivation despite negative affect valence. *Journal of Personality and Social Psychology, 74*, 1310–1316.

Harmon-Jones, E., & Sigelman, J. D. (2001). State anger and prefrontal brain activity: Evidence that insult-related relative left prefrontal activity is associated with experienced anger and aggression. *Journal of Personality and Social Psychology, 80*, 797–803.

Jamison, K. R. (1996). *Touched with fire: Manic-depressive illness and the artistic temperament.* New York: Free Press.

Johnson, S. L. (2005). Mania and dysregulation in goal pursuit: A review. *Clinical Psychology Review, 25*, 241–262.

Johnson, S. L., Cueller, A. K., Ruggero, C., Winett-Perlman, C., Goodnick, P., White, R., et al. (2008). Life events as predictors of mania and depression in bipolar I disorder. *Journal of Abnormal Psychology, 117*, 268–277.

Johnson, S. L., Sandrow, D., Meyer, B., Winters, R., Miller, I., Solomon, D., et al. (2000). Increases in manic symptoms after life events involving goal attainment. *Journal of Abnormal Psychology, 109*, 721–727.

Kennedy, N., Boydell, J., Kalidindi, S., Fearon, P., Jones, P. B., van Os, J., et al. (2005). Gender differences in incidence and age at onset of mania and bipolar disorder over a 35-year period in Camberwell, England. *American Journal of Psychiatry, 162*, 257–262.

Kessler, R. C., Rubinow, D. R., Holmes, C., Abelson, J. M., & Zhao, S. (1997). The epidemiology of DSM-III-R bipolar I disorder in a general population survey. *Psychological Medicine, 27,* 1079–1089.

Kupfer, D. J., Frank, E., Grochocinski, V. J., Cluss, P. A., Houck, P. R., & Stapf, D. A. (2002). Demographic and clinical characteristics of individuals in a bipolar disorder case registry. *Journal of Clinical Psychiatry, 63,* 120–125.

Kutcher, S., Robertson, H. A., & Bird, D. (1990). Premorbid functioning in adolescent onset bipolar I disorder: A preliminary report from an ongoing study. *Journal of Affective Disorders, 51,* 137–144.

Kwapil, T. R., Miller, M. B., Zinser, M. C., Chapman, L. J., & Eckblad, M. (2000). A longitudinal study of high scorers on the Hypomanic Personality Scale. *Journal of Abnormal Psychology, 109,* 222–226.

Lagace, D. C., & Kutcher, S. P. (2005). Academic performance of adolescents with bipolar disorder. *Directions in Psychiatry, 25,* 111–117.

Leibenluft, E. (1996). Women with bipolar illness: Clinical and research issues. *American Journal of Psychiatry, 153,* 163–173.

Leibenluft, E., Charney, D. S., & Pine, D. S. (2003). Researching the pathophysiology of pediatric bipolar disorder. *Biological Psychiatry, 53,* 1009–1020.

Lozano, B. E., & Johnson, S. L. (2001). Can personality traits predict increases in manic and depressive symptoms? *Journal of Affective Disorders, 63,* 103–111.

Malkoff-Schwartz, S., Frank, E., Anderson, B. P., Hlastala, S. A., Luther, J. F., Sherrill, J. T., et al. (2000). Social rhythm disruption and stressful life events in the onset of bipolar and unipolar episodes. *Psychological Medicine, 30,* 1005–1010.

Malkoff-Schwartz, S., Frank, E., Anderson, B. P., Sherrill, J. T., Siegel, L., Patterson, D., et al. (1998). Stressful life events and social rhythm disruption in the onset of manic and depressive bipolar episodes: A preliminary investigation. *Archives of General Psychiatry, 55,* 702–707.

McGuffin, P., Rijsdijk, F., Andrew, M., Sham, P., Katz, R., & Cardno, A. (2003). The heritability of bipolar affective disorder and the genetic relationship to unipolar depression. *Archives of General Psychiatry, 60,* 497–502.

Merikangas, K. R., Chakravarti, A., Moldin, S. O., Araj, H., Blangero, J. C., Burmeister, M., et al. (2002). Future of genetics of mood disorders research. *Biological Psychiatry, 52,* 457–477.

Meyer, B., Johnson, S. L., & Winters, R. (2001). Responsiveness to threat and incentive in bipolar disorder: Relations of the BIS/BAS scales with symptoms. *Journal of Psychopathology and Behavioral Assessment, 23,* 133–143.

Mick, E., Biederman, M. D., Faraone, S. V., Murray, K., & Wozniak, J. (2003). Defining a developmental subtype of bipolar disorder in a sample of nonreferred adults by age of onset. *Journal of Child and Adolescent Psychopharmacology, 13,* 453–462.

Miller, A., & Tomarken, A. J. (2001). Task-dependent changes in frontal brain asymmetry: Effects of incentive cues, outcome expectancies, and motor responses. *Psychophysiology, 38,* 500–511.

Monk, T. H., Flaherty, J. F., Frank, E., Hoskinson, K., & Kupfer, D. J. (1990). The Social Rhythm Metric: An instrument to quantify the daily rhythms of life. *Journal of Nervous and Mental Disease, 178,* 120–126.

Neeren, A. M., Alloy, L. B., & Abramson, L. Y. (2008). History of parenting and bipolar spectrum disorders. *Journal of Social and Clinical Psychology, 27,* 1021–1044.

Nolen-Hoeksema, S., Morrow, J., & Fredrickson, B. L. (1993). Response styles and the duration of episodes of depressed mood. *Journal of Abnormal Psychology, 101,* 20–28.

Nusslock, R., Abramson, L. Y., Harmon-Jones, E., Alloy, L. B., & Coan, J. A. (2009). Psychoso-cial interventions for bipolar disorder: Perspective from the Behavioral Approach System (BAS) dysregulation theory. *Clinical Psychology: Science and Practice, 16,* 449–469.

Nusslock, R., Abramson, L. Y., Harmon-Jones, E., Alloy, L. B., & Hogan, M. E. (2007). A goal-striving life event and the onset of bipolar episodes: Perspective from the behav-ioral approach system (BAS) dysregulation theory. *Journal of Abnormal Psychology, 116,* 105–115.

Nusslock, R., Alloy, L. B., Abramson, L. Y., Harmon-Jones, E., & Hogan, M. E. (2008). Impair-ment in the achievement domain in bipolar spectrum disorders: Role of behavioral approach system (BAS) hypersensitivity and impulsivity. *Minerva Pediatrica, 60,* 41–50.

Parker, G. (1983). Parental "affectionless control" as an antecedent to adult depression. *Archives of General Psychiatry, 34,* 138–147.

Peterson, C. K., Shackman, A. J., & Harmon-Jones, E. (2008). The role of asymmetrical corti-cal activity in aggression. *Psychophysiology, 45,* 86–92.

Petterson, U. (1977). Manic-depressive illness: Investigation of social factors. *Acta Psychiatrica Scandinavica, 269,* 43–54.

Rasgon, N., Bauer, M., Grof, P., Gyulai, L., Elman, S., Glenn, T., et al. (2005). Sex-specific self-reported mood changes by patients with bipolar disorder. *Journal of Psychiatric Research, 39,* 77–83.

Richards, R., Kinney, D. K., Lunde, I., Benet, M., & Merzel, A. P. (1988). Creativity in manic-depressives, cyclothymes, their normal relatives, and control subjects. *Journal of Abnor-mal Psychology, 97,* 281–288.

Rosenberg, D., & Lewis, D. (1995). Postnatal maturation of the dopaminergic innervation of monkey prefrontal and motor cortices: A tyrosine hydroxylase immunohistochemical analysis. *Journal of Comparative Neurology, 358,* 383–400.

Salavert, J., Caseras, X., Torrubia, R., Furest, S., Arranz, B., Duenas, R., et al. (2007). The functioning of the behavioral activation and inhibition systems in bipolar I euthymic patients and its influence in subsequent episodes over an 18-month period. *Personality and Individual Differences, 42,* 1323–1331.

Shen, G. C., Alloy, L. B., Abramson, L. Y., & Sylvia, L. G. (2008). Social rhythm regularity and the onset of affective episodes in bipolar spectrum individuals. *Bipolar Disorders, 10,* 520–529.

Simeonova, D. I., Chang, K. D., Strong, C., & Ketter, T. A. (2005). Creativity in familial bipolar disorder. *Journal of Psychiatric Research, 39,* 623–631.

Sisk, C., & Foster, D. (2004). The neural basis of puberty and adolescence. *Nature Neurosci-ence, 7,* 1040–1047.

Sisk, C., & Zehr, J. (2005). Pubertal hormones organize the adolescent brain and behavior. *Frontiers in Neuroendocrinology, 26,* 163–174.

Sobotka, S. S., Davidson, R. J., & Senulis, J. A. (1992). Anterior brain asymmetries in response to reward and punishment. *Electroencephalography and Clinical Neurophysiology, 83,* 236–247.

Spear, L. P. (2000). The adolescent brain and age-related behavioral manifestations. *Neurosci-ence Biobehavioral Review, 24,* 417–463.

Spitzer, R. L., & Endicott, J. (1978). *Schedule for Affective Disorders and Schizophrenia, Change version.* New York: Biometrics Research Division, Evaluation Section, New York State Psychiatric Institute.

Spitzer, R. L., Endicott, J., & Robins, E. (1978). *Research diagnostic criteria (RDC) for a selected group of functional disorders* (3rd ed.). New York: New York Psychiatric Institute.

Steinberg, L. (2008). A social neuroscience perspective on adolescent risk-taking. *Develop-mental Review, 28,* 78–106.

Steinberg, L., Graham, S., O'Brien, L., Woolard, J., Cauffman, E., & Banich, M. (2009). Age differences in future orientation and delay discounting. *Child Development, 80,* 28–44.

Strakowski, S. M., DelBello, M. P., Fleck, D. E., & Arndt, S. (2000). The impact of substance abuse on the course of bipolar disorder. *Biological Psychiatry, 48,* 477–485.

Strober, M., Morrell, W., Burroughs, J., Lampert, C., Danforth, H., & Freeman, R. (1988). A family study of bipolar I disorder in adolescence: Early onset of symptoms linked to increased familial loading and lithium resistance. *Journal of Affective Disorders, 15,* 255–268.

Suominen, K., Mantere, O., Valtonen, H., Arvilommi, P., Leppamaki, S., Paunio, T., et al. (2007). Early age at onset of bipolar disorder is associated with more severe clinical features but delayed treatment seeking. *Bipolar Disorders, 9,* 698–705.

Sutton, S. K., & Davidson, R. J. (1997). Prefrontal brain asymmetry: A biological subtrate of the behavioral approach and inhibition systems. *Psychological Science, 8,* 204–210.

Swann, A. C., Dougherty, D. M., Pazzaglia, P. J., Pham, M., Steinberg, J. L., & Moeller, F. G. (2005). Increased impulsivity associated with severity of suicide attempt history in patients with bipolar disorder. *American Journal of Psychiatry, 162,* 1680–1687.

Swann, A. C., Moeller, F., Steinberg, J. L., Schneider, L., Barrat, E. S., & Doughterty, D. M. (2007). Manic symptoms and impulsivity during bipolar depressive episodes. *Bipolar Disorders, 9,* 206–212.

Sylvia, L. G., Alloy, L. B., Hafner, J. A., Gauger, M. C., Verson, K., & Abramson, L. Y. (2009). Life events and social rhythms in bipolar spectrum disorders: A prospective study. *Behavior Therapy, 40,* 131–141.

Torrubia, R., Avila, C., Molto, J., & Caseras, X. (2001). The Sensitivity to Punishment and Sensitivity to Reward Questionnaire (SPSRQ) as a measure of Gray's anxiety and impulsivity dimensions. *Personality and Individual Differences, 31,* 837–862.

Tsuchiya, K. J. (2004). Higher socio-economic status of parents may increase risk for bipolar disorder in the offspring. *Psychological Medicine, 34,* 787–793.

Urosevic, S., Abramson, L. Y., Alloy, L. B., Nusslock, R., Harmon-Jones, E., Bender, R., et al. (2009). *Increased rates of behavioral approach system (BAS) activating and deactivating, but not goal-attainment, events in bipolar spectrum disorders.* Manuscript under review.

Urosevic, S., Abramson, L. Y., Harmon-Jones, E., & Alloy, L. B. (2008). Dysregulation of the behavioral approach system (BAS) in bipolar spectrum disorders: Review of theory and evidence. *Clinical Psychology Review, 28,* 1188–1205.

Wagner, C. A., Alloy, L. B., & Abramson, L. Y. (2009). *Parenting, behavioral approach system (BAS)—relevant cognitive styles, and diagnosis and course of bipolar spectrum disorders.* Manuscript submitted for publication.

Weissman, A., & Beck, A. T. (1978). *Development and validation of the Dysfunctional Attitudes Scale: A preliminary investigation.* Paper presented at the annual meeting of the American Educational Research Association, Toronto, Ontario, Canada.

Weissman, M. M., Bland, R. C., Canino, G. J., Faravelli, C., Greenwald, S., Hwu, H. G., et al. (1996). Cross-national epidemiology of major depression and bipolar disorder. *Journal of the American Medical Association, 276,* 293–299.

CHAPTER 7

A Developmental Perspective on the Course of Bipolar Disorder in Adulthood

Joseph F. Goldberg

The longitudinal course of illness for patients with bipolar disorder (BD) is remarkably heterogeneous. Extreme examples range from individuals who experience single (or relatively few) affective episodes who then enter and remain fully in remission to those who encounter multiple relapses, residual subsyndromal symptoms, complex comorbidities, and persistent psychosocial impairment. Some individuals respond dramatically to a single pharmacotherapy trial or specific medication regimen, whereas others undergo iterative trials that yield little benefit against persistent symptoms. The purpose of this chapter is to examine determinants of the course of BD in adulthood as a possible window for understanding the development and progression of the illness process itself. Because longitudinal course of illness represents a key facet for corroborating the validity of a diagnostic construct (Robins & Guze, 1970), outcome data offer a promising source for clues about the more fundamental pathogenesis of the disease.

The chapter provides an overview of illness course to serve as a focal point for understanding multifinality, followed by a discussion of constructs that influence illness course, such as personality structure, locus of control, resilience to stress, and temperamental traits such as impulsivity. Protective factors and risk factors are then reviewed for affective relapse and functional outcome, including genetic, neurotrophic, environmental, and psychosocial considerations. Finally, unresolved controversies and directions for future research are described regarding the developmental determinants of longitudinal course and outcome.

COURSE OF ILLNESS

Kraepelin's (1921) early distinction between manic–depressive illness and dementia praecox hinged on an overall better prognosis, with less psychosocial impairment and more typical interepisode recovery, in the former than latter. More recent prospective studies have challenged this dichotomy. By comparison to modern-day schizophrenia, individuals with BD are less likely to encounter pervasive impairment with a progressively deteriorating course, although many patients experience persistent problems with work and social adjustment long after resolution of an affective episode (Tohen et al., 2000), even after their first lifetime manic episode (Strakowski et al., 1998).

Despite Kraepelin's (1921) original view that manic–depressive illness generally held a favorable prognosis, modern-day studies suggest that consistent, long-term remission is uncommon. Notably, over a 10-year prospective follow-up, our group found that only 10% of patients with BD had consistently good overall functioning and symptomatic remission at each of four assessment points across the study period, in contrast to 28% of patients with unipolar nonpsychotic depression (Goldberg & Harrow, 2004). Elsewhere, in the National Institute of Mental Health (NIMH) Collaborative Depression Study (CDS), a sizable minority of subjects with BD (20%) had persistent affective symptoms throughout the entire year preceding their 15-year follow-up (Coryell et al., 1998). Similarly, findings from a 15-year prospective follow-up study based in Taiwan found poor long-term overall outcome in 17% of subjects (Tsai et al., 2001).

DEVELOPMENTAL CONSIDERATIONS IN THE MULTIFINALITY OF POOR OUTCOME

Numerous factors contribute to the multifinality of outcome states in BD, often involving complex interrelationships. Perhaps one of the most fundamental considerations in the development and progression of multiple affective recurrences is the propensity for repetitive episodes to occur with increasing facility and progressively shorter intermorbid intervals once the illness has become established. As originally described by Post (1992) and discussed further in Post and Miklowitz (Chapter 12, this volume), models of behavioral sensitization and kindling have been suggested to explain the generation and propagation of affective recurrences, with a progressively decremental importance attached to environmental stresses as successive episodes ensue with increasing spontaneity. A related tenet involves the hypothesis that individuals with BD develop a progressively increasing vulnerability to relatively minor levels of stress as the illness progresses (i.e., stress sensitization).

It should be noted that the kindling model remains a nonhomologous analogy borrowed from the presumed mechanism of recurrent seizures in epilepsy and has not been demonstrated in vivo with respect to a measurable focus of brain activity. However, there is at least some evidence showing a decremental association between stressful life events and successive episodes in major depressive disorder that is moderated by genetic risk (i.e., probands with higher genetic risk for depression, as reflected by concordance or discordance for depression in a monozygotic or dizygotic twin, are more likely to have spontaneous episodes) (Kendler, Thornton, & Gardner, 2001). On the other hand, life stresses of high intensity may be associated with a substantially greater hazard for affective relapse than seen with low-intensity stresses in patients with BD (Ellicott, Hammen, Gitlin, Brown, & Jamison, 1990). An association between stressful life events and relapse in BD can also occur independent of episode number (Cohen, Hammen, Henry, & Daley, 2004; Dienes, Hammen, Henry, Cohen, & Daley, 2006). Furthermore, at least one study has found that recurrence is more rapid among patients with highly chronic BD after a life event (Hammen & Gitlin, 1997).

Symptomatic relapses and recurrences may not necessarily occur in tandem with poor psychosocial functioning. A number of longitudinal studies have observed that disproportionate levels of social impairment and work disability may persist many months after resolution of an index manic or depressive episode (e.g., Tohen et al., 2000). Reasons for poor functional outcome despite syndromic or symptomatic recovery are many, and include the persistence of residual or subthreshold affective (especially depressive) symptoms (Altshuler et al., 2006; Simon, Bauer, Ludman, Operskalski, & Unützer, 2007), trait cognitive deficits (especially poor attentional processing; Mur, Portella, Martínez-Arán, Pifarré, & Vieta, 2008), and comorbid psychiatric or substance use disorders (Otto et al., 2006; Tohen, Waternaux, & Tsuang, 1990) or personality disorders (Loftus & Jaeger, 2006).

Complex forms of illness, such as BD with comorbid Axis I or II disorders, tend to be associated with more severe and frequent affective episodes, alongside poorer response to treatments (McElroy et al., 2001). From the standpoint of multifinality, preillness characteristics that encompass temperament, personality, and other early traits represent fundamental factors that can elevate risk or confer protection against poor outcome. The development of personality structure during childhood and adolescence represents a unique challenge in understanding both the phenotype and clinical course of BD. Affective symptoms first occur before the age of 18 in the vast majority of individuals in whom BD develops (Perlis et al., 2004), coincident with the time frame for traversing stage-salient developmental tasks, developing appropriate object relations, and effectively negotiating developmental transitions. Clinically, it can be extremely difficult to discriminate between maladaptive interpersonal behavioral patterns that are best attributable to personality structure versus the developmental effects of a chronic, recurrent mood disorder that may have begun in childhood or adolescence.

Although few longitudinal studies have attempted to assess the stability of personality traits over time in people with BD, a number of studies have examined personality disorders as comorbid phenomena (rather than differential diagnoses in themselves). Clinically important comorbid personality disorders are thought to arise in about one-third to one-half of adults with DSM-IV (American Psychiatric Association, 1994) bipolar I or II disorder (Uçok, Karaveli, Kundakçi, & Yazici, 1998), and their presence may impede syndromic recovery following an index manic episode, independent of treatment adherence (Dunayevich et al., 2000), as well as contribute to an increased risk for suicidal behavior (Garno, Goldberg, Ramirez, & Ritzler, 2005a; Uçok et al., 1998). Comorbid personality disorders also may directly contribute to poor treatment adherence (Colom et al., 2000).

A useful consideration involves recognizing the developmental time frames in which both BD and personality disorders are most likely to have their onset. For example, because polarity conversions from unipolar depression to BD become increasingly rare beyond young adulthood or early-middle adulthood (Goldberg, Harrow, & Whiteside, 2001), the incidence of new-onset BD among young adult with established personality disorders is relatively low (Goldberg & Garno, 2009; Gunderson et al., 2006). Less well explored from a developmental perspective is the role of temperamental factors from infancy through early childhood that help to shape subsequent personality structure among individuals who eventually have a manic or hypomanic episode. Behavioral disinhibition and poor emotional regulation have been suggested as two specific temperamental indicators for children at increased risk for developing BD (Hirshfeld-Becker et al., 2003), although the long-term prognostic relevance of these markers has not yet been examined.

Normal Developmental Processes and Adult Course of Illness

The appropriate negotiation and resolution of stage-salient tasks during development may contribute directly to disease characteristics of BD (e.g., affect regulation, dysfunctional attitudes) as well as indirectly through the personal skills necessary for competent disease management and resilience to stress (Cicchetti & Toth, 1995; Luthar, Cicchetti, & Becker, 2000). Some of these skills include self-regulatory competence, coping styles such as distress tolerance, effective problem solving, internal versus external locus of control and attributional style, adopting help-seeking versus help-rejecting stances toward the sick role, recognizing versus denying symptoms, and medication adherence. Disease management skills are reflected in the degree of activity or passivity with which patients approach affective recurrences. By way of example, the passive and externalizing statement "My medications have stopped working" contrasts with the internalized locus of control statement "I may be relapsing because I've taken my medications erratically and have resumed drinking alcohol and smoking marijuana." Development of an internal versus external locus of control likely contributes to adopting a more active versus passive stance in managing one's illness.

Trait impulsivity is evident across illness phases of BD, including euthymia (Swann, Pazzaglia, Nichols, Dougherty, & Moeller, 2003), and has been implicated in treatment nonadherence as well as various complications of BD, such as substance abuse (Swann, Dougherty, Pazzaglia, Pham, & Moeller, 2004) and severe suicide attempts (Swann et al., 2005). Its developmental origins arise at least in part through child–caregiver interactions, child temperament, and child cognitive skills (Olson, Bates, Sandy, & Schilling, 2002). The capacity for delayed gratification and inhibitory control also derives from the formation of secure attachments and the quality of early parent–child interactions (Olson, Bates, & Bayles, 1990). Developmental competence in these areas may be prerequisite to the ability to tolerate distress, negotiate risks, and resolve social conflicts effectively. Problem-focused and task-oriented coping styles are probably more effective than emotion-oriented or avoidance coping styles in preventing affective relapse (Christensen & Kessing, 2005). Deficits in these disease management skills, along with the capacity for resiliency in response to stress, represent important mediators of longitudinal course and outcome in BD. Risk factors for the initial onset and subsequent recurrence of affective episodes in BD are summarized in Table 7.1.

PREDICTORS OF OUTCOME IN FIRST-EPISODE STUDIES

Outcome data are now available from several prospective follow-up studies of patients with BD following a first lifetime manic episode. A methodological advantage of first-episode studies is the unique opportunity to examine mediational processes associated with early recurrences before the emergence of chronicity and its potential influence on outcome, such as demoralization after multiple treatment failures or the socioeconomic and psychosocial consequences of job losses or the loss of social supports. Although naturalistic outcome studies do not control a priori for treatment assignment, many have utilized multiple regression to adjust statistically for the effects of relevant potential confounding factors, such as age at illness onset, treatment adherence, and the presence of subsyndromal mood symptoms. For example, in the Canadian Systematic Treatment Optimization Program for Early Mania project, functional disability 6 months after an initial manic episode was most strongly predicted by residual depressive symptoms (either syndromal or subsyndromal) (Kauer-Sant'Anna, Bond, Lam, & Yatham, 2009) while controlling for sex, education, age at onset, length of illness, and current manic or depressive symptoms.

Prevalence rates of functional disability after a first lifetime mania parallel those seen in multiepisode cohorts. Thus, in the McLean–Harvard First Episode Mania Study, only 43% of patients achieved functional recovery 2 years after their initial manic episode (Tohen et al., 2003); both older age and shorter duration of index hospitalization predicted recovery. Similarly, among 134 individuals hospitalized for a first manic episode at the University of Cincinnati Hospital, functional recovery occurred after 1 year in only 24% (Keck et al., 1998). In this latter study group, shorter duration of illness and full treatment adherence were the best predictors of syndromic recovery; higher social class was a strong predictor of symptomatic and functional outcome. Finally, 12 months after a first

TABLE 7.1. Risk Factors for Affective Episodes: Evidence at Illness Onset versus Recurrence

Variable	Data in illness onset	Data in recurrence
Stressful life events	In the original model of kindling (Post, 1992), life stresses posited to be a more likely precipitant of early rather than later episodes.	Contemporary studies suggest an association between life stresses and affective recurrences independent of episode number (Dienes et al., 2006; Hlastala et al., 2000) or medication adherence (Johnson & Miller, 1997).
Severe childhood abuse	Birth cohort studies reveal increased risk among survivors of childhood sexual abuse for development of depression and suicidal behaviors (Fergusson, Horwood, & Lynskey, 1996).	Associated with more depressive (Brown et al., 2005) or total affective (Nolen et al., 2004) recurrences as well as more prevalent rapid cycling (Garno et al., 2005b; Leverich et al., 2002) than in patients with BD without childhood abuse histories.
Molecular genetic factors, including anticipation and gene × environment interactions	Polymorphisms of the serotonin transporter and catechol-O-methyltransferase genes associated with vulnerability to initial episodes, especially in conjunction with life stresses (Mandelli et al., 2007; Zalsman et al., 2006).	Preliminary data suggest risk alleles associated with antidepressant-associated mania (Mundo et al., 2001).
Family history	Parental or grandparental mania has been associated with polarity conversion from unipolar depression to BD in subjects with prepubescent major depression (Geller, Zimerman, Williams, Bolhofner, & Craney, 2001).	Family history of BD has been associated with increased likelihood of multiple episodes (Winokur et al., 1994).
Maladaptive personality traits	Cluster B personality disorder traits among unipolar depressed patients were predictive of eventual polarity conversion to BD (Holma, Melartin, Holma, & Isometsä, 2008). Neuroticism associated with onset of unipolar depression but inconclusive evidence for personality traits associated with lifetime onset of mania (Christensen & Kessing, 2006).	Introversion and obsessionality interact with stressful events to increase the risk of affective relapse (Swendsen, Hammen, Heller, & Gitlin, 1995). Indirect associations also exist between personality disorders and relapse (e.g., poorer treatment adherence [Colom et al., 2000]).
Alcohol/ substance abuse comorbidity	Lower prevalence of alcohol/substance use disorders in first episode mania (~33%; Baethge et al., 2005) than in multiepisode patients.	Comorbid alcohol use disorders conferred approximate fourfold increased risk for syndromic recurrence after a first lifetime hospitalized manic or mixed episode (DelBello et al., 2007). Cannabis

(cont.)

TABLE 7.1. *(cont.)*

Variable	Data in illness onset	Data in recurrence
Alcohol/ substance abuse comorbidity *(cont.)*		use among patients with BD appears associated with rapid cycling (Strakowski et al., 2007). Even remitted substance use disorders appear associated with longer time to remission from an acute mood episode and more time spent with subthreshold affective symptoms (Guadiano, Uebelacker, & Miller, 2008).
Psychosis	Psychotic depression may increase the likelihood for polarity conversion from unipolar to bipolar (Goldberg et al., 2001).	Mood-congruent psychosis in a first lifetime mania predicted mania recurrence (Tohen et al., 2003).
Sleep deprivation and other chronobiological events	Sleep deprivation and sleep reduction may represent a "final common pathway" for inducing mania (Wehr, Sack, & Rosenthal, 1987).	Dysregulation of sleep patterns may contribute fundamentally to affective relapse (Harvey, 2008); sleep disturbance has been identified as the most common prodrome of mania (Jackson, Cavanagh, & Scott, 2003).
High levels of expressed emotion (EE) and family interpersonal factors; family and caregiver burden	Unknown whether high intrafamily EE is associated with initial illness precipitation or earlier age at onset.	Low maternal warmth associated with mania relapse and more weeks ill with manic episodes at 2-year (Geller et al., 2002), 4-year (Geller, Tillman, Craney, & Bolhofner, 2004), and 8-year follow-up in children with bipolar I disorder (Geller, Tillman, Bolhofner, & Zimerman, 2008). Caregivers' emotional overinvolvement significantly predicts affective relapse at 15-month follow-up (Perlick et al., 2004). High intrafamily EE associated with increased relapse rates in BD (Miklowitz, Goldstein, Nuechterlein, Snyder, & Mintz, 1988).
Mood destabilization secondary to medications (e.g., antidepressants, steroids)	Unknown whether mania precipitated by medications is more common at illness onset versus later in the course of patients with established BD.	Rapid cycling has been associated with antidepressant use in some studies (Azorin et al., 2008; Schneck et al., 2008), although causal relationships remain uncertain.

(cont.)

TABLE 7.1. *(cont.)*

Variable	Data in illness onset	Data in recurrence
Residual affective symptoms after an index episode	First-episode mania studies have not, as yet, identified unique prodromal symptoms that antecede a first lifetime mania. It is unknown whether residual depressive symptoms in initially unipolar patients increase the likelihood for a first lifetime mania.	In STEP-BD, residual manic symptoms associated with faster time to manic/hypomanic/mixed recurrence; residual manic or depressive symptoms associated with faster time to depressive recurrence (Perlis et al., 2006). In the NIMH CDS, residual affective symptoms more than tripled the time until a next mood episode (Judd et al., 2008).
Delayed treatment initiation	Prolonged duration of untreated illness, or the passage of multiple episodes, may diminish responsivity to lithium (Franchini et al., 1999; Gelenberg et al., 1989). Inappropriate initial treatments (with consequent prolonged time until beginning mood-stabilizing agents) may independently contribute to poorer outcome (Ghaemi et al., 2000).	Delayed mood stabilizer initially associated with poorer psychosocial functioning, more hospitalizations, and increased risk for suicide attempts (Goldberg & Ernst, 2002).
Early age at onset	Prepubertal (Geller et al., 2001) or adolescent (Goldberg et al., 2001) major depression associated with eventual polarity conversion to BD.	More extensive anxiety and substance use comorbidity, more recurrences, shorter periods of euthymia, greater likelihood for suicide attempts, and increased risk for rapid cycling (Goldberg & Ernst, 2004b; Perlis et al., 2004).
Bipolar II subtype	No reported differences in age at onset between bipolar I and II disorders (Suominen et al., 2007).	Patients with bipolar II disorder spend about 40% more time with depressive symptoms than do those with bipolar I disorder (Mantere et al., 2008).
Endocrinopathies (e.g., hypothyroidism)	Adrenocorticotropic hyperactivity may predispose to the development of mood disorders by mediating physiological response to stress (Heim & Nemeroff, 2001).	Subclinical hypothyroidism has been linked with rapid cycling (Bauer, Whybrow, & Winokur, 1990).

Note. NIMH CDS, National Institute of Mental Health Collaborative Depression Study; STEP-BD, Systematic Treatment Enhancement Program for Bipolar Disorder.

lifetime hospitalized psychotic mania within a Swiss cohort, 40% had not recovered symptomatically and 66% failed to regain premorbid levels of functioning by 12 months (Conus et al., 2006). Age at intake, family history of BD, comorbid substance abuse, and recovery status after 6 months were the best predictors of 12-month functional outcomes. Predictors of outcome following a first manic episode may thus be heterogeneous but often involve clinical features related to brevity of illness duration, milder severity, and the absence of complicating factors such as treatment nonadherence or comorbidity.

RISK FACTORS FOR POOR FUNCTIONAL OUTCOMES

The most commonly cited mediators of relapse include poor adherence to existing treatment (Tsai et al., 2001), a history of multiple episodes (Nolen et al., 2004), and incomplete remission with residual symptoms (Perlis et al., 2006). A summary of outcome predictors identified in the literature on BD is presented in Table 7.2. A number of these factors warrant more detailed discussion with respect to their developmental implications.

Childhood Trauma and Abuse

Convergent findings from several large independent studies suggest that childhood physical, emotional, or sexual abuse is reported by about half of adults with BD (Brown, McBride, Bauer, Williford, & Cooperative Studies Program 430 Study Team, 2005; Garno, Goldberg, Ramirez, & Ritzler, 2005b; Leverich et al., 2002). Childhood abuse among individuals who develop BD, in turn, has been associated with a range of poor outcome states, including multiple depressive episodes (Brown et al., 2005), comorbid alcohol abuse (Brown et al., 2005), and a higher likelihood of attempting suicide (Brown et al., 2005). Early life adversity also may serve to moderate the effects of stressful life events on the risk for affective recurrence in BD (Dienes et al., 2006). Proposed mechanisms by which severe childhood abuse histories contribute to the development and expression of eventual mood disorders include altered physiological response to stress (including hyperactivity of the hypothalamic–pituitary–adrenocortical axis) (Heim & Nemeroff, 2001; see also Cicchetti, Rogosch, Gunnar, & Toth, in press), neuroanatomic structural abnormalities (e.g., diminished hippocampal volume; Vythilingam et al., 2002), and impaired development of the capacity for affect regulation, executive function, resiliency, and social competence (Martel et al., 2007).

Comorbid Axis I Disorders

More than half of individuals with bipolar I or II disorder have at least one additional psychiatric diagnosis (McElroy et al., 2001). The development of comorbid psychopathology in the longitudinal course of BD reflects multifinality with

TABLE 7.2. Predictors of Outcome in Bipolar Disorder: Evaluating the Evidence

Variable	Studies finding significant association with poor outcome	Studies finding no significant association or negative association with poor outcome
Early age at illness onset	• Tohen et al. (2000) • Meeks (1999) (in a cohort of older adults with BD, effect of age at onset was mediated by number of depressive episodes) • Carter, Mundo, Parikh, & Kennedy (2003) (increased risk for rapid cycling, comorbid anxiety and substance use disorders, suicide attempts) • Perlis et al. (2004) (increased risk for comorbid anxiety and substance use disorders, affective recurrences, and suicide attempts) • Goldberg & Ernst (2004b) (increased risk for comorbid substance abuse and rapid cycling) • Lin et al. (2006) (increased risk for comorbid alcohol and substance use disorders, rapid cycling, and suicide attempts) • Pope, Dudley, & Scott (2007) (later age at onset associated with better social functioning) • Goldberg et al. (2009) (increased likelihood of comorbid borderline personality disorder) • Goldstein & Levitt (2006) (increased likelihood of comorbid antisocial personality disorder)	• Coryell et al. (1998) • Nolen et al. (2004) • Tsai et al. (2001) (in a Taiwanese cohort, early age at onset was associated with better outcome at 15-year follow-up) • Goldberg & Ernst (2004b) (no increased risk for suicide attempts)
Gender	• Tohen et al. (1990) (men had *poorer* outcomes than women in a 4-year U.S.-based prospective study) • Tsai et al. (2001) (men had *better* outcomes than women in a 15-year Taiwanese follow-up study)	• Coryell et al. (1998) (no association)
Marital status	• Tohen et al. (2000) (married patients with first-episode mania had faster syndromal recovery)	• Coryell et al. (1998) (no association)
Poor premorbid adjustment	• Goldberg & Ernst (2004a) (poor childhood and adolescent adjustment associated with later development of rapid cycling, comorbid alcohol or substance abuse, and suicide attempts) • Bromet et al. (1996) • Brieger, Röttig, Röttig, Marneros, & Priebe (2007) • Tabarés-Seisdedos et al. (2008) • Pope et al. (2007) (premorbid neuroticism associated with poor social functioning)	
Comorbid personality disorders	• Kay, Altshuler, Ventura, & Mintz (2002) (poorer work functioning) • Garno et al. (2005a) (increased risk for suicidal behavior) • Loftus & Jaeger (2006) (poorer work, residential, and social/leisure functioning at 1-year follow-up)	

(cont.)

TABLE 7.2. *(cont.)*

Variable	Studies finding significant association with poor outcome	Studies finding no significant association or negative association with poor outcome
Severe childhood abuse	• Leverich et al. (2002, 2003); Garno et al. (2005b) (increased risk for suicide attempts) • Neria, Bromet, Carlson, & Naz (2005) (lower remission rates following a first hospitalization for mania in patients with histories of assaultive trauma)	
Socioeconomic status (SES)	• Keck et al. (1998) (faster and more extensive recovery from a first lifetime mania in higher-SES subjects) • Tohen et al. (2003) (lower premorbid occupational status associated with recurrent mania after a first lifetime manic episode) • DelBello et al. (2007) (low SES was one among several predictors of poor syndromic recovery after a first hospitalized adolescent mania)	• Nolen et al. (2004) (no association)
Alcohol abuse/ dependence	• Tohen et al. (1990) • Winokur et al. (1994) (better outcome if alcoholism precedes BD than vice versa) • Nolen et al. (2004) • DelBello et al. (2007) • Coryell et al. (1998) (observed univariate association with poor outcome at 15-year follow-up loses significance in multivariate model) • Cardoso et al. (2008)	
Drug abuse/ dependence	• Less extensive recovery and poorer psychosocial functioning with current or past substance abuse than no substance abuse comorbidity (Weiss et al., 2005) • Conus et al. (2006) (drug abuse associated with poorer functional outcome 12 months after a first lifetime hospitalized psychotic mania) • Mazza et al. (2009) (poorer social function over 12 months' follow-up in patients with BD with vs. without drug abuse/dependence) • Conus et al. (2006)	
Medical comorbidity	• Pirraglia et al. (2009) (physical illness burden rather than number of medical comorbidities predicted poor outcome over 3 years)	
Cognitive deficits	• Martínez-Arán et al. (2004) (verbal memory impairment was associated with poor global functioning and longer illness duration independent of subsyndromal affective symptoms)	

(cont.)

TABLE 7.2. *(cont.)*

Variable	Studies finding significant association with poor outcome	Studies finding no significant association or negative association with poor outcome
	• Impaired attentional processing associated with work disability at 2-year follow-up (Mur et al., 2008) • Martino et al. (2009) (deficits in verbal memory, attention and executive function predicted global functioning at 1-year outcome independent of depressive symptoms)	
Psychosis	• Tohen et al. (1990) • Tohen, Tsuang, & Goodwin (1992) (mood-incongruent and first-rank psychotic features associated with shorter time in remission at 4-year follow-up) • Strakowski et al. (2000) (poorer overall functioning 1 year after a first manic episode in patients with, vs. without, mood-incongruent psychosis) • Van Riel et al. (2008) (extent of delusions and hallucinations at baseline associated with chronicity of mania at 1-year follow-up)	
Subsyndromal depressive symptoms	• Kauer-Sant'Anna et al. (2009) (subsyndromal depressive features associated with poor functioning 6 months after a first lifetime mania) • Judd et al. (2005) (subsyndromal depression, but not mania or hypomania, linked with functional impairment at 20-year follow-up in patients with bipolar I or II) • Altshuler et al. (2006) (subsyndromal depression associated with impaired social, work, and home functioning roles) • Martino et al. (2009)	

respect to the emergence and progression of an especially complex and phenotypically heterogeneous form of illness. Less often, comorbidity can also reflect equifinality when substance misuse or other Axis I psychiatric disorders precede the onset of BD but nonetheless have outcomes similar to those seen in patients with BD without comorbidities. It remains a subject of speculation as to whether the co-occurrence of BD with common comorbidities, notably alcohol use disorders and anxiety disorders, represents different manifestations of a common underlying disease process (i.e., homotypic continuity) versus greater diversity in longitudinal disease progression (i.e., heterotypic continuity). At least one-third of first-episode mania patients have a history of alcohol or substance abuse (Baethge et al., 2005), although outcome data beyond 1 year are not yet available for first-episode mania patients with versus without comorbid disorders or for patients with BD who develop comorbidities early versus late in their course of illness. Generally, 1-year outcomes are better when BD arises later in life and when a first episode of mania follows rather than precedes the onset of alcohol or substance use disorders (Strakowski et al., 2005).

Apart from comorbid substance use disorders, anxiety disorders are perhaps the most frequently occurring comorbidity, arising in half or more of patients with BD (Grant et al., 2005). The implications of comorbid anxiety on treatment and clinical course have only recently begun to receive empirical study. Comorbid panic disorder has been linked with a higher number of mood episodes (Toniolo, Caetano, da Silva, & Lafer, 2009). Anxiety disorders, in general, were associated with fewer days well, a diminished likelihood for recovery from depression, earlier relapse, and greater functional impairment among participants in the Systematic Treatment Enhancement Program for Bipolar Disorder cohort (Otto et al., 2006). Conceptually, one might speculate that prominent anxiety features could adversely affect the course of BD by disrupting emotional processing, executive function, and related aspects of central nervous system homeostasis.

Rapid Cycling

Originally defined based on its association with poor outcome during lithium maintenance therapy (Dunner & Fieve, 1974), the construct of rapid cycling has since become a focus of tremendous interest in the nosology, treatment, and prognosis of BD. Contemporary prospective studies suggest that the DSM-IV course specifier of rapid cycling (i.e., ≥ four episodes per year) is more likely a transient rather than an enduring phenomenon (Coryell et al., 2003), one that may emerge at any point in the course of illness. Other authors have argued that very frequent episodes are more likely an end result of poorly treated illness, particularly in connection with the hypothesis that antidepressant use may accelerate cycling frequency (Azorin et al., 2008; Ghaemi, Boiman, & Goodwin, 2000). Although the latter perspective remains controversial, there is at least some evidence that a predisposition to frequent episodes is more apparent in certain subgroups of individuals with BD (notably, women and those with an earlier age at illness onset) (Schneck et al., 2004). Rapid cycling also represents both a predictor of later functional or syndromal outcome as well as an outcome state in itself.

Time Spent with Affective Symptoms

Several lines of evidence point to the duration of time spent with manic or depressive symptoms as a robust predictor of hospitalizations or functional impairment. For example, in the NIMH CDS, when examining 15 independent variables involving various aspects of affective switch (e.g., depressive-to-manic vs. manic-to-depressive polarity, polyphasic episodes), severity of episodes, numbers of episodes, or age at onset or comorbid substance abuse, only the number of weeks with manic/hypomanic/mixed or depressive symptoms significantly predicted future illness burden (Mysels et al., 2007). Although the course of BD is affected by multiple risk and protective factors, the prior course of illness is still a robust predictor of future illness course, an example of homotypic continuity.

Poor Functioning Predicts Poor Functioning

Most prospective longitudinal outcome studies of BD have found that poor outcome at earlier time points strongly predicts poor outcome at later assessments. This is evident at 6- and 12-month follow-ups in first-episode mania patients (Conus et al., 2006), 10-year outcome in the Chicago Follow-up Study (Goldberg & Harrow, 2004), and 15-year outcome in the NIMH CDS cohort (Coryell et al., 1998). Similarly, in the Chicago Follow-up Study (Goldberg & Harrow, 2004), sustained remission at 7½- and 10-year assessments was best predicted by having achieved symptomatic and functional remission at earlier follow-ups, suggesting that early recovery after an index manic episode may be among the most critical indicators for anticipating a favorable long-term prognosis. Thus, there is evidence for homotypic continuity in the course of BD: the expression of similar symptoms or behaviors at different phases of development (Cicchetti & Toth, 1998). Research has not clarified, however, whether these symptoms and behaviors have the same meaning at different phases of the illness.

RISK FACTORS IN THE SYMPTOMATIC COURSE OF BIPOLAR DISORDER

When analyzing the complex pathways by which poor-outcome states may arise, it is readily apparent that variables associated with persistent relapse or functional impairment are interrelated. Colinearity, hierarchical relationships, chronological relationships, and complex interactions all bear on the prediction of recovery, relapse, and psychosocial outcome. Several examples follow.

- Early age at onset has been implicated with a multitude of complications, comorbidities, and negative outcome states related to BD (see Table 7.2), many of which involve colinear variables. For example, comorbid substance abuse (Leverich et al., 2002) and comorbid cluster B personality traits (Garno et al., 2005a; Leverich et al., 2002), both associated with early age at onset, are also both associated with suicidality in BD. Early onset is associated with poor outcome as well as delayed treatment seeking (Suominen et al., 2007); in turn, the latter may diminish treatment responsiveness (Franchini, Zanardi, Smeraldi, & Gasparini, 1999; Gelenberg et al., 1989).
- The adverse effects of comorbid alcohol or substance abuse on outcome in BD appear to be more dramatic when the onset of BD precedes the onset of alcohol

or substance abuse rather than the reverse (Strakowski et al., 2005). Interestingly, the negative effect of comorbid substance use disorders on outcome in BD dissipates after controlling for early age at onset of BD (Fossey et al., 2006).

• Cognitive deficits, particularly involving verbal memory, attentional processing, and executive function, are intrinsic aspects of BD that may predict occupational or other functional impairment (see Table 7.2). Multiple affective episodes (especially depressions) are associated with both worsening cognitive function (Robinson & Ferrier, 2006) and poorer functional outcome (Nolen et al., 2004).

• Childhood trauma, itself associated with greater affective morbidity and cycling frequency (see Table 7.2), has been shown to predict cognitive dysfunction (Savitz, van der Merwe, Stein, Solms, & Ramesar, 2008) and multiple adult psychiatric comorbidities (Brown et al., 2005; Leverich et al., 2003), all of which, in turn, may increase the likelihood of frequent relapse, poor recovery, and functional disability.

• The presence of comorbid psychiatric or substance use disorders is associated with poorer functional outcome (Otto et al., 2006), although comorbidly ill patients may also be less likely to receive adequate pharmacotherapy for BD (Simon et al., 2004).

• Mood-incongruent psychosis is associated with poor functional outcome (see Table 7.2) and also with poor treatment adherence (Miklowitz, 1992); poor treatment adherence is a widely recognized predictor of relapse and poor functional outcome (Tsai et al., 2001).

• Rapid cycling, a predictor of high relapse rates and poor functional outcome, has been linked with histories of childhood abuse and with comorbid substance abuse (Kupka et al., 2005), both of which are themselves predictors of poor outcome. Moreover, there remains considerable debate about the extent to which rapid cycling more likely arises *because of* excessive antidepressant use (Ghaemi et al., 2000) or persists *despite* antidepressant use (Goldberg, 2008).

• Family and caregiver burden is a correlate of functional outcome as well as medication adherence among patients with BD (Perlick et al., 2004). It is uncertain whether relapse and poor outcome are driven directly by family members' affective response or whether medication nonadherence is a mediator of family members' emotional overinvolvement. Path analyses indicate significant independent effects of caregiver emotional overinvolvement and of medication nonadherence on relapse risk at a 15-month follow-up (Perlick et al., 2004).

When multiple risk factors for poor outcome are identifiable, it may be difficult to pinpoint the relative contribution or magnitude of effect of a given risk factor relative to another. That is, it is often uncertain when an additive, hierarchical, or synergistic model is more likely to account for high relapse rates and poor psychosocial functioning and whether all identifiable risk factors warrant equal weighting to account for the observable variation in outcome. For example, when examining the total number of mood episodes at 1-year follow-up in the Stanley Foundation Bipolar Network, an initial model identified four significant outcome predictors (family history of drug abuse, self-reported history of childhood abuse, age at onset, and comorbid substance abuse) that together accounted for 15% or less of the variance in outcome. Including prior illness variables (e.g., number of episodes) and illness state at study entry increased the proportion of explained variance to 42%.

It is also unknown whether predictors of short-term outcome remain equally robust as predictors of long-term outcome or whether outcome predictors of child or adolescent BD differ from those of adult BD. One example of the latter involves gender in adolescent mania, insofar as boys appear twice as likely as girls to recover symptomatically from a first manic episode (DelBello, Hansemann, Adler, Fleck, & Strakowski, 2007). Yet gender differences have not been reported in rates of symptomatic remission from adult mania. In the National Epidemiologic Survey on Alcohol and Related Conditions, BD had an earlier age at onset in men than women (Grant et al., 2005), perhaps suggesting that age at onset moderates the effects of gender on longitudinal outcome (see Table 7.2).

Another consideration is whether novel factors may emerge as significant correlates of long-term outcome that may not be as evident in short-term follow-ups. Examples include the development of later-life comorbid medical conditions (Pirraglia, Biswas, Kilbourne, Fenn, & Bauer, 2009) or existential despair and demoralization in the setting of multiple relapses and failed life expectations (Ghaemi, 2007; Goldberg & Harrow, 2005).

PROTECTIVE FACTORS

When considering the stage-salient tasks of normal development, risk and protective factors likely involve psychological, psychosocial, and neurobiological underpinnings. Protective factors are discussed next.

Neurotrophic Factors

A number of intracellular molecules or proteins that promote neuronal survival have been identified that represent putative targets of psychotropic medications and, furthermore, may be relevant to affective resilience following a manic or depressive episode. One such protein, bcl-2-associated athanogene (*BAG1*), has been shown in preclinical studies to enhance recovery from amphetamine-induced hyperlocomotion in animal studies of mania as well as diminish anxious behavior and helplessness in laboratory paradigms (Maeng et al., 2008). Preclinical studies also show that mood-stabilizing medications increase the production of brain-derived neurotrophic factor (BDNF), another protein necessary for neuronal viability (Chang, Rapoport, Rao, 2009; Pandey, Rizavi, Dwivedi, & Pavuluri, 2008). Inasmuch as low BDNF levels may be associated with rapid cycling in BD (Müller et al., 2006), its upregulation may represent a protective factor against affective episodes and possible disease progression.

Allostatic Load and Resilience

As originally described by McEwen and Stellar (1993), *allostatic load* refers to physiological responses to stress and the capacity to maintain homeostasis. Dysfunctional allostasis (allostatic overload) occurs in the form of physiological maladaptations to chronic stress, as reflected by neuroendocrine (e.g., hypercortisolemia associated with loss of hippocampal volume) (McEwen, 1999, 2001), immunological, cardiovascular (Schwartz et al., 2003), or other organ system dysfunction. Insofar as multiple affective episodes constitute physiological stress, resilience entails the capacity to habituate to repeated stresses without compensatory neurophysiological hyperactivity (e.g., abnormal hypercortisolemia), thereby protecting neural circuitry involved in cognitive function and affective regulation.

Exaggerated Response to Emotional Stimuli

Functional imaging studies using sad mood induction paradigms suggest that some individuals with BD may have an increased vulnerability to emotional provocation (as demonstrated by decreased blood flow in the orbitofrontal cortex [OFC]), coupled with increased activity in the dorsal anterior cingulate gyrus (Krüger et al., 2006). By contrast, unaffected siblings of patients with BD more often tend to have increased (rather than decreased) blood flow in medial frontal cortex (a region involved with emotional processing), suggesting a possible compensatory response that could help to counter emotional vulnerability and provide an element of resilience in the setting of emotional distress. Thus, decreased OFC blood flow in the setting of emotional stress could neurobiologically predispose vulnerable individuals to persistent or highly recurrent affective symptoms. In contrast, a patient with multiple risk factors (e.g., dysfunctional allostasis, low BDNF) may be protected from poor outcomes through increased OFC blood flow. In this respect, prefrontal cortical blood flow patterns may pose either risk factors or protective factors with respect to multifinality of outcomes.

Gene × Environment Interactions

Multiple genes of small effect are thought to contribute to the development and progression of BD through identifiable environmental interactions (Willcutt & McQueen, Chapter 8, this volume). Less well established is the potential bidirectionality of environmental factors influencing genotypes or the extent to which maturation of the nervous system could alter genetic vulnerability, an example of "probabilistic epigenesis" (Gottlieb, 2007). Among candidate genes implicated in both disease susceptibility and course of illness, a polymorphic variant in the serotonin transporter (5-HTT) gene (locus *SLC6A4*) has been associated with an increased vulnerability for depressive episodes to occur in the context of multiple adverse life stresses. In general population studies, the so-called long variant of the *SLC6A4* locus has been shown to confer protection against the development of depressive episodes (Caspi et al., 2003; Wilhelm et al., 2006). Association studies involving 5-HTT and outcome specifically in probands with BD have not been reported, other than a possible association between the *SLC6A4* short variant and the development of rapid cycling (Rousseva et al., 2003). Evidence also suggests that among healthy volunteers presence of the short variant of the serotonin transporter gene is associated with a diminished capacity to generate and use effective coping strategies and problem-solving skills (Wilhelm et al., 2007), which may, in turn, contribute to work and social dysfunction.

A further example of genetic vulnerability to recurrent mood disorders involves physiological responses to life stresses. Several identified single nucleotide polymorphisms in the corticotropin-releasing hormone type I receptor gene (*CRHR1*) appear to moderate the risk for developing depressive episodes among general medical patients with histories of childhood abuse (Bradley et al., 2008). Potential specificity of such findings to individuals with BD has not yet been examined.

TREATMENT EXPOSURE IN RELATION TO THE MULTIFINALITY OF BIPOLAR OUTCOMES

What factors contribute to the heterogeneity of outcome states after accounting for baseline characteristics? By and large, the effects of treatment and environmental or psychosocial supports are among the most salient factors that have been shown to influence outcome. These include the following.

Exposure to Antidepressants and Other Possible Mood Destabilizers

The circumstances under which antidepressants may exert beneficial versus adverse effects on the clinical course of BD remain highly controversial (Carlson et al., 2007; Ghaemi et al., 2000). Antidepressant use has never been shown to *reduce* the frequency of episodes of either polarity among individuals with rapid cycling, and there is at least naturalistic evidence to show association (if not causality) between long-term antidepressant use and more frequent episodes (Schneck et al., 2008). There is also some suggestion that delaying the initiation of antidepressants after initial illness onset in BD may help to reduce the likelihood of later developing rapid cycling (Goldberg & Ernst, 2004b).

Antidepressants have come to represent one element from among several additional factors collectively that may be described as mood *destabilizers*. Exogenous factors other than antidepressants that may induce mania, or cycle acceleration, may include sleep deprivation and other chronobiological or circadian events (e.g., crossing multiple time zones during air travel), alcohol or substance misuse, and a poor capacity to manage life stresses. By contrast, extended bed rest with darkness has been described as a chronobiological intervention that may help to stabilize high recurrence rates associated with rapid-cycling BD (Wehr et al., 1998).

Choice of Mood-Stabilizing Agents

Although lithium and certain anticonvulsant medications are broadly regarded as mood stabilizers for which clinicians often assume comparable efficacy, findings from clinical trials as well as effectiveness-based studies point to fundamental differences among the agents that may contribute importantly to differential treatment outcome. For example, outcomes during lithium maintenance therapy appear more favorable when it is begun within the first few episodes, when manias precede rather than follow depressions, when "classical" manias occur more often than mixed episodes, when there is a family history of BD, when rapid cycling is absent, and when comorbid conditions such as substance use disorders are absent (Goldberg, Harrow, & Leon, 1996). Lamotrigine, by comparison, appears to exert a more robust prophylactic effect against recurrent depressions than manias (Goodwin et al., 2004) and as such may be an especially appropriate agent in patients who may be more prone to recurrent depressions than manias (Goldberg et al., 2009). Divalproex may have a more robust effect than lithium among patients with multiple prior episodes (Swann, Bowden, Calabrese, Dilsaver, & Morris, 1999) or mixed episodes (Swann et al., 1997). Matching appropriate pharmacotherapies to their corresponding clinical profiles may, at least in principle, help to promote better outcomes.

Acquisition and Integration of Patient Self-Management Skills and Psychoeducation

In the Department of Veterans Affairs Cooperative Studies Program, patients with BD who were randomized to receive a skills-based self-management intervention had better outcomes (measured as reduced weeks spent with an affective episode, social role functioning, quality of life, and treatment satisfaction) compared with those receiving usual care (Bauer et al., 2006). The skills intervention focused on illness management skills, group psychoeducation, access to care, and facilitated clinician decision support. Acquisition of structured disease management skills may thus represent a protective factor from the standpoint of multifinality of outcomes.

Caregiver Psychoeducation

Familiarization with disease management skills as a protective factor does not pertain solely to patients themselves. It is now well recognized that BD is associated with substantial family and caregiver burden (Perlick et al., 2004). Compared with usual treatment, patients with BD whose caregivers undergo a formal series of psychoeducation modules have a significantly longer time until a manic/hypomanic (but not depressive) relapse (Reinares et al., 2008).

Poor Treatment Adherence

High treatment adherence was the strongest predictor of outcome over a long-term (15-year) period in a Taiwanese sample with BD (Tsai et al., 2001). Treatment nonadherence also has been linked with poor syndromic recovery after an initial manic episode among adolescents (DelBello et al., 2007) and adults (Keck et al., 1998).

Utilization of Evidence-Based Psychotherapies

In addition to hastening time to recovery from acute depressive episodes in BD, adjunctive structured psychotherapies such as cognitive-behavioral therapy, interpersonal/social rhythm therapy, and family-focused therapy have also been shown to improve functional outcomes beyond the effects seen with pharmacotherapy alone (Miklowitz, 2008). The mechanisms of these treatments, whether they reduce risk factors, enhance protection, or both, deserve clarification.

PREDICTION AT THE INDIVIDUAL LEVEL: MOVING TOWARD PERSONALIZED TREATMENT

Despite the extensive database of both univariate predictors of outcome as well as hierarchies based on regression models, remarkably little is known about how and why a unique course of illness unfolds for a given individual. For example, not all patients who receive long-term antidepressants develop rapid cycling, and it is difficult to predict in any individual whether rapid cycling will endure. Similarly, alcohol abuse or dependence arises in a substantial proportion of individuals with BD, but protective factors against the development of "problem drinking" (i.e., factors that may permit "healthy drinking") are subject to speculation. Likewise, what intrinsic factors predispose versus protect against postpartum mood episodes in high-risk women with known BD? In older adults with BD, a history of multiple episodes may predispose to an increased risk for the eventual development of dementia, by 6% with every successive episode, according to findings from a 29-year case registry in Denmark (Kessing & Andersen, 2004). Yet protective factors against marked cognitive decline despite multiple episodes are relatively unknown.

With respect to treatment outcome, some patients may be more likely to respond robustly and completely to certain agents, such as lithium, at least in part because of familial or genetic underpinnings (Grof et al., 2002). However, there are as yet no definitive or reliable markers by which to anticipate short- or long-term response to any psychotropic medication, often making longitudinal treatment more of a trial-and-error succession than a series of biologically informed decisions. Refinement of illness phenotypes and endophenotypes may ultimately help to improve treatment specificity and reduce the extreme variability now evident in course and outcome.

CONCLUSIONS AND FUTURE DIRECTIONS

The ability to prognosticate illness course and outcome with greater reliability remains an elusive goal in the individualized treatment of BD. Future research strides will no doubt depend in part on expectations from personalized medicine and related genetic or neurobiological methods to anticipate the likelihood of response to specific interventions. Greater insights from developmental predictors of outcome will likely enhance such efforts, particularly as a means to better stratify disease status from the time of illness onset. Table 7.2 summarizes a number of known factors related to illness onset and relapse for which developmental windows (e.g., exposure to childhood vs. adolescent or adult trauma; intrafamily expressed emotion in early vs. middle or late childhood) may bear on the course and outcome of BD.

One important area for future research involves the elucidation of homotypic versus heterotypic continuity in explaining common comorbidities in people with BD. For example, although alcohol and substance use disorders often arise in half or more of individuals with BD, they tend to follow a course separate from that of BD in about half of dual-diagnosis cases (Strakowski et al., 1998). Little is known about factors that increase the risk for (or protect against) the development of alcohol and substance use disorders in people with BD. In men without BD, behaviorally aggressive traits along with paternal alcoholism confer increased risk for the development of more severe, so-called type B or type II alcoholism in a model described as the Apollonian–Dionysian taxonomy (Carpenter & Hasin, 2001). Such developmental classification schemes for susceptibility to alcoholism have not as yet been investigated in people with BD. Furthermore, comorbid substance use disorders do not appear to arise simply as a function of severity of affective symptoms, which would suggest a uniform underlying cause, nor are they an inevitable or predictable consequence of BD, which would suggest homotypic continuity. Nonetheless, substance misuse and BD may share certain common dimensions of psychopathology, such as impulsivity or a poor capacity to self-regulate internal affective states. Further longitudinal research on such comorbid conditions may help to identify clues about possible shared pathophysiological mechanisms leading to phenotypic heterogeneity.

Another key direction for future investigation involves efforts to better identify neurobiological, psychosocial, and other factors associated with resilience. Current knowledge identifies the high prevalence of adverse early life events, intrafamilial high expressed emotion, allostatic overload, or even poor treatment response for many individuals with BD; yet, from the standpoint of multifinality, little is known about which individuals who encounter trauma or other forms of adversity may be at greater or lesser risk for developing poor-outcome states. Notably, a very limited number of polymorphic loci have been shown to moderate the risk for relapse in major depressive disorder in the setting of multiple life stresses (Caspi et al., 2003) or the potential for antidepressants to destabilize mood (Mundo, Walker, Cate, Macciardi, & Kennedy, 2001). A greater understanding of developmental mechanisms of BD will likely emerge from the identification of other risk alleles as well as loci that may confer protection against outcome states such as violent suicidal behavior, affective dysregulation, cognitive decline, or medication response.

Finally, from the standpoint of primary prevention, there is a compelling need for further studies of populations at high risk for developing BD before the onset of symptoms. Children of affected parents, especially those from genetically dense pedigrees, remain an especially critical study population for better determining prodromal phases of illness as well as the diversity of initial states that can eventually converge in common outcome states (i.e., equifinality). Endophenotypic approaches may be especially valuable for the detection of "soft signs" for developing BD in this regard, such as deficits in the capacity for facial recognition (Brotman et al., 2008), impaired probabilistic reversal in learning paradigms involving reward and punishment (Gorrindo et al., 2005), and related aspects of social cognition (e.g., pragmatic judgment of language and response flexibility) (McClure et al., 2005). Although such traits may not, in themselves, represent modifiable risk factors for disease progression, they may help to corroborate diagnoses of early-onset BD and thereby facilitate early intervention as a means to diminish the risk for poor treatment outcome.

REFERENCES

Altshuler, L. L., Post, R. M., Black, D. O., Keck, P. E., Jr., Nolen, W. A., Frye, M. A., et al. (2006). Subsyndromal depressive symptoms are associated with functional impairment in patients with bipolar disorder: Results of a large, multi-site study. *Journal of Clinical Psychiatry, 67,* 1551–1560.

American Psychiatric Association. (1994). *Diagnostic and statistical manual of mental disorders* (4th ed.). Washington, DC: Author.

Azorin, J. M., Kaladjian, A., Adida, M., Hantouche, E. G., Hameg, A., Lancrenon, S., et al. (2008). Factors associated with rapid cycling in bipolar I manic patients: Findings from a French national study. *CNS Spectrums, 13,* 780–787.

Baethge, C., Baldessarini, R. J., Khalsa, H. M., Hennen, J., Salvatore, P., & Tohen, M. (2005). Substance abuse in first-episode bipolar I disorder: Indications for early intervention. *American Journal of Psychiatry, 162,* 1008–1010.

Bauer, M. S., McBride, L., Williford, W. O., Glick, H., Kinosian, B., Altshuler, L., et al. (2006). Collaborative care for bipolar disorder: Part II. Impact on clinical outcome, function, and costs. *Psychiatric Services, 57,* 937–945.

Bauer, M. S., Whybrow, P. C., & Winokur, A. (1990). Rapid cycling bipolar affective disorder: I. Association with grade I hypothyroidism. *Archives of General Psychiatry, 47,* 427–432.

Bradley, R. G., Binder, E. B., Epstein, M. P., Tang, Y., Nair, H. P., Liu, W., et al. (2008). Influence of child abuse on adult depression: Moderation by the corticotrophin-releasing hormone receptor gene. *Archives of General Psychiatry, 65,* 190–200.

Brieger, P., Röttig, S., Röttig, D., Marneros, S., & Priebe, S. (2007). Dimensions underlying outcome criteria in bipolar I disorder. *Journal of Affective Disorders, 99,* 1–7.

Bromet, E. J., Jandorf, L., Fennig, S., Lavelle, J., Kovasznay, B., Ram, R., et al. (1996). The Suffolk County Mental Health Project: Demographic, pre-morbid and clinical correlates of 6-month outcome. *Psychological Medicine, 26,* 953–962.

Brotman, M. A., Guyer, A. E., Lawson, E. S., Horsey, S. E., Rich, B. A., Dickstein, D. P., et al. (2008). Facial emotion labeling deficits in children and adolescents at risk for bipolar disorder. *American Journal of Psychiatry, 165,* 385–390.

Brown, G. R., McBride, L., Bauer, M. S., Williford, W. O., & Cooperative Studies Program 430 Study Team. (2005). Impact of childhood abuse on the course of bipolar disorder: A replication study in U.S. veterans. *Journal of Affective Disorders, 89,* 57–67.

Cardoso, B. M., Kauer Sant'Anna N., Dias, V. V., Andreazza, A. C., Ceresér, K. M., & Kapczinski, F. (2008). The impact of co-morbid alcohol use disorder in bipolar patients. *Alcohol, 42,* 451–457.

Carlson, G. A., Finch, S. J., Fochtmann, L. J., Ye, Q., Wang, Q., Naz, B., et al. (2007). Antidepressant-associated switches from depression to mania in severe bipolar disorder. *Bipolar Disorders, 9,* 851–859.

Carpenter, K. M., & Hasin, D. S. (2001). Reliability and discriminant validity of the type I/II and type A/B alcoholic subtype classifications in untreated problem drinkers: A test of the Apollonian- Dionysian hypothesis. *Drug and Alcohol Dependence, 63,* 51–67.

Carter, T. D., Mundo, E., Parikh, S. V., & Kennedy, J. L. (2003). Early age at onset as a risk factor for poor outcome of bipolar disorder. *Journal of Psychiatric Research, 37,* 297–303.

Caspi, A., Sugden, K., Moffitt, T. E., Taylor, A., Craig, I. W., Harrington, H., et al. (2003). Influence of life stress on depression: Moderation by a polymorphism in the 5-HTT gene. *Science, 301,* 386–389.

Chang, Y. C., Rapoport, S. I., & Rao, J. S. (2009). Chronic administration of mood stabilizers upregulates BDNF and bcl-2 expression levels in rat prefrontal cortex. *Neurochemical Research, 34,* 536–541.

Christensen, M. V., & Kessing, L. V. (2005). Clinical use of coping in affective disorder: A critical review of the literature. *Clinical Practice and Epidemiology in Mental Health, 1,* 20.

Christensen, M. V., & Kessing, L. V. (2006). Do personality traits predict first onset in depressive and bipolar disorder? *Nordic Journal of Psychiatry, 60,* 79–88.

Cicchetti, D., Rogosch, F. A., Gunnar, M. R., & Toth, S. L. (in press). The differential impacts of early abuse on internalizing problems and diurnal cortisol activity in school-aged children. *Child Development.*

Cicchetti, D., & Toth, S. L. (1995). Developmental psychopathology and disorders of affect. In D. Cicchetti & D. J. Cohen (Eds.), *Developmental psychopathology: Risk, disorder, and adaptation* (Vol. 2, pp. 369–420). New York: Wiley.

Cicchetti, D., & Toth, S. L. (1998). The development of depression in children and adolescents. *American Psychologist, 53,* 221–241.

Cohen, A. N., Hammen, C., Henry, R. M., & Daley, S. E. (2006). Effects of stress and social support on recurrence in bipolar disorder. *Journal of Affective Disorders, 82,* 143–147.

Colom, F., Vieta, E., Martínez-Arán, A., Reinares, M., Benabarre, A., & Gastó, C. (2000). Clinical factors associated with treatment noncompliance in euthymic bipolar patients. *Journal of Clinical Psychiatry, 61,* 549–555.

Conus, P., Cotton, S., Abdel-Baki, A., Lambert, M., Berk, M., & McGorry, P. D. (2006). Symptomatic and functional outcome 12 months after a first episode of psychotic mania: Barriers to recovery in a catchment area sample. *Bipolar Disorders, 8,* 221–231.

Coryell, W., Solomon, D., Turvey, C., Keller M., Leon, A., Endicott, J., et al. (2003). The long-term course of rapid-cycling bipolar disorder. *Archives of General Psychiatry, 60,* 914–920.

Coryell, W., Turvey, C., Endicott, J., Leon, A. C., Mueller, T., Solomon, D., et al. (1998). Bipolar I affective disorder: Predictors of outcome after 15 years. *Journal of Affective Disorders, 50,* 109–116.

DelBello, M. P., Hansemann, P., Adler, C. M., Fleck, D. E., & Strakowski, S. M. (2007). Twelve-month outcome of adolescents with bipolar disorder following first hospitalization for a manic or mixed episode. *American Journal of Psychiatry, 164,* 582–590.

Dienes, K. A., Hammen, C., Henry, R. M., Cohen, A. N., & Daley, S. E. (2006). The stress sensitization hypothesis: Understanding the course of bipolar disorder. *Journal of Affective Disorders, 95(1–3),* 43–49.

Dunayevich, E., Sax, K. W., Keck, P. E., Jr., McElroy, S. L., Sorter, M. T., McConville, B. J., et al. (2000). Twelve-month outcome in bipolar patients with and without personality disorders. *Journal of Clinical Psychiatry, 61,* 134–139.

Dunner, D. L., & Fieve, R. R. (1974). Clinical factors in lithium carbonate prophylaxis failure. *Archives of General Psychiatry, 30,* 228–233.

Ellicott, A., Hammen, C., Gitlin, M., Brown, G., & Jamison, K. (1990). Life events and the course of bipolar disorder. *American Journal of Psychiatry, 147,* 1194–1198.

Fergusson, D. M., Horwood, L. J., & Lynskey, M. T. (1996). Childhood sexual abuse and psychiatric disorder in young adulthood: II. Psychiatric outcomes of childhood sexual abuse. *Journal of the American Academy of Child and Adolescent Psychiatry, 35,* 1365–1374.

Fossey, M. D., Otto, M. W., Yates, W. R., Wisniewski, S. R., Gyulai, L., Allen, M. H., et al. (2006). Validation of the distinction between primary and secondary substance use disorder in patients with bipolar disorder: Data from the first 1000 STEP-BD participants. *American Journal of Addictions, 15,* 138–143.

Franchini, L., Zanardi, R., Smeraldi, E., & Gasparini, M. (1999). Early onset of lithium prophylaxis as a predictor of good long-term outcome. *European Archives of Psychiatry and Clinical Neuroscience, 249,* 227–230.

Garno, J. L., Goldberg, J. F., Ramirez, P. M., & Ritzler, B. A. (2005a). Bipolar disorder with comorbid cluster B personality features: Impact on suicidality. *Journal of Clinical Psychiatry, 66,* 339–345.

Garno, J. L., Goldberg, J. F., Ramirez, P. M., & Ritzler, B. A. (2005b). Impact of childhood abuse on the clinical course of bipolar disorder. *British Journal of Psychiatry, 186,* 121–125.

Gelenberg, A. J., Kane, J. M., Keller, M. B., Lavori, P., Rosenbaum, J. F., Cole, K., et al. (1989). Comparison of standard and low serum levels of lithium for maintenance treatment of bipolar disorder. *New England Journal of Medicine, 321,* 1389–1493.

Geller, B., Craney, J. L., Bolhofner, K., Nickelsburg, M. J., Williams, M., & Zimerman, B. (2002). Two-year prospective follow-up of children with a prepubertal and early adolescent bipolar disorder phenotype. *American Journal of Psychiatry, 159,* 927–933.

Geller, B., Tillman, R., Bolhofner, K., & Zimerman, B. (2008). Child bipolar I disorder: Prospective continuity with adult bipolar I disorder; characteristics of second and third episodes; predictors of 8-year outcome. *Archives of General Psychiatry, 65,* 1125–1133.

Geller, B., Tillman, R., Craney, J. L., & Bolhofner, K. (2004). Four-year prospective outcome and natural history of mania in children with a prepubertal and early adolescent bipolar disorder phenotype. *Archives of General Psychiatry, 61,* 459–467.

Geller, B., Zimerman, B., Williams, M., Bolhofner, K., & Craney, J. L. (2001). Bipolar disorder at prospective follow-up of adults who had prepubertal major depressive disorder. *American Journal of Psychiatry, 158*, 125–127.

Ghaemi, S. N. (2007). Feeling and time: The phenomenology of mood disorders, depressive realism, and existential psychotherapy. *Schizophrenia Bulletin, 33*, 122–130.

Ghaemi, S. N., Boiman, E. E., & Goodwin, F. K. (2000). Diagnosing bipolar disorder and the effect of antidepressants: A naturalistic study. *Journal of Clinical Psychiatry, 61*, 804–808.

Goldberg, J. F. (2008). Antidepressant prescribing and rapid cycling. *American Journal of Psychiatry, 165*, 1048–1049.

Goldberg, J. F., Calabrese, J. R., Saville, B. R., Frye, M. A., Ketter, T. A., Suppes, T., et al. (2009). Mood destabilization during acute and continuation phase treatment for bipolar I disorder with lamotrigine or placebo. *Journal of Clinical Psychiatry, 70*, 1273–1280.

Goldberg, J. F., & Ernst, C. L. (2002). Features associated with the delayed initiation of mood stabilizers at illness onset in bipolar disorder. *Journal of Clinical Psychiatry, 63*, 985–991.

Goldberg, J. F., & Ernst, C. L. (2004a). Clinical correlates of childhood and adolescent adjustment in adult patients with bipolar disorder. *Journal of Nervous and Mental Disease, 192*, 187–192.

Goldberg, J. F., & Ernst, C. L. (2004b). Clinical features related to age at onset in bipolar disorder. *Journal of Affective Disorders, 82*, 21–27.

Goldberg, J. F., & Garno, J. L. (2009). Age at onset of bipolar disorder and risk for comorbid borderline personality disorder. *Bipolar Disorders, 11*, 205–208.

Goldberg, J. F., & Harrow, M. (2004). Consistency of remission and outcome in bipolar and unipolar mood disorders: A 10-year prospective follow-up. *Journal of Affective Disorders, 81*, 123–131.

Goldberg, J. F., & Harrow, M. (2005). Subjective life satisfaction and objective functional outcome in bipolar and unipolar mood disorders: A longitudinal analysis. *Journal of Affective Disorders, 89*, 79–89.

Goldberg, J. F., Harrow, M., & Leon, A. C. (1996). Lithium treatment of bipolar disorders under naturalistic follow-up conditions. *Psychopharmacology Bulletin, 32*, 47–54.

Goldberg, J. F., Harrow, M., & Whiteside, J. E. (2001). Risk for bipolar illness in patients initially hospitalized for unipolar depression. *American Journal of Psychiatry, 158*, 1265–1270.

Goldstein, B. I., & Levitt, A. J. (2006). Further evidence for a developmental subtype of bipolar disorder defined by age at onset: Results from the National Epidemiologic Survey on Alcohol and Related Conditions. *American Journal of Psychiatry, 163*, 1633–1636.

Goodwin, G. M., Bowden, C. L., Calabrese, J. R., Grunze, H., Kasper, S., White, R., et al. (2004). A pooled analysis of 2 placebo-controlled 18-month trials of lamotrigine and lithium maintenance in bipolar I disorder. *Journal of Clinical Psychiatry, 65*, 432–441.

Gorrindo, T., Blair, R. J. R., Budhani, S., Dickstein, D. P., Pine, D. S., & Leibenluft, E. (2005). Deficits on a probabilistic response-reversal task in patients with pediatric bipolar disorder. *American Journal of Psychiatry, 162*, 1975–1977.

Gottlieb, G. (2007). Probabilistic epigenesist. *Developmental Science, 10*, 1–11.

Grant, B. F., Stinson, F. S., Hasin, D. S., Dawson, D. A., Chou, S. P., Ruan, W. J., et al. (2005). Prevalence, correlates, and comorbidity of bipolar I disorder and axis I and II disorders: Results from the National Epidemiological Survey on Alcohol and Related Conditions. *Journal of Clinical Psychiatry, 60*, 1205–1215.

Grof, P., Duffy, A., Cavazzoni, P., Grof, E., Garnham, J., MacDougall, M., et al. (2002). Is response to prophylactic lithium a familial trait? *Journal of Clinical Psychiatry, 63*, 942–947.

Guadiano, B. A., Uebelacker, L. A., & Miller, I. W. (2008). Impact of remitted substance use disorders on the future course of bipolar I disorder: Findings from a clinical trial. *Psychiatry Research, 160,* 63–71.

Gunderson, J. G., Weinberg, I., Daversa, M. T., Kuppenbender, K. D., Zanarini, M. C., Shea, M. T., et al. (2006). Descriptive and longitudinal observations on the relationship of borderline personality disorder and bipolar disorder. *American Journal of Psychiatry, 163,* 1173–1178.

Hammen, C., & Gitlin, M. (1997). Stress reactivity in bipolar patients and its relation to prior history of disorder. *American Journal of Psychiatry, 154,* 856–857.

Harvey, A. G. (2008). Sleep and circadian rhythms in bipolar disorder: Seeking synchrony, harmony, and regulation. *American Journal of Psychiatry, 165,* 820–829.

Heim, C., & Nemeroff, C. B. (2001). The role of childhood trauma in the neurobiology of mood and anxiety disorders: Preclinical and clinical studies. *Biological Psychiatry, 49,* 1023–1039.

Hirschfeld-Becker, D. R., Biederman, J., Calltharp, S., Rosenbaum, E. D., Faraone, S. V., & Rosenbaum, J. F. (2003). Behavioral inhibition and disinhibition as hypothesized precursors to psychopathology: Implications for pediatric bipolar disorder. *Biological Psychiatry, 53,* 985–999.

Hlastala, S. A., Frank, E., Kowalski, J., Sherrill, J. T., Tu, X. M., Anderson, B., et al. (2000). Stressful life events, bipolar disorder, and the "kindling model." *Journal of Abnormal Psychology, 109,* 777–786.

Holma, K. M., Melartin, T. K., Holma, I. A., & Isometsä, E. T. (2008). Predictors for switch from unipolar major depressive disorder to bipolar disorder type I or II: A 5-year prospective study. *Journal of Clinical Psychiatry, 69,* 1267–1275.

Jackson, A., Cavanagh, J., & Scott, J. (2003). A systematic review of manic and depressive prodromes. *Journal of Affective Disorders, 74,* 209–217.

Johnson, S. L., & Miller, I. (1997). Negative life events and time to recovery from episodes of bipolar disorder. *Journal of Abnormal Psychology, 106,* 449–457.

Judd, L. L., Akiskal, H. S., Schettler, P. J., Endicott, J., Leon, A. C., Solomon, D. A., et al. (2005). Psychosocial disability in the course of bipolar I and II disorders: A prospective, comparative, longitudinal study. *Archives of General Psychiatry, 62,* 1322–1330.

Judd, L. L., Schettler, P. J., Akiskal, H. S., Coryell, W., Leon, A. C., Maser, J. D., et al. (2008). Residual symptom recovery from major affective episodes in bipolar disorders and rapid episode relapse/recurrence. *Archives of General Psychiatry, 65,* 386–394.

Kauer-Sant'Anna, M., Bond, D. J., Lam, R. W., & Yatham, L. N. (2009). Functional outcomes in first-episode patients with bipolar disorder: A prospective study from the Systematic Treatment Optimization Program for Early Mania Project. *Comprehensive Psychiatry, 50,* 1–8.

Kay, J. H., Altshuler, L. L., Ventura, J., & Mintz, J. (2002). Impact of axis II comorbidity of bipolar illness in men: A retrospective chart review. *Bipolar Disorders, 4,* 237–242.

Keck, P. E., Jr., McElroy, S. L., Strakowski, S. M., West, S. A., Sax, K. W., Hawkins, J. M., et al. (1998). 12-month outcome of patients with bipolar disorder following hospitalization for a manic or mixed episode. *American Journal of Psychiatry, 155,* 646–652.

Kendler, K. S., Thornton, L. M., & Gardner, C. O. (2001). Genetic risk, number of previous depressive episodes, and stressful life events in predicting onset of major depression. *American Journal of Psychiatry, 158,* 582–586.

Kessing, L. V., & Andersen, P. K. (2004). Does the risk of developing dementia increase with the number of episodes in patients with depressive disorder and in patients with bipolar disorder? *Journal of Neurology, Neurosurgery, and Psychiatry, 75,* 1662–1666.

Kraepelin, E. (1921). *Manic depressive insanity and paranoia* (G. M. Robertson, Ed. & R. M. Barclay, Trans.). Edinburgh, UK: Livingstone.

Krüger, S., Alda, M., Young, L. T., Goldapple, K., Parikh, S., & Mayberg, H. S. (2006). Risk and resilience markers in bipolar disorder: Brain responses to emotional challenge in bipolar patients and their healthy siblings. *American Journal of Psychiatry, 163*, 257–264.

Kupka, R. W., Luckenbaugh, D. A., Post, R. M., Suppes, T., Altshuler, L. L., Keck, P. E., Jr., et al. (2005). Comparison of rapid-cycling and non-rapid-cycling bipolar disorder based on prospective mood ratings in 539 outpatients. *American Journal of Psychiatry, 162*, 1273–1280.

Leverich, G. S., Altshuler, L. L., Frye, M. A., Suppes, T., Keck, P. E., Jr., McElroy, S. L., et al. (2003). Factors associated with suicide attempts in 648 patients with bipolar disorder in the Stanley Foundation Bipolar Network. *Journal of Clinical Psychiatry, 64*, 506–515.

Leverich, G. S., McElroy, S. L., Suppes, T., Keck, P. E., Jr., Denicoff, K. D., Nolen, W. A., et al. (2002). Early physical and sexual abuse associated with an adverse course of bipolar illness. *Biological Psychiatry, 51*, 288–297.

Lin, P. I., McInnis, M. G., Potash, J. B., Willour, V., MacKinnon, D. F., DePaulo, J. R., et al. (2006). Clinical correlates and familial aggregation of age at onset in bipolar disorder. *American Journal of Psychiatry, 163*, 240–246.

Loftus, S. T., & Jaeger, J. (2006). Psychosocial outcome in bipolar I patients with a personality disorder. *Journal of Nervous and Mental Disease, 194*, 967–970.

Luthar, S. S., Cicchetti, D., & Becker, B. (2000). The construct of resilience: A critical evaluation and guidelines for future work. *Child Development, 71*, 543–562.

Maeng, S., Hunsberger, J. G., Pearson, B., Yuan, P., Wang, Y., Wei, Y., et al. (2008). BAG1 plays a critical role in regulating recovery from both manic-like and depression-like behavioral impairments. *Proceedings of the National Academy of Sciences, 105*, 8766–8771.

Mandelli, L., Serretti, A., Marino, E., Pirovano, A., Calati, R., & Colombo, C. (2007). Interaction between serotonin transporter gene, catechol-O-methyltransferase gene and stressful life events in mood disorders. *International Journal of Neuropsychopharmacology, 10*, 437–447.

Mantere, O., Suominen, K., Valtonen, H. M., Arvilommi, P., Leppämäki, S., Melartin, R., et al. (2008). Differences in outcome of DSM-IV bipolar I and II disorders. *Bipolar Disorders, 10*, 413–425.

Martel, M. M., Nigg, J. T., Wong, M. M., Fitzgerald, H. E., Jester, J. M., Puttler, L. I., et al. (2007). Childhood and adolescent resiliency, regulation, and executive functioning in relation to adolescent problems and competence in a high-risk sample. *Developmental Psychopathology, 19*, 541–563.

Martínez-Arán, A., Vieta, E., Colom, F., Torrent, C., Sánchez-Moreno, J., Reinares, M., et al. (2004). Cognitive impairment in euthymic bipolar patients: Implications for clinical and functional outcome. *Bipolar Disorders, 6*, 224–232.

Martino, D. J., Marengo, E., Igoa, A., Scápola, M., Ais, E. D., Perinot, L., et al. (2009). Neurocognitive and symptomatic predictors of functional outcome in bipolar disorders: A prospective 1 year follow up study. *Journal of Affective Disorders, 116*(1–2), 37–42.

Mazza, M., Mandelli, L., Di Nicola, M., Harnic, D., Catalano, V., Tedeschi, D., et al. (2009). Clinical features, response to treatment and functional outcome of bipolar disorder patients with and without comorbid substance use disorder: 1-year follow-up. *Journal of Affective Disorders, 115*(1–2), 27–35.

McClure, E. B., Treland, J. E., Snow, J., Schmajuk, M., Dickstein, D. P., Towbin, K. E., et al. (2005). Deficits in social cognition and response flexibility in pediatric bipolar disorder. *American Journal of Psychiatry, 162*, 1644–1651.

McElroy, S. L., Altshuler, L. L., Suppes, T., Keck, P. E., Jr., Frye, M. A., Denicoff, K. D., et al. (2001). Axis I psychiatric comorbidity and its relationship to historical illness variables in 288 patients with bipolar disorder. *American Journal of Psychiatry, 158*, 420–426.

McEwen, B. S. (1999). Stress and hippocampal plasticity. *Annual Review of Neuroscience, 22,* 105–122.

McEwen, B. S. (2001). Plasticity of the hippocampus: Adaptation to chronic stress and allostatic load. *Annals of the New York Academy of Science, 933,* 265–277.

McEwen, B. S., & Stellar, E. (1993). Stress and the individual. Mechanisms leading to disease. *Archives of Internal Medicine, 153,* 2093–2101.

Meeks, S. (1999). Bipolar disorder in the latter half of life: symptom presentation, global functioning and age at onset. *Journal of Affective Disorders, 52,* 161–167.

Miklowitz, D. (1992). Longitudinal outcome and medication noncompliance among manic patients with and without mood-incongruent psychotic features. *Journal of Nervous and Mental Disease, 180,* 703–711.

Miklowitz, D. (2008). Adjunctive psychotherapy for bipolar disorder: State of the evidence. *American Journal of Psychiatry, 165,* 1408–1419.

Miklowitz, D. J., Goldstein, M. J., Nuechterlein, K. H., Snyder, K. S., & Mintz, J. (1988). Family factors and the course of bipolar affective disorder. *Archives of General Psychiatry, 45,* 225–231.

Müller, D. J., de Luca, V., Sicard, T., King, N., Strauss, J., & Kennedy, J. L. (2006). Brain-derived neurotrophic factor (BDNF) gene and rapid-cycling bipolar disorder: Family-based association study. *British Journal of Psychiatry, 189,* 317–323.

Mundo, E., Walker, M., Cate, T., Macciardi, F., & Kennedy, J. L. (2001). The role of serotonin transporter protein gene in antidepressant-induced mania in bipolar disorder: Preliminary findings. *Archives of General Psychiatry, 58,* 539–544.

Mur, M., Portella, M. J., Martínez-Arán, A., Pifarré, J., & Vieta, E. (2008). Long-term stability of cognitive impairment in bipolar disorder: A 2-year follow-up study of lithium-treated euthymic bipolar patients. *Journal of Clinical Psychiatry, 69,* 712–719.

Mysels, D. J., Endicott, J., Nee, J., Maser, J. D., Solomon, D., Coryell, W., et al. (2007). The association between course of illness and subsequent morbidity in bipolar I disorder. *Journal of Psychiatric Research, 41,* 80–89.

Neria, Y., Bromet, E. J., Carlson, G. A., & Naz, B. (2005). Assaultive trauma and illness course in psychotic bipolar disorder: Findings from the Suffolk County Mental Health Project. *Acta Psychiatric Scandinavica, 111,* 380–383.

Nolen, W. A., Luckenbaugh, D. A., Altshuler, L. L., Suppes, T., McElroy, S. L., Frye, M. A., et al. (2004). Correlates of 1-year prospective outcome in bipolar disorder: Results from the Stanley Foundation Bipolar Network. *American Journal of Psychiatry, 161,* 1447–1454.

Olson, S. L., Bates, J. E., & Bayles, K. (1990). Early antecedents of childhood impulsivity: The role of parent–child interaction, cognitive competence, and temperament. *Journal of Abnormal Child Psychology, 18,* 317–334.

Olson, S. L., Bates, J. E., Sandy, J. M., & Schilling, E. M. (2002). Early developmental precursors of impulsive and inattentive behavior: From infancy to middle childhood. *Journal of Child Psychology and Psychiatry, 43,* 435–447.

Otto, M. W., Simon, N. M., Wisniewski, S. R., Miklowitz, D. J., Kogan, J. N., Reilly-Harrington, N. A., et al. (2006). Prospective 12-month course of bipolar disorder in out-patients with and without comorbid anxiety disorders. *British Journal of Psychiatry, 189,* 20–25.

Pandey, G. N., Rizavi, H. S., Dwivedi, Y., & Pavuluri, M. N. (2008). Brain-derived neurotrophic factor gene expression in pediatric bipolar disorder: Effects of treatment and clinical response. *Journal of the American Academy of Child and Adolescent Psychiatry, 47,* 1077–1085.

Perlick, D. A., Rosenheck, R. A., Clarkin, J. F., Maciejewski, P. K., Sirey, J., Struening, E., et al. (2004). Impact of family burden and affective response on clinical outcome among patients with bipolar disorder. *Psychiatric Services, 55,* 1029–1035.

Perlis, R. H., Miyahara, S., Marangell, L. B., Wisniewski, S. R., Ostacher, M., DelBello, M. P., et al. (2004). Long-term implications of early onset in bipolar disorder: Data from the first 1000 participants in the Systematic Treatment Enhancement Program for Bipolar Disorder (STEP-BD). *Biological Psychiatry, 55*, 875–881.

Perlis, R. H., Ostacher, M. J., Patel, J. K., Marangell, L. B., Zhang, H., Wisniewski, S. R., et al. (2006). Predictors of recurrence in bipolar disorder: Primary outcomes from the Systematic Treatment Enhancement Program for Bipolar Disorder (STEP-BD). *American Journal of Psychiatry, 163*, 217–224.

Pirraglia, P. A., Biswas, K., Kilbourne, A. M., Fenn, H., & Bauer, M. S. (2009). A prospective study of the impact of comorbid medical disease on bipolar disorder outcomes. *Journal of Affective Disorders, 115*(3), 355–359.

Pope, M., Dudley, R., & Scott, J. (2007). Determinants of social functioning in bipolar disorder. *Bipolar Disorders, 9*, 38–44.

Post, R. M. (1992). Transduction of psychosocial stress into the neurobiology of recurrent affective disorder. *American Journal of Psychiatry, 149*, 999–1010.

Reinares, M., Colom, F., Sánchez-Moreno, J., Torrent, C., Martínez-Arán, A., Comes, M., et al. (2008). Impact of caregiver group psychoeducation on the course and outcome of bipolar patients in remission: A randomized controlled trial. *Bipolar Disorders, 10*, 511–519.

Robins, E., & Guze, S. B. (1970). Establishment of diagnostic validity in psychiatric illness: Its application to schizophrenia. *American Journal of Psychiatry, 126*, 983–987.

Robinson, L. J., & Ferrier, I. N. (2006). Evolution of cognitive impairment in bipolar disorder: A systematic review of cross-sectional evidence. *Bipolar Disorders, 8*, 103–116.

Rousseva, A., Henry, C., van den Bulke, D., Fournier, G., Laplanche, J. L., Leboyer, M., et al. (2003). Antidepressant-induced mania, rapid cycling and the serotonin transporter gene polymorphism. *Pharmacogenomics, 3*, 101–104.

Savitz, J. B., van der Merwe, L., Stein, D. J., Solms, M., & Ramesar, R. S. (2008). Neuropsychological task performance in bipolar spectrum illness: Genetics, alcohol abuse, medication and childhood trauma. *Bipolar Disorders, 10*, 479–494.

Schneck, C. D., Miklowitz, D. J., Calabrese, J. R., Allen, M. H., Thomas, M. R., Wisniewski, S. R., et al. (2004). Phenomenology of rapid-cycling bipolar disorder: Data from the first 500 participants in the Systematic Treatment Enhancement Program. *American Journal of Psychiatry, 161*, 1902–1908.

Schneck, C. D., Miklowitz, D. J., Miyahara, S., Araga, M., Wisniewski, S., Gyulai, L., et al. (2008). The prospective course of rapid-cycling bipolar disorder: Findings from the STEP-BD. *American Journal of Psychiatry, 165*, 370–377.

Schwartz, A. R., Gerin, W., Davidson, K. W., Pickering, T. G., Brosschot, J. F., Thayer, J. F., et al. (2003). Toward a causal model of cardiovascular responses to stress and the development of cardiovascular disease. *Psychosomatic Medicine, 65*, 22–35.

Simon, G. E., Bauer, M. S., Ludman, E. J., Operskalski, B. H., & Unützer, J. (2007). Mood symptoms, functional impairment, and disability in people with bipolar disorder: Specific effects of mania and depression. *Journal of Clinical Psychiatry, 68*, 1237–1245.

Simon, N. M., Otto, M. W., Weiss, R. D., Bauer, M. S., Miyahara, S. R., Thase, M. E., et al. (2004). Pharmacotherapy for bipolar disorder and comorbid conditions: Baseline data from STEP-BD. *Journal of Clinical Psychopharmacology, 24*, 512–520.

Strakowski, S. M., DelBello, M. P., Fleck, D. E., Adler, C. M., Anthenelli, R. M., Keck, P. E., Jr., et al. (2005). Effects of co-occurring alcohol abuse on the course of bipolar disorder following a first hospitalization for mania. *Archives of General Psychiatry, 62*, 851–858.

Strakowski, S. M., DelBello, M. P., Fleck, D. E., Adler, C. M., Anthenelli, R. M., Keck, P. E., Jr., et al. (2007). Effects of co-occurring cannabis use disorders on the course of bipolar disorder after a first hospitalization for mania. *Archives of General Psychiatry, 64*, 57–64.

Strakowski, S. M., Keck, P. E., Jr., McElroy, S. L., West, S. A., Sax, K. W., Hawkins, J. M., et al. (1998). Twelve-month outcome after a first hospitalization for affective psychosis. *Archives of General Psychiatry, 55,* 49–55.

Strakowski, S. M., Williams, J. R., Sax, K. W., Fleck, D. E., DelBello, M. P., & Bourne, M. L. (2000). Is impaired outcome following a first manic episode due to mood-incongruent psychosis? *Journal of Affective Disorders, 61,* 87–94.

Suominen, K., Mantere, O., Valtonen, H., Arvilommi, P., Leppämäki, S., Paunio, T., et al. (2007). Early age at onset of bipolar disorder is associated with more severe clinical features but delayed treatment seeking. *Bipolar Disorders, 9,* 698–705.

Swann, A. C., Bowden, C. L., Calabrese, J. R., Dilsaver, S. C., & Morris, D. D. (1999). Differential effect of number of previous episodes of affective disorder on response to lithium or divalproex in acute mania. *American Journal of Psychiatry, 156,* 1264–1266.

Swann, A. C., Bowden, C. L., Morris, D., Calabrese, J. R., Petty, F., Small, J., et al. (1997). Depression during mania. Treatment response to lithium or divalproex. *Archives of General Psychiatry, 54,* 37–42.

Swann, A. C., Dougherty, D. M., Pazzaglia, P. J., Pham, M., & Moeller, F. G. (2004). Impulsivity: A link between bipolar disorder and substance abuse. *Bipolar Disorders, 6,* 204–212.

Swann, A. C., Dougherty, D. M., Pazzaglia, P. J., Pham, M., Steinberg, J. L., & Moeller, F. G. (2005). Increased impulsivity associated with severity of suicide attempt history in patients with bipolar disorder. *American Journal of Psychiatry, 162,* 1680–1687.

Swann, A. C., Pazzaglia, P., Nichols, A., Dougherty, D. M., & Moeller, F. G. (2003). Impulsivity and phase of illness in bipolar disorder. *Journal of Affective Disorders, 73,* 105–111.

Swendsen, J., Hammen, C., Heller, T., & Gitlin, M. (1995). Correlates of stress reactivity in patients with bipolar disorder. *American Journal of Psychiatry, 152,* 795–797.

Tabarés-Seisdedos, R., Balanzá-Martínez, V., Sánchez-Moreno, J., Martínez-Arán, A., Salazar-Fraile, J., Selva-Vera, G., et al. (2008). Neurocognitive and clinical predictors of functional outcome in patients with schizophrenia and bipolar I disorder at one-year follow-up. *Journal of Affective Disorders, 109,* 286–299.

Tohen, M., Hennen, J., Zarate, C. M., Jr., Baldessarini, R. J., Strakowski, S. M., Stoll, A. L., et al. (2000). Two-year syndromal and functional recovery in 219 cases of first-episode major affective disorder with psychotic features. *American Journal of Psychiatry, 157,* 220–228.

Tohen, M., Tsuang, M. T., & Goodwin, D. C. (1992). Prediction of outcome in mania by mood-congruent or mood-incongruent psychotic features. *American Journal of Psychiatry, 149,* 1580–1584.

Tohen, M., Waternaux, C. M., & Tsuang, M. T. (1990). Outcome in mania: A 4-year prospective follow-up of 75 patients utilizing survival analysis. *Archives of General Psychiatry, 47,* 1106–1111.

Tohen, M., Zarate, C. A., Jr., Hennen, J., Khalsa, H. M., Strakowski, S. M., Gebre-Medhin, P., et al. (2003). The McLean–Harvard First-Episode Mania Study: Prediction of recovery and first recurrence. *American Journal of Psychiatry, 160,* 2099–2107.

Toniolo, R. A., Caetano, S. C., da Silva, P. V., & Lafer, B. (2009). Clinical significance of lifetime panic disorder in the course of bipolar disorder type I. *Comprehensive Psychiatry, 50,* 9–12.

Tsai, S. M., Chen, C., Kuo, C., Lee, J., Lee, H., & Strakowski, S. M. (2001). 15-year outcome of treated bipolar disorder. *Journal of Affective Disorders, 63,* 215–220.

Uçok, A., Karaveli, D., Kundakçi, T., & Yazici, O. (1998). Comorbidity of personality disorders with bipolar mood disorders. *Comprehensive Psychiatry, 39,* 72–74.

Van Riel, W. G., Vieta, E., Martínez-Arán, A., Haro, J. M., Bertsch, J., Reed, C., et al. (2008). Chronic mania revisited: Factors associated with treatment non-response during prospective follow-up of a large European cohort (EMBLEM). *World Journal of Biological Psychiatry, 9,* 313–320.

Vythilingam, M., Heim, C., Newport, J., Miller, A. H., Anderson, E., Bronen, R., et al. (2002). Childhood trauma associated with smaller hippocampal volume in women with major depression. *American Journal of Psychiatry, 159,* 2072–2080.

Wehr, T. A., Sack, D. A., & Rosenthal, N. E. (1987). Sleep reduction as a final common pathway in the genesis of mania. *American Journal of Psychiatry, 144,* 201–204.

Wehr, T. A., Turner, E. H., Shimada, J. H., Loew, C. H., Barker, C., & Leibenluft, E. (1998). Treatment of rapidly cycling bipolar patient by extended bed rest and darkness to stabilize the timing and duration of sleep. *Biological Psychiatry, 43,* 822–828.

Weiss, R. D., Ostacher, M. J., Otto, M. W., Calabrese, J. R., Fossey, M., Wisniewski, S. R., et al. (2005). Does recovery from substance abuse matter in patients with bipolar disorder? *Journal of Clinical Psychiatry, 66,* 730–735.

Wilhelm, K., Siegel, J. E., Finch, A. W., Hadzi-Pavlovic, D., Mitchell, P. B., Parker, G., et al. (2007). The long and the short of it: Associations between 5-HTT genotypes and coping with stress. *Psychosomatic Medicine, 69,* 614–620.

Winokur, G., Coryell, W., Akiskal, H. S., Endicott, J., Keller, M., & Mueller, T. (1994). Manic-depressive (bipolar) disorder: The course in light of a prospective ten-year follow-up of 131 patients. *Acta Psychiatrica Scandinavica, 89,* 102–110.

Zalsman, G., Huang, Y.-Y., Oquendo, M. A., Burke, A. K., Hu, X.-Z., Brent, D. A., et al. (2006). Association of a triallelic serotonin transporter gene promoter region (5-HTTLPR) polymorphism with stressful life events and severity of depression. *American Journal of Psychiatry, 163,* 1588–1593.

PART III

ETIOLOGY/RISK AND PROTECTIVE MECHANISMS

CHAPTER 8

Genetic and Environmental Vulnerability to Bipolar Spectrum Disorders

Erik Willcutt and Matt McQueen

The past two decades have yielded an exponential increase in research examining the genetic and environmental factors that affect individual differences in mood regulation and increase susceptibility to bipolar disorder (BD) and other mood disorders. This rapid accumulation of new knowledge has demonstrated the potential impact of behavioral and molecular genetic methods. However, the complicated and sometimes contradictory results that have emerged from these studies also illustrate the complexity of the etiological pathways to BD and underscore how much remains to be learned.

This chapter is divided into five sections. The first sets the stage for the remainder of the chapter by summarizing a recent paradigm shift in the conceptualization of theoretical models of BD and other psychopathologies. We then describe how etiologically informative studies can help to answer important questions about the nature of BD, using the specific example of the current controversy regarding the nature of the relation between pediatric-onset BD (PBD) and adult-onset BD. In this section, we describe five developmental models that have been proposed to explain this association. The third section summarizes family, adoption, and twin studies of adult-onset bipolar spectrum disorders and PBD, and the fourth section reviews studies that attempted to identify specific genetic and environmental risk factors that increase susceptibility to BD. The final section of the chapter summarizes the implications of these etiologically informative studies for the five competing developmental models of BD introduced in the second section and describes several areas in which additional research is needed.

A PARADIGM SHIFT FROM SINGLE-CAUSE MODELS TO MULTIFACTORIAL ETIOLOGICAL MODELS

A fundamental criticism of molecular genetic studies of BD and virtually all other mental disorders has been the inconsistent replication of initial positive results. This issue is dramatically illustrated by the recent findings of the SzGene project, a meta-analysis of more than 1,000 studies of genetic risk factors for schizophrenia (Allen et al., 2008). The meta-analysis revealed that of the 516 different genes tested for association with schizophrenia by at least one study, only four displayed "strong epidemiological credibility."

The poor reproducibility of initial positive findings has been attributed to a variety of sources of variability among studies. These include small samples sizes, differences in study design and sampling procedures, variability in the specific criteria used to define BD, and differences in the populations from which samples were drawn (e.g., Faraone, Glatt, & Tsuang, 2003; Ioannidis, Ntzani, Trikalinos, & Contopoulos-Ioannidis, 2001).

Although each of these factors almost certainly contributes to the inconsistent results obtained in molecular genetic studies of BD, an important alternative explanation may also play a role. During the latter half of the 20th century, conceptual models of mental disorders were guided by the classical disease formulation set out in diagnostic manuals. This theoretical approach typically implicated simple linear pathways with a single genetic or environmental risk factor that was necessary and sufficient to cause all cases of the disorder. Models that proposed a 1:1 relation between a specific cause and a disorder were optimal for conditions that were caused by a single gene, such as Huntington's disease and phenylketonuria (although even in these cases the etiology is far more complex than was initially understood). In contrast, an increasing literature suggests that these models do not provide a satisfactory account of BD or other mental disorders.

In addition to the inconsistent replication and small effect sizes of the genetic risk factors that were first identified, models that posit a single cause were challenged further when subsequent studies identified new risk factors for the disorder. Single-cause models also struggled to account for the striking heterogeneity among individuals within each diagnostic category, the pervasive comorbidity between different disorders, and the fact that many individuals with a putative causal risk factor did not meet criteria for any disorder. Taken together, these results precipitated a major reconceptualization of theoretical models of mental disorders. Rather than attempting to identify a single necessary and sufficient cause that is specific to each disorder, more recent theoretical models explicitly hypothesize that BD and other mental disorders are heterogeneous conditions that arise from the additive and interactive effects of multiple genetic and environmental risk factors at different phases of development (e.g., Faraone, Perlis, et al., 2005; Pennington, 2006; Willcutt, Sonuga-Barke, Nigg, & Sergeant, 2008).

Two specific examples help to illustrate how a multifactorial etiology could lead to BD. Independent pathway models suggest that distinct sets of risk factors independently lead to the development of BD, a phenomenon known as *equifinality* (e.g., Curtis & Cicchetti, 2003). Therefore, independent pathway models propose etiological subtypes within the overall population of individuals with BD. In contrast, quantitative trait models suggest that BD arises from the additive and interactive effects of multiple genetic and environmental risk factors. Each risk factor increases susceptibility to BD by a small amount, but none are necessary or sufficient to cause BD in isolation (see Willcutt et al., 2008, for a more detailed discussion of these models and their implications).

Multifactorial models may be able to account for several results that could not be explained by earlier models that proposed that BD arose from a single necessary and sufficient cause. Most relevant to this chapter, multifactorial models suggest that the effect sizes of genetic risk loci or environmental risk factors are likely to be relatively small. If this is correct, even "true positive" results may replicate inconsistently because of the low statistical power of most studies to detect a specific small effect. The quantitative trait model also offers an explanation for the wide range of severity within the bipolar I diagnosis as well as the fact that many individuals at risk for bipolar I develop a less severe bipolar spectrum disorder such as cyclothymia or BD not otherwise specified rather than bipolar I. Finally, multifactorial models may help to explain why some risk factors for BD are also risk factors for other conditions with multifactorial etiologies, leading to the frequent comorbidity between BD and a wide range of other mental disorders.

COMPETING MODELS OF THE RELATION BETWEEN PEDIATRIC-ONSET BIPOLAR DISORDER AND ADULT-ONSET BIPOLAR DISORDER: IMPLICATIONS OF ETIOLOGICALLY INFORMATIVE STUDIES

As reviewed in more detail elsewhere in this volume, one of the most important ongoing controversies in the BD literature involves the nature and validity of PBD and its relation with adult-onset BD. The optimal test of the continuity or discontinuity of PBD versus adult-onset BD will come from longitudinal studies that follow children diagnosed with PBD into adulthood. Until those data are available, etiologically informative methods may provide important information relevant to this question. In this section, we describe five competing theoretical models of the relation between PBD and adult-onset BD. We then systematically review studies of the etiology of PBD and adult-onset BD. In the concluding section of the chapter, we examine the implications of these results for each of the five theories that have been proposed to explain the relation between PBD and adult-onset BD.

Model 1: Pediatric-Onset Bipolar Disorder Is Not a Valid Diagnosis

Some authors in the popular press have argued that PBD does not exist and that children diagnosed with PBD are simply displaying the exuberant behavior of normal children. The criteria that must be met for a mental disorder to be considered valid have been the focus of considerable discussion (e.g., Cantwell, 1980; Wakefield, 1999; Widiger & Clark, 2000), and a comprehensive description of all facets of this debate is beyond the scope of this chapter. The hypothesis that PBD does not exist, however, hinges on a straightforward question: Do the symptoms of PBD lead to significant impairment in important domains of functioning that is sufficiently severe to warrant intervention?

The reviews in several other chapters in this volume indicate that children with PBD experience significant impairment. In comparison to children without PBD, those with PBD exhibit pronounced difficulties in peer and family relationships, significant academic impairment, and higher rates of comorbidity with substance use disorders, disruptive disorders, and other diagnoses. Children with PBD are also more likely to be hospitalized and are at significantly higher risk for suicide attempts and completions. Finally, studies of neuropsychological functioning indicate that children with PBD exhibit a range of neurocognitive weaknesses that include slow and inconsistent cognitive processing speed, difficulty inhibiting inappropriate behaviors, and difficulty retaining and manipulating new information in memory.

These data strongly suggest that, although the optimal diagnostic classification is not straightforward, most children who are diagnosed with PBD experience significant difficulty in a wide range of functional domains. Therefore, we can reject the hypothesis that the PBD diagnosis mislabels children who are simply exuberant and are not experiencing clinically significant impairment. We turn next to five more plausible hypotheses regarding the relation between PBD and adult-onset BD.

Model 2: Pediatric-Onset Bipolar Disorder and Adult-Onset Bipolar Disorder Are a Single Developmental Disorder

This parsimonious model suggests that there is full developmental continuity between PBD and adult-onset BD, such that PBD is simply the early developmental manifestation of adult bipolar I (e.g., Chang, 2007; Geller et al., 2006). This model is supported by studies that suggest that both PBD and adult-onset BD are characterized by similar core symptoms such as emotional lability as well as by self-report data suggesting that 20–40% of adults with BPD experienced their first episode during childhood (e.g., Perlis et al., 2009). In contrast, many adults with BPD report onset of symptoms after puberty (Manchia et al., 2008; Perlis et al.,

TABLE 8.1. Results at Each Level of Analysis That Would Support the Six Competing Models of Pediatric-Onset Bipolar Disorder and Its Relation with Adult-Onset Bipolar Disorder

Model	Level of analysis				
	Symptoms and impairment	Familial rate of BD	Familial rate of other disorders	Heritability	Environmental and genetic risk factors
PBD is an invalid diagnosis.	PBD = Cont	PBD = Cont	PBD = Cont	ABD > PBD	Only for adult
PBD and ABD are a single disorder.	ABD = PBD > Cont	ABD = PBD > Cont	ABD = PBD > Cont	ABD = PBD	ABD = PBD > Cont
PBD and ABD are distinct disorders.	PBD ≠ ABD	ABD > PDB = Cont	PBD ≠ ABD	PBD ≠ ABD	PBD ≠ ABD
PBD is a severe form of ABD.	PBD > ABD > Cont	PBD > ABD > Cont	PBD > ABD > Cont	PBD > ABD	PBD > ABD > Cont
Comorbidity subtype: BD + ADHD[a]	BD + ADHD ≠ BD − ADHD	BD + ADHD ≠ BD − ADHD	ADHD: BD + ADHD > BD − ADHD	BD + ADHD ≠ BD − ADHD	BD + ADHD ≠ BD − ADHD

Note. PBD, pediatric-onset bipolar disorder; ABD, adult-onset bipolar disorder; Cont, control group. BD, bipolar disorder; ADHD, attention-deficit/hyperactivity disorder.
[a]Although BD + ADHD is used as the specific example, the same predictions would hold for subtypes defined by comorbidity with anxiety, psychosis, or any other disorder.

2009), arguing against a single developmental pathway that accounts for all cases. In etiologically informative studies, the single-disorder model would be supported if PBD and adult-onset BD are associated with the same pattern of impairment, similar familial risk, and similar rates of specific genetic and environmental risk factors (Table 8.1).

Model 3: Pediatric-Onset Bipolar Disorder and Adult-Onset Bipolar Disorder Are Distinct Disorders

The distinct disorders hypothesis is another highly parsimonious model that suggests that PBD and adult-onset BD are completely separate and unrelated disorders. In contrast to model 1, the distinct disorders model does not imply that children who receive a diagnosis of PBD are clinically unimpaired. Instead, this model suggests that symptoms that have been classified as PBD may be attributable to a different condition that is unrelated to adult-onset BD, such as severe attention-deficit/hyperactivity disorder (ADHD) or aggressive conduct disorder (e.g., McClellan, Kowatch, & Findling, 2007).

The distinct disorders model predicts that the rate of bipolar I will be higher in the biological family members of probands with adult-onset BD than families of children with PBD. Moreover, if PBD is a completely separate condition, the rate of bipolar I in families of children with PBD should not differ from the rate in families of a comparison sample without BD. In contrast, the biological family members of children with PBD may exhibit elevated rates of disorders other than BD (e.g., higher rates of antisocial behavior if the optimal diagnostic classification is early-onset aggressive conduct disorder). Finally, the distinct disorders model would be supported if PBD and adult-onset BD are associated with different genetic and environmental risk factors and distinct profiles of functional impairment.

Model 4: Severity Gradient

The severity gradient model suggests that PBD is a more severe form of adult-onset BD that has an earlier and more severe onset because of a stronger loading from the same overall pool of genetic and environmental risk factors (e.g., Geller & Tillman, 2005). The plausibility of the severity gradient hypothesis is supported by studies that show that early onset is associated with greater severity in BD and a variety of other disorders, including mental disorders such as schizophrenia (Luoma, Hakko, Ollinen, Jarvelin, & Lindeman, 2008) and conduct disorder (e.g., Moffitt et al., 1993) and other conditions such as breast cancer (e.g., Claus, Risch, & Thompson, 1990).

The severity gradient model would be supported if PBD is associated with qualitatively similar but quantitatively more severe functional and neurocognitive impairment than adult-onset BD. Similarly, this model predicts that rates of BD will be higher in the families of probands with PBD versus adult-onset BD, and that genetic or environmental risk factors will have larger effects in groups with PBD versus adult-onset BD.

Model 5: Comorbid Subtype

Comorbidity, the co-occurrence of two or more disorders in the same individual, is the rule rather than the exception for bipolar spectrum disorders. In a meta-analytic review of studies of PBD, Kowatch, Youngstrom, Danielyan, and Findling (2005) reported that nearly two-thirds met criteria for ADHD (40–90%; $M = 62\%$), more than half met criteria for oppositional defiant disorder (ODD; 25–79%; $M = 53\%$), and a significant minority met criteria for conduct disorder (CD; 10–37%; $M = 19\%$). Both adult-onset and PBD also frequently co-occur with a range of anxiety disorders such as panic disorder, obsessive–compulsive disorder, generalized anxiety disorder, and social phobia (e.g., Brotman et al., 2007; Doughty, Wells, Joyce, Olds, & Walsh, 2004; Henin et al., 2005; Kessler, Avenevoli, Ries, & Merikangas, 2001; Kowatch et al., 2005; Pini et al., 1997), and approximately half of all individuals with BD experience significant psychotic symptoms during their lifetime (e.g., Dunayevich & Keck, 2000; Kowatch et al., 2005).

Comorbidity with several of these disorders appears to impact the clinical presentation of individuals with BD. In comparison to individuals with BD alone, individuals with comorbid ADHD or psychotic features have an earlier age of onset, more chronic course, and more severe functional and neuropsychological impairment (e.g., Coryell et al., 2001; Glahn et al., 2007; Nierenberg et al., 2005). Individuals with BD and ADHD are more likely to be nonresponders to lithium therapy (Strober et al., 1998), and comorbidity with CD or posttraumatic stress disorder is associated with higher rates of substance use and abuse (e.g., Goldstein et al., 2008).

On the basis of these findings, some authors have suggested that etiological subtypes of BD may be identified based on comorbidity with disorders such as ADHD or panic disorder (e.g., Faraone, Biederman, Mennin, Wozniak, & Spencer, 1997; Faraone, Biederman, Wozniak, et al., 1997; Masi et al., 2007). The comorbid subtype model suggests that when BD occurs with a specific comorbid disorder, it is a distinct disorder that is due to different etiological influences than BD without the comorbid disorder. If this model is correct, the comorbid subtype should be transmitted separately from BD alone in families, may show differential heritability, and should have a distinct profile of risk factors and clinical correlates.

THE ETIOLOGY OF BIPOLAR DISORDER

Individuals cannot be randomly assigned to different environmental or genetic backgrounds. Therefore, family, adoption, and twin studies take advantage of naturally occurring events to estimate the magnitude of genetic and environmental influences on a trait or disorder (for a detailed description of these methods, see Faraone, Tsuang, & Tsuang, 1999; Plomin, DeFries, McClearn, & McGuffin, 2001).

Family Studies

Family studies test whether the rate of a disorder is significantly higher in biological family members of individuals with the disorder than in family members of individuals without the diagnosis. If the disorder occurs more frequently in family members of individuals with the disorder, this suggests that familial factors increase susceptibility for the disorder. Family data can also be used to examine diagnostic heterogeneity by testing for differences in familiality in subgroups of interest within the overall disorder.

Overview of Family Studies and Implications for Developmental Models of Bipolar Disorder

More than 20 family studies demonstrate that first-degree biological family members of individuals with adult-onset BD are approximately 10 times more likely to meet criteria for BD than individuals in the general population (see comprehensive review by Smoller & Finn, 2003). Similarly, siblings and parents of children with PBD have a rate of BD that is three to 10 times higher than that in the parents of clinically referred children without BD and 10 to 20 times higher than the base rate of BD in the population (e.g., Brotman et al., 2007; Faraone, Biederman, Mennin, et al., 1997; Faraone, Biederman, & Monuteaux, 1997; Faraone, Biederman, Wozniak, et al., 2001; Geller et al., 2006; Pavuluri, Henry, Nadimpalli, O'Connor, & Sweeney, 2006; Strober et al., 1988). This overall pattern of results across studies clearly demonstrates a strong familial component to BD. Several subsequent studies have extended these findings to examine the familial continuity between PBD and adult-onset BD.

AGE OF ONSET

The high familiality in populations with PBD suggests that the etiology of BD may vary as a function of age of onset. This hypothesis has received additional support from family studies that subdivided groups with adult-onset BD into early onset versus late onset. Although the specific definition of early-onset BD was variable (most often late adolescence or early adulthood), these studies consistently found that the familial risk for BD was at least two to four times higher in the early-onset group (e.g., Geller et al., 2006; Lewinsohn, Klein, & Seeley, 2000; Rice et al., 1987; Strober et al., 1988). Moreover, when Lin and colleagues (2006) subdivided their sample into three groups that included an early-onset group with a first episode before 21 years of age, they found that family members of each type of proband tended to fall into the same age of onset categorization if they met criteria for BD. These results suggest that the early-onset group may be a useful group for molecular genetic studies (e.g., Faraone et al., 2003).

DEVELOPMENT OF CHILDREN AT RISK FOR BIPOLAR DISORDER

Two specific types of family studies are especially important for models of the relation between PBD and adult-onset BD. First, the studies summarized previously found significant elevations of bipolar I in the adult family members of probands with PBD, suggesting that PBD and adult-onset BD I are due at least in part to a common risk diathesis (e.g., Geller et al., 2006). The second set of studies examined the rate of PBD in children at risk for BD because of a parent who meets criteria for BD in adulthood (see reviews by DelBello & Geller, 2001; Jones & Bentall, 2008). By the end of childhood, the rate of bipolar spectrum disorders in the at-risk group (4–13%) was significantly higher than the estimated base rate of bipolar spectrum disorders in children (Chang, Steiner, & Ketter, 2000; Duffy, Alda, Crawford, Milin, & Grof, 2007; Duffy, Grof, Kutcher, Robertson, & Alda, 2001; Henin et al., 2005; Hillegers et al., 2005; Hirshfeld-Becker et al., 2006), and up to 50% of the children of parents with BD met criteria for a major mood disorder by adulthood (e.g., Chang et al., 2000).

Familial Associations with Other Disorders

OTHER MOOD DISORDERS

In addition to the elevated rates of BD described in the previous section, the systematic review by Smoller and Finn (2003) reported a 14-fold increase in risk for unipolar depression in the families of adult probands with BD. Similarly, children with at least one parent who met criteria for BD are significantly more likely to meet criteria for major depressive disorder (MDD) than children of parents without BD (18–43% vs. 0–8%; e.g., Duffy et al., 2007; Henin et al., 2005). In contrast to the pattern in families of individuals with BD, the biological family members of probands with MDD are at dramatically increased risk for MDD (up to 18 times higher than in families of individuals without MDD) but only a slightly increased risk for BD (Smoller & Finn, 2003).

Although some cases of MDD in these family studies may eventually meet criteria for BD, these data suggest that familial BD is associated with increased risk for both BD and unipolar mood disorders. One set of familial risk factors may increase susceptibility to general mood dysregulation that may be expressed as unipolar depression or BD, and a second set of risk factors may specifically increase susceptibility to mania.

DISRUPTIVE BEHAVIOR DISORDERS

Parental BPD is associated bidirectionally with childhood ADHD (Faraone, Biederman, Mennin, & Russell, 1998). Children of adults with BD are three to five times more likely to meet criteria for ADHD or ODD than children of parents without BD (e.g., Chang et al., 2000; Duffy et al., 2007; Henin et al., 2005; Hirshfeld-Becker et al., 2006), and relatives of children with ADHD have twice the risk of BD than relatives of children without ADHD (Faraone et al., 2001; Geller et al., 2006). The disruptive disorders may also be markers for important differences in familiality in groups with BD. For example, Geller and colleagues (2006) found that risk for bipolar I was five to seven times higher in first-degree biological relatives of children with bipolar I and a comorbid disruptive behavior disorder (ADHD, ODD, or CD) than in relatives of probands with bipolar I alone. This study and others (e.g., Sachs, Baldassano, Truman, & Guille, 2000) also reported that children of parents with both BD and ADHD had an earlier onset of BD than children of parents with BD without ADHD, and Duffy and colleagues (2007) found that children of a parent with BD were only at higher risk for ADHD if the parent was a nonresponder to lithium treatment.

ANXIETY DISORDERS

Studies of adults with BD suggest that BD and panic disorder are often transmitted together in families (e.g., Doughty et al., 2004). Similarly, children of parents with BD exhibit higher rates of a range of anxiety-related disorders and phenotypes, including separation anxiety disorder (18–27% vs. 0–5%), generalized anxiety disorder (9–18% vs. 1–9%), and obsessive-compulsive disorder (3–9% vs. 0–1%), suggesting that anxiety disorders and bipolar spectrum disorders share some familial risk (e.g., Henin et al., 2005; Hirshfeld-Becker et al., 2006).

Conclusions from Family Studies of Bipolar Disorder

Bipolar spectrum disorders are highly familial and share some familial risk factors with frequent comorbid conditions such as disruptive disorders and anxiety disorders. We turn next to studies that tested the extent to which this increased familial risk is attributable to genetic or environmental influences.

Adoption Studies

Significant familiality provides necessary support for the hypothesis that a disorder may be partially attributable to genetic influences but does not provide sufficient evidence by itself. Because members of biological families living in the same home share both genetic and family environmental influences, adoption and twin studies are necessary to disentangle the relative contributions of genetic and environmental influences.

The biological relatives of an individual who is adopted at birth are genetically related to the individual but do not experience the same environmental influences (other than factors that influence both mother and child during pregnancy). In contrast, adoptive relatives live in the same family environment but are biologically unrelated to the proband. Therefore, the relative influence of genes and family environment can be estimated by comparing the prevalence of a disorder among adoptive and biological relatives of individuals with the disorder. If a disorder is due to genetic factors, the biological relatives of individuals with the disorder should exhibit a higher rate of the disorder than the population base rate, whereas an elevated rate of the disorder among adoptive relatives suggests that family environmental influences play a role in the etiology of the disorder.

The adoption study design is elegant and has provided important data for some disorders (e.g., Cadoret, Leve, & Devor, 1997), but two specific constraints have limited the utility of these studies. First, adoptive parents may not be representative of the overall population of parents because of the laudable desire of adoption agencies to place adopted children in an optimal environment with high-functioning parents with access to extensive resources (e.g., Plomin et al., 2001). Second, and most important, in societies in which adoption records are closed, it is often quite difficult to obtain information regarding the biological relatives of individuals who are adopted. As a result, at least in part, of these constraints, only two adoption studies of bipolar spectrum disorders have been completed, one in the 1970s (Mendlewicz & Rainier, 1977) and one in the 1980s (Wender et al., 1986). Both studies provided important converging evidence implicating genetic risk for BD, a finding that is consistent with the results of the twin studies described in the subsequent section.

Twin Studies

By comparing the similarity of monozygotic (MZ) twins, who share all of their genes, and dizygotic (DZ) twins, who share half of their segregating genes on average, twin analyses provide direct estimates of the extent to which a disorder or trait is due to genetic or environmental influences (e.g., Plomin et al., 2001). The most straightforward test for genetic influences on a clinical diagnosis is a comparison of the rate of concordance in pairs of MZ versus DZ twins. If the disorder is influenced by genes, the proportion of MZ pairs who both meet criteria for the disorder will be higher than the proportion of DZ pairs who are concordant for the disorder.

Convincing evidence suggests that BD and virtually all other psychological disorders are influenced by both genetic and environmental risk factors (e.g., Plomin et al., 2001). Therefore, although the simplicity of a comparison of concordance rates is appealing, the primary question of interest is no longer whether BD is due to nature or nurture. Instead, Neale, Boker, Xie, and Maes (2002) and others have developed maximum likelihood methods that provide quantitative estimates of the relative impact of genetic influences, environmental influences, and their interaction. Rather than comparing rates of concordance for the diagnosis between MZ and DZ twins, these methods compare the correlations between MZ and DZ pairs, typically on dimensional measures of symptoms of BD.

Basic twin models estimate three parameters. *Heritability* is the proportion of the total phenotypic variance in a trait that is attributable to genetic influences. The proportion of variance resulting from environmental factors is subdivided to distinguish two types of environmental influences. *Shared environmental influences* are environmental factors that increase the similarity of individuals within a family in comparison to unrelated individuals in the population. These effects may potentially include environmental influences within the home or any other shared experiences such as mutual friends or shared teachers. In contrast, *nonshared environmental influences* are environmental factors that affect just one twin. These risk factors could include a head injury or other accident, exposure to a traumatic event, or physical or sexual abuse (if the other twin was not similarly exposed).

Twin Studies of Adult-Onset Bipolar Spectrum Disorders

Twin studies of bipolar spectrum disorders in adults are summarized in Table 8.2. All studies of adult bipolar I found that the rate of concordance was higher

TABLE 8.2. Twin Studies of Adult-Onset Bipolar Spectrum Disorders

Study	Proband diagnosis[nt]	Co-twin diagnosis[nt]	Number of pairs MZ	DZ	Probandwise concordance MZ	DZ	Heritability	Shared environment	Nonshared environment
Bipolar I only									
Bertelson et al. (1977)	BD I	BD I	34	37	62%	8%	.59	.00	.41
Edvardsen et al. (2008)	BD I	BD I	8	13	25%	0%	.73	.00	.27
Kieseppa et al. (2004)	BD I	BD I	7	18	43%	6%	.93	.00	.07
McGuffin et al. (2003)	BD I	BD I	30	37	40%	5%	.85	.00	.15
Bipolar spectrum									
Tsuang & Faraone (1990)[a]	UD or BD I	UD or BP I	195	255	78%	29%	.63	.00	.37
Bertelson et al. (1977)	UD or BD I	UD or BP I	55	52	67%	20%	.59	.00	.41
Edvardsen et al. (2008)	BD I or II	BD I or II	21	25	38%	8%	.77	.00	.23
Edvardsen et al. (2008)	BD I or II, CT	BD I or II, CT	26	27	43%	11%	.71	.00	.29
Kendler et al. (1995)	BD I	BD I	13	22	39%	5%	.79	.00	.21
Kieseppa et al. (2004)	BD I, SZ	BD I, SZ	8	19	50%	5%	.93	.00	.07
Kieseppa et al. (2004)	BD I, SZ	BD I or II, SZ, CT, UD	8	19	75%	11%	—[nr]	—[nr]	—[nr]
McGuffin et al. (2003)	BD I or II, SZ, CT, UD	BD I or II, SZ, CT, UD	30	37	67%	19%			

Note. BD I, bipolar disorder I; BD II, bipolar disorder II; UD, unipolar depression; CT, cyclothymia; SZ, schizoaffective disorder, bipolar type.
[a]Tsuang and Faraone (1990) summarized results from 11 early twin studies that did not distinguish between bipolar disorder and unipolar depression.

among MZ pairs (25–62%; weighted M = 48%) than same-sex DZ pairs (0–8%; weighted M = 6%), providing strong evidence that bipolar I is influenced by genes. A similar pattern is apparent in studies that used a broader definition of bipolar spectrum disorders (69% MZ, 23% DZ across samples). Heritability estimates are consistently high for both bipolar I (weighted mean h^2 = .75) and the broader bipolar spectrum phenotypes (weighted mean h^2 = .71), indicating clearly that genetic influences play an important role in the development of bipolar spectrum disorders. On the other hand, MZ correlations were less than 1.0 and MZ concordance rates were less than 100% in all studies, indicating that bipolar spectrum disorders are also influenced by the environment. All of the twin studies found that the variance that was not accounted for by genetic influences was attributable to nonshared environmental influences (weighted mean e^2 = .25 and .29, respectively bipolar I and bipolar spectrum phenotypes), and shared environmental influences were not significant in any study. These results suggest that familial influences that affect both twins do not play a strong role in the etiology of the initial diagnosis of BD, although these factors may still be important moderators of severity and risk of recurrence.

Twin Studies of Pediatric-Onset Bipolar Disorder

Mania was not measured directly in any of the large-scale twin studies of childhood disorders conducted to date, precluding a direct estimate of genetic and environmental influences on PBD. Therefore, several groups examined a specific profile on the Child Behavior Checklist (CBCL; Achenbach, 1991), a widely used parent rating scale, to obtain indirect evidence that may be informative regarding the etiology of PBD.

In a meta-analysis of all studies of PBD that administered the CBCL, Mick, Biederman, Pandina, and Faraone (2003) found that PBD is correlated with a CBCL profile characterized by significant elevations on the Anxious/Depressed, Attention Problems, and Aggressive Behavior subscales (CBCL-PBD profile). Subsequent studies replicated the association between mania or hypomania and the CBCL-PBD profile in additional samples and with more sophisticated statistical approaches (Diler, Uguz, Seydaoglu, & Avci, 2008; Faraone, Althoff, et al., 2005; Youngstrom, Youngstrom, & Starr, 2005), and the external validity of the profile was supported by significant associations with important correlates such as suicidal ideation, decreased need for sleep, and hypersexuality (Althoff, Rettew, Faraone, Boomsma, & Hudziak, 2006; Holtmann et al., 2007).

Although these initial studies suggest that the CBCL-PBD profile is correlated with PBD, it is not associated with PBD in all samples (Volk & Todd, 2007). In addition, a less severe form of the profile has been reported in groups with ADHD and CD, suggesting that this profile may also not be specific to PBD (Mick et al., 2003). These mixed results suggest that additional research is needed to test the predictive power and discriminant validity of the CBCL-PBD profile (Youngstrom et al., 2005). Nonetheless, because PBD has not been measured directly in

TABLE 8.3. Twin Studies of the CBCL-PBD Profile

Study	Heritability	Shared environment	Nonshared environment
Althoff et al. (2006)	.53–.87	.00	.17–.47
Hudziak et al. (2005)	.59–.68	.18–.30	.14–.17
Volk & Todd (2007)	.67	.00	.33
Colorado twins	.57–.68	.00	.32–.43

large twin samples, analyses of individual differences on the CBCL-PBD profile may provide useful preliminary information regarding the etiology of this closely related construct.

Four large twin studies all suggest that individual differences in CBCL-PBD scores are moderately to highly heritable (h^2 = .53–.87; Table 8.3), and Boomsma and colleagues (2006) found that the profile had high stability that was primarily attributable to genetic influences. In three of the four samples, nonshared environmental influences accounted for all of the environmental variance, whereas Hudziak, Althoff, Derks, Faraone, and Boomsma (2005) reported small but significant shared environmental influences.

Summary of Behavioral Genetic Studies

Family, adoption, and twin studies indicate that adult-onset bipolar I is familial and highly heritable. Although no twin studies have measured PBD, indirect evidence regarding the genetic and environmental etiology of PBD is provided by studies of CBCL-PBD profile scores, dimensional measures of constructs such as irritability and emotional lability, and symptoms of childhood disorders such as ADHD, ODD, and internalizing disorders that are frequently comorbid with PBD. Heritability estimates were moderate to high in nearly all studies of each of these constructs. In combination with the high familiality of PBD and high heritability of adult-onset BD, the additional circumstantial evidence from these three lines of research strongly suggests that PBD is significantly heritable.

Twin studies consistently indicate that nonshared environmental influences play a role in BD, whereas estimates of shared environmental influences were not significant in any twin study. Somewhat surprisingly, the absence of shared environmental influences argues against theories that suggest that BD is due in part to environmental risk factors that might be expected to influence both twins similarly, such as family cohesion and discord. We discuss several potential explanations for this result in more detail later in the chapter, including the possibility that family discord may affect one twin more than the other even if both are similarly exposed. We turn next to studies that have attempted to identify the specific environmental or genetic factors that increase the likelihood that a child will develop BD.

Molecular Genetic Studies

Although an estimated 99% of the DNA sequence that comprises the human genetic code is identical in all humans, the genetic sequence varies at millions of locations across the human genome. Some of these sequence differences lead to individual differences in protein production, which may then lead to individual differences in neural development or adult brain functioning if the sequence difference is in a gene that is expressed in the central nervous system.

Previous studies have used three primary methods to attempt to identify individual differences in the genetic sequence (polymorphisms) that increase susceptibility to BD. Because space constraints preclude a detailed description of these methods, in this section we provide a brief overview of each approach and refer the interested reader to one of several volumes that provide more comprehensive coverage (e.g., Faraone et al., 1999; Plomin et al., 2001).

Candidate Genes

The candidate gene approach is a specific subset of genetic association analysis, which is described in more detail in a subsequent section. A candidate gene study investigates the role of a specific gene that has been targeted because it influences a physiological substrate that is known to be associated with the disorder of interest. For example, because the neurotransmitters dopamine, serotonin, and norepinephrine are known to play an important role in the regulation of mood, many studies of BD have examined polymorphisms in genes that influence these neurotransmitter systems in the brain. By comparing the frequency of the different alleles, or forms, of a polymorphism in a candidate gene in groups of individuals with and without BD, it is possible to test whether any of the alleles are associated with significantly increased risk for BD.

The relative ease and minimal expense involved in carrying out a small case–control candidate gene study has facilitated a vast number of reports of associations between specific candidate gene polymorphisms and risk for BD (Allen et al., 2008; Bertram, McQueen, Mullin, Blacker, & Tanzi, 2007). Although many initial positive results have failed to replicate in subsequent studies, a number of genes have been implicated as risk factors for BD via meta-analyses. These genes include the serotonin transporter (Lasky-Su, Faraone, Glatt, & Tsuang, 2005), brain-derived neurotrophic factor (BDNF) (Kremeyer et al., 2006; Neves-Pereira et al., 2002; Sklar et al., 2002), d-amino acid oxidase activator (Detera-Wadleigh & McMahon, 2006), the monoamine oxidase A gene (e.g., Muller et al., 2007), and the gene encoding 5,10-methylenetetrahydrofolate reductase (Gilbody, Lewis, & Lightfoot, 2007).

CANDIDATE GENE STUDIES OF PEDIATRIC-ONSET BIPOLAR DISORDER

Only a handful of studies have tested for association between candidate genes and PBD. Geller and colleagues found no association between PBD and polymorphisms in the catechol-O-methyltransferase gene (Geller & Cook, 2000) or the gene for the serotonin transporter (Geller & Cook, 1999). In contrast, their group reported a significant association between PBD and both the BDNF gene (Geller et al., 2004) and the glutamate decarboxylase 1 (GD1) gene (Geller, Tillman, Bolhofner, Hennessy, & Cook, 2008), and Mick and colleagues (2008) reported an association between PBD and a polymorphism in the dopamine transporter gene.

In summary, results of candidate gene studies are inconsistent for both adult-onset BD and PBD, but these findings highlight several genes that may increase risk for BD. These findings suggest that the candidate gene approach is a potentially useful technique to identify genes that increase susceptibility to BD. On the other hand, the effect size of each of these polymorphisms is relatively small, the majority of the genetic variance in BD remains unexplained, and current knowledge regarding the pathophysiology of BD is insufficient to identify all plausible candidate genes. Therefore, we turn next to two different approaches that have been used to screen the entire genome or a targeted region of a specific chromosome to identify additional genes that increase susceptibility to BD.

Linkage Analysis: Using Family Data to Screen the Genome

All cells in the human body with the exception of gamete (sperm and egg) cells contain two full sets of the 23 human chromosomes. Gamete cells contain only one of each chromosome so that after fertilization the new embryo will have the full complement of 46 chromosomes (23 different chromosomes, with one copy of each inherited from the mother and one from the father). During meiosis parental cells with two copies of each chromosome divide to create gamete cells with a single set of the 23 chromosomes. Prior to dividing, homologous chromosomes line up next to each other, and one chromosome from each pair is included in each new gamete cell. However, a child typically does not inherit an ancestral chromosome in its entirety. Instead, when homologous chromosomes line up during meiosis, they physically cross over one another and in the process break and rejoin with the other chromosome. As a result of this *recombination*, the offspring inherits a combination of segments from the two original chromosomes of the parent.

Linkage analysis is based on the extent to which risk alleles for a disorder at an unknown chromosomal location co-occur with specific alleles at a marker locus whose location in the genome is known (e.g., Plomin et al., 2001). If the marker locus and the gene that increases susceptibility to the disorder are close together on the same chromosome, recombination is unlikely to occur between the two loci, and their alleles are likely to be transmitted together from parent to child. In contrast, if the marker locus and the susceptibility locus are on different chromosomes or are far apart on the same chromosome, recombination will frequently separate the marker allele from the risk allele at the susceptibility locus, and alleles at the two loci will be transmitted independently. Thus, linkage is indicated if a specific marker allele co-occurs with the disorder in a family significantly more often than expected by chance.

LINKAGE STUDIES OF BIPOLAR DISORDER

There have been more than 40 linkage studies of adult-onset BD and one linkage study of the CBCL-PBD phenotype (McGough et al., 2008). At least one of these studies has implicated at least one region of nearly every chromosome (Baron, 2002). However, very few of these positive results remained significant after correcting for the thousands of statistical tests that are required to screen the entire genome, and independent replication across studies is rare. These inconsistent results suggest that some initial findings are almost certainly false positives, but others may be true positives with small effect sizes. In an attempt to disentangle these two possibilities and synthesize existing results, three meta-analyses of linkage studies of BD have been published (Badner & Gershon, 2002; McQueen et al., 2005; Segurado et al., 2003).

Segurado and colleagues (2003) used a rank-based binning procedure to conduct a meta-analysis of 18 linkage studies of BD. Their results revealed no evidence of significant linkage across the genome, although a region of chromosome 9p achieved the highest statistical significance. In contrast, using a method that combines p values from different studies, Badner and Gershon (2002) reported significant evidence for linkage on chromosomes 13q and 22q. The linkage result on chromosome 13q is further supported by other studies not included in the Badner and Gershon meta-analysis (Craddock & Forty, 2006; Craddock, O'Donovan, & Owen, 2005; Lambert et al., 2005).

The most comprehensive effort involved pooling the data from 11 linkage studies of BD (McQueen et al., 2005). In this study, linkage to regions of chromosomes 6q (for bipolar I) and 8q (for bipolar I and bipolar II) were significant even after correcting for the multiple tests conducted across the genome, whereas chromosome 9p (for bipolar I) was found to be suggestive. Chromosome 6q has been further implicated in independent studies that were not included in the meta-analysis by McQueen et al., including a Danish sample (Ewald, Flint, Kruse, & Mors, 2002) and a Swedish sample (Venken et al., 2005). Chromosome 8q has not been identified in additional studies of BD but has been shown to be significantly linked to schizophrenia in a meta-analysis by Badner and Gershon (2002).

Genomewide Association Studies

Classical linkage analysis is optimized for categorical disorders that are influenced by major genes that account for a large proportion of the variance in the phenotype of interest. As noted previously, a growing consensus suggests that genetic risk for disorders such as BD is likely to represent the combined effects of multiple genes that each have small effects in isolation. Therefore, the current generation of molecular genetic studies has turned to a more powerful population-based method, genetic association analysis, as an alternative to the family-based linkage approach.

Similar to linkage analysis, association analysis is based on the extent to which a disorder co-occurs with a specific allele at a marker locus with a known genomic location. However, in contrast to the linkage method, which tests for a correlation between a marker allele and the disorder in a few generations of a family, association analysis tests whether a specific allele at a marker locus co-occurs with the disorder in the entire population. A significant association indicates that a gene that increases susceptibility to the disorder is so close to the marker locus that recombination has rarely occurred between the two loci even in the hundreds or thousands of generations represented in the population. Because the same marker allele is associated with the disorder in all families, a significant association may indicate that the marker allele has a functional effect that leads to the disorder. However, a more likely outcome is that the marker is simply close to the gene that influences the disorder, and additional work will need to be done to identify the functional genetic variant.

In comparison to linkage analysis, one major advantage of the association approach is its ability to detect modest genetic effects. Until very recently, however, prohibitive genotyping costs meant that association analyses were restricted to small-scale approaches that usually involved candidate genes or fine mapping of specific regions of an individual chromosome identified by linkage analysis. More recently, the cost and practicality of conducting a genomewide association (GWA) study have approached manageable levels due to the development of an automated system that can quickly genotype up to 1 million single nucleotide polymorphism (SNP) markers in each individual. Nonetheless, the statistical considerations (i.e., adjusting p values for hundreds of thousands to millions of comparisons) remain a daunting challenge.

There have been three GWA studies conducted on BD to date (Baum et al., 2008; Sklar et al., 2008; Wellcome Trust Case Control Consortium [WTCCC], 2007). The first study used a DNA pooling strategy with 1,233 cases and 1,439 controls that identified a SNP located in the diacylglycerol kinase eta (DGKH) gene on chromosome 13 (Baum et al., 2008). In 2007 the WTCCC conducted a GWA study on 1,868 cases and 2,939 controls and identified a locus in a region on chromosome 16p12. The third GWA study of 1,461 cases and 2,008 controls identified yet another different SNP in the myosin 5B (MYO5B) gene on chromosome 18 (Sklar et al., 2008). Each of the GWA study groups then teamed up to combine all available data in a meta-analytic fashion to conduct the largest GWA analysis of a psychiatric disorder to date (Ferreira et al., 2008). This collaborative effort combined data across the available studies, resulting in 4,387 BD cases and 6,209 controls. The strongest association signals arising from this effort did not identify any of the previously reported GWA study association reports. Rather, the strongest association signal was found in the ankyrin G (ANK3) gene on chromosome 10q21, an adaptor protein that is postulated to be involved in the regulation of the assembly of voltage-gated sodium channels.

Summary of Molecular Genetic Studies of Bipolar Disorder

Candidate gene and genomewide linkage and association studies clearly support two important conclusions: (1) Multiple genes are involved in the etiology of BD and (2) no single genetic risk factor is a necessary or sufficient cause of BD. The relatively weak convergence across studies suggests that additional research is need to clarify the inconsistent results that emerge both within each type of study and across these levels of analysis. In light of the complexity of these results, it is not surprising that BD is a heterogeneous disorder that may arise from multiple etiological pathways. In the final section of the chapter, we discuss methods that may help to refine the phenotype to improve the replicability of molecular genetic results. In the next section, we turn to studies that examined specific environmental influences that increase risk for BD.

Environmental Risk Factors

In addition to strong genetic influences, twin and family studies suggest that non-shared environmental risk factors increase susceptibility to BD. Previous studies have focused primarily on prenatal and perinatal complications and later social factors in the family and broader social environment.

Prenatal Risk Factors

Although some previous studies have suggested that prenatal or perinatal complications may be a risk factor for BD, a recent systematic review found no evidence of elevated birth complications in individuals who developed BD (Scott, McNeill, Cavanagh, Cannon, & Murray, 2006). The only study that has examined birth complications in PBD found that, although no specific prenatal complication was significantly associated with increased risk for PBD, children with PBD were more likely to have experienced at least one of several potential prenatal complications that were measured (Pavuluri et al., 2006). Additional research is needed to clarify the relation between birth complications and BD, but any effect of these complications is likely to be small.

Family Environment

As reviewed in detail elsewhere in this volume, families of individuals with BD report lower family cohesion, greater conflict, and more frequent expressed emotion (e.g., Chang, Blasey, Ketter, & Steiner, 2001; Geller et al., 2000; Miklowitz, 2007). Individuals with BD also often have poorer social skills and fewer friends than their peers (Geller et al., 2000). Pinpointing the direction of causation of these difficulties is extremely difficult because they could potentially play a causal role in the development of BD or may simply arise as a secondary consequence of BD symptoms. Whichever of these possibilities is correct, family conflict and more general social difficulties are likely to exacerbate the symptoms of BD by causing stress that interacts with genetic vulnerabilities.

The importance of familial risk factors may seem to contradict results from twin studies, which suggest that shared environmental influences are not an important part of the etiology of BD. However, at least three plausible explanations may account for this finding. First, existing twin studies included a relatively small number of twins with BD and may not have had adequate power to detect shared environmental influences. Second, some studies suggest that familial factors may be more important for maintenance and recurrence of BD than for the initial onset of the disorder (e.g., Miklowitz, 2004), in which case the family influences could be missed by twin studies that used lifetime history of BD as their primary measure. Third, by definition, shared environmental influences are environmental influences that affect both twins similarly and cause them to be more similar to one another than to others in the population. Any differences in parental behavior toward the two twins, or even differences in the twins' perception and response to the same parental behavior, may lead to differences between the twins that would be identified as nonshared environmental variance.

Conclusions from Etiologically Informative Studies

Family and twin studies clearly show that BD is highly familial and heritable. Current data suggest that BD is caused by the combination of multiple genetic and environmental risk factors, each of which has a relative small effect that is neither necessary nor sufficient to cause the development of BD in isolation. Moreover, it is likely that interactions among these risk factors may contribute to susceptibility to BD, and the nature and strength of these interactions are likely to change over the course of development. To fully understand the complex etiology of BD, future studies will require measuring multiple genetic or environmental risk factors in a single well-characterized sample of individuals with BD. Multivariate analyses can then be used to estimate the relative contribution of each genetic or environmental factor to the development of BD and to test whether each of these influences acts independently of the others or interacts with other influences to increase susceptibility to BD.

IMPLICATIONS FOR DEVELOPMENTAL MODELS OF BIPOLAR DISORDER

Table 8.4 summarizes the key points of this review, and Table 8.5 summarizes the implications of the review for the five models described at the beginning of the chapter. Perhaps most importantly, results across virtually all levels of analysis

TABLE 8.4. Key Conclusions from Etiologically Informative Studies

1. Pediatric-onset bipolar disorder is a valid disorder that is associated with significant social, academic, and neuropsychological impairment.

2. Bipolar disorder is a heterogeneous condition that arises from the additive and interactive effects of multiple genetic and environmental risk factors at different points in development.

3. Etiologically informative studies suggest that pediatric-onset bipolar disorder is related to adult-onset bipolar disorder, but may be most strongly associated with the most severe manifestation of bipolar disorder in adults.

4. Bipolar disorder is strongly influenced by genes, but only a subset of the specific genes that increase risk for bipolar disorder have been identified.

5. Environmental risk factors also play an important role in the development of bipolar disorder, and may be especially important predictors of relapse.

indicate that children who receive a diagnosis of PBD exhibit significant impairment in academic, social, and neuropsychological functioning. These difficulties are strongly familial and almost certainly influenced by genes. These converging results provide strong evidence against the hypothesis that PBD is an invalid diagnosis that mislabels children who are not experiencing significant difficulties.

Two other models can also be rejected, at least in their strongest form. The distinct disorders model suggests that PBD and adult-onset BD are completely separate disorders, whereas the single-disorder model argues that they are simply the same disorder measured at different points in development. The fact that families of children with PBD exhibit higher rates of bipolar I and II argues against the hypothesis that PBD and bipolar I are distinct disorders (e.g., Pavuluri et al., 2006), as does the qualitative similarity of the symptoms, impairment, comorbidities, and other clinical correlates exhibited by individuals with PBD and adult-onset BD. In contrast, some quantitative differences are apparent between the two groups. In comparison to adult-onset BD, PBD is more strongly familial and is associated with greater impairment in a subset of domains of functioning. Therefore, although existing data suggest that PBD and adult-onset BD are more similar than different, quantitative differences in familiality and severity may have important implications for future genetic studies.

Geller and colleagues (2006) have suggested that PBD is indeed related to adult-onset bipolar I but propose that, within the overall bipolar I category, there is a continuum of severity that is highly correlated with age of symptom onset. The authors suggest that PBD is at the severe end of this continuum and is, therefore, most strongly associated with the most severe form of the adult-onset illness, characterized by rapid cycling with only brief intervals of healthy functioning between episodes. The severity gradient hypothesis is at least partially supported across nearly all levels of analysis that we have reviewed (see Table 8.4). In comparison to adult-onset BD, individuals with PBD more frequently experience rapid cycling and mixed mood states, have higher rates of comorbidity with ADHD and anxiety disorders, and exhibit prominent irritability,

TABLE 8.5. Summary and Implications for Developmental Models of Pediatric-Onset Bipolar Disorder and Adult-Onset Bipolar Disorder

	Summary of results of previous studies	Summary of evidence for or against each model[a]				
		Invalid diagnosis	Single disorder	Distinct disorders	Severity gradient	ADHD subtype
Symptoms and correlates						
Symptoms	Many similarities between PBD, ABD, BD + ADHD; PBD, BD + ADHD = more frequent rapid cycling/mixed state	↓↓	↓	⇅	↑	↑
Comorbidity	Similar overall; rates of comorbid ADHD, anxiety, SUD, LD: PBD > ABD; rates of comorbid SUD, CD: BD + ADHD > BD − ADHD	↓↓	↓	⇅	↑↑	↑
Functional impairment	Similar impairment in ABD, PBD; PBD and BD + ADHD more severe on some measures	↓↓	⇅	⇅	↑↑	↑
Cognitive functioning	Similar deficits in ABD, PBD; PBD and BD + ADHD more severe on some measures	↓↓	⇅	⇅	↑↑	↑
Psychopathology in family members						
Rate of BD	PBD > ABD > Cont; BD + ADHD > BD − ADHD	↓↓	↓	↓	↑↑	↑
Rate of ADHD	PBD > ABD > Cont; BD + ADHD > BD − ADHD > Cont	↓↓	↓	↓	↑	↑
Rate of other disorders	Generally similar; PBD > ABD for suicidality, substance abuse	↓↓	↓	↓	↑	↑
Genetic and environmental risk factors						
Heritability	High for ABD I, ABD spectrum, CBCL-PBD profile	↓↓	↑	↓	⇅	—
Candidate genes	Small effects for both ABD and PBD	—	⇅	⇅	↓	—
Genomewide scans	Small effects for ABD and CBCL-PBD measure	—	—	—	↓	—
Environmental factors	Small effects for ABD and PBD	—	—	—	↓	—

Note. PBD, pediatric-onset bipolar disorder; ABD, adult-onset bipolar disorder; ADHD, attention-deficit/hyperactivity disorder; Cont, control group; SUD, substance use disorder; LD, learning disability; CD, conduct disorder; CBCL, Child Behavior Checklist.
[a]Symbols indicate evidence for or against each model at that level of analysis. ↓↓ = strong evidence against the model, ↓ = moderate evidence against the model, ⇅ = mixed evidence, ↑ = moderate support, ↑↑ = strong support, — = neutral/provides no information about the model.

increased suicidality, and greater risk for substance use and abuse (Birmaher & Axelson, 2006; Faedda, Baldessarini, Glovinsky, & Austin, 2004; Lin et al., 2006; Nwulia et al., 2007). The one exception to this pattern is the failure to find larger effects in the genomewide linkage scan using the CBCL-PBD phenotype than were obtained in genomewide studies of adult-onset BD, but this may reflect small sample sizes or the fact that the CBCL-PBD phenotype is a correlate of PBD rather than a direct measure.

The final model proposed that comorbidity with ADHD or another disorder may be a marker for an etiological subtype of BD. This hypothesis received mixed support in our review. Comorbidity with ADHD is associated with more frequent mixed and rapid-cycling episodes, stronger familiality, higher rates of CD and other psychopathology, and greater neuropsychological impairment in some studies. In contrast, rates of ADHD were higher in families of individuals with BD than families of controls even if the proband did not have comorbid ADHD, arguing against a strict subtype hypothesis. Nonetheless, the overall pattern of results suggests that the presence of ADHD moderates the clinical severity and etiology of PBD.

Summary

A definitive answer regarding the relation between PBD and adult-onset BD will emerge from longitudinal studies that follow children diagnosed with PBD into adulthood, but these data are still several years away. Based on current evidence, the best fitting model suggests that PBD falls at the severe end of a continuum of susceptibility that includes adult-onset BD. Existing data clearly show that most children who receive a diagnosis of PBD experience impairment across a wide range of domains of functioning. These difficulties lead to significant distress and are sufficiently severe to warrant treatment.

CLINICAL IMPLICATIONS

There is currently no valid genetic test for BD, and it is unlikely that a definitive diagnostic test will be developed in the near future. As we have seen in the studies described in this chapter, BD and most other mental disorders have a polygenic, multifactorial etiology in which symptoms arise from the additive and interactive effects of multiple genetic and environmental risk factors at different phases of development. Because each risk factor is likely to confer only a small increase in susceptibility to BD, no specific risk factor will have sufficient predictive power to be used as a diagnostic measure.

Even if behavioral and molecular genetic studies do not identify a genetic test for BD, these methods may still have important clinical benefits. It may eventually be possible to develop probabilistic risk profiles based on genetic background, family history, environmental circumstances, and other factors to identify those who may benefit from primary prevention or early intervention techniques. For example, if a perinatal screening revealed significant genetic susceptibility to BD, psychoeducational consultation and structured assistance with child behavior management techniques could be provided to reduce the probability that these risk factors would lead to the development of BD. Similarly, by providing a better understanding of the underlying pathophysiology of BD, molecular genetic techniques may inform the development of tertiary pharmacological or psychosocial treatments that directly target the physiological and psychological mechanisms that are compromised in BD (e.g., Cicchetti & Gunnar, 2008).

FUTURE DIRECTIONS

In this final section, we describe several ways that the next generation of etiologically informative studies may help to continue to refine our understanding of BD. The chapter then concludes with a call for increased multidisciplinary collaboration among researchers investigating the genetic and environmental risk factors, pathophysiology, and clinical diagnosis and treatment of BD.

Additional Molecular Genetic Studies of Pediatric-Onset Bipolar Disorder

Only a handful of molecular genetic studies of PBD have emerged to date. Additional studies are needed to confirm and refine the susceptibility loci identified in these initial studies. In addition, genomewide scans are needed to identify additional quantitative trait loci that have not yet been identified by previous candidate gene studies. Both of these approaches require large samples to obtain sufficient statistical power, suggesting that collaborative studies that combine samples across multiple sites may be most effective.

Endophenotypes

Despite the high heritability of BD, the establishment of replicated genetic risk factors has been elusive in comparison to other disorders with somewhat lower heritability, such as reading disorder, obesity, and breast cancer (Farooqi & O'Rahilly, 2005; Fisher & DeFries, 2002; Frayling et al., 2007; Hebebrand, Friedel, Schauble, Geller, & Hinney, 2003; Herbert et al., 2006; Lasky-Su et al., 2008; Locatelli, Lichtenstein, & Yashin, 2004; Willcutt, Pennington, Olson, & DeFries, 2007). One contributing factor to the success of studies of these other disorders has been the use of endophenotype measures in addition to categorical diagnoses. Endophenotypes are quantitative measures of pathophysiological processes that may mediate the relation between a specific gene and the observed symptoms of a disorder (e.g., Burmeister, McInnis, & Zollner, 2008; Cannon, Gasperoni, van Erp, & Rosso, 2001; Gottesman & Gould, 2003).

Because an endophenotype is more proximal to the functional gene product than the symptoms of the disorder, these refined phenotypes may increase statistical power to detect genetic risk factors. Proof of principal is provided by several other disorders. For example, studies of reading disability obtained stronger evidence of linkage for measures of several specific reading-related language processes than for an overall reading composite measure (e.g., Fisher & DeFries, 2002). Similarly, studies of schizophrenia found the strongest association between the α7-nicotinic cholinergic receptor gene and a specific phenotype characterized by failure to habituate to repeated auditory stimuli in an event-related potential paradigm (e.g., Freedman et al., 2000).

Initial studies provide preliminary support for a diverse range of potential endophenotypes that have been proposed for BD, including cyclotaxia (mood dysregulation at the subsyndromal level, abnormal regulation of circadian rhythms, response to medication, neuropsychological functioning, and differences in brain structure and function; e.g., Bearden & Freimer, 2006; Findling et al., 2005; Lenox, Gould, & Manji, 2002). These data suggest that endophenotypes may be useful tools to identify novel risk factors for BD. In addition, endophenotype measures may help to specify the physiological effects of genes that have been identified with other methods, facilitating the development of comprehensive models of the pathophysiology of BD.

Gene × Environment and Gene × Gene Interactions

The latest generation of studies has already taken an important next step by moving beyond simple linear models of genetic and environmental influences to test for interactions between genetic and environmental risk and protective factors (Cicchetti, 2007). The potential utility of this approach was recently demonstrated in a genome scan study of BD (Abou et al., 2007). The authors found significant gene × gene interactions between a genetic locus on chromosomes 2 and loci on chromosomes 6 and 15. These significant interactions indicate that the effect of each genetic locus depends in part on the alleles that the individual had at the genetic loci on the other chromosomes. Similarly, gene × environment interactions have been identified for related disorders such as major depression (e.g., Caspi et al., 2003), suggesting that additional research is warranted to test for interactions in samples with BD.

Copy Number Variation

Copy number variants (CNVs) are segments of DNA that repeat multiple times in specific locations in the genome. The number of times that the sequence repeats varies between individuals (Iafrate et al., 2004; Sebat et al., 2004). Although CNVs were not examined systematically in early molecular genetic studies of BD, recent studies implicate CNV in schizophrenia (Walsh et al., 2008; Xu et al., 2008) and autism (Sebat et al., 2007). Studies of these two disorders also provide preliminary evidence that at least some of these CNVs are de novo mutations, meaning that they are random DNA mutations that are not inherited from either parent. Based on this initial evidence suggesting that CNVs may play a role in the etiology of mental disorders, systematic evaluations of CNVs at the whole-genome scale have begun in earnest (Komura et al., 2006; Redon et al., 2006; Sebat et al., 2007). To date, no published studies have evaluated this type of genetic variation as a risk factor for BD, but studies are currently underway.

CONCLUSION:
THE NEED FOR EXPANDED MULTIDISCIPLINARY COLLABORATIONS

The groundbreaking studies reviewed in this chapter have provided critical information regarding the etiology of BD and also underscore how much remains to be learned. One of the most important lessons provided by these results is the conclusion that nearly all molecular genetic studies of BD conducted to date were severely underpowered. It is now clear that many of the procedures for gene localization described in this chapter will require extremely large samples (5,000–10,000 individuals or more), which is simply not feasible for a single laboratory to collect in isolation. Therefore, multisite collaborations will play an increasingly important role in the next generation of molecular genetic studies of BD.

On the other hand, procedures for DNA collection and genetic analysis continue to become more automated and efficient, making it relatively inexpensive to collect and store DNA as part of studies with a primary focus on clinical aspects of BD. After molecular genetic studies identify specific genes that increase risk for BD, the stored DNA samples can be used to genotype these loci, and the genotype information can be incorporated in analyses of clinical questions. These analyses are likely to facilitate extraordinary collaborative synergy between genetic researchers and investigators focusing on the clinical aspects of BD, strengthening the quality of research in both domains.

REFERENCES

Abou, J. R., Fuerst, R., Kaneva, R., Orozco, D. G., Rivas, F., Mayoral, F., et al. (2007). The first genomewide interaction and locus-heterogeneity linkage scan in bipolar affective disorder: Strong evidence of epistatic effects between loci on chromosomes 2q and 6q. *American Journal of Human Genetics, 81*, 974–986.

Achenbach, T. M. (1991). *Manual for the Child Behavior Checklist/ 4-18 and 1991 Profile*. Burlington: University of Vermont Department of Psychiatry.

Allen, N. C., Bagade, S., McQueen, M. B., Ioannidis, J. P. A., Kavvoura, F. K., Khoury, M. J., et al. (2008). Systematic meta-analyses and field synopsis of genetic association studies in schizophrenia: The SzGene database. *Nature Genetics, 40*, 827–834.

Althoff, R. R., Rettew, D. C., Faraone, S. V., Boomsma, D. I., & Hudziak, J. J. (2006). Latent class analysis shows strong heritability of the Child Behavior Checklist—Juvenile Bipolar Phenotype. *Biological Psychiatry, 60*, 903–911.

Badner, J. A., & Gershon, E. S. (2002). Meta-analysis of whole-genome linkage scans of bipolar disorder and schizophrenia. *Molecular Psychiatry, 7*, 405–411.

Baron, M. (2002). Manic-depression genes and the new millennium: Poised for discovery. *Molecular Psychiatry, 7*, 342–348.

Baum, A. E., Akula, N., Cabanero, M., Cardona, I., Corona, W., Klemens, B., et al. (2008). A genome-wide association study implicates diacylglycerol kinase eta (DGKH) and several other genes in the etiology of bipolar disorder. *Molecular Psychiatry, 13*, 197–207.

Bearden, C. E., & Freimer, N. B. (2006). Endophenotypes for psychiatric disorders: Ready for primetime? *Trends in Genetics, 22*, 306–313.

Bertelsen, A., Harvald, B., & Hauge, M. (1977). A Danish twin study of manic-depressive disorders. *British Journal of Psychiatry, 130*, 330–351.

Bertram, L., McQueen, M. B., Mullin, K., Blacker, D., & Tanzi, R. E. (2007). Systematic meta-analyses of Alzheimer disease genetic association studies: The AlzGene database. *Nature Genetics, 39*, 17–23.

Birmaher, B., & Axelson, D. (2006). Course and outcome of bipolar spectrum disorder in children and adolescents: A review of the existing literature. *Development and Psychopathology, 18*, 1023–1035.

Boomsma, D. I., Rebollo, I., Derks, E. M., van Beijsterveldt, T. C., Althoff, R. R., Rettew, D. C., et al. (2006). Longitudinal stability of the CBCL-juvenile bipolar disorder phenotype: A study in Dutch twins. *Biological Psychiatry, 60*, 912–920.

Brotman, M. A., Kassem, L., Reising, M. M., Guyer, A. E., Dickstein, D. P., Rich, B. A., et al. (2007). Parental diagnoses in youth with narrow phenotype bipolar disorder or severe mood dysregulation. *American Journal of Psychiatry, 164*, 1238–1241.

Burmeister, M., McInnis, M. G., & Zollner, S. (2008). Psychiatric genetics: Progress amid controversy. *Nature Reviews Genetics, 9*, 527–540.

Cadoret, R. J., Leve, L. D., & Devor, E. (1997). Genetics of aggressive and violent behavior. *Psychiatric Clinics of North America, 20*, 301–322.

Cannon, T. D., Gasperoni, T. L., van Erp, T. G., & Rosso, I. M. (2001). Quantitative neural indicators of liability to schizophrenia: Implications for molecular genetic studies. *American Journal of Medical Genetics, 105*, 16–19.

Cantwell, D. P. (1980). The diagnostic process and diagnostic classification in child psychiatry—DSM-III. *Journal of the American Academy of Child and Adolescent Psychiatry, 19*, 345–355.

Caspi, A., Sugden, K., Moffitt, T. E., Taylor, A., Craig, I. W., Harrington, H., et al. (2003). Influence of life stress on depression: Moderation by a polymorphism in the 5-HTT gene. *Science, 301*, 386–389.

Chang, K. (2007). Adult bipolar disorder is continuous with pediatric bipolar disorder. *Canadian Journal of Psychiatry, 52*, 418–425.

Chang, K. D., Blasey, C., Ketter, T. A., & Steiner, H. (2001). Family environment of children and adolescents with bipolar parents. *Bipolar Disorders, 3*, 73–78.

Chang, K. D., Steiner, H., & Ketter, T. A. (2000). Psychiatric phenomenology of child and adolescent bipolar offspring. *Journal of the American Academy of Child and Adolescent Psychiatry, 39*, 453–460.

Cicchetti, D. (2007). Gene-environment interaction. *Developmental Psychopathology, 19*, 957–959.

Cicchetti, D., & Gunnar, M. R. (2008). Integrating biological measures into the design and evaluation of preventive interventions. *Developmental Psychopathology, 20*, 737–743.

Claus, E. B., Risch, N. J., & Thompson, W. D. (1990). Using age of onset to distinguish between subforms of breast cancer. *Annals of Human Genetics, 54,* 169–177.

Coryell, W., Leon, A. C., Turvey, C., Akiskal, H. S., Mueller, T., & Endicott, J. (2001). The significance of psychotic features in manic episodes: A report from the NIMH collaborative study. *Journal of Affective Disorders, 67,* 79–88.

Craddock, N., & Forty, L. (2006). Genetics of affective (mood) disorders. *European Journal of Human Genetics, 14,* 660–668.

Craddock, N., O'Donovan, M. C., & Owen, M. J. (2005). The genetics of schizophrenia and bipolar disorder: Dissecting psychosis. *Journal of Medical Genetics, 42,* 193–204.

Curtis, W. J., & Cicchetti, D. (2003). Moving research on resilience into the 21st century: Theoretical and methodological considerations in examining the biological contributors to resilience. *Developmental Psychopathology, 15,* 773–810.

DelBello, M. P., & Geller, B. (2001). Review of studies of child and adolescent offspring of bipolar parents. *Bipolar Disorders, 3,* 325–334.

Detera-Wadleigh, S. D., & McMahon, F. J. (2006). G72/G30 in schizophrenia and bipolar disorder: Review and meta-analysis. *Biological Psychiatry, 60,* 106–114.

Diler, R. S., Uguz, S., Seydaoglu, G., & Avci, A. (2008). Mania profile in a community sample of prepubertal children in Turkey. *Bipolar Disorders, 10,* 546–553.

Doughty, C. J., Wells, J. E., Joyce, P. R., Olds, R. J., & Walsh, A. E. (2004). Bipolar-panic disorder comorbidity within bipolar disorder families: A study of siblings. *Bipolar Disorder, 6,* 245–252.

Duffy, A., Alda, M., Crawford, L., Milin, R., & Grof, P. (2007). The early manifestations of bipolar disorder: A longitudinal prospective study of the offspring of bipolar parents. *Bipolar Disorders, 9,* 828–838.

Duffy, A., Grof, P., Kutcher, S., Robertson, C., & Alda, M. (2001). Measures of attention and hyperactivity symptoms in a high-risk sample of children of bipolar parents. *Journal of Affective Disorders, 67,* 159–165.

Dunayevich, E., & Keck, P. E., Jr. (2000). Prevalence and description of psychotic features in bipolar mania. *Current Psychiatry Reports, 2,* 286–290.

Edvardsen, J., Torgersen, S., Røysamb, E., Lygren, S., Skre, I., Onstad, S., et al. (2008). Heritability of bipolar spectrum disorders. Unity or heterogeneity? *Journal of Affective Disorders, 106,* 229–240.

Ewald, H., Flint, T., Kruse, T. A., & Mors, O. (2002). A genome-wide scan shows significant linkage between bipolar disorder and chromosome 12q24.3 and suggestive linkage to chromosomes 1p22-21, 4p16, 6q14-22, 10q26 and 16p13.3. *Molecular Psychiatry, 7,* 734–744.

Faedda, G. L., Baldessarini, R. J., Glovinsky, I. P., & Austin, N. B. (2004). Pediatric bipolar disorder: Phenomenology and course of illness. *Bipolar Disorders, 6,* 305–313.

Faraone, S. V., Althoff, R. R., Hudziak, J. J., Monuteaux, M., & Biederman, J. (2005). The CBCL predicts DSM bipolar disorder in children: A receiver operating characteristic curve analysis. *Bipolar Disorders, 7,* 518–524.

Faraone, S. V., Biederman, J., Mennin, D., & Russell, R. (1998). Bipolar and antisocial disorders among relatives of ADHD children: Parsing familial subtypes of illness. *American Journal of Medical Genetics. Part B, Neuropsychiatric Genetics, B81,* 108–116.

Faraone, S. V., Biederman, J., Mennin, D., Wozniak, J., & Spencer, T. (1997). Attention-deficit hyperactivity disorder with bipolar disorder: A familial subtype? *Journal of the American Academy of Child and Adolescent Psychiatry, 36,* 1378–1387.

Faraone, S. V., Biederman, J., & Monuteaux, M. C. (2001). Attention deficit hyperactivity disorder with bipolar disorder in girls: Further evidence for a familial subtype? *Journal of Affective Disorders, 64,* 19–26.

Faraone, S. V., Biederman, J., Wozniak, J., Mundy, E., Mennin, D., & O'Donnell, D. (1997). Is comorbidity with ADHD a marker for juvenile-onset mania? *Journal of the American Academy of Child and Adolescent Psychiatry, 36*, 1046–1055.

Faraone, S. V., Glatt, S. J., Su, J., & Tsuang, M. T. (2004). Three potential susceptibility loci shown by a genome-wide scan for regions influencing the age at onset of mania. *American Journal of Psychiatry, 161*, 625–630.

Faraone, S. V., Glatt, S. J., & Tsuang, M. T. (2003). The genetics of pediatric-onset bipolar disorder. *Biological Psychiatry, 53*, 970–977.

Faraone, S. V., Perlis, R. H., Doyle, A. E., Smoller, J. W., Goralnick, J. J., Holmgren, M. A., et al. (2005). Molecular genetics of attention-deficit/hyperactivity disorder. *Biological Psychiatry, 57*, 1313–1323.

Faraone, S. V., Tsuang, M. T., & Tsuang, D. W. (1999). *Genetics of mental disorders: What practitioners and students need to know.* New York: Guilford Press.

Farooqi, I. S., & O'Rahilly, S. (2005). New advances in the genetics of early onset obesity. *International Journal of Obesity, 29*, 1149–1152.

Ferreira, M. A., O'Donovan, M. C., Meng, Y. A., Jones, I. R., Ruderfer, D. M., Jones, L., et al. (2008). Collaborative genome-wide association analysis supports a role for ANK3 and CACNA1C in bipolar disorder. *Nature Genetics, 40*, 1056–1058.

Findling, R. L., Youngstrom, E. A., McNamara, N. K., Stansbrey, R. J., Demeter, C. A., Bedoya, D., et al. (2005). Early symptoms of mania and the role of parental risk. *Bipolar Disorders, 7*, 623–634.

Fisher, S. E., & DeFries, J. C. (2002). Developmental dyslexia: Genetic dissection of a complex cognitive trait. *Nature Reviews: Neuroscience, 3*, 767–780.

Frayling, T. M., Timpson, N. J., Weedon, M. N., Zeggini, E., Freathy, R. M., Lindgren, C. M., et al. (2007). A common variant in the FTO gene is associated with body mass index and predisposes to childhood and adult obesity. *Science, 316*, 889–894.

Freedman, R., Adams, C. E., Adler, L. E., Bickford, P. C., Gault, J., Harris, J. G., et al. (2000). Inhibitory neurophysiological deficit as a phenotype for genetic investigation of schizophrenia. *American Journal of Medical Genetics, 97*, 58–64.

Geller, B., Badner, J. A., Tillman, R., Christian, S. L., Bolhofner, K., & Cook, E. H., Jr. (2004). Linkage disequilibrium of the brain-derived neurotrophic factor Val66Met polymorphism in children with a prepubertal and early adolescent bipolar disorder phenotype. *American Journal of Psychiatry, 161*, 1698–1700.

Geller, B., Bolhofner, K., Craney, J. L., Williams, M., DelBello, M. P., & Gundersen, K. (2000). Psychosocial functioning in a prepubertal and early adolescent bipolar disorder phenotype. *Journal of the American Academy of Child and Adolescent Psychiatry, 39*, 1543–1548.

Geller, B., & Cook, E. H., Jr. (1999). Serotonin transporter gene (HTTLPR) is not in linkage disequilibrium with prepubertal and early adolescent bipolarity. *Biological Psychiatry, 45*, 1230–1233.

Geller, B., & Cook, E. H., Jr. (2000). Ultradian rapid cycling in prepubertal and early adolescent bipolarity is not in transmission disequilibrium with val/met COMT alleles. *Biological Psychiatry, 47*, 605–609.

Geller, B., Tillman, R., Bolhofner, K., Hennessy, K., & Cook, E. H., Jr. (2008). GAD1 single nucleotide polymorphism is in linkage disequilibrium with a child bipolar I disorder phenotype. *Journal of Child and Adolescent Psychopharmacology, 18*, 25–29.

Geller, B., Tillman, R., Bolhofner, K., Zimerman, B., Strauss, N. A., & Kaufmann, P. (2006). Controlled, blindly rated, direct-interview family study of a prepubertal and early-adolescent bipolar I disorder phenotype: Morbid risk, age at onset, and comorbidity. *Archives of General Psychiatry, 63*, 1130–1138.

Gilbody, S., Lewis, S., & Lightfoot, T. (2007). Methylenetetrahydrofolate reductase (MTHFR) genetic polymorphisms and psychiatric disorders: A HuGE review. *American Journal of Epidemiology, 165*, 1–13.

Glahn, D. C., Bearden, C. E., Barguil, M., Barrett, J., Reichenberg, A., Bowden, C. L., et al. (2007). The neurocognitive signature of psychotic bipolar disorder. *Biological Psychiatry, 62*, 910–916.

Goldstein, B. I., Strober, M. A., Birmaher, B., Axelson, D. A., Esposite-Smythers, C., Goldstein, T. R., et al. (2008). Substance use disorders among adolescents with bipolar spectrum disorders. *Bipolar Disorders, 10*, 469–478.

Gottesman, I. I., & Gould, T. D. (2003). The endophenotype concept in psychiatry: Etymology and strategic intentions. *American Journal of Psychiatry, 160*, 636–645.

Hebebrand, J., Friedel, S., Schauble, N., Geller, F., & Hinney, A. (2003). Perspectives: Molecular genetic research in human obesity. *Obesity Reviews, 4*, 139–146.

Henin, A., Biederman, J., Mick, E., Sachs, G. S., Hirshfeld-Becker, D. R., Siegel, R. S., et al. (2005). Psychopathology in the offspring of parents with bipolar disorder: A controlled study. *Biological Psychiatry, 58*, 554–561.

Herbert, A., Gerry, N. P., McQueen, M. B., Heid, I. M., Pfeufer, A., Illig, T., et al. (2006). A common genetic variant is associated with adult and childhood obesity. *Science, 312*, 279–283.

Hillegers, M. H., Reichart, C. G., Wals, M., Verhulst, F. C., Ormel, J., & Nolen, W. A. (2005). Five-year prospective outcome of psychopathology in the adolescent offspring of bipolar parents. *Bipolar Disorders, 7*, 344–350.

Hirshfeld-Becker, D. R., Biederman, J., Henin, A., Faraone, S. V., Dowd, S. T., De Petrillo, L. A., et al. (2006). Psychopathology in the young offspring of parents with bipolar disorder: A controlled pilot study. *Psychiatry Research, 145*, 155–167.

Holtmann, M., Bölte, S., Goth, K., Döpfner, M., Plück, J., Huss, M., et al. (2007). Prevalence of the Child Behavior Checklist-pediatric bipolar disorder phenotype in a German general population sample. *Bipolar Disorders, 9*, 895–900.

Hudziak, J. J., Althoff, R. R., Derks, E. M., Faraone, S. V., & Boomsma, D. I. (2005). Prevalence and genetic architecture of Child Behavior Checklist-juvenile bipolar disorder. *Biological Psychiatry, 58*, 562–568.

Iafrate, A. J., Feuk, L., Rivera, M. N., Listewnik, M. L., Donahoe, P. K., Qi, Y., et al. (2004). Detection of large-scale variation in the human genome. *Nature Genetics, 36*, 949–951.

Ioannidis, J. P., Ntzani, E. E., Trikalinos, T. A., & Contopoulos-Ioannidis, D. G. (2001). Replication validity of genetic association studies. *Nature Genetics, 29*, 306–309.

Jones, S. H., & Bentall, R. P. (2008). A review of potential cognitive and environmental risk markers in children of bipolar parents. *Clinical Psychology Review, 28*, 1083–1095.

Kendler, K. S., Pedersen, N. L., Neale, M. C., & Mathe, A. A. (1995). A pilot Swedish twin study of affective illness including hospital- and population-ascertained subsamples: Results of model fitting. *Behavior Genetics, 25*, 217–232.

Kessler, R. C., Avenevoli, S., & Ries Merikangas, K. (2001). Mood disorders in children and adolescents: An epidemiologic perspective. *Biological Psychiatry, 49*, 1002–1014.

Kieseppa, T., Partonen, T., Haukka, J., Kaprio, J., & Lonnqvist, J. (2004). High concordance of bipolar I disorder in a nationwide sample of twins. *American Journal of Psychiatry, 161*, 1814–1821.

Komura, D., Shen, F., Ishikawa, S., Fitch, K. R., Chen, W. W., Zhang, J., et al. (2006). Genome-wide detection of human copy number variations using high-density DNA oligonucleotide arrays. *Genome Research, 16*, 1575–1584.

Kowatch, R. A., Youngstrom, E. A., Danielyan, A., & Findling, R. L. (2005). Review and meta-analysis of the phenomenology and clinical characteristics of mania in children and adolescents. *Bipolar Disorders, 7,* 483–496.

Kremeyer, B., Herzberg, I., Garcia, J., Kerr, E., Duque, C., Parra, V., et al. (2006). Transmission distortion of BDNF variants to bipolar disorder type I patients from a South American population isolate. *American Journal of Medical Genetics. Part B, Neuropsychiatric Genetics, 141B,* 435–439.

Lambert, D., Middle, F., Hamshere, M. L., Segurado, R., Raybould, R., Corvin, A., et al. (2005). Stage 2 of the Wellcome Trust UK-Irish bipolar affective disorder sibling-pair genome screen: Evidence for linkage on chromosomes 6q16-q21, 4q12-q21, 9p21, 10p14-p12 and 18q22. *Molecular Psychiatry, 10,* 831–841.

Lasky-Su, J., Lyon, H. N., Emilsson, V., Heid, I. M., Molony, C., Raby, B. A., et al. (2008). On the replication of genetic associations: Timing can be everything! *American Journal of Human Genetics, 82,* 849–858.

Lasky-Su, J. A., Faraone, S. V., Glatt, S. J., & Tsuang, M. T. (2005). Meta-analysis of the association between two polymorphisms in the serotonin transporter gene and affective disorders. *American Journal of Medical Genetics. Part B, Neuropsychiatric Genetics, 133B,* 110–115.

Lenox, R. H., Gould, T. D., & Manji, H. K. (2002). Endophenotypes in bipolar disorder. *American Journal of Medical Genetics. Part B, Neuropsychiatric Genetics, B114,* 391–406.

Lewinsohn, P. M., Klein, D. N., & Seeley, J. R. (2000). Bipolar disorder during adolescence and young adulthood in a community sample. *Bipolar Disorders, 2,* 281–293.

Lin, P. I., McInnis, M. G., Potash, J. B., Willour, V., Mackinnon, D. F., DePaulo, J. R., et al. (2006). Clinical correlates and familial aggregation of age at onset in bipolar disorder. *American Journal of Psychiatry, 163,* 240–246.

Locatelli, I., Lichtenstein, P., & Yashin, A. I. (2004). The heritability of breast cancer: A Bayesian correlated frailty model applied to Swedish twins data. *Twin Research, 7,* 182–191.

Luoma, S., Hakko, H., Ollinen, T., Jarvelin, M. R., & Lindeman, S. (2008). Association between age at onset and clinical features of schizophrenia: The Northern Finland 1966 birth cohort study. *European Psychiatry, 23,* 331–335.

Manchia, M., Lampus, S., Chillotti, C., Sardu, C., Ardau, R., Severino, G., et al. (2008). Age at onset in Sardinian bipolar I patients: Evidence for three subgroups. *Bipolar Disorders, 10,* 443–446.

Masi, G., Perugi, G., Millepiedi, S., Toni, C., Mucci, M., Bertini, N., et al. (2007). Clinical and research implications of panic-bipolar comorbidity in children and adolescents. *Psychiatry Research, 153,* 47–54.

McClellan, J., Kowatch, R., & Findling, R. L. (2007). Practice parameter for the assessment and treatment of children and adolescents with bipolar disorder. *Journal of the American Academy of Child and Adolescent Psychiatry, 46,* 107–125.

McGough, J. J., Loo, S. K., McCracken, J. T., Dang, J., Clark, S., Nelson, S. F., et al. (2008). CBCL Pediatric Bipolar Disorder Profile and ADHD: Comorbidity and quantitative trait loci analysis. *Journal of the American Academy of Child and Adolescent Psychiatry, 47,* 1151–1157.

McGuffin, P., Rijsdijk, F., Andrew, M., Sham, P., Katz, R., & Cardno, A. (2003). The heritability of bipolar affective disorder and the genetic relationship to unipolar depression. *Archives of General Psychiatry, 60,* 497–502.

McQueen, M. B., Devlin, B., Faraone, S. V., Nimgaonkar, V. L., Sklar, P., Smoller, J. W., et al. (2005). Combined analysis from eleven linkage studies of bipolar disorder provides strong evidence of susceptibility loci on chromosomes 6q and 8q. *American Journal of Human Genetics, 77*, 582–595.

Mendlewicz, J., & Rainier, J. (1977). Adoption study supporting genetic transmission in manic depressive illness. *Nature, 268*, 327–329.

Mick, E., Biederman, J., Pandina, G., & Faraone, S. V. (2003). A preliminary meta-analysis of the Child Behavior Checklist in pediatric bipolar disorder. *Biological Psychiatry, 53*, 1021–1027.

Mick, E., Kim, J. W., Biederman, J., Wozniak, J., Wilens, T., Spencer, T., et al. (2008). Family based association study of pediatric bipolar disorder and the dopamine transporter gene (SLC6A3). *American Journal of Medical Genetics. Part B, Neuropsychiatric Genetics, 147B*, 1182–1185.

Miklowitz, D. J. (2004). The role of family systems in severe and recurrent psychiatric disorders: A developmental psychopathology view. *Development and Psychopathology, 16*, 667–688.

Miklowitz, D. J. (2007). The role of the family in the course and treatment of bipolar disorder. *Current Directions in Psychological Science, 16*, 192–196.

Moffitt, T. E. (1993). Adolescence-limited and life-course persistent antisocial behavior: A developmental taxonomy. *Psychological Review, 100*, 674–701.

Muller, D. J., Serretti, A., Sicard, T., Tharmalingam, S., King, N., Artioli, P., et al. (2007). Further evidence of MAO-A gene variants associated with bipolar disorder. *American Journal of Medical Genetics. Part B, Neuropsychiatric Genetics, 144B*, 37–40.

Neale, M. C., Boker, S. M., Xie, G., & Maes, H. H. (2002). *Mx: Statistical modeling* (6th ed.). Richmond: Virginia Commonwealth University Department of Psychiatry.

Neves-Pereira, M., Mundo, E., Muglia, P., King, N., Macciardi, F., & Kennedy, J. L. (2002). The brain-derived neurotrophic factor gene confers susceptibility to bipolar disorder: Evidence from a family-based association study. *American Journal of Human Genetics, 71*, 651–655.

Nierenberg, A. A., Miyahara, S., Spencer, T., Wisniewski, S. R., Otto, M. W., Simon, N., et al. (2005). Clinical and diagnostic implications of lifetime attention-deficit/hyperactivity disorder comorbidity in adults with bipolar disorder: Data from the first 1000 STEP-BD participants. *Biological Psychiatry, 57*, 1467–1473.

Nwulia, E. A., Miao, K., Zandi, P. P., Mackinnon, D. F., DePaulo, J. R., Jr., & McInnis, M. G. (2007). Genome-wide scan of bipolar II disorder. *Bipolar Disorders, 9*, 580–588.

Pavuluri, M. N., Henry, D. B., Nadimpalli, S. S., O'Connor, M. M., & Sweeney, J. A. (2006). Biological risk factors in pediatric bipolar disorder. *Biological Psychiatry, 60*, 936–941.

Pennington, B. F. (2006). From single to multiple deficit models of developmental disorders. *Cognition, 101*, 385–413.

Perlis, R. H., Dennehy, E. B., Miklowitz, D. J., DelBello, M. P., Ostacher, M., Calabrese, J. R., et al. (2009). Retrospective age at onset of bipolar disorder and outcome during two-year follow-up: Results from the STEP-BD study. *Bipolar Disorders, 11*(4), 391–400.

Pini, S., Cassano, G. B., Simonini, E., Savino, M., Russo, A., & Montgomery, S. A. (1997). Prevalence of anxiety disorders comorbidity in bipolar depression, unipolar depression and dysthymia. *Journal of Affective Disorders, 42*, 145–153.

Plomin, R., DeFries, J. C., McClearn, G. E., & McGuffin, P. (2001). *Behavioral genetics* (4th ed.). New York: Freeman.

Redon, R., Ishikawa, S., Fitch, K. R., Feuk, L., Perry, G. H., Andrews, T. D., et al. (2006). Global variation in copy number in the human genome. *Nature, 444*, 444–454.

Rice, J., Reich, T., Andreasen, N. C., Endicott, J., Van Eerdewegh, M., Fishman, R., et al.

(1987). The familial transmission of bipolar illness. *Archives of General Psychiatry, 44*, 441–447.

Sachs, G. S., Baldassano, C. F., Truman, C. J., & Guille, C. (2000). Comorbidity of attention deficit hyperactivity disorder with early- and late-onset bipolar disorder. *American Journal of Psychiatry, 157*, 466–468.

Scott, J., McNeill, Y., Cavanagh, J., Cannon, M., & Murray, R. (2006). Exposure to obstetric complications and subsequent development of bipolar disorder: Systematic review. *British Journal of Psychiatry, 189*, 3–11.

Sebat, J., Lakshmi, B., Malhotra, D., Troge, J., Lese-Martin, C., Walsh, T., et al. (2007). Strong association of de novo copy number mutations with autism. *Science, 316*, 445–449.

Sebat, J., Lakshmi, B., Troge, J., Alexander, J., Young, J., Lundin, P., et al. (2004). Large-scale copy number polymorphism in the human genome. *Science, 305*, 525–528.

Segurado R., Detera-Wadleigh, S. D., Levinson, D. F., Lewis, C. M., Gill, M., Nurnberger, J. I., Jr., et al. (2003). Genome scan meta-analysis of schizophrenia and bipolar disorder: Part III. Bipolar disorder. *American Journal of Human Genetics, 73*, 49–62.

Sklar, P., Gabriel, S. B., McInnis, M. G., Bennett, P., Lim, Y. M., Tsan, G., et al. (2002). Family-based association study of 76 candidate genes in bipolar disorder: BDNF is a potential risk locus. Brain-derived neutrophic factor. *Molecular Psychiatry, 7*, 579–593.

Sklar, P., Smoller, J. W., Fan, J., Ferreira, M. A., Perlis, R. H., Chambert, K., et al. (2008). Whole-genome association study of bipolar disorder. *Molecular Psychiatry, 13*, 558–569.

Smoller, J. W., & Finn, C. T. (2003). Family, twin, and adoption studies of bipolar disorder. *American Journal of Medical Genetics. Part C, Seminars in Medical Genetics, 123C*, 48–58.

Strober, M., DeAntonio, M., Schmidt-Lackner, S., Freeman, R., Lampert, C., & Diamond, J. (1998). Early childhood attention deficit hyperactivity disorder predicts poorer response to acute lithium therapy in adolescent mania. *Journal of Affective Disorders, 51*, 145–151.

Strober, M., Morrell, W., Burroughs, J., Lampert, C., Danforth, H., & Freeman, R. (1988). A family study of bipolar I disorder in adolescence. Early onset of symptoms linked to increased familial loading and lithium resistance. *Journal of Affective Disorders, 15*, 255–268.

Tsuang, M. T., & Faraone, S. V. (1990). *The genetics of mood disorders.* Baltimore: Johns Hopkins University Press.

Venken, T., Claes, S., Sluijs, S., Paterson, A. D., van Duijn, C., Adolfsson, R., et al. (2005). Genomewide scan for affective disorder susceptibility loci in families of a northern Swedish isolated population. *American Journal of Human Genetics, 76*, 237–248.

Volk, H. E., & Todd, R. D. (2007). Does the Child Behavior Checklist juvenile bipolar disorder phenotype identify bipolar disorder? *Biological Psychiatry, 62*, 115–120.

Wakefield, J. C. (1999). Evolutionary versus prototype analyses of the concept of disorder. *Journal of Abnormal Psychology, 108*, 374–399.

Walsh, T., McClellan, J. M., McCarthy, S. E., Addington, A. M., Pierce, S. B., Cooper, G. M., et al. (2008). Rare structural variants disrupt multiple genes in neurodevelopmental pathways in schizophrenia. *Science, 320*, 539–543.

Wellcome Trust Case Control Consortium. (2007). Genome-wide association study of 14,000 cases of seven common diseases and 3,000 shared controls. *Nature, 447*, 661–678.

Wender, P. H., Kety, S. S., Rosenthal, D., Schulsinger, F., Ortmann, J., & Lunde, I. (1986). Psychiatric disorders in the biological and adoptive families of adopted individuals with affective disorders. *Archives of General Psychiatry, 43*, 923–929.

Widiger, T. A., & Clark, L. A. (2000). Toward *DSM-V* and the classification of psychopathology. *Psychological Bulletin, 126*, 946–963.

Willcutt, E. G., Pennington, B. F., Olson, R. K., & DeFries, J. C. (2007). Understanding comorbidity: A twin study of reading disability and attention-deficit/hyperactivity disorder. *American Journal of Medical Genetics. Part B, Neuropsychiatric Genetics, 144B,* 709–714.

Willcutt, E. G., Sonuga-Barke, E. J. S., Nigg, J. T., & Sergeant, J. A. (2008). Recent developments in neuropsychological models of childhood psychiatric disorders. *Advances in Biological Psychiatry, 24,* 195–226.

Xu, B., Roos, J. L., Levy, S., van Rensburg, E. J., Gogos, J. A., & Karayiorgou, M. (2008). Strong association of de novo copy number mutations with sporadic schizophrenia. *Nature Genetics, 40,* 880–885.

Youngstrom, E., Youngstrom, J. K., & Starr, M. (2005). Bipolar diagnoses in community mental health: Achenbach Child Behavior Checklist profiles and patterns of comorbidity. *Biological Psychiatry, 58,* 569–575.

CHAPTER 9

Neurodevelopment in Bipolar Disorder

A Neuroimaging Perspective

David E. Fleck, Michael A. Cerullo, Jayasree Nandagopal,
Caleb M. Adler, Nick C. Patel, Stephen M. Strakowski,
and Melissa P. DelBello

There has been increasing interest in the neurobiology of bipolar disorder (BD) because of the variable phenotypic expression of this illness across the life span. Relative to adults with BD, there are higher rates of mixed episodes, rapid cycling, and comorbid attention-deficit/hyperacticity disorder (ADHD), oppositional defiant disorder, and conduct disorder in affected youth (Pavuluri, Birmaher, & Naylor, 2005). Factors associated with longer illness duration such as co-occurring substance use disorders, illness progression, number of affective episodes, medication exposure, and medical comorbidities may also contribute to the disparity in clinical presentation between adults and youth with BD. However, it is still unclear to what extent clinical differences in symptom manifestation between child- and adult-onset bipolar disorder reflect biological or environmentally driven changes in neural development or how biology and environment interact to predispose an individual to neuropathology.

By studying the neural circuitry of youth and adults with BD using noninvasive neuroimaging techniques such as structural and functional magnetic resonance imaging (MRI/fMRI), diffusion tensor imaging (DTI), and magnetic resonance spectroscopy (MRS), crucial insights into the pathogenesis of this disorder are now coming to light. Neuroimaging is beginning to uncover patterns of similarities and differences between childhood- and adult-onset BD and is helping to determine whether pediatric BD is continuous with adult BD or whether it represents a distinct subtype of the illness. Neuroimaging holds promise not only for defining developmental changes that occur in BD over time but also for identifying early trait characteristics to facilitate timely diagnosis and treatment and perhaps eventually the prediction of onset, treatment response, and illness course of BD.

THE ANTERIOR LIMBIC NETWORK

There are several neural circuits that subserve emotional and cognitive homeostasis in healthy individuals. Prefrontal-striatal-thalamic circuits have been implicated in socioemotional behavior and higher order cognition (Lichter & Cummings, 2001), whereas medial temporal structures are thought to play a primary role in emotional regulation, reward, and memory (Phillips, Drevets, Rauch, & Lane, 2003). Figure 9.1 depicts a network of prefrontal-subcortical circuits and its intersection with the temporal-limbic circuit to form an extended anterior limbic network (ALN) responsible for maintaining emotional and cognitive homeostasis

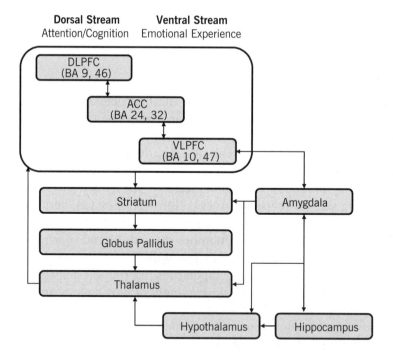

FIGURE 9.1. Simplified anatomy of the anterior-limbic network, including behaviorally relevant frontal-subcortical circuits [dorsolateral prefrontal cortex (DLPFC), ventrolateral prefrontal cortex (VLPFC), and anterior cingulate cortex (ACC)] and intersections with the temporal-limbic circuit (hippocampus, hypothalamus, and thalamus) and the hippocampal–amygdala complex. The cognitive stream (dorsal stream) and emotional stream (ventral stream) are thought to be integrated in ACC.

(Nauta, 1971; Ongur & Price, 2000). Prefrontal regions of the ALN continually monitor internal and external sensory information in order to iteratively modulate emotional and social behavior.

Normal neural development of the ALN is typically characterized by peaks in prefrontal gray matter during childhood followed by decreases through adolescence and early adulthood. Regions of prefrontal association cortex involved in the integration of primary and higher order functions (e.g., dorsolateral prefrontal cortex [DLPFC] and ventrolateral prefrontal cortex [VLPFC]) and related subcortical structures involved in movement, attention, and affect (e.g., striatum, globus pallidus) are among the last to mature in preadolescents (Geidd, 2008). White matter tracts connecting prefrontal cortex with subcortical structures and connecting the two cerebral hemispheres via the corpus callosum show a reciprocal pattern, with increasing volumes occurring throughout childhood and adolescence, likely indicating structural and functional increases in connectivity (Geidd, 2008). The amygdala and hippocampus also increase in volume through adolescence, but these changes are more likely to be gender specific with the amygdalar increase occurring in males and the hippocampal increase in females (Geidd et al., 1996). Indeed, gender differences are common in neural development, with males typically lagging behind females in maturation time for most regional volumes.

Functional neuroimaging studies suggest that the developmental trajectory of cortical control systems (i.e., primarily frontal lobe attentional systems that constrain more automatic processes of subcortex) may account for the higher incidence of risk-taking behaviors during adolescence. In typical development there appears to be a shift away from diffuse prefrontal lobe activation to more focal recruitment (Casey, Getz, & Galvan, 2008), which may impart greater top-down control and fewer risk-taking behaviors over time. However, a variety of influences may disrupt the efficiency of cortical control systems during adolescence. For instance, Hare and colleagues (2008) demonstrated that adolescents, but not children or adults, show exaggerated amygdala activity on an emotional go/no-go task and less functional connectivity between ventral prefrontal cortex and amygdala, consistent with a release from cortical inhibition. The relative failure to habituate the amygdala response with repeated exposures was related to greater anxiety (Hare et al., 2008).

Beyond demonstrating the developmental importance of the ALN, neuroimaging research also suggests that the affective and cognitive symptoms characterizing BD arise from dysfunction within the ALN (Ketter et al., 2002; Strakowski, DelBello, & Adler, 2005). Similar to the explanation for risk-taking behaviors in normally developing adolescent samples, emotional and cognitive dysregulation in BD are also hypothesized to arise from a lack of inhibitory control by orbital, inferior, or dorsolateral prefrontal cortex on subcortical and medial temporal structures within the ALN, especially the hippocampal–amygdala complex. Abnormal processing of emotional stimuli in adults with BD has been related to dysfunction between prefrontal regions and the amygdala relative to healthy comparison subjects (Altshuler, Bookheimer, & Proenza, 2005; Altshuler, Bookheimer,

& Townsend, 2005). Additionally, a small study of cortical development in pediatric BD both before and after illness onset found increased cortical gray matter in left temporal cortex and decreased bilateral gray matter in the anterior cingulate cortex (ACC) (Gogtay et al., 2007), a region purported to integrate emotional and cognitive processes (Yamasaki, LaBar, & McCarthy, 2002). In fact, numerous lines of evidence from various imaging modalities support the conclusion that ALN abnormalities underlie the pathophysiology of BD in both children and adults as described next. Although there are a number of neural circuits that are strongly tied to the ALN, and might be considered to comprise it (not the least of these involve cerebellar inputs that influence ALN function; see DelBello, Strakowski, Zimmerman, Hawkins, & Sax, 1999; Mills, DelBello, Adler, & Strakowski, 2005), we limit our discussion to structures within an anatomically narrow definition of the ALN (see Figure 9.1).

DEVELOPMENTAL PSYCHOPATHOLOGY AND BRAIN IMAGING

Although there is now good evidence for ALN involvement in both normal and abnormal neural development, how genetics, experience, and the interaction of these factors influence the course of development remains a complicated issue. Brain abnormalities can occur during early or late neurodevelopment and adversely influence structural and functional integrity at later stages (Cicchetti & Thomas, 2008). Genetic and environmental influences determine not only the onset of developmental abnormalities but also whether or not they are accommodated by new growth or functional connectivity (even that not conforming to typical developmental patterns). On the one hand, additional or alternate brain regions or structures can be recruited to preserve normal brain function, whereas chronic, stable network dysfunction often results in psychopathology (Cicchetti & Thomas, 2008). One of the enduring questions of developmental psychopathology is why individuals are more or less "resilient" to genetic and psychosocial stressors that produce and propagate brain abnormalities (Cicchetti & Blender, 2006). Neuroimaging techniques are not yet sensitive enough to address resilience on an individual level. Nonetheless, age-dependent changes in relation to genotype, phenotype (e.g., clinical symptoms), and endophenotype (e.g., cognitive markers) as well as measures of environment context (e.g., current stress) have been observed at the group level.

Because neuroimaging techniques are still relatively new, there is considerable work to be done to prospectively document the longitudinal course of normal developmental and much more so the altered developmental trajectory of BD. Multiple levels of analysis considering biological, psychological, and environmental processes will be necessary to appropriately interpret developmental neuroimaging data in the future (Cicchetti & Blender, 2006), while much of the extant neuroimaging data focus primarily on biological processes. Currently, when differences in brain structure or function are observed between studies of children and adults, it is difficult to ascertain whether they reflect a normal, neuroprotective, or pathological developmental process. By incrementally examining both normal and pathological brain development across the age range, neuroimaging researchers are beginning to address these questions. However, it is only through longitudinal research addressing both genetic and environmental influences that we will eventually come to a useful model of pathological emotional and cognitive neural processing in BD that will allow for the attribution of cause and effect and, eventually, preventive measures.

With these caveats in mind, in subsequent sections, we compare and contrast neuroimaging studies of adults and children/adolescents with BD, relative to healthy individuals, in an attempt to flesh out differences in neural structure and function that are most likely to be reliable and developmentally relevant. In making qualitative comparisons between primarily cross-sectional studies of child- and adult-onset BD, there is danger of overinterpretation because it is not possible to determine the cause of any difference (i.e., genetic, environmental, or both). However, this approach allows us to draw some tentative conclusions to guide future longitudinal studies adopting a developmental psychopathology perspective. We focus on the most consistent neurodevelopmental distinctions between child- and adult-onset BD in each of four neuroimaging modalities, including MRI, DTI, fMRI, and MRS.

NEUROIMAGING OF CHILD- AND ADULT-ONSET BIPOLAR DISORDER

Volumetric Magnetic Resonance Imaging

Volumetric MRI, also called morphometric or structural MRI, consists of a set of techniques to examine the anatomic structure of the brain. Unlike computed tomography, volumetric MRI does not use ionizing radiation. Instead, it relies on the different properties of various tissue types to generate a three-dimensional static image. There are two main approaches to volumetric MRI of the brain: region-of-interest (ROI) analysis and voxel-based morphometry (VBM). ROI analysis is performed by isolating specific regions of the brain by "tracing" them either manually or through an automated procedure. The total volume of these regions is then calculated and compared among different experimental groups or conditions of interest. This type of analysis is potentially very time consuming and can generally only be used to examine a relatively few a priori defined brain regions. With VBM, every voxel in the brain is examined in an automated procedure. VBM picks up volume differences through the entire brain in very rapid fashion despite the large volume of data input. However, this method is potentially less sensitive to regional differences in small subcortical structures relative to ROI analysis.

The ongoing development and more routine use of higher field-strength magnets than those typically used for clinical purposes (e.g., 3 and 4 Tesla vs. 1.5 Tesla) and multicoil receivers continue to advance the field. With all other variables being equal (e.g., gradient strength), high-field-strength magnets allow superior

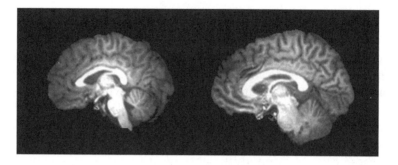

FIGURE 9.2. A T1-weighted anatomic rendering of a midsagittal brain slice from a healthy 11-year-old (left) relative to that of a healthy adult (right). Note that smaller brain volumes in children interfere with the ability to "normalize" child and adult data into the same sterotactic space.

quality of neuroanatomical images with resolution in the submillimeter range by delivering images with improved contrast-to-noise ratio. This resolution provides superior boundary demarcation between gray and white matter, which will be essential for continued improvement in automatic VBM gray–white segmentation algorithms. The use of multicoil receivers too can improve resolution and reduce imaging time to allow visualization of even more subtle structural changes, reduce costs, and improve patient comfort. Figure 9.2 depicts an anatomic rendering of a midsagittal brain slice from a healthy 11-year-old relative to that of a healthy adult and demonstrates the resolution of a high-field-strength 4-Tesla magnet.

Several similarities emerge in volumetric MRI studies comparing either adults or youth with BD with healthy comparison subjects. Both age groups generally have a greater incidence of white matter hyperintensities, either normal or increased striatal (and globus pallidus) volumes, and reduced prefrontal cortical volumes (Adler, DelBello, & Strakowski, 2006; DelBello, Adler, & Strakowski, 2006). However, the greatest developmental differences occur in a single neuroanatomic structure: the amygdala.

Amygdala Volume

The most important neurodevelopmental distinction in the volumetric MRI literature to date has been the finding of reduced amygdala volume in youth with BD relative to normal or enlarged amygdala volume in adults with BD (Pfeifer, Welge, Strakowski, Adler, & DelBello, 2008). In studies involving pediatric bipolar samples reduced amygdala volume has been the most consistent neuroanatomical finding (Blumberg, Kaufman, et al. 2003; Chen et al., 2004; DelBello, Zimmerman, Mills, Getz, & Strakowski, 2004; Dickstein et al., 2005; Frazier et al., 2005). In contrast, studies of individuals with adult-onset BD have found either increased (Altshuler et al., 2000; Brambilla et al., 2003; Frangou, 2005; Strakowski et al., 1999) or normal (Strakowski et al., 2002; Swayze, Andreasen, Alliger, Yuh,

& Ehrhardt, 1992) amygdala volume relative to healthy comparison subjects. It is still unclear what influence a narrow (bipolar I only) versus broad definition (bipolar I, II, and not otherwise specified) of BD might have on developmental distinctions in amygdala volume, which warrants further research.

Smaller amygdala volumes have also been noted in youth with BD who have a parent with BD (Chang et al., 2005) and in first-episode patients (Rosso et al., 2007). These findings suggest that amygdala volume deficits are a consequence of events occurring just before or very early in the illness course and might be useful as an illness biomarker. However, studies of children at familial risk for developing BD generally do not demonstrate a significant decrease in amygdala volume (e.g., Blumberg, Kaufman et al., 2003; Chen et al., 2004; Singh, DelBello, Adler, Stanford, & Strakowski, 2008), so the use of reduced amygdala size as a risk biomarker of incipient mania prior to illness onset is more tenuous.

Chen and colleagues (2004) observed that amygdala size is positively correlated with age in adolescents with BD, but negatively correlated with age in healthy adolescents, suggesting abnormal amygdala development in BD. This result provides further evidence that reduced amygdala size may represent an early illness biomarker that is developmentally specific to childhood-onset BD. This may also represent a disease-specific finding, as reduced amygdala volumes have not been associated with other childhood psychopathologies such as ADHD and autism (Filipek et al., 1997; Schumann et al., 2004). It has also been reported that amygdala size is negatively associated with antidepressant exposure and duration of illness (DelBello et al., 2004) but positively associated with lithium or divalproex exposure in pediatric samples (Chang et al., 2005), possibly indicating that antidepressants (and increased illness duration) potentiate the risk of amygdala reductions while lithium and mood stabilizers protect against volume loss in pediatric BD.

Diffusion Tensor Imaging

DTI is a newer magnetic resonance-based technique that utilizes measurements of in vivo water diffusion to examine white matter integrity. Water diffusion within white matter tracts is strongly influenced by specific structural features, including the myelin sheath and the tightly packed nature of the axonal bundle (Beaulieu, 2002). In the absence of any constraints on diffusion, the volume over which water molecules diffuse would form a sphere. The structure of normal white matter, however, results in a more rapid diffusion along the axis of the tract. This relative freedom of movement in only one direction gives rise to a nonisotropic (i.e., anisotropic) diffusion pattern (Beaulieu, 2002). Fractional anisotropy is a measure derived from the ratio between water molecule movement parallel with and perpendicular to the axonal tract that has been widely used by psychiatric researchers. Decreased fractional anisotropy may represent axonal pathology such as neuropathic changes, a loss of bundle coherence (i.e., less tightly packed fibers), or a disruption in axonal organization (Foong et al., 2002). The trace apparent diffusion coefficient (TADC) is another value derived from measurements of water diffusion in white matter tracts that has been widely used by psychiatric investigators. Increased TADC is thought to reflect a decrement in impediments to the movement of water molecules in and around the white matter tract and has been observed with axonal demyelization, axonal loss, and edema (Beaulieu, 2002).

For the most part, BD researchers have been concerned with white matter tracts originating within frontal cortex. Elsewhere in the brain, DTI findings either have been inconsistent or lack replication. One exception is the corpus callosum, where Wang, Kalmar, and colleagues (2008) recently identified reduced fractional anisotropy in the anterior portion of corpus callosum in adult patients with BD. This is consistent with another finding of reduced corpus callosum anisotropy in adult patients, possibly indicating altered interhemispheric connectivity (Yurgelun-Todd, Silveri, Gruber, Rohan, & Pimentel, 2007). Additionally, reduced fractional anisotropy has been reported in temporal cortex (Bruno, Cercignani, & Ron, 2008), posterior cingulate (Wang, Jackowski, et al., 2008), and subcortical white matter (Haznedar et al., 2005). By contrast, diffusivity changes have not been widely identified outside of frontal-subcortical white matter tracts (Beyer et al., 2005; Houenou et al., 2007; Yurgelun-Todd et al., 2007). Because of the greater reliability of frontal-subcortical DTI findings and the neurodevelopmental implication that frontal-subcortical white matter abnormalities underlie a behavioral "disconnection syndrome" involving disinhibition and risk-taking behaviors, we focus on these circuits.

Frontal–Subcortical White Matter Tracts

DTI has only been used to examine frontal-subcortical white matter tracts in individuals with BD over the last few years, and findings have been mixed. Several investigators have reported reduced fractional anisotropy, suggesting neuropathic changes in anterior prefrontal white matter tracts (Adler, Holland, et al., 2004; Wang, Jackowski, et al., 2008), whereas other investigators have reported either a lack of anisotropy differences in prefrontal white matter (Beyer et al., 2005; Bruno et al., 2008; Haznedar et al., 2005; Yurgelun-Todd et al., 2007) or increased fractional anisotropy (Versace et al., 2008). The areas involved do not entirely overlap, so it is unclear to what extent discrepant findings between studies may reflect methodological differences. Similarly, frontal-subcortical diffusivity has been found to be both increased in adult patients with BD (Beyer et al., 2005; Bruno et al., 2008) or unchanged (Adler, Holland, et al., 2004; Yurgelun-Todd et al., 2007). Nonetheless, a pattern is beginning to emerge suggesting frontal-subcortical network dysfunction in adults with BD.

Only two DTI studies have been conducted examining children and adolescents with BD, but the findings are relatively consistent. Adler, Adams, and colleagues (2006) studied a small group of bipolar and healthy youth ranging in age from 10 to 18 years. Patients with BD were experiencing their first documented manic or mixed episode when they were scanned. Findings mirrored the results obtained in older patients: Fractional anisotropy was reduced in anterior white matter tracts while TADC was unchanged. In an additional analysis of posterior white matter tracts, no between-group differences in either fractional anisotropy or TADC were found (Adler, Adams, et al., 2006). Frazier and colleagues (2007) studied a somewhat younger group of children with BD. Decreased fractional anisotropy was again observed in superior-frontal white matter tracts in addition to orbitofrontal white matter and corpus callosum. Moreover, fractional anisotropy values did not correlate with age. Frazier and colleagues extended their study to include a group of high-risk children who showed similar but smaller differences in fractional anisotropy compared with healthy comparison subjects. The combination of reduced fractional anisotropy values in acute and at-risk children independent of age may suggest that these findings are developmental in origin. The combination of reduced fractional anisotropy without changes in the TADC also suggests that frontal white matter abnormalities in young patients with BD may represent axonal disorganization rather than frank axonal loss (Adler, Adams, et al., 2006).

These findings are not pathognomonic for BD. Changes in anisotropy and diffusivity have also been observed in patients with other affective and psychotic disorders, including major depressive disorder and schizophrenia (Kyriakopoulos, Bargiotas, Barker, & Frangou, 2008; Zou et al., 2008). Many of these changes suggest similar pathology in frontal-subcortical tracts consistent with the elements of overlapping symptomatology observed between BD and both major depressive disorder and schizophrenia.

Although relatively sparse, the DTI data to date suggest that white matter pathology in frontal-subcortical tracts involved in neural networking between portions of the prefrontal cortex and subcortical and limbic structures is present across bipolar age groups. Furthermore, white matter abnormalities in these pathways may be intrinsic to BD, rather than the result of neurodevelopmental changes. This inference is supported by the lack of correlation between DTI measures and illness duration in children and adults (Bruno et al., 2008; Frazier et al., 2007). Further DTI studies in BD across the life span will be needed to further clarify the developmental nature of white matter abnormalities and their role in bipolar symptomatology.

Functional Magnetic Resonance Imaging

In contrast to structural brain imaging techniques, functional imaging allows for examination of brain activity. fMRI has the advantage over positron emission tomography (PET) and single-photon emission computed tomography (SPECT) of not requiring the use of ionizing radiation. fMRI also provides much greater spatial resolution than PET and SPECT. fMRI builds on the basic principles of MRI and adds an additional step that allows brain activation to be inferred from changes in the blood-oxygenation-level dependent (BOLD) response. The BOLD effect occurs because the magnetic properties of hemoglobin differ depending on whether the molecule is oxygenated or deoxygenated. Because active brain regions have an increased rate of neural firing, they recruit more blood flow, and this is detected via the BOLD response. fMRI has the additional advantage of requiring little special equipment outside a standard MRI machine. Disadvantages of fMRI include a slow temporal resolution, on the order of seconds, and a potential loss of signal along air–tissue interfaces.

Previous fMRI studies in adults or adolescents with BD have frequently found altered activation in the striatum and amygdala (e.g., Altshuler, Bookheimer, et al., 2005; Blumberg, Kaufman, et al., 2003; Chang et al., 2004; Lawrence et al., 2004; Rich et al., 2006). Increased striatal and amygdala activation in both adolescent and adult populations may represent a core feature of the illness occurring across the life span. Activation patterns in prefrontal regions, on the other hand, are more likely to show discrepancies between child and adult studies.

Prefrontal Cortical Activation

fMRI studies of individuals with BD have been conducted in samples of early and midadolescents as well as adults. Adults and adolescents with BD share a pattern of abnormal brain activation in the DLPFC, a region implicated in sustained attention and working memory performance. However, the direction of activation differences has been variable in both age ranges. In euthymic adolescents with BD, Chang and colleagues (2004) found increased activation in the left DLPFC during a visuospatial working memory task, and Nelson and colleagues (2007) found increased DLPFC activation during successful motor inhibition. However, Pavuluri, O'Connor, Harral, and Sweeney (2008) found decreased DLPFC activation during the matching of negative words in a group of euthymic adolescent patients relative to a group of demographically matched healthy controls.

In adults, Adler, Holland, Schmithorst, Tuchfarber, and Strakowski (2004) found increased DLPFC activation in euthymic individuals with BD during a working memory task. Compared with adults with major depressive disorder, Lawrence and colleagues (2004) found that patients with BD during a depressive episode had increased DLPFC activation when viewing sad faces. However, Yurgelun-Todd and colleagues (2000) showed decreased activation of the DLPFC while viewing fearful faces regardless of mood state, and Kronhaus and colleagues (2006) found decreased activation in the DLPFC during a Stroop color–word task in euthymic patients. For the most part, these activation patterns cannot be fully attributed to differences in the severity of mood symptoms, because these studies (with the exception of Lawrence et al., 2004) were conducted with euthymic samples.

In ventral regions of the prefrontal cortex, necessary for coordinating effortful motor responses, inhibition, and mood regulation, adolescent patients with BD tend to show decreased activation, while the pattern of activation in adults is less consistent. A number of adolescent studies have found decreased activation in VLPFC regardless of mood state. Adler and colleagues (2005) found decreased VLPFC activation in subjects with manic BD and comorbid ADHD compared with those with manic BD without comorbid ADHD during a sustained attention task. Pavuluri, O'Connor, Harral, and Sweeney (2007) showed that euthymic adolescents with BD had decreased VLPFC activation while viewing angry and happy faces and matching negative words (Pavuluri et al., 2008). Although Blumberg, Martin, and colleagues (2003) showed no difference in VLPFC activation during a color-naming Stroop task in adolescent subjects, rostroventral prefrontal cortex activation correlated positively with age in healthy comparison participants, but not in adolescents with BD, suggesting a possible failure of normal development in this region in adolescents with BD.

In adults, the findings in the VLPFC have been mixed, with certain studies finding decreased activation (Blumberg, Leung, et al., 2003; Kronhaus et al., 2006; Lagopoulos, Ivanovski, & Malhi, 2007; Malhi et al., 2004) and others showing increased activation (Lawrence et al., 2004; Strakowski, Adler, Holland, Mills, & DelBello, 2004). Because activation differences in VLPFC have been observed in both syndromatic and euthymic patients, it is difficult to rectify this discrepancy, but one possibility is that VLPFC overactivation represents a dysfunction of inhibitory cognitive control, especially in unmedicated patients with BD (Strakowski et al., 2004).

The fMRI data to date suggest the possibility of abnormal prefrontal function. Adults and adolescents with BD share a pattern of abnormal brain activation in the DLPFC. However, the extent and direction of activation differences have been variable. In ventral regions of the prefrontal cortex, adolescents with BD may show somewhat less activation than controls, whereas the pattern of activation in adults is less consistent. In general, activation in dorsal and ventral prefrontal regions appears to be more abnormal in adults than in adolescents compared with age-matched controls, suggesting the possibility that prefrontal dysfunction is a sign of disease progression and is, therefore, greater in older patients. However, variability in mood state and medications, among other confounding factors, limits the comparability and interpretation of most fMRI studies of BD.

Magnetic Resonance Spectroscopy

MRS provides information about the in vivo concentrations of neurochemicals in localized brain regions, thereby allowing evaluation of neurochemical abnormalities representative of bipolar pathophysiology, neurochemical effects of psychotropic medications, and potential neurochemical markers of treatment response. MRS can be used to detect the spectra from any number of isotopes. For instance, lithium (^{7}Li) MRS studies have demonstrated that brain-to-serum lithium concentration ratios may be affected by age (Moore et al., 2002), which has implications for the dosing of lithium carbonate for patients with BD across the life span. However, most studies of pediatric BD have used proton (^{1}H) MRS, so we limit our discussion to this technique primarily.

In ^{1}H MRS, signals from small neurochemical concentrations (measured in parts per million [ppm]) are detected in a large concentration of water in a localized region of the brain, known as a voxel, over a narrow frequency range. Figure 9.3 demonstrates the localized spectrum from a single voxel within the anterior cingulate of a patient with BD using ^{1}H MRS. As depicted in Figure 9.3, neurochemicals typically evaluated using ^{1}H MRS include *N*-acetyl aspartate (NAA), *myo*-inositol (mI), choline-containing compounds (Cho), creatine/creatine phosphate (Cr), and glutamate/glutamine/gamma-aminobutyric acid (Glx). *Myo*-inositol is especially relevant to the study of BD. It is a sugar involved in a number of biological processes, including cellular second messenger signaling pathways. One of these signaling pathways is the phosphoinositide cycle, where lithium is purported to exert its mood-stabilizing effects through inhibition of inositol monophosphastase (IMPase). This pharmacological activity is believed to result in decreased mI concentrations and, in turn, a reduction in overactive neuronal signaling (Allison & Stewart, 1971; Berridge, 1989), which may be a mechanism of action by which lithium exerts a mood-stabilizing effect.

In both adults and youth with BD, several ^{1}H MRS similarities have been reported. Among the most frequently reported findings in each age group are decreased NAA levels. Although this may indicate alterations in neuronal integ-

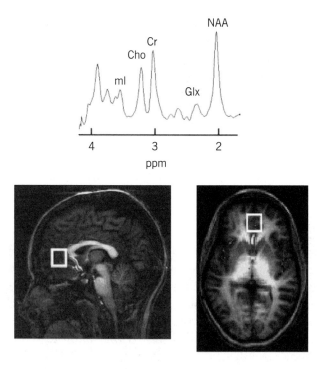

FIGURE 9.3. A 2 × 2 × 2 cm voxel placed at the anterior cingulate guided by a T1-weighted scout image. An example of the localized spectrum from the single-voxel region of the anterior cingulate in a patient with BD using a PRESS sequence. (NAA, *N*-acetyl aspartate; Cr, creatine/creatine phosphate; Cho, choline-containing compounds; MI, *myo*-inositol; Glx, glutamate/glutamine/gamma-aminobutyric acid)

rity or mitochondrial function across the entire age spectrum, contributions from ongoing neurodevelopmental processes during adolescence, namely pruning and arborization, may be confounding factors that artificially deflate NAA concentrations in younger patients. Relative to neurochemical similarities across the age range such as decreased NAA, differences are less common. However, in contrast to adults, children and adolescents with BD may have increased prefrontal mI levels.

Myo-*Inositol*

MRS studies of individuals with BD have been conducted across much of the age range from childhood through midadulthood. Proton MRS studies of adults with BD have not supported the hypothesis of elevated mI concentrations contributing to the neuropathophysiology of the illness. Localized mI levels or mI/Cr ratios in euthymic (Bruhn et al., 1993; Scherk et al., 2007, 2008; Silverstone et al., 2002; Winsberg et al., 2000), manic (Cecil, DelBello, Morey, & Strakowski, 2002; Frey et al., 2005; Frye, Thomas, et al., 2007), and depressed (Dager et al., 2004; Frye, Watzl, et al., 2007; Moore et al., 2000) adults with BD are similar to those in healthy comparison subjects. Previous or current psychotropic medication use, including lithium, was common in these studies, thereby making it difficult to determine whether alterations in mI concentrations were normalized with mood-stabilizing medications. However, a study of medication-free adults with BD reported unaltered mI levels in the left DLPFC (Frey et al., 2007). Left DLPFC mI concentrations did positively correlate with length of illness, suggesting that mI levels in this region may be a marker of chronicity (Frey et al., 2007).

In contrast to studies of adults with BD, those of children and adolescents with BD report elevated prefrontal mI concentrations, specifically in the medial prefrontal cortex of high-risk euthymic (Cecil, DelBello, Sellars, & Strakowski, 2003) and acutely manic children and adolescents (Davanzo et al., 2001, 2003). Although this may represent an early, specific biomarker of BD, several other studies have failed to identify such abnormalities in dorsolateral and medial prefrontal cortex mI levels or mI/Cr ratios in children with BD (Chang et al., 2003; Gallelli et al., 2005; Moore et al., 2007; Olvera et al., 2007) or at risk for BD (Gallelli et al., 2005).

Lithium's Influence on Myo-*Inositol*

Based on lithium's activity on the phosphoinositide cycle, investigations of lithium's in vivo effects on mI have been of interest. Sharma, Venkatasubramanian, Barany, and Davis (1992) reported increased mI/Cr in the basal ganglia of adults with BD who were stable on lithium compared with healthy controls. Two ^{1}H MRS studies have examined the temporal effects of lithium on mI in adults with bipolar depression. In a study by Moore and colleagues (1999), acute (5–7 days) and chronic (3–4 weeks) lithium treatment resulted in decreased frontal lobe mI concentrations compared with baseline. When corrections for multiple comparisons were applied, the observed decreases did not remain significant. Friedman and colleagues (2004) reported increases in regional gray matter mI concentrations with chronic lithium administration, supporting the hypothesis that extended lithium exposure may increase IMPase activity (Kaya, Resmi, Ozerdem, Guner, & Tunca, 2004). Several MRS studies of lithium in healthy adult volunteers reported no effect on brain mI concentrations (Silverstone, Hanstock, Fabian, Staab, & Allen, 1996; Silverstone, Hanstock, & Rotzinger, 1999), indicating that lithium-induced changes in mI may be specific to individuals with BD.

The effects of lithium on mI concentrations have also been studied in children with mania and adolescents with bipolar depression. Davanzo and colleagues (2001) reported a significant reduction in anterior cingulate cortex mI/Cr following 7 days of lithium treatment; this occurred specifically in subjects who achieved symptom response. Patel and colleagues (2006) investigated the acute (1 week) and chronic (6 weeks) effects of lithium on prefrontal cortex mI in adolescents with bipolar depression. Although mI concentrations in these regions at weeks 1 and 6 were not significantly different from those at baseline, mI concentrations at week 6 were elevated compared with those at week 1 in the medial and right lateral ventral prefrontal cortices (Patel et al., 2006). This finding is consistent with the study by Friedman and colleagues (2004) in adult bipolar depression and suggests that chronic treatment may increase IMPase activity and subsequently mI concentrations.

In general, then, children and adolescents with BD may have elevated prefrontal mI concentrations relative to adults with BD, specifically in the medial prefrontal cortex (although some studies fail to identify such abnormalities in the dorsolateral and medial prefrontal cortex of affected or at risk children). Therefore, although mI abnormalities may be somewhat specific to youth with BD, the penetrance of mI abnormalities in these patients may be incomplete.

DISCUSSION

The extant neuroimaging literature suggests that a number of neurodevelopmental differences exist between patients with pediatric- and adult-onset BD. These include, but are not limited to, (1) reduced amygdala volume in youth with BD relative to normal or enlarged amygdala volume in adults with BD, (2) loss of white matter coherence in tracks innervating prefrontal cortex that may be developmental in nature, (3) greater functional abnormalities in certain prefrontal regions in adults with BD relative to youth with BD, and (4) elevated prefrontal mI concentrations in youth with BD relative to adults with BD. Although many of these neuroimaging results need further replication, and the exact interpretation and significance of these findings are not fully understood, they do have important implications for our understanding of neurodevelopment in BD.

Neurodevelopmental Perspectives

The onset of BD commonly occurs during a neurodevelopmentally sensitive period, which may have significant long-term implications for brain maturation (DelBello, Adler, & Strakowski, 2006). As described, white matter connectivity between prefrontal cortical regions and subcortical structures increases throughout childhood and adolescence (Geidd, 2008). During childhood and preadolescence, prefrontal gray matter increases may represent a period of arborization during which new neuronal connections are being generated. Because this process is dynamic, the impact of the timing of illness onset on development may be substantial. For instance, if illness onset occurs during periods of heavy arborization in childhood, connections with DLPFC responsible for attentional processing may be reduced, leading to functional abnormalities in prefrontal-subcortical circuits (DelBello et al., 2006). This possibility might explain the high rate of co-occurring ADHD in early-onset BD. Similarly, decreases in ventromedial-amygdala connectivity necessary for emotional processing might explain the more severe mood dysregulation often observed in pediatric-onset BD as characterized by a chronic, mixed episode and rapid-cycling presentation relative to the more biphasic presentation of adult-onset BD (Geller & Luby, 1997; Pavuluri et al., 2005). Underlying differences in developmental connectivity may also explain reported differences in pharmacological response between child and adult patients. Alternatively, if neural connections are already in place before illness onset as in most adults, pruning (where neural connections are refined through elimination) may allow for neural reorganization to compensate for processing deficiencies by diverting them to secondary cortical regions outside of the ALN (e.g., Strakowski et al., 2004).

Clinical and Neuroimaging Considerations

Several potential confounding factors need to be considered when implementing developmental neuroimaging studies and interpreting the resultant data. First, the heart and respiration rates of children are significantly faster than in adults. Therefore, these physiological variables should be collected and considered as sources of potential error before the final analysis (Kotsoni, Byrd, & Casey, 2006). Second, a smaller brain volume in children and adolescents calls into question the ability to "normalize" their data into the same sterotactic space as used for adults (see Figure 9.2). This is a particular concern for young children. Third, because children often approach cognitive tasks differently than adults, it is difficult to say with any certainty whether or not they are using similar strategies or perceive the task to be similarly difficult in fMRI studies. Such concerns can generally be addressed by a number of techniques such as manipulating task difficulty and effort in the design of the task, equating group performance either methodologically or through post hoc group selection, and correlating or covarying age and performance (Kotsoni et al., 2006).

Clinically speaking, it is relatively rare to have a homogenous patient sample. Most studies of BD include heterogeneous patient samples that may also be diagnosed with other DSM-IV Axis I disorders, which is particularly relevant to pediatric samples. The most common comorbid condition in pediatric BD is ADHD. This is significant because when Adler and colleagues (2005) compared patients with BD with and without comorbid ADHD they found different patterns of brain activation. Those subjects with comorbid ADHD showed increased activation in the parietal and temporal gyrus as well as decreased activation in the VLPFC and anterior cingulate cortex. Leibenluft and colleagues (2007) also found differences in patients with BD with comorbid ADHD. Compared with subjects without ADHD, those with comorbid ADHD also exhibited decreased activation in the VLPFC. Decreased frontal lobe activation in the comorbid condition may reflect a loss of frontal control of attention, but it is yet to be determined whether this relates to decreased frontal arborization or other structural abnormalities. Beyond ADHD, in the pediatric population other common comorbid illnesses include anxiety disorders; the effect of anxiety disorders on brain structure and activation can be profound. For example, Thomas and colleagues (2001) have reported a strong positive correlation between self-perceived anxiety levels and amygdala activation, which has implications for findings of increased amygdala activation in fMRI studies of individuals with BD.

Of course, medications may also affect neurophysiology. Many of the neuroimaging studies included patients with BD on various psychotropic medications. Additionally, most of these studies did not include enough medication-free subjects to adequately control for these effects. In addition to current medication status, prior psychotropic medication exposure is another potential confound. Finally, mood state and symptom severity at the time of the scan as well as illness duration, number of affective episodes, and pubertal status are possible confounding variables. Although it is often impossible to remove the effects of these variables, appropriate care in study design such as a priori power analyses to ensure adequate sample size and the collection of secondary assessments (e.g., related physiological, clinical and symptom measures) can limit the effects of extraneous variables or allow for their statistical control during the analysis.

FUTURE DIRECTIONS

Neuroimaging studies have been important in advancing our understanding of developmental differences in BD. Although most of the data indicate abnormalities within the ALN across development in BD, certain findings highlight pediatric- and adult-onset differences. The interpretation of these differences is still under debate, but continual progress in the field of neuroimaging will eventually aid our understanding of the significance of developmental differences in brain structure and function. In the meantime, to further characterize pediatric BD and identify disease-specific and risk biomarkers, additional longitudinal neuroimaging studies are warranted. Longitudinal studies of at-risk and early-onset patients into adulthood, although conceptually and methodologically difficult to conduct, will be of paramount importance. Additionally, further development of age-appropriate cognitive paradigms for fMRI is especially needed. Specifically, tasks that target behaviorally relevant characteristics of BD, including mood dysregulation, impulsivity, risk taking, and impaired sustained attention, are needed, as are those tasks that target neurophysiologically relevant brain regions such as the prefrontal cortex, amygdala, and striatum. Finally, neuroimaging research can be used to (1) compare specific mood states in terms of cognition and brain function, (2) identify cognitive and neuroimaging endophenotypes to guide genetics research, and (3) identify targets for the treatment and prevention of BD.

For our part, we are conducting a number of systematic treatment studies of previously unmedicated, early-course adolescent and adult patients with BD using repeated neuroimaging assessments as part of the newly initiated University of Cincinnati Bipolar Disorder Imaging and Treatment Research Center. The use of a longitudinal design, as well as an extended age range, will allow examination of possible differences in medication effects and predictors of medication response both within and between various age strata. Additionally, we are examining neurochemical and neurofunctional predictors of developing BD in those at familial risk. This work, along with other large-scale neurodevelopmental studies currently underway in other research groups across the country and around the world, offers great promise not only for our understanding of neuropathology but also for new treatment options to help ameliorate the symptoms of BD.

REFERENCES

Adler, C., DelBello, M., Mills, N., Schmithorst, V., Holland, S., & Strakowski, S. (2005). Comorbid ADHD is associated with altered patterns of neuronal activation in adolescents with bipolar disorder performing a simple attention task. *Bipolar Disorders, 7,* 577–588.

Adler, C., Holland, S., Schmithorst, V., Tuchfarber, M., & Strakowski, S. (2004). Changes in neuronal activation in patients with bipolar disorder during performance of a working memory task. *Bipolar Disorders, 6,* 540–549.

Adler, C. M., Adams, J., DelBello, M. P., Holland, S. K., Schmithorst, V., Levine, A., et al. (2006). Evidence of white matter pathology in first-episode manic adolescents with bipolar disorder: A diffusion tensor imaging study. *American Journal of Psychiatry, 163,* 322–324.

Adler, C. M., DelBello, M. P., & Strakowski, S. M. (2006). Brain network dysfunction in bipolar disorder. *CNS Spectrums, 11,* 312–320.

Adler, C. M., Holland, S. K., Schmithorst, V., Wilke, M., Weiss, K. L., Pan, H., et al. (2004). Abnormal frontal white matter tracts in bipolar disorder: A diffusion tensor imaging study. *Bipolar Disorders, 6,* 197–203.

Allison, J. H., & Stewart, M. A. (1971). Reduced brain inositol in lithium-treated rats. *Nature New Biology, 233,* 267–268.

Altshuler, L., Bookheimer, S., Proenza, M. A., Townsend, J., Sabb, F., Firestine, A., et al. (2005). Increased amygdala activation during mania: A functional magnetic resonance imaging study. *American Journal of Psychiatry, 162,* 1211–1213.

Altshuler, L. L., Bartzokis, G., Grieder, T., Curran, J., Jimenez, T., Leight, K., et al. (2000). An MRI study of temporal lobe structures in men with bipolar disorder or schizophrenia. *Biological Psychiatry, 48,* 147–162.

Altshuler, L. L., Bookheimer, S. Y., Townsend, J., Proenza, M. A., Eisenberger, N., Sabb, F., et al. (2005). Blunted activation in orbitofrontal cortex during mania: A functional magnetic resonance imaging study. *Biological Psychiatry, 58,* 763–769.

Beaulieu, C. (2002). The basis of anisotropic diffusion in the nervous system—A technical review. *NMR in Biomedicine, 15,* 435–55.

Berridge, M. J. (1989). The Albert Lasker Medical Awards: Inositol trisphosphate, calcium, lithium, and cell signaling. *Journal of the American Medical Association, 262,* 1834–1841.

Beyer, J. L., Taylor, W. D., MacFall, J. R., Kuchibhatla, M., Payne, M. E., Provenzale, J. M., et al. (2005). Cortical white matter microstructural abnormalities in bipolar disorder. *Neuropsychopharmacology, 30,* 2225–2229.

Blumberg, H., Leung, H., Skudlarski, P., Lacadie, C., Fredericks, C., Harris, B., et al. (2003). A functional magnetic resonance imaging study of bipolar disorder. *Archives of General Psychiatry, 60,* 601–609.

Blumberg, H., Martin, A., Kaufman, J., Leung, H., Skudlarski, P., Lacadie, C., et al. (2003). Frontostriatal abnormalities in adolescents with bipolar disorder: Preliminary observations from functional MRI. *American Journal of Psychiatry, 160,* 1345–1347.

Blumberg, H. P., Kaufman, J., Martin, A., Whiteman, R., Zhang, J. H., Gore, J. C., et al. (2003). Amygdala and hippocampal volumes in adolescents and adults with bipolar disorder. *Archives of General Psychiatry, 60,* 1201–1208.

Brambilla, P., Harenski, K., Nicoletti, M., Sassi, R. B., Mallinger, A. G., Frank, E., et al. (2003). MRI investigation of temporal lobe structures in bipolar patients. *Journal of Psychiatry Research, 37,* 287–295.

Bruhn, H., Stoppe, G., Staedt, J., Merboldt, K. D., Hanicke, W., & Frahm, J. (1993). Quantitative proton MRS in vivo shows cerebral *myo*-inositol and cholines to be unchanged in manic-depressive patients treated with lithium. *Proceedings of the Society for Magnetic Resonance Medicine, 1543.*

Bruno, S., Cercignani, M., & Ron, M. A. (2008). White matter abnormalities in bipolar disorder: A voxel-based diffusion tensor imaging study. *Bipolar Disorders, 10,* 460–468.

Casey, B. J., Getz, S., & Galvan, A. (2008). The adolescent brain. *Developmental Review, 28,* 62–77.

Cecil, K. M., DelBello, M. P., Morey, R., & Strakowski, S. M. (2002). Frontal lobe differences in bipolar disorder as determined by proton MR spectroscopy. *Bipolar Disorders, 4,* 357–365.

Cecil, K. M., DelBello, M. P., Sellars, M. C., & Strakowski, S. M. (2003). Proton magnetic resonance spectroscopy of the frontal lobe and cerebellar vermis in children with a mood disorder and a familial risk for bipolar disorders. *Journal of Child and Adolescent Psychopharmacology, 13,* 545–555.

Chang, K., Adleman, N., Dienes, K., Barnea-Goraly, N., Reiss, A., & Ketter, T. (2003). Decreased N-acetylaspartate in children with familial bipolar disorder. *Biological Psychiatry, 53,* 1059–1065.

Chang, K., Adleman, N., Dienes, K., Simeonova, D., Menon, V., & Reiss, A. (2004). Anomalous prefrontal-subcortical activation in familial pediatric bipolar disorder. *Archives of General Psychiatry, 61,* 781–792.

Chang, K., Karchemskiy, A., Barnea-Goraly, N., Garrett, A., Simeonova, D. I., & Reiss, A. (2005). Reduced amygdalar gray matter volume in familial pediatric bipolar disorder. *Journal of the American Academy of Child and Adolescent Psychiatry, 44,* 565–573.

Chen, B. K., Sassi, R., Axelson, D., Hatch, J. P., Sanches, M., Nicoletti, M., et al. (2004). Cross-section study of abnormal amygdala development in adolescents and young adults with bipolar disorder. *Biological Psychiatry, 56*, 399–405.

Cicchetti, D., & Blender, J. A. (2006). A multiple-levels-of-analysis perspective on resilience: Implications for the developing brain, neural plasticity, and preventive interventions. *Annals of the New York Academy of Science, 1094*, 248–258.

Cicchetti, D., & Thomas, K. M. (2008). Imaging brain systems in normality and psychopathology. *Development and Psychopathology, 20*, 1023–1027.

Dager, S. R., Friedman, S. D., Parow, A., Demopulos, C., Stoll, A. L., Lyoo, I. K., et al. (2004). Brain metabolic alterations in medication-free patients with bipolar disorder. *Archives of General Psychiatry, 61*, 450–458.

Davanzo, P., Thomas, M. A., Yue, K., Oshiro, T., Belin, T., Strober, M., et al. (2001). Decreased anterior cingulate myo-inositol/creatine spectroscopy resonance with lithium treatment in children with bipolar disorder. *Neuropsychopharmacology, 24*, 359–369.

Davanzo, P., Yue, K., Thomas, M. A., Belin, T., Mintz, J., Venkatraman, T. N., et al. (2003). Proton magnetic resonance spectroscopy of bipolar disorder versus intermittent explosive disorder in children and adolescents. *American Journal of Psychiatry, 160*, 1442–1452.

DelBello, M. P., Adler, C. M., & Strakowski, S. M. (2006). The neurophysiology of childhood and adolescent bipolar disorder. *CNS Spectrums, 11*, 298–311.

DelBello, M. P., Strakowski, S. M., Zimmerman, M. E., Hawkins, J. M., & Sax, K. W (1999). MRI analysis of the cerebellum in bipolar disorder: A pilot study. *Neuropsychopharmacology, 21*, 63–68.

DelBello, M. P., Zimmerman, M. E., Mills, N. P., Getz, G. E., & Strakowski, S. M. (2004). Magnetic resonance imaging analysis of amygdala and other subcortical brain regions in adolescents with bipolar disorder. *Bipolar Disorders, 6*, 143–152.

Dickstein, D. P., Milham, M. P., Nugent, A. C., Drevets, W. C., Charney, D. S., Pine, D. S., et al. (2005). Frontotemporal alterations in pediatric bipolar disorder: Results of a voxel-based morphometry study. *Archives of General Psychiatry, 62*, 734–741.

Filipek, P. A., Semrud-Clikeman, M., Steingard, R. J., Renshaw, P. F., Kennedy, D. N., & Biederman, J. (1997). Volumetric MRI analysis comparing subjects having attention-deficit hyperactivity disorder with normal controls. *Neurology, 48*, 589–601.

Foong, J., Symms, M. R., Barker, G. J., Maier, M., Miller, D. H., & Ron, M. A. (2002). Investigating regional white matter in schizophrenia using diffusion tensor imaging. *NeuroReport, 13*, 333–336.

Frangou, S. (2005). The Maudsley Bipolar Disorder Project. *Epilepsia, 46*, 19–25.

Frazier, J. A., Breeze, J. L., Papadimitriou, G., Kennedy, D. N., Hodge, S. M., Moore, C. M., et al. (2007). White matter abnormalities in children with and at risk for bipolar disorder. *Bipolar Disorders, 9*, 799–809.

Frazier, J. A., Chiu, S., Breeze, J. L., Makris, N., Lange, N., Kennedy, D. N., et al. (2005). Structural brain magnetic resonance imaging of limbic and thalamic volumes in pediatric bipolar disorder. *American Journal of Psychiatry, 162*, 1256–1265.

Frey, B. N., Folgierini, M., Nicoletti, M., Machado-Vieira, R., Stanley, J. A., Soares, J. C., et al. (2005). A proton magnetic resonance spectroscopy investigation of the dorsolateral prefrontal cortex in acute mania. *Human Psychopharmacology, 20*, 133–139.

Frey, B. N., Stanley, J. A., Nery, F. G., Monkul, E. S., Nicoletti, M. A., Chen, H. H., et al. (2007). Abnormal cellular energy and phospholipid metabolism in the left dorsolateral prefrontal cortex of medication-free individuals with bipolar disorder: An in vivo 1H MRS study. *Bipolar Disorders, 9*(Suppl. 1), 119–127.

Friedman, S. D., Dager, S. R., Parow, A., Hirashima, F., Demopulos, C., Stoll, A. L., et al. (2004). Lithium and valproic acid treatment effects on brain chemistry in bipolar disorder. *Biological Psychiatry, 56*, 340–348.

Frye, M. A., Thomas, M. A., Yue, K., Binesh, N., Davanzo, P., Ventura, J., et al. (2007). Reduced concentrations of N-acetylaspartate (NAA) and the NAA-creatine ratio in the basal ganglia in bipolar disorder: A study using 3-Tesla proton magnetic resonance spectroscopy. *Psychiatry Research, 154,* 259–265.

Frye, M. A., Watzl, J., Banakar, S., O'Neill, J., Mintz, J., Davanzo, P., et al. (2007). Increased anterior cingulate/medial prefrontal cortical glutamate and creatine in bipolar depression. *Neuropsychopharmacology, 32,* 2490–2499.

Gallelli, K. A., Wagner, C. M., Karchemskiy, A., Howe, M., Spielman, D., Reiss, A., et al. (2005). N-acetylaspartate levels in bipolar offspring with and at high-risk for bipolar disorder. *Bipolar Disorders, 7,* 589–597.

Geidd, J. N. (2008). The teen brain: Insights from neuroimaging. *Journal of Adolescent Health, 42,* 335–343.

Geidd, J. N., Vaituzis, A. C., Hamburger, S. D., Lange, N., Rajapakse, J. C., Kaysen, D., et al. (1996). Quantitative MRI of the temporal lobe, amygdala, and hippocampus in normal human development: Ages 4–18 years. *Journal of Comparative Neurology, 366,* 223–230.

Geller, B., & Luby J. (1997). Child and adolescent bipolar disorder: A review of the past 10 years. *Journal of the American Academy of Child and Adolescent Psychiatry, 37,* 1168–1176.

Gogtay, N., Ordonez, A., Herman, D. H., Hayashi, K. M., Greenstein, D., Vaituzis, C., et al. (2007). Dynamic mapping of cortical development before and after the onset of pediatric bipolar illness. *Journal of Child Psychology and Psychiatry, 48,* 852–862.

Hare, T. A., Tottenham, N., Galvan, A., Voss, H. U., Glover, G. H., & Casey, B. J. (2008). Biological substrates of emotional reactivity and regulation in adolescents during an emotional go-no go task. *Biological Psychiatry, 63,* 927–934.

Haznedar, M. M., Roversi, F., Pallanti, S., Baldini-Rossi, N., Schnur, D. B., Licalzi, E. M., et al. (2005). Fronto-thalamo-striatal gray and white matter volumes and anisotropy of their connections in bipolar spectrum illnesses. *Biological Psychiatry, 57,* 733–742.

Houenou, J., Wessa, M., Douaud, G., Leboyer, M., Chanraud, S., Perrin, M., et al. (2007). Increased white matter connectivity in euthymic bipolar patients: Diffusion tensor tractography between the subgenual cingulate and the amygdalo-hippocampal complex. *Molecular Psychiatry, 12,* 1001–1010.

Kaya, N., Resmi, H., Ozerdem, A., Guner, G., & Tunca, Z. (2004). Increased inositol-monophosphatase activity by lithium treatment in bipolar patients. *Progress in Neuropsychopharmacology and Biological Psychiatry, 28,* 521–527.

Ketter, T. A., Wang, P. W., Dieckmann, N. F., Lembke, A., Becker, O. V., & Camilleri, C. (2002). Brain anatomic circuits and the pathophysiology of affective disorders. In J.C. Soares (Ed.), *Brain imaging in affective disorders* (pp. 79–118). New York: Marcel Dekker.

Kotsoni, E., Byrd, D., & Casey, B. J. (2006). Special considerations for functional magnetic resonance imaging of pediatric populations. *Journal of Magnetic Resonance Imaging, 23,* 877–886.

Kronhaus, D., Lawrence, N., Williams, A., Frangou, S., Brammer, M., Williams, S., et al. (2006). Stroop performance in bipolar disorder: Further evidence for abnormalities in the ventral prefrontal cortex. *Bipolar Disorders, 8,* 28–39.

Kyriakopoulos, M., Bargiotas, T., Barker, G. J., & Frangou, S. (2008). Diffusion tensor imaging in schizophrenia. *European Psychiatry, 23,* 255–273.

Lagopoulos, J., Ivanovski, B., & Malhi, G. (2007). An event-related functional MRI study of working memory in euthymic bipolar disorder. *Journal of Psychiatry and Neuroscience, 332,* 174–184.

Lawrence, N., Williams, A., Surguladze, V., Giampietro, V., Brammer, M., Andrew, C., et al. (2004). Subcortical and ventral prefrontal cortical neural responses to facial expressions distinguish patients with bipolar disorder and major depression. *Biological Psychiatry*, 55, 578–587.

Leibenluft, E., Rich, B., Vinton, D., Nelson, E., Fromm, S., Berghorst, L., et al. (2007). Neural circuitry engaged during unsuccessful motor inhibition in pediatric bipolar disorder. *American Journal of Psychiatry*, 164, 52–60.

Lichter, D. G., & Cummings, J. L. (2001). Introduction and overview. In D. G. Lichter & J. L. Cummings (Eds.), *Frontal–subcortical circuits in psychiatric and neurological disorders* (pp. 1–43). New York: Guilford Press.

Malhi, G., Lagopoulos, J., Sachdev, P., Mitchell, P., Ivanovski, B., & Parker, G. (2004). Cognitive generation of affect in hypomania: An fMRI study. *Bipolar Disorders*, 6, 271–285.

Mills, N. P., DelBello, M. P., Adler, C. M., & Strakowski, S. M. (2005). MRI analysis of cerebellar vermal abnormalities in bipolar disorder. *American Journal of Psychiatry*, 162, 1530–1532.

Moore, C. M., Breeze, J. L., Gruber, S. A., Babb, S. M., Frederick, B. B., Villafuerte, R. A., et al. (2000). Choline, myo-inositol and mood in bipolar disorder: A proton magnetic resonance spectroscopic imaging study of the anterior cingulate cortex. *Bipolar Disorders*, 2, 207–216.

Moore, C. M., Demopulos, C. M., Henry, M. E., Steingard, R. J., Zamvil, L., Katic, A., et al. (2002). Brain-to-serum lithium ratio and age: An in vivo magnetic resonance spectroscopy study. *American Journal of Psychiatry*, 159, 1240–1242.

Moore, C. M., Frazier, J. A., Glod, C. A., Breeze, J. L., Dieterich, M., Finn, C. T., et al. (2007). Glutamine and glutamate levels in children and adolescents with bipolar disorder: A 4.0-T proton magnetic resonance spectroscopy study of the anterior cingulate cortex. *Journal of the American Academy of Child and Adolescent Psychiatry*, 46, 524–534.

Moore, G. J., Bebchuk, J. M., Parrish, J. K., Faulk, M. W., Arfken, C. L., Strahl-Bevacqua, J., et al. (1999). Temporal dissociation between lithium-induced changes in frontal lobe myo-inositol and clinical response in manic-depressive illness. *American Journal of Psychiatry*, 156, 1902–1908.

Nauta, W. J. H. (1971). The problem of the frontal lobe: A reinterpretation. *Journal of Psychiatry Research*, 8, 167–187.

Nelson, E., Vinton, D., Berghorst, L., Towbin, K., Hommer, R., Dickstein, D., et al. (2007). Brain systems underlying response flexibility in healthy and bipolar adolescents: An event-related fMRI study. *Bipolar Disorders*, 9, 810–819.

Olvera, R. L., Caetano, S. C., Fonseca, M., Nicoletti, M., Stanley, J. A., Chen, H. H., et al. (2007). Low levels of N-acetyl aspartate in the left dorsolateral prefrontal cortex of pediatric bipolar patients. *Journal of Child and Adolescent Psychopharmacology*, 17, 461–473.

Ongur, D., & Price, J. L. (2000). The organization of networks within the orbital and medial prefrontal cortex of rats, monkeys, and humans. *Cerebral Cortex*, 10, 206–219.

Patel, N. C., DelBello, M. P., Cecil, K. M., Adler, C. M., Bryan, H. S., Stanford, K. E., et al. (2006). Lithium treatment effects on myo-inositol in adolescents with bipolar depression. *Biological Psychiatry*, 60, 998–1004.

Pavuluri, M., O'Connor, M., Harral, E., & Sweeney, J. (2007). Affective neural circuitry during facial emotion processing in pediatric bipolar disorder. *Biological Psychiatry*, 62, 158–167.

Pavuluri, M., O'Connor, M., Harral, E., & Sweeney, J. (2008). An fMRI study of the interface between affective and cognitive neural circuitry in pediatric bipolar disorder. *Psychiatry Research: Neuroimaging*, 162, 244–255.

Pavuluri, M. N., Birmaher, B., & Naylor, M. W. (2005). Pediatric bipolar disorder: A review of the past 10 years. *Journal of the American Academy of Child and Adolescent Psychiatry*, 44, 846–871.

Pfeifer, J. C., Welge, J., Strakowski, S.M., Adler, C. M., & DelBello, M. P. (2008). Meta-analysis of amygdala volumes in children and adolescents with bipolar disorder. *Journal of the American Academy of Child and Adolescent Psychiatry, 47,* 1289–1298.

Phillips, M. L., Drevets, W. C., Rauch, S. L., & Lane, R. (2003). Neurobiology of emotion perception: II. Implications for major psychiatric disorders. *Biological Psychiatry, 54,* 515–528.

Rich, B. A., Vinton, D. T., Roberson-Nay, R., Hommer, R. E., Berghorst, L. H., McClure, E. B., et al. (2006). Limbic hyperactivation during processing of neutral facial expressions in children with bipolar disorder. *Proceedings of the National Academy of Science USA, 103,* 8900–8905.

Rosso, I. M., Killgore, W. D., Cintron, C. M., Gruber, S. A., Tohen, M., & Yurgelun-Todd, D. A. (2007). Reduced amygdala volumes in first-episode bipolar disorder and correlation with cerebral white matter. *Biological Psychiatry, 61,* 743–749.

Scherk, H., Backens, M., Schneider-Axmann, T., Kemmer, C., Usher, J., Reith, W., et al. (2008). Neurochemical pathology in hippocampus in euthymic patients with bipolar I disorder. *Acta Psychiatrica Scandinavica, 117,* 283–288.

Scherk, H., Backens, M., Schneider-Axmann, T., Usher, J., Kemmer, C., Reith, W., et al. (2007). Cortical neurochemistry in euthymic patients with bipolar I disorder. *World Journal of Biological Psychiatry, 13,* 1–10.

Schumann, C. M., Hamstra, J., Goodlin-Jones, B. L., Lotspeich, L. J., Kwon, H., Buonocore, M. H., et al. (2004). The amygdala is enlarged in children but not adolescents with autism: The hippocampus is enlarged at all ages. *Journal of Neuroscience, 24,* 6392–6401.

Sharma, R., Venkatasubramanian, P. N., Barany, M., & Davis, J. M. (1992). Proton magnetic resonance spectroscopy of the brain in schizophrenic and affective patients. *Schizophrenia Research, 8,* 43–49.

Silverstone, P. H., Hanstock, C. C., Fabian, J., Staab, R., & Allen, P. S. (1996). Chronic lithium does not alter human myo-inositol or phosphomonoester concentrations as measured by 1H and 31P MRS. *Biological Psychiatry, 40,* 235–246.

Silverstone, P. H., Hanstock, C. C., & Rotzinger, S. (1999). Lithium does not alter the choline/creatine ratio in the temporal lobe of human volunteers as measured by proton magnetic resonance spectroscopy. *Journal of Psychiatry and Neuroscience, 24,* 222–226.

Silverstone, P. H., Wu, R. H., O'Donnell, T., Ulrich, M., Asghar, S. J., & Hanstock, C. C. (2002). Chronic treatment with both lithium and sodium valproate may normalize phosphoinositol cycle activity in bipolar patients. *Human Psychopharmacology, 17,* 321–327.

Singh, M. K., DelBello, M. P., Adler, C. M., Stanford, K. E., & Strakowski, S. M. (2008). Neuroanatomical characterization of child offspring of bipolar parents. *Journal of the American Academy of Child and Adolescent Psychiatry, 47,* 526–531.

Strakowski, S. M., Adler, C. M., Holland, S. K., Mills, N., & DelBello, M. P. (2004). A preliminary fMRI study of sustained attention in euthymic, unmedicated bipolar disorder. *Neuropsychopharmacology, 29,* 1734–1740.

Strakowski, S. M., DelBello, M. P., & Adler, C. M. (2005). The functional neuroanatomy of bipolar disorder: A review of neuroimaging findings. *Molecular Psychiatry, 10,* 105–116.

Strakowski, S. M., DelBello, M. P., Sax, K. W., Zimmerman, M. E., Shear, P. K., Hawkins, J. M., et al. (1999). Brain magnetic resonance imaging of structural abnormalities in bipolar disorder. *Archives of General Psychiatry, 56,* 254–260.

Strakowski, S. M., DelBello, M. P., Zimmerman, M. E., Getz, G. E., Mills, N. P., Ret, J., et al. (2002). Ventricular and periventricular structural volumes in first- versus multiple-episode bipolar disorder. *American Journal of Psychiatry, 159,* 1841–1847.

Swayze, V. W., Andreasen, N. C., Alliger, R. J., Yuh, W. T., & Ehrhardt, J. C. (1992). Subcortical and temporal structures in affective disorder and schizophrenia: A magnetic resonance imaging study. *Biological Psychiatry, 31,* 221–240.

Thomas, K. M., Drevets, W. C., Dahl, R. E., Ryan, N. D., Birmaher, B., Eccard, C. H., et al. (2001). Amygdala response to fearful faces in anxious and depressed children. *Archives of General Psychiatry, 58,* 1057–1063.

Versace, A., Almeida, J. R., Hassel, S., Walsh, N. D., Novelli, M., Klein, C. R., et al. (2008). Elevated left and reduced right orbitomedial prefrontal fractional anisotropy in adults with bipolar disorder revealed by tract-based spatial statistics. *Archives of General Psychiatry, 65,* 1041–1052.

Wang, F., Jackowski, M., Kalmar, J. H., Chepenik, L. G., Tie, K., Qiu, M., et al. (2008). Abnormal anterior cingulum integrity in bipolar disorder determined through diffusion tensor imaging. *British Journal of Psychiatry, 193,* 126–129.

Wang, F., Kalmar, J. H., Edmiston, E., Chepenik, L. G., Bhagwagar, Z., Spencer, L., et al. (2008). Abnormal corpus callosum integrity in bipolar disorder: A diffusion tensor imaging study. *Biological Psychiatry, 64,* 730–733.

Winsberg, M. E., Sachs, N., Tate, D. L., Adalsteinsson, E., Spielman, D., & Ketter, T. A. (2000). Decreased dorsolateral prefrontal N-acetyl aspartate in bipolar disorder. *Biological Psychiatry, 47,* 475–481.

Yamasaki, H., LaBar, K. S., & McCarthy, G. (2002). Dissociable prefrontal brain systems for attention and emotion. *Proceedings of the National Academy of Science USA, 99,* 11447–11451.

Yurgelun-Todd, D., Gruber, S., Kanayama, G., Killgore, W., Baird, A., & Young, A. (2000). fMRI during affect discrimination in bipolar affective disorder. *Bipolar Disorders, 2,* 237–248.

Yurgelun-Todd, D. A., Silveri, M. M., Gruber, S. A., Rohan, M. L., & Pimentel, P. J. (2007). White matter abnormalities observed in bipolar disorder: A diffusion tensor imaging study. *Bipolar Disorders, 9,* 504–512.

Zou, K., Huang, X., Li, T., Gong, Q., Li, Z., Ou-yang, L., et al. (2008). Alterations of white matter integrity in adults with major depressive disorder: A magnetic resonance imaging study. *Journal of Psychiatry and Neuroscience, 33,* 525–530.

CHAPTER 10

Adolescent-Onset Bipolar Spectrum Disorders

A Cognitive Vulnerability–Stress Perspective

Lauren B. Alloy, Lyn Y. Abramson, Patricia D. Walshaw,
Jessica Keyser, and Rachel K. Gerstein

Little work has examined the co-influence of cognitive, psychosocial, and neu-robiological factors in vulnerability to bipolar disorder (BD) and its course and phenomenology, particularly in the context of an understanding of normative developmental processes. In this chapter, we present a cognitive vulnerability–stress perspective on the development and characteristics of adolescent bipolar spectrum disorders informed by research on normative adolescent brain, cognitive, and emotional/motivational development. BDs form a continuum or spectrum of severity from the milder subsyndromal cyclothymia to bipolar II disorder to full-blown bipolar I disorder (Akiskal, Djenderedjian, Rosenthal, & Khani, 1977; Akiskal, Khani, & Scott-Strauss, 1979; Cassano et al., 1999; Depue et al., 1981; Goodwin & Jamison, 2007). Moreover, milder forms of BD often progress to the more severe forms (e.g., Akiskal et al., 1977, 1979; Birmaher et al., 2006; Shen, Alloy, Abramson, & Sylvia, 2008), providing support for the spectrum concept of BD. Thus, we consider the full range of bipolar spectrum disorders in this chapter. However, whether findings reported for individuals with milder disorders in the bipolar spectrum generalize to those with bipolar I disorder must be examined specifically.

We begin by discussing three clinical phenomena of BD associated with the transitional period of adolescence: adolescent onset or exacerbation, gender differences, and specific symptom presentations. We present the cognitive vulnerability–transactional stress model of unipolar depression and its extension to bipolar spectrum disorders. The extension of this model to BDs includes a recognition that the cognitive styles and life events involved in the cognitive

282

vulnerability–stress combination for bipolar conditions are related to behavioral approach system (BAS) dysregulation (see Alloy, Abramson, Urosevic, Nusslock, & Jager-Hyman, Chapter 6, this volume). We review evidence that life events, cognitive vulnerability, the cognitive vulnerability–stress combination, and developmental experiences of poor parenting and maltreatment featured in the BAS-relevant cognitive vulnerability–stress model play a role in the onset and course of BDs. We then apply the cognitive vulnerability–stress model to an understanding of adolescent onset/exacerbation, gender differences, and adolescent phenomenology of BD. Finally, we further elaborate this application of the model by embedding it in the contexts of normative adolescent cognitive (executive functioning) and brain development, normative adolescent development of the stress-emotion and reward systems, and genetic predisposition. *We suggest that increased brain maturation and accompanying increases in executive functioning, along with augmented neural and behavioral stress sensitivity and reward sensitivity during adolescence, combine with the cognitive vulnerability–stress model to explain the high-risk period for onset or exacerbation of BD, gender differences, and unique symptom presentation during adolescence.*

AGE OF ONSET, GENDER DIFFERENCES, AND PHENOMENOLOGY IN BIPOLAR SPECTRUM DISORDERS

Adolescence is a developmental period characterized by large transitions in neurobiological, psychological, and social role functioning. Although the median age of onset for bipolar I and II disorders ranges from 17 to 31 years, the first peak in rates of BD is between ages 15 and 19 (Burke, Burke, Regier, & Rao, 1990; Kennedy et al., 2005; Kessler, Rubinow, Holmes, Abelson, & Zhao, 1997; Kupfer et al., 2002; Weissman et al., 1996). Weissman and colleagues (1996) refer to this 4-year period as the "hazard period" for BD. Indeed, admixture analyses indicate that there are three high-risk periods in onset of BD, with the earliest around midadolescence (Bellivier, Golmard, Henry, Leboyer, & Schurhoff, 2001; Bellivier et al., 2003). Moreover, childhood- or adolescent-onset BD is associated with a worse course, greater comorbidity, and greater familial loading than adult-onset BD (e.g., Carter, Mundo, Parikh, & Kennedy, 2003; Ernst & Goldberg, 2004; Mick, Biederman, Faraone, Murray, & Wozniak, 2003). Thus, adolescence is a critical developmental period constituting an "age of risk" during which bipolar conditions may initially become manifest, "consolidate," and often progress to a more severe course. Although recent research has demonstrated the existence of prepubertal-onset bipolar disorder (see Meyer & Carlson, Chapter 2, and Youngstrom, Chapter 3, this volume), in this chapter we focus on the adolescent hazard period for onset of BD.

There are gender differences in the onset and course of bipolar spectrum disorders. Although men and women have similar overall prevalence of bipolar spectrum disorders, the course of BD in women is more often characterized by primarily depressive episodes (e.g., bipolar II), whereas the course in men is more likely to be marked by hypomania/mania (e.g., Angst, 1978; Leibenluft, 1996; Rasgon et al., 2005; Robb, Young, Cooke, & Joffe, 1998; Roy-Byrne, Post, Uhde, Porcu, & Davis, 1985; Viguera, Baldessarini, & Tondo, 2001). This is similar to the robust gender difference found for unipolar depression (e.g., Nolen-Hoeksema, 1990). Men also have an earlier onset of BD than women, and men's first episode is more likely to be hypomanic/manic, whereas women's first episode is more likely to be depressed (Burke et al., 1990; Kawa et al., 2005; Kennedy et al., 2005; Robb et al., 1998; Viguera et al., 2001). Moreover, prepubertal-onset cases of BD are overwhelmingly male, whereas there is a more even gender distribution in adolescent-onset BD (Biederman et al., 2005; Geller et al., 1995; Hendrick, Altshuler, Gitlin, Delrahim, & Hammen, 2000).

Third, with respect to phenomenology, some studies find that children and adolescents with BD experience more mixed states, rapid cycling, greater dysphoria and irritability, and greater chronicity than adults (Biederman et al., 2005; Geller et al., 1995; Geller, Tillman, Craney, & Bolhofner, 2004; Leibenluft, Charney, & Pine, 2003; Mick et al., 2003; Strober et al., 1988). Juvenile BD is also associated with high comorbidity with attention-deficit/hyperactivity disorder that may continue into adolescence (Geller et al., 1998; Leibenluft et al., 2003; Wozniak et al., 1995), and symptoms of ADHD are often the first signs of psychopathology in offspring of parents with BD (Chang, Steiner, & Ketter, 2000; DelBello & Geller, 2001). Thus, BD in childhood and adolescence appears to be characterized by considerable depression, irritability, and attention problems.

MECHANISMS FOR THE ADOLESCENT ONSET AND GENDER DIFFERENCES IN BIPOLAR SPECTRUM DISORDERS

Why might adolescence be an "age of risk" for onset of bipolar spectrum disorders, especially for females? A cognitive vulnerability–transactional stress model may be plausible in explaining why many individuals with a bipolar diathesis have an onset of BD during adolescence because some of the key etiological factors featured in the theory (e.g., cognitive vulnerability, stress, rumination, future expectancies) have just become developmentally operative during this period as a result of normative brain maturation and cognitive (e.g., growth in executive functions), emotional (e.g., increase in biological "stress sensitivity"), and motivational (e.g., increase in biological "reward sensitivity") development.

Cognitive Vulnerability–Transactional Stress Model of Depression

There has been growing interest in the role of cognition and life events in BDs over the past two decades (for reviews, see Alloy, Abramson, et al., 2005; Alloy, Reilly-Harrington, et al., 2005; Alloy, Abramson, Neeren, et al., 2006; Alloy, Abramson, Walshaw, et al., 2006). Many studies of cognition and life stress in BD have been guided by extensions of the cognitive vulnerability–stress models of unipolar depression (Abramson, Metalsky, & Alloy, 1989; Beck, 1987); thus, we provide a brief description of the cognitive vulnerability–transactional stress model of depression here (see Figure 10.1).

The cognitive vulnerability–transactional stress model of depression (Alloy & Abramson, 2007; Hankin & Abramson, 2001) was influenced by transactional models in developmental psychopathology. Transactional developmental psychopathology models emphasize the importance of bidirectional influences between risk factors and psychopathological outcomes. That is, maladaptive developmental outcomes can, in turn, create the conditions that further contribute to their onset, maintenance, and worsening. The cognitive vulnerability–transactional stress model is a developmentally sensitive elaboration of two cognitive theories of depression: hopelessness theory (Abramson et al., 1989) and Beck's (1987) cognitive theory of depression. When they confront negative events, individuals with negative cognitive styles are more likely to become depressed than nonvulnerable individuals because they tend to make negative inferences about the causes, consequences, or self-implications of the events. An individual exhibiting such cognitive vulnerability who gets rejected by a lover may attribute this event to stable, global causes (e.g., unlovability) and infer that he or she never will get married and is worthless. This model is a classic vulnerability–stress model because negative cognitive styles (the vulnerability) contribute to depression in the presence, but not the absence, of negative events (the stress). In addition, the cognitive vulnerability × stress combination leads to depression onset through mediation by negative cognitions such as hopelessness. Furthermore, increases in depression or cognitive vulnerability itself can contribute to the creation of further dependent, negative life events through a transactional process, which, in turn, maintains or worsens the depression.

Recently, we (Abramson et al., 2002; Alloy & Abramson, 2007) elaborated the model to include rumination in the causal chain. Rumination is another cognitive factor important in depression onset and course (Nolen-Hoeksema, 1991, 2000; Spasojevic & Alloy, 2001) as well as in gender differences in depression (Nolen-Hoeksema & Jackson, 2001). When a negative event occurs, it is adaptive to turn attention to the event, find a resolution, and then continue goal-directed behavior (the self-regulatory cycle; Carver & Scheier, 1998). Selective attention remains focused on the negative event until it is resolved by generating a solution to the problem, decreasing the event's importance, or distracting attention away from it. We hypothesized that, because of their negative inferences, cognitively vulnerable individuals would have difficulty with all three exits. For example, no solution is readily available if a cognitively vulnerable adolescent attributes not getting a date to "ugliness." Instead, these individuals' attention becomes "stuck" on negative cognitive content because the inferences they generate in response to negative events only lead to further perceived problems (e.g., "No one will want to be with me because I am so ugly") rather than to resolutions. Such self-regulatory perseveration (Pyszczynski & Greenberg, 1987) constitutes rumination because selec-

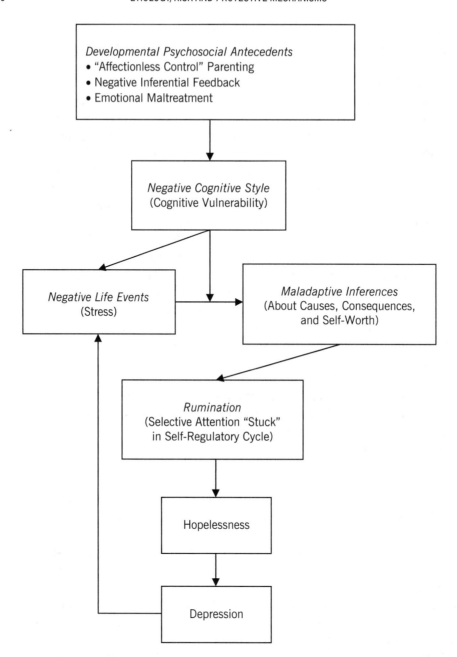

FIGURE 10.1. The cognitive vulnerability–transactional stress model of depression. The causal relations proposed in the model are described throughout the chapter.

tive attention remains focused on negative content, which, in turn, should result in the spiral into clinical depression. This self-regulatory perspective, then, highlights rumination as mediating the effects of cognitive vulnerability on depression (see Figure 10.1).

Evidence for the Cognitive Vulnerability–Transactional Stress Model of Depression

Much empirical evidence supports the cognitive vulnerability–transactional stress model of depression (for reviews, see Abramson et al., 2002; Alloy & Abramson, 2007; Alloy, Abramson, Safford, & Gibb, 2005; Alloy, Abramson, Whitehouse, et al., 2006; Hankin & Abramson, 2001). We briefly review major relevant findings here.

In the Temple–Wisconsin Cognitive Vulnerability to Depression Project (Alloy & Abramson, 1999; Alloy et al., 2000; Alloy, Abramson, Whitehouse, et al., 2006), ethnically diverse male and female university freshmen (n = 349) at a major "age of risk" for depression were followed for 5.5 years. They were selected to be at high risk (HR; n = 173) or low risk (LR; n = 176) for depression based on the presence versus absence of negative cognitive styles (negative inferential styles and dysfunctional attitudes) and were nondepressed with no other Axis I psychiatric disorders at the outset of the study. Consistent with the cognitive vulnerability hypothesis, Alloy, Abramson, Whitehouse, and colleagues (2006) found that among individuals with no history of depression, HR participants were more likely than LR participants to have a first onset of major depression, minor depression, and hopelessness depression (odds ratios = 5.6–11.7). These findings are especially important because they are based on a truly prospective test, uncontaminated by history of depression. HR participants also were more likely than LR participants to develop recurrences of major depression, minor depression, and hopelessness depression (odds ratios = 3.1–4.1; Alloy, Abramson, Whitehouse, et al., 2006). In addition, the HR group was more likely than the LR group to exhibit suicidal ideation and attempts during the follow-up, mediated by hopelessness (Abramson et al., 1998). These results indicate that negative cognitive styles indeed confer vulnerability to clinically significant depression and suicidality.

Rumination

Consistent with the hypothesis that rumination is a form of "self-regulatory perseveration," Spasojevic and Alloy (2001) found that a ruminative response style mediated the association between cognitive risk status and the development of prospective onsets of MD. Also, Robinson and Alloy (2003) suggested that rumination would exacerbate negative cognitive styles, such that cognitively HR individuals who tend to ruminate on their negative cognitions when stressful life events occur (stress-reactive rumination) would be more likely to become depressed. Consistent with this proposed extension, HR participants who were also high in stress-reactive rumination were more likely to have a history of major depression and hopelessness depression and prospective onsets of major depression and hopelessness depression than were HR participants low in stress-reactive rumination or LR participants with high or low stress-reactive rumination levels (Alloy et al., 2000; Robinson & Alloy, 2003). Thus, rumination may act as both a mediator and moderator of the effects of cognitive vulnerability.

Congruent with the vulnerability–stress component of the model, in studies of depressive symptoms and major depressive episodes among adolescents and young adults, we (for reviews, see Abramson et al., 2002; Alloy & Abramson, 2007; Alloy, Abramson, Safford, et al., 2005; Alloy, Abramson, Whitehouse, et al., 2006; Hankin & Abramson, 2001) found that negative cognitive styles interacted with negative life events to predict prospective increases in depressive symptoms and episodes. Moreover, the cognitive vulnerability × stress interaction was mediated by hopelessness (Alloy & Clements, 1998). Consistent with the transactional (stress-generation) hypothesis of the model, Safford, Alloy, Abramson, and Crossfield (2007) also found that, controlling for current and past depression, HR participants, particularly females, generated more negative events dependent on their behavior than LR participants, increasing the likelihood that their vulnerability will be translated into depression. Thus, cognitively vulnerable individuals generate more negative events and then interpret them more negatively as well (i.e., a "two-hit" model).

Familial Socialization

Familial socialization practices and early life experiences may contribute to the development of cognitive vulnerability to depression (see Figure 10.1 and Alloy et al., 2004, for a review). For example, the inferential feedback parents give their children about causes and consequences of negative events in the child's life may lead the child to develop cognitive styles consistent with their parents' inferential feedback. Negative parenting practices, such as "affectionless control" (Parker, 1983), may also contribute to the development of cognitive vulnerability to depression in offspring. Supporting both the feedback and parenting hypotheses, Alloy and colleagues (2001) found that parents of HR participants provided more negative inferential feedback about causes and consequences of negative events that happened to their child than did parents of LR participants. Also, fathers of HR participants showed less warmth than did fathers of LR participants. Moreover, negative parental inferential feedback and fathers' low warmth predicted prospective onsets of depressive episodes in their offspring during the follow-up, mediated by the offspring's cognitive risk status (Alloy et al., 2001).

Maltreatment

A developmental history of maltreatment may also contribute to the origins of cognitive vulnerability to depression (Rose & Abramson, 1992). In particular, emotional abuse may be especially likely to lead to development of negative cognitive styles because the depressive cognitions (e.g., "You're so stupid; you'll never amount to anything") are directly supplied to the child by the abuser (see Figure 10.1). Consistent with this hypothesis, Gibb and colleagues (2001a, 2001b) found that HR participants reported more emotional, but not physical or sexual, maltreatment than LR participants. Controlling for initial depressive symptoms, a history of emotional maltreatment predicted onsets of major depression, hopelessness depression, and levels of suicidal ideation across the prospective follow-up, mediated by participants' cognitive vulnerability and hopelessness. In addition, controlling for parents' depression, cognitive styles, and abuse, peer victimization was also associated with HR status (Gibb, Abramson, & Alloy, 2004), suggesting that the association of emotional maltreatment with cognitive vulnerability is not entirely due to genetic effects or a generally negative family environment. Finally, Liu, Alloy, Abramson, Iacoviello, and Whitehouse (2009) found that increased levels of emotional maltreatment assessed prospectively predicted a shorter time to onset of depressive episodes during the follow-up.

The Cognitive Vulnerability–Stress Perspective Applied to Bipolar Spectrum Disorders

The success of the cognitive vulnerability–transactional stress model in contributing to the understanding of unipolar depression led to the extension of this model to BDs (see Alloy, Abramson, Neeren, et al., 2006; Alloy, Abramson, Urosevic, et al., 2005; Alloy, Abramson, Walshaw, et al., 2006; Alloy, Reilly-Harrington, et al., 2005). In particular, this model may help explain bipolar mood episodes when integrated with theorizing (e.g., Alloy, Abramson, Urosevic, Bender, & Wagner, 2009; Depue & Iacono, 1989; Depue, Krauss, & Spoont, 1987; Urosevic, Abramson, Harmon-Jones, & Alloy, 2008) that individuals with BD possess a hypersensitive BAS, a motivational system involved in goal seeking and attainment of reward. There is also recent evidence that cognitive styles of individuals with BD are characterized by distinctive BAS-relevant features of autonomy, perfectionism, and goal striving (see "Multifinality: Cognitive Styles and Bipolar Spectrum Disorders" section later) as well as evidence that bipolar mood episodes are triggered by BAS-relevant life events (see "Multifinality: Life Events and Bipolar Spectrum Disorders" section).

BAS-relevant cognitive styles involving high self-standards, self-criticism, and perfectionism may combine with negative events that deactivate the BAS (e.g., irrevocable failures or losses) to increase the likelihood of bipolar depression. The effects of this cognitive vulnerability–stress combination on depressive symptoms should be mediated by rumination and hopelessness, with subsequent disengagement from goals. These same perfectionistic, goal-striving BAS-relevant cognitive styles may combine with BAS-activating positive life events (e.g., goal attainments, rewards) or BAS-activating negative life events (e.g., goal obstacles that can be overcome, anger-inducing events) to increase the likelihood of hypomanic/manic episodes. Negative events have been found to trigger manic as well as depressive episodes among individuals with BD (see "Multifinality: Life Events and Bipolar Spectrum Disorders" section). Moreover, negatively valenced anger-inducing events, in particular, have been associated with BAS activation and hypomanic symptoms (Carver, 2004; Harmon-Jones & Allen, 1998; Harmon-Jones & Sigelman, 2001; Harmon-Jones et al., 2002; Harmon-Jones, Sigelman, Bohlig, & Harmon-Jones, 2003). From a cognitive vulnerability–stress perspective, individuals with BD with a predominantly manic/hypomanic course are likely to create and be exposed to frequent BAS-activating positive and negative life events. Self-focused attentional processes such as "basking," the positive counterpart to rumination (Segerstrom, Stanton, Alden, & Shortridge, 2003), and cognitions such as hope and self-efficacy that promote goal striving and attainment, should mediate the effect of the combination of cognitive vulnerability and BAS-activating events on the development of hypomanic/manic symptoms. Indeed, positive repetitive thought such as basking or rumination has recently been found to promote positive affect and hypomanic/manic symptoms (Feldman, Joorman, & Johnson, 2008; Hughes, Alloy, Choi, Goldstein, & Black, 2009; Johnson, McKenzie, & McMurrich, 2008; Segerstrom et al., 2003). Given that the same BAS-relevant cognitive styles may contribute risk to both depression and hypomania/mania in individuals with BD, certain kinds of negative events (e.g., failures that can be remediated, goal obstacles) could trigger a mixture of depressive, hypomanic/manic, and irritable symptoms (i.e., mixed states), and daily variations in life events could lead to alternations between depression and hypomania/mania (i.e., rapid cycling). Indeed, from the cognitive perspective, the dysfunctional cognitive styles characterizing individuals at risk for BD "transforms the normally mild effects of events into periods of dysregulation. That is, the biobehavioral systems of bipolar-prone individuals will be more perturbed by stimuli of both positive and negative valence" (Depue et al., 1987, pp. 118–119).

In accord with our findings (Safford et al., 2007) indicating that cognitive vulnerability itself, controlling for current and past depression, leads to stress generation, the transactional part of the cognitive vulnerability–transactional stress perspective suggests a two-hit model for BD in which individuals with maladaptive BAS-relevant cognitive styles not only react more strongly to relevant life events but also are exposed to such events more frequently (via event generation). This, in turn, may precipitate bipolar mood episodes. Consistent with this hypothesis, we found that individuals with bipolar II and cyclothymia do, in fact, generate both BAS-activating and BAS-deactivating events more than controls (Urosevic et al., 2009).

Evidence for the Cognitive Vulnerability–Stress Model of Bipolar Spectrum Disorders

We briefly review evidence for the role of life events, cognitive/personality styles, and their interaction in the onset, course, and expression of bipolar spectrum disorders. We also review the evidence for the role of negative parenting and maltreatment histories in BDs, developmental factors that have been found to contribute to cognitive vulnerability and unipolar depression.

Multifinality: Life Events and Bipolar Spectrum Disorders

The concept of multifinality in the developmental literature refers to the principle that the same or similar initial conditions can lead to different outcomes. Based on recent reviews of the association between life events and BD (Alloy, Abramson, Neeren, et al., 2006; Alloy, Abramson, Urosevic, et al., 2005; Alloy, Abramson, Walshaw, et al., 2006; Alloy, Reilly-Harrington, et al., 2005; Johnson, 2005), individuals with bipolar spectrum disorders experience increased life events before onset of mood episodes. Moreover, consistent with an extension of the multifinality phenomenon, many studies have found that negative life events appear to trigger both hypomanic/manic and depressive episodes of individuals with BD. Thus, similar risk factors (negative life events) may lead to different types of mood episodes among individuals with BD. We briefly review the more methodologically limited retrospective studies first, followed by the stronger prospective studies. We then consider whether specific BAS-relevant life events or events at earlier points in the course of BD are particularly likely to trigger mood episodes and whether bipolar symptoms lead to generation of BAS-relevant life events as well, relevant to the transactional part of the model.

In evaluating the life events and BD literature, several methodological limitations should be considered (see Alloy, Abramson, Urosevic, et al., 2005, for review). First, many life event studies use retrospective designs, which could lead to "effort after meaning" bias (Brown & Harris, 1978) in recall of the pre-episode environment by individuals with BD. Retrospective designs also make it difficult to determine whether life events are causes or consequences of bipolar symptoms. Related to this, many studies have not differentiated between events that are independent of or dependent on people's behavior. This is important because individuals with BDs may generate life stressors as well as react to them. Second, some studies rely on self-report life event measures, which can lead to different subjective interpretations of what experiences count as an instance of a particular life event category. Moreover, use of self-report compounds the potential problem of mood-based report biases in studies that do not control for the mood state of individuals with BD at the time of their life event reports. Thus, studies that use interviewer assessments of events should be given greater weight. Third, many studies do not distinguish between the depressive and manic/hypomanic episodes of individuals with BD; thus, it is not possible to examine polarity-specific effects. In addition, some studies do not include an appropriate control group, and others use hospital admission or the start of a treatment regimen as the time of episode onset, which does not necessarily correspond well with the actual time of episode onset. Finally, many studies include small samples with insufficient power to examine event–disorder relationships.

With these limitations in mind, retrospective studies have found that, among individuals with BD, first and subsequent episodes are preceded by the occurrence of stressful events, including those rated as independent of their behavior. Five retrospective studies that used life events interviews to specifically examine independent stressors in the onsets of manic episodes (Bebbington et al., 1993; Chung, Langeluddecke, & Tennant, 1986; Joffe, MacDonald, & Kutcher, 1989; Kennedy, Thompson, Stancer, Roy, & Persad, 1983; Sclare & Creed, 1990) found that manic patients experienced more independent negative events prior to episode onset than controls or in comparison with periods after episode onset (although the effect was not statistically significant in Chung et al., 1986). However, none of these studies investigated whether particular types of negative events are important in onsets of manic vs. depressive episodes.

Although several of the methodologically sounder prospective studies found that patients diagnosed as bipolar I (Ellicott, Hammen, Gitlin, Brown, & Jamison, 1990; Hammen & Gitlin, 1997; Hunt, Bruce-Jones, & Silverstone, 1992) and as subsyndromal bipolar (Lovejoy & Steuerwald, 1997) relapsed at a significantly higher rate following a period of many negative events than following low-stress periods, others either did not obtain this stress-relapse effect (McPherson, Herbison, & Romans, 1993) or only obtained the effect for women (Christensen et al., 2003) or only for certain types of stressful events (Hall, Dunner, Zeller, & Fieve, 1977; Pardoen et al., 1996). Specifically, patients with BD who had a hypomanic/manic relapse had a greater number of work-related stressors (Hall et al., 1977) or marital stressors (Pardoen et al., 1996) prior to the relapse than did nonrelapsers. Johnson and Miller (1997) also reported that inpatients with bipolar I who experienced a severe, independent event during the index episode took three times longer to recover than those who did not experience a severe, independent event.

Recent evidence suggests that particular types of life events are associated with occurrences of mood episodes in individuals with BD. Relevant to our integration of the cognitive vulnerability–stress model with a BAS perspective, three prospective studies found that BAS-activating life events involving goal attainment or goal striving are especially likely to trigger hypomanic/manic episodes or symptoms in individuals with BD. In two studies, Johnson, Sandrow, and colleagues (2000), and Johnson and colleagues (2008) found that goal attainment events predicted increases in manic but not depressive symptoms among patients with bipolar I over a prospective follow-up, whereas general positive events did not. Similarly, Nusslock, Abramson, Harmon-Jones, Alloy, and Hogan (2007) reported that individuals with bipolar II or cyclothymic disorders were significantly more likely to develop new onsets of hypomanic, but not depressive, episodes during a goal-striving period (final exams) compared with a prior control period. In addition, as noted earlier, BAS-activating negative events such as anger-inducing events have also been associated with hypomanic symptoms (Carver, 2004; Harmon-Jones et al., 2002). Prospective studies have not yet examined whether negative events that involve BAS deactivation specifically predict the depressive episodes of individuals with BD; however, BAS-deactivation events (e.g., losses and failures) have predicted unipolar depressive episodes.

BAS-relevant events not only may be more likely to trigger mood episodes but may also occur at a higher rate in individuals with BDs as a result of stress-generation (e.g., Hammen, 1991) processes. Although two prior studies (Grandin, Alloy, & Abramson, 2007; Hammen, 1991) did not find much evidence for stress generation in individuals with bipolar I or spectrum disorders, these studies had a number of methodological limitations and, in particular, did not examine the generation of BAS-relevant events specifically (Bender, Alloy, Sylvia, Urosevic, & Abramson, 2009). In contrast, in a prospective study, Urosevic and colleagues (2009) reported that individuals with bipolar spectrum disorders (bipolar II and cyclothymia) generated both BAS-activation and BAS-deactivation events at significantly greater rates than matched normal controls. Similarly, in another prospective study of individuals with bipolar II and cyclothymia, Bender and colleagues (2009) found that hypomanic symptoms predicted greater subsequent occurrence of BAS-relevant positive and negative achievement events in males, whereas depressive symptoms predicted the greater occurrence of positive and negative interpersonal events in females. These gender differences in the effects of hypomanic and depressive symptoms on the generation of life events may help to explain why BD in males typically has a more hypomanic/manic course, whereas in women's BD it typically has a more depressive course.

Some evidence suggests that life events may be more likely to trigger early than later bipolar mood episodes. In his "kindling" model, Post (1992) hypothesized that mood episodes become increasingly autonomous with each recurrence such that psychosocial stressors are less likely to precipitate episodes that occur later than early in the course of disorder. Although five retrospective studies (Ehnvall & Agren, 2002; Glassner & Haldipur, 1983; Glassner, Haldipur, & Dessauersmith, 1979; Johnson, Andersson-Lundman, Asberg-Wistedt, & Mathe, 2000; Perris, 1984) claimed to obtain results consistent with the kindling effect, these studies did not distinguish between "stress sensitization" and "stress autonomy" interpretations of the kindling effect (see Monroe & Harkness, 2005). To distinguish between these alternative forms of kindling effects, studies must examine major and minor events separately, and the impact versus frequency of these events, relative to the onset of mood episodes. The retrospective studies to date have not done this. Furthermore, Hlastala and colleagues (2000) found that age, rather than the number of previous episodes, predicted stress level in pre-onset, but not control, periods. They suggested that the aging process rather than illness progression might account for prior studies' apparent support for the kindling model. In a prospective study, Hammen and Gitlin (1997) found that compared with patients with bipolar I disorder with few past episodes, those who had many past episodes were more likely to experience a severe negative event prior to relapse and to relapse more quickly. In addition, Coryell and colleagues (2003) reported that rapid cycling did not accelerate over a 13-year follow-up in patients with bipolar I or II disorder. Consequently, although retrospective studies suggest that life events may play a larger role in triggering mood episodes earlier than later in the course of BD or at an earlier age, the prospective studies to date fail to support the kindling model.

In summary, the evidence to date suggests that life events may contribute proximal risk to onsets and relapses/recurrences of mood episodes in individuals with bipolar spectrum disorders, with onsets early in the disorder's course or at an earlier age perhaps being particularly responsive to life events. Given the extensive literature on the role of stress as a precipitant of unipolar depression, it is not surprising that negative events may trigger bipolar depressive episodes. However, negative events also appear to be relevant to precipitating hypomanic/manic episodes. Further research is needed to determine whether particular kinds of negative events that deactivate the BAS (e.g., definite failure or loss) precipitate depression, whereas BAS-activating negative events (e.g., goal obstacles, anger-evoking events) trigger hypomania/mania, particularly in combination with cognitive styles that are BAS relevant (see Alloy et al., Chapter 6, this volume). In addition, there is evidence that positive events such as achievements and upcoming goals could activate the BAS-relevant cognitive styles of individuals with BD and, in turn, lead to hypomanic/manic symptoms. Bipolar symptoms themselves appear to generate BAS-relevant events, which, in turn, can further worsen the course of BD.

Multifinality: Cognitive Styles and Bipolar Spectrum Disorders

Recent reviews of the association between cognitive styles and BD (Alloy, Abramson, Neeren, et al., 2006; Alloy, Abramson, Urosevic, et al., 2005; Alloy, Abramson, Walshaw, et al., 2006; Alloy, Reilly-Harrington, et al., 2005) concluded that current mood state and the type of cognitive style assessment (explicit or implicit measures) influence the observed cognitive styles of individuals with BD. Several studies find that individuals with BD exhibit underlying cognitive patterns as negative as those of unipolar depressed persons but with unique BAS-relevant features. However, they sometimes present themselves positively on explicit cognitive style measures. Moreover, consistent with the general principle of multifinality, there is some evidence that similar maladaptive cognitive styles, particularly in combination with relevant life events, predict prospectively both depressive and hypomanic/manic episodes or symptoms. Again, a similar risk factor (maladaptive cognitive styles) is associated with differential mood episodes.

A central methodological issue in this literature is the need to establish the nature of cognitive styles in individuals with BD independent of mood states and symptoms of the disorder (Alloy, Abramson, Neeren, et al., 2006; Alloy, Abramson, Urosevic, et al., 2005; Alloy, Abramson, Walshaw, et al., 2006; Alloy, Reilly-Harrington, et al., 2005). Studies have addressed this issue by controlling statistically for concurrent moods and symptoms, by examining cognitions among remitted or euthymic individuals with BD, by comparing individuals with BD in depressive versus manic episodes, or by conducting within-subject longitudinal studies of the same individuals with BD in different mood states. Other study limitations in this literature include failure to take medication status into account, absence of control groups, unvalidated cognitive measures, undiagnosed samples, and small sample sizes.

When assessed in a current depressive episode, cross-sectional studies of individuals with bipolar I and bipolar spectrum disorders find that their cognitive styles are as negative as those of unipolar depressed individuals and more negative than those of normal comparison groups (Hill, Oei, & Hill, 1989; Hollon, Kendall, & Lumry, 1986; Reilly-Harrington, Alloy, Fresco, & Whitehouse, 1999; Rosenfarb, Becker, Khan, & Mintz, 1998; but see Donnelly & Murphy, 1973, for an exception). Similarly, in cross-sectional studies of student samples, although high hypomanic tendencies were associated with positive cognitive styles on explicit measures, they were related to negative cognitive styles on implicit measures (Bentall & Thompson, 1990; French, Richards, & Scholfield, 1996; Meyer & Krumm-Merabet, 2003; but see Thompson & Bentall, 1990, for an exception).

The results of studies that examine cognitive styles of remitted or euthymic individuals with BD are mixed. Five studies (Hollon et al., 1986; MacVane, Lange, Brown, & Zayat, 1978; Pardoen, Bauwens, Tracy, Martin, & Mendlewicz, 1993; Reilly-Harrington et al., 1999; Tracy, Bauwens, Martin, Pardoen, & Mendlewicz, 1992) using primarily explicit measures obtained little evidence of negative cognitions in the remitted state among participants with bipolar I and bipolar spectrum disorders compared with normal controls. In contrast, six other studies (Alloy et al., 2008; Alloy, Reilly-Harrington, Fresco, Whitehouse, & Zechmeister, 1999; Lam, Wright, & Smith, 2004; Rosenfarb et al., 1998; Scott, Stanton, Garland, & Ferrier, 2000; Winters & Neale, 1985), also using mostly explicit measures of cognition, did find negative cognitive styles among individuals with remitted bipolar I and bipolar spectrum disorders. Of particular relevance to our integration of the cognitive vulnerability–stress model with a BAS perspective, four of these studies (Alloy et al., 2008; Lam et al., 2004; Rosenfarb et al., 1998; Scott et al., 2000) converged on the finding that euthymic individuals with bipolar I and bipolar spectrum disorders exhibit a unique profile of negative cognitive styles characterized by perfectionism, self-criticism, autonomy, and goal striving (consistent with the high drive/incentive motivation associated with high BAS sensitivity) but not by maladaptive dependency and attachment attitudes typically observed among unipolar depressed individuals. Similarly, Goldberg, Gerstein, Wenze, Welker, and Beck (2008) also found that perfectionism, but not approval seeking, was elevated in manic outpatients with bipolar I relative to controls.

Although three cross-sectional studies comparing individuals with bipolar I in different mood states (Ashworth, Blackburn, & McPherson, 1982; Hayward, Wong, Bright, & Lam, 2002; Murphy et al., 1999) found more positive cognitive styles in manic than depressed individuals with BD, Scott and Pope (2003) observed more negative cognitive styles in hypomanic individuals compared with those who were remitted bipolar. Lyon, Startup, and Bentall (1999) found that manic patients showed underlying negative cognitive styles on implicit measures, although they exhibited positive cognitive styles on explicit questionnaire measures. Only three studies to date investigated the stability of cognitive patterns across different mood states within the same individuals with BD in longitudinal designs. Whereas Ashworth, Blackburn, and McPherson (1985) observed that explicit self-esteem reverted to normal levels when previously depressed or manic patients with bipolar I disorder recovered, Alloy and colleagues (1999) found that attributional styles and dysfunctional attitudes were stable across cyclothymic participants' mood swings. Eich, Macaulay, and Lam (1997) observed that mood-dependent recall was common to both depressed and manic states, but patients with bipolar I generated more positive than negative autobiographical events when manic and more negative than positive events when depressed.

Cognitive styles have also been examined as predictors of bipolar course in five longitudinal studies. Whereas Scott and Pope (2003) found that negative self-esteem was the most robust predictor of relapse at 12-month follow-up among hypomanic patients with BD, two studies of patients with bipolar I found that negative automatic thoughts (Johnson & Fingerhut, 2004) and low self-esteem (Johnson, Meyer, Winett, & Small, 2000) predicted depressive, but not manic, symptoms over prospective follow-up. Two longitudinal studies specifically examined whether cognitive styles with BAS relevance predicted bipolar mood symptoms or episodes. Lozano and Johnson (2001) found that the BAS-relevant trait of achievement-striving predicted increases in manic symptoms over 6 months in patients with bipolar I. Similarly, Alloy and colleagues (2009) reported that BAS-relevant cognitive styles of self-criticism and autonomy predicted prospective onsets of hypomanic/manic and depressive episodes among individuals with bipolar II and cyclothymia, whereas cognitive styles involving dependency and sociotropy did not.

Cognitive Vulnerability–Stress Prediction of Bipolar Spectrum Disorders

To date, six studies, all using explicit measures of cognitive style, have examined the cognitive vulnerability–stress hypothesis for BD. Only one of these studies explicitly examined BAS-relevant cognitive styles. Swendsen, Hammen, Heller, and Gitlin (1995) found that patients with remitted bipolar I disorder who relapsed were distinguished from those who did not by interactions of stressful events with both obsessionality and extraversion. Three studies tested Beck's (1987) event congruence, vulnerability–stress hypothesis for sociotropic and autonomous cognitive styles in which the experience of stressful events congruent with one's style (interpersonal events for sociotropic individuals and achievement events for autonomous individuals) should lead to an onset or exacerbation of symptoms. Hammen and colleagues (Hammen, Ellicott, & Gitlin, 1992; Hammen, Ellicott, Gitlin, & Jamison, 1989) reported that the interaction of sociotropy and negative interpersonal events (although a nonsignificant trend in Hammen et al., 1989) predicted symptom severity, but not symptom onset, in individuals with bipolar I disorder. The autonomy × negative achievement events interaction did not predict symptom severity. Francis-Raniere, Alloy, and Abramson (2006) found that in individuals with bipolar spectrum disorder (bipolar II and cyclothymia), controlling for initial symptoms and the total events experienced, a BAS-relevant self-critical, perfectionistic cognitive style interacted with self-criticism-relevant negative or positive events, respectively, to predict prospective increases in depressive or hypomanic symptoms.

Two studies examined attributional style and dysfunctional attitudes in cognitive vulnerability × stress interactions for BD. Consistent with hopelessness theory (Abramson et al., 1989), Alloy and colleagues (1999) found that a negative attributional style for negative events at time 1 (euthymic state) interacted with subsequent negative events to predict increases in depressive symptoms, and a positive attributional style for positive events combined with subsequent positive events to predict increases in hypomanic symptoms in individuals with cyclothymia or hypomania. Dysfunctional attitudes × life events did not predict depressive or hypomanic symptoms. In a large sample of individuals with unipolar, bipolar I, bipolar II, and cyclothymic disorders, Reilly-Harrington and colleagues (1999) found that controlling for initial symptoms, time 1 negative attributional styles, dysfunctional attitudes, and negative self-referent information processing each interacted significantly with subsequent negative life events to predict increases in depressive symptoms and, within the bipolar group, manic symptoms.

Whereas Alloy and colleagues (1999) found that positive life events combined with positive attributional styles to predict increases in hypomanic symptoms, Reilly-Harrington and colleagues (1999) found that it was negative events combined with negative cognitive styles that predicted manic symptoms. It may be that Reilly-Harrington and colleagues' sample was more severe, including primarily participants with bipolar II as well as some with bipolar I disorder, whereas Alloy and colleagues' sample included individuals with milder cyclothymic and hypomanic disorders. Given that individuals with bipolar I and with bipolar II disorders have a course that includes major depressive episodes, they may be more responsive to negative life events. Alternatively, the particular types of negative events experienced by participants in the two studies may be critical for whether such events would precipitate hypomanic/manic symptoms. Negative events that activate the BAS (e.g., challenges that can be overcome; anger-inducing events) may be more likely to trigger hypomania/mania. Clearly, more work is needed to understand the conditions under which positive versus negative events and positive versus negative cognitive styles provide risk for hypomania/mania.

In sum, there is some evidence that individuals with BDs possess underlying maladaptive cognitive styles, consistent with an extension of cognitive theories of unipolar depression to BD. However, the strength of the observed association between negative cognitive styles and BD may depend on whether the measures of cognition are explicit or implicit and the current mood state of individuals with BD. Moreover, compared with individuals with unipolar depression, the cognitive styles of persons with BD appear to be more uniquely characterized by goal striving, perfectionism, self-criticism, and autonomy, features characteristic of high BAS sensitivity, rather than dependency, attachment and sociotropy. In addition, there is evidence that cognitive styles alone, and particularly in combination with relevant life events, prospectively predict the course of bipolar depression and more mixed evidence that they predict the course of bipolar mania/hypomania. Further longitudinal studies are needed to test the cognitive vulnerability–stress hypothesis for BD and, in particular, whether BAS-relevant cognitive styles specifically in combination with BAS-activating and deactivating life events increase prediction of mania/hypomania and depression, respectively. It is also important to examine whether findings reported for individuals with milder disorders in the bipolar spectrum generalize to individuals with bipolar I disorder.

Developmental Factors and Bipolar Spectrum Disorders

A growing research literature has begun to address the role of negative parenting practices, family factors such as high expressed emotion (EE; high criticism and emotional overinvolvement from family members), and maltreatment histories in risk for and the course of BDs. Thus, we briefly review parenting, EE, and maltreatment research in BD.

Important methodological limitations in both the parenting and maltreatment literatures make it difficult to draw firm conclusions regarding the role of these developmental factors in the onset, expression, and course of BD (Alloy, Abramson, Neeren, et al., 2006; Alloy, Abramson, Urosevic, et al., 2005; Alloy, Abramson, Walshaw, et al., 2006; Alloy, Reilly-Harrington, et al., 2005; Alloy, Abramson, Smith, Gibb, & Neeren, 2006). First, the vast majority of studies asked adults with BD to recall their childhood histories; thus, these retrospective studies cannot determine whether developmental factors were a cause or a consequence of the bipolarity. Indeed, only three studies have even attempted to examine whether these developmental factors preceded the onset of the BD and thus could have contributed to the bipolarity. Second, most studies do not control for mood states of participants with BD at the time their childhood histories are assessed; consequently, reporting biases associated with current mood cannot be ruled out in most cases. In addition, some studies do not include an appropriate control group, and the operationalizations of parenting and maltreatment histories differ widely across studies, with some studies using measures of questionable reliability and validity (e.g., only one- or two-item indicators of childhood history). Finally, with few exceptions, these studies do not attempt to rule out third variable explanations, such as shared genes, for the association between reported familial environment and BD. Thus, it is important to keep these caveats in mind as we briefly review evidence on the developmental histories of individuals with BD.

Most studies of parenting examined whether parents of individuals with BD were characterized by low care or warmth and high overprotection or psychological control, a pattern referred to as "affectionless control" by Parker (1983). Although four retrospective studies of adults (Cooke, Young, Mohri, Blake, & Joffe, 1999; Joyce, 1984; Parker, 1979; Perris, Arrindell, Van der Ende, & Knorr, 1986) found no differences between the reported parenting of bipolar and comparison groups, Joyce (1984) and Cooke and colleagues (1999) observed that negative parenting practices were associated with greater severity and a worse course of bipolar I disorder (e.g., more hospitalizations for both depression and mania and a greater history of suicide attempts). In contrast, three other methodologically stronger studies (Geller et al., 2000; Neeren, Alloy, & Abramson, 2008; Rosenfarb, Becker, & Khan, 1994) did find greater affectionless control in the parenting reportedly received by participants with bipolar I and bipolar spectrum disorders relative to controls. In addition, in one prospective study of youth with BD followed for 4 years, low maternal warmth predicted faster relapse after recovery from mania (Geller et al., 2004). Moreover, Wagner, Alloy, and Abramson (2009) suggested that parenting that is overly critical may be especially likely to contribute to the development of a self-critical, perfectionistic cognitive style in offspring, a style shown to be specific to BD. Controlling for family history of mood disorders and depressive and hypomanic/manic symptoms, Wagner and colleagues found that higher reported critical parenting from both parents was associated with cognitive styles of higher perfectionism and autonomy but not with cognitive styles of approval seeking or sociotropy, among individuals with bipolar II and cyclothymic disorders.

Studies of family members' EE and BD are related to the work on parenting. Cross-sectional studies of EE found that, compared with patients with bipolar I and with low EE relatives, those whose relatives made more critical or intrusive comments had higher hostility/suspicion (Miklowitz, Goldstein, & Nuechterlein, 1995), greater distress (Koenig, Sachs-Ericsson, & Miklowitz, 1997), and more manic symptoms and a trend toward more depressive symptoms (Simoneau, Miklowitz, & Saleem, 1998). Moreover, in prospective studies, high EE in relatives predicted a worse course of BD, specifically predicting relapse (Miklowitz, Goldstein, Nuechterlein, Snyder, & Mintz, 1988; Rosenfarb et al., 2001), depressive but not manic relapse (Yan, Hammen, Cohen, Daley, & Henry, 2004), worse functioning (O'Connell, Mayo, Flatow, Cuthbertson, & O'Brien, 1991), and increased morbidity (hospital admissions, symptoms, additional medications; Priebe, Wildgrube, & Muller-Oerlinghausen, 1989).

Six retrospective studies examined the maltreatment histories (and other childhood stressors) of individuals with BD with no normal control group. Two of these compared patients with unipolar and bipolar disorders on overall trauma exposure and posttraumatic stress disorder (PTSD) (Mueser et al., 1998) or on a single-item measure of combined abuse (Wexler, Lyons, Lyons, & Mazure, 1997) and found that patients with unipolar disorder had higher rates of PTSD or childhood abuse than patients with bipolar I disorder. However, two other studies observed that patients with bipolar I did report higher rates of either physical

(Levitan et al., 1997) or sexual (Hyun, Friedman, & Dunner, 2000) abuse than depressed patients with unipolar disorder. Two additional studies found an association between childhood maltreatment history and a worse course of bipolar I disorder, including the presence of auditory hallucinations (Hammersley et al., 2003) and higher incidence of Axis I and II comorbidity, early (≤14) age of onset, faster cycling frequencies, increased suicide attempts, and increased severity of mania (Leverich et al., 2002; Post & Leverich, 2006).

Finally, three studies included normal comparison groups in their examination of BD and childhood stressors. Coverdale and Turbott (2000) found that a combined measure of childhood physical and sexual abuse did not differ between patients and controls, but more patients reported both forms of abuse as adults (≥ age 16) than controls. However, patients with BD comprised only 15.6% of the patient sample. Controlling for current depressive and manic symptoms and family history of mood disorder, Neeren and colleagues (2008) found that bipolar II and cyclothymic individuals reported more childhood physical abuse from mothers and more childhood emotional abuse from both parents before the age of onset of their BD than did demographically matched normal controls (before the same age). Similarly, once controlling for current depressive and manic symptoms and family history of mood disorder, Grandin and colleagues (2007) reported that independent childhood stressors (including abuse) occurring before the age of onset were associated with bipolar spectrum (bipolar II or cyclothymia) status. Moreover, higher numbers of pre-onset childhood stressors actually predicted an earlier age of onset.

In summary, there is some suggestion that the histories of individuals with BD are characterized by parenting involving low care and high overprotection, high criticism, and childhood abuse, but the evidence is inconsistent (for more details, see reviews by Alloy, Abramson, Neeren, et al., 2006; Alloy, Abramson, Walshaw, et al., 2006; Alloy, Reilly-Harrington, et al., 2005). There is better evidence that high EE, negative or critical parenting, and maltreatment histories may be associated with the tendency of individuals with BD to be perfectionistic and to self-criticize as well as an earlier age of onset, rapid cycling, and a worse course of BD, the type of phenomenology observed in individuals with childhood- or adolescent-onset BD.

APPLICATION OF THE COGNITIVE VULNERABILITY–STRESS PERSPECTIVE TO THE ADOLESCENT ONSET, GENDER DIFFERENCES, AND PHENOMENOLOGY OF BIPOLAR SPECTRUM DISORDERS

The five constructs in the cognitive vulnerability–transactional stress model are life events, cognitive vulnerability, rumination/basking, cognitive vulnerability × stress interaction, and hopelessness versus hope and self-efficacy. If the model explains why adolescence is a high-risk period for onset of BD, especially for girls, as well as the mixed presentation of bipolarity in adolescence involving depression, irritability, and attention problems, then increases in the operation or "consolidation" of any of the five constructs in the model should be associated with the occurrence of these developmental phenomena (onset, gender differences, and phenomenology).

Prior research documents a developmentally normative rise in the number of negative life events after age 13 for both boys and girls (Garber, Keiley, & Martin, 2002; Gest, Reed, & Masten, 1999) but especially for adolescent girls (Ge, Lorenz, Conger, Elder, & Simons, 1994). This normative increase in adolescent events could include both BAS-activating and deactivating negative events and could contribute to the initial onset of bipolar mood episodes in adolescence. In addition, adolescence is also a period that offers increased opportunities and greater expectations for individual achievement (Steinberg et al., 2006). Such goal striving and attainment could trigger initial onset of hypomania/mania in adolescents, as reviewed previously (Johnson, Sandrow, et al., 2000, 2008; Nusslock et al., 2007), particularly in those with maladaptive BAS-relevant cognitive styles. In addition, irrevocable failures to achieve desired goals could precipitate initial onsets of depression. Moreover, adolescents with bipolar spectrum disorders were also found to generate BAS-activating and -deactivating events at a higher rate than controls (Urosevic et al., 2009; transactional stress component); depressed, adolescent girls with bipolar spectrum disorder generated more interpersonal positive and negative events, whereas hypomanic adolescent boys with bipolar spectrum disorder generated more achievement-oriented positive and negative events (Bender et al., 2009). Such stress-generation processes may also help to explain the relative predominance of manic/hypomanic versus depressive episodes in the course of BDs in males versus females.

To more fully understand the role of life events in contributing to the onset and course of adolescent BD, future studies must remedy problems associated with prior life events research (e.g., poor sensitivity in dating event and symptom onset) and examine the same youth longitudinally, thereby permitting construction of individual trajectories of growth in stress across adolescence and comparison of such trajectories with those for bipolar symptoms and episodes. It is also important to determine whether the cognitive factors unique to the cognitive vulnerability–stress model show relevant developmental changes that proximally precede the onset of BD, and whether they are relevant to the emergence of gender differences in symptoms among adolescents.

Some evidence suggests that cognitive vulnerability may "consolidate" (relative stability over time and consistency across situations) by adolescence and thus be accessible for the cognitive vulnerability × stress interaction (Cole et al., 2008; Gibb & Alloy, 2006; Gibb et al., 2006). Longitudinal studies of second to ninth graders found that attributional style became more stable in the later grades and interacted with stress to predict depression in older but not younger children (Cole et al., 2008; Gibb & Alloy, 2006; Nolen-Hoeksema, Girgus, & Seligman,

1992; Turner & Cole, 1994). Also, given the achievement of formal operations and increases in future orientation beginning in adolescence, adolescents can experience hopelessness or hope, a mediating link in the chain culminating in depression or hypomania/mania. Moreover, decreases in attributional optimism as children transition into adolescence suggest that cognitive vulnerability may increase during this transition and, in turn, contribute to depression or hypomania/mania onset in adolescence (Mezulis, Abramson, Hyde, & Hankin, 2004).

Developmental increases in cognitive vulnerability may also contribute to the greater predominance of depression in females' BD beginning in adolescence. Girls show greater rumination on negative affect than boys postpuberty but not before (Broderick, 1998; Smith, Floyd, Alloy, Hughes, & Neeren, 2009). Adolescent females also exhibit more negative cognitive styles than adolescent males (Hankin & Abramson, 2002), and in three cross-sectional studies, adolescent girls' more negative cognitive styles and rumination mediated the gender difference in depressive symptoms (Floyd, Alloy, Smith, Neeren, & Thorell, 2009; Hankin & Abramson, 2002; Smith et al., 2009). Thus, adolescent girls may exhibit greater cognitive vulnerability than adolescent boys, which could contribute both to the gender difference in adolescent unipolar depression and perhaps the greater propensity for a depressive course in BD among adolescent females.

The cognitive vulnerability–stress model suggests that a history of maladaptive inferential feedback about the causes and consequences of stressful events from family and peers should contribute to the development of cognitive vulnerability. Consistent with this hypothesis, negative inferential feedback from parents during childhood (Alloy et al., 2001) and from current members of the support network (Panzarella, Alloy, & Whitehouse, 2006) predicted negative cognitive styles and prospective depression onset in adolescence. Negative inferential feedback from others may be the milder end of a continuum of negative emotional feedback with emotional abuse at the extreme end (Alloy et al., 2001, 2004). Rose and Abramson (1992) hypothesized that recurrent childhood abuse, particularly emotional abuse, would lead to the development of cognitive vulnerability. We found support for this hypothesis with both retrospective studies in late adolescents (Gibb et al., 2001a, 2001b, 2004; Spasojevic & Alloy, 2002) and prospective studies in children and late adolescents (Gibb et al., 2006; Liu et al., 2009).

Negative inferential and emotional feedback from others may be especially likely to be internalized in adolescence and contribute to the formation of cognitive vulnerability. Peers become increasingly important beginning in early adolescence (Harris, 1995; Steinberg, 2002), and rates of negative emotional feedback from peers, including teasing, harassment, rejection, and derogation (i.e., "relational aggression"; Crick & Grotpeter, 1996), rise at this time, especially among adolescent girls. Thus, negative emotional feedback from peers in particular, may contribute to the adolescent onset of BD or the exacerbation of bipolar symptoms with initial onset in childhood, the emergence of gender differences in symptom course, and dysphoric and irritable symptom presentations (see Liu & Kaplan, 1999).

EMBEDDING THE COGNITIVE VULNERABILITY–STRESS PERSPECTIVE IN A NORMATIVE ADOLESCENT BRAIN AND COGNITIVE DEVELOPMENT CONTEXT

According to developmental psychopathologists (Cicchetti & Rogosch, 2002; Steinberg, 2002; Steinberg et al., 2006) and developmental neuroscientists (Casey, Tottenham, Liston, & Durston, 2005; Walker, Sabuwalla, & Huot, 2004), it is crucial to study psychopathology in adolescence in the context of normative adolescent cognitive and brain development. Thus, an understanding of BD in adolescence from a cognitive vulnerability–transactional stress perspective should proceed with an explicit recognition of the brain maturation and concomitant cognitive capacities and attainments of the adolescent. Brain development and cognitive maturation occur concurrently in childhood and adolescence (Casey, Giedd, & Thomas, 2000; Sowell, Thompson, & Toga, 2007; Spear, 2007). Placed in such a normative adolescent brain and cognitive development context, some of the key etiological factors in the cognitive vulnerability–stress model (e.g., cognitive vulnerability, rumination/basking, future expectations) have just become developmentally operative during adolescence as a result of normative brain maturation and concomitant cognitive development (see Figure 10.2).

Contemporary neuroimaging methods have provided evidence of linkages between changes in structural architecture and functional organization of the developing brain and increases in cognitive competencies (e.g., Casey, Galvan, & Hare, 2005; Casey, Tottenham, et al., 2005). Longitudinal magnetic resonance imaging (MRI) studies show that cognitive milestones in development parallel the sequence in which the cortex matures (Giedd, 2004; Gogtay et al., 2004; Sowell et al., 2007). Motor and sensory systems mature earliest and higher order association areas, such as the prefrontal cortex (PFC), that integrate sensorimotor processes and control executive functions such as self-regulation, attention, working memory, planning, and decision making mature more slowly, and not completely, until early adulthood (Casey, Galvin, & Hare, 2005; Casey, Tottenham, et al., 2005; Gogtay et al., 2004; Sowell et al., 2007). During adolescence, in parallel, PFC white matter volume increases, reflecting ongoing myelination of axons (e.g., Casey, Tottenham, et al., 2005; Giedd et al., 1999; Gogtay et al., 2004), and PFC gray matter volume decreases (Casey, Galvin, & Hare, 2005; Giedd, 2004; Gogtay et al., 2004; Sowell et al., 2007), involving synaptic pruning and the elimination of connections (e.g., Casey, Tottenham, et al., 2005; Giedd et al., 1996), suggesting that connections are being fine-tuned with the elimination of extra synapses and strengthening of relevant connections (Casey, Tottenham, et al., 2005).

In addition, there are sex differences in PFC maturation. Females show smaller increase of PFC white matter volume and smaller loss of PFC gray matter volume compared with males as a function of age and pubertal status (De Bellis et al., 2001; Giedd et al., 1999). Normal pubertal development is associated with large increases in sex hormones and glucocorticoids (Walker et al., 2004), which influence brain maturation (De Bellis et al., 2001; Walker et al., 2004), in part

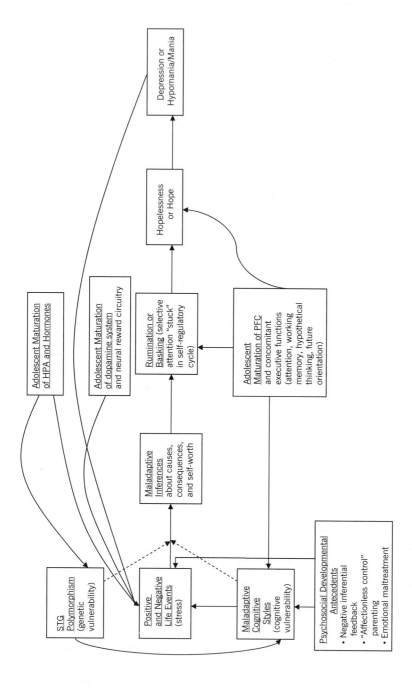

FIGURE 10.2. An integrated biological and cognitive vulnerability–transactional stress model of bipolar disorder in the context of normative adolescent brain and cognitive development, emotional/motivational development, and genetic predisposition. The causal relations proposed in the model are described throughout the chapter. Dashed arrows indicate interactive effects; thus, the model includes both cognitive vulnerability × stress and genetic vulnerability × stress interactions. Solid arrows indicate direct effects. (STG, serotonin transporter gene; HPA, hypothalamic–pituitary–adrenal; PFC, prefrontal cortex.)

through their effects on gene expression (Walker et al., 2004). Thus, the high-risk period for onset of BD that occurs in adolescence may be related to the maturational changes in the adolescent brain and the later age of onset of BD for females, and the greater depressive course among females may be associated with the sex differences in adolescent brain development.

Performance on cognitive tasks is correlated with the developmental changes in cortical development (e.g., Casey, Tottenham, et al., 2005). The fine-tuning of PFC structural architecture during adolescence observed in MRI studies is associated functionally with a shift from diffuse recruitment of cortical regions by children performing executive function tasks to more focal recruitment of PFC regions specifically implicated in cognitive control by adolescents (see Paus, 2005, for a review). That is, a reorganization of frontally based neural executive systems involved in affect and self-regulation occurs in adolescence (Leibenluft et al., 2003). On the basis of this work, we hypothesize that four cognitive competencies (attention, working memory, hypothetical thinking/decision making, and future orientation) attained during adolescence and linked to maturation of the PFC are cognitive developmental "prerequisites" for the cognitive vulnerability × stress interaction to "pack its punch" in contributing to onset of bipolar mood episodes. Ironically, adolescents' increased cognitive competence and brain maturation may come with a cost. It puts them at greater risk for mood disorder than they were in childhood.

Earlier, we argued that attention is a self-regulatory mechanism in the causal chain of the cognitive vulnerability–stress model (Abramson et al., 2002; Alloy & Abramson, 2007). Cognitively vulnerable individuals can become stuck in the self-regulatory cycle with their attention focused on affectively laden cognitions as they attempt to cope with life events that activate their cognitive styles (i.e., ruminating on failures and losses or basking in goal attainments). An implication is that a cognitively vulnerable individual must achieve sufficient attentional competence in order for the cognitive vulnerability × stress interaction to lead to full-blown depression or hypomania/mania. For example, a cognitively vulnerable child who has not yet developed sufficient competence in selective and sustained attention may make negative inferences for a negative event but will not remain focused on such inferences and not be as likely to suffer their depressive effects. We suggest that emerging normative cognitive development of self-regulatory executive functions (i.e., sustained and selective attention and executive control over attentional switching) is a prerequisite for adolescents to engage in attempts to self-regulate affect and thus for full-blown rumination or basking to occur (Alloy & Abramson, 2007). With developmental maturation of the medial PFC and anterior cingulate cortex (ACC), attentional processes become more efficient with age and continue to develop through adolescence (Botvinik, Braver, Barch, Carter, & Cohen, 2001; Casey et al., 1997). Moreover, studies of normative development suggest that emotion regulation mechanisms are dependent on attentional regulation and control (Leibenluft et al., 2003). The maturation of attention in adolescence and the link between attentional control and emotion regulation is relevant to adolescent onset or exacerbation of BD and may help explain the attentional difficulties and frequent comorbidity with ADHD observed among adolescents with BD (Leibenluft et al., 2003). Thus, as attentional executive control develops during adolescence, recursive thinking (rumination or basking) in an effort to regulate affect and the cognitive vulnerability × stress interaction can more fully contribute to onset of mood episodes.

Similarly, normative development of dorsolateral PFC and working memory (Owen, 2000) is essential for maintaining information and the present context in mind (Cohen & Servan-Schreiber, 1992; Kimberg & Farah, 1993) and thus is also an important cognitive capacity underlying self-regulation and affect regulation. Therefore, increases in working memory skills should also be a prerequisite for adolescents to more fully engage in self-regulation and rumination or basking.

Hypothetical thinking also increases in adolescence. Adolescents develop greater competence in viewing situations from multiple perspectives, generating options, and anticipating potential consequences of decisions (Keating, 2005). Increased competency in hypothetical thinking and decision making is also influenced by PFC maturation and should be a prerequisite for generating implications of life events and for experiencing hopelessness or hope (Steinberg, 2002). In addition, in order to experience hopelessness or hope, the proximal cause of depressive or hypomanic/manic symptoms in the cognitive vulnerability–stress model, children must develop the normative capacity to think about the future, also a likely outgrowth of PFC maturation.

Prefrontal Executive Functioning in Bipolar Spectrum Disorders

Is abnormal functioning of the PFC and the executive control it serves implicated in BD? We briefly review neuroimaging and neuropsychological studies of executive function (see Walshaw, Alloy, & Sabb, in press, for a more complete review) involved in attentional control and working memory that suggest PFC and ACC abnormalities in BD that may be relevant to the operation of maladaptive cognitive styles and self-regulatory processes featured in the cognitive vulnerability–stress model of BD.

Histopathological and morphometric studies of the cerebral lobes suggest structural abnormalities of the PFC (Cotter et al., 2002; Drevets et al., 1997; Haznedar et al., 2005; Lopez-Larson, DelBello, Zimmerman, Schwiers, & Strakowski, 2002; Ongur, Drevets, & Price, 1998; Rajkowska, Halaris, & Selemon, 2001) and ACC (Benes, Vincent, & Todtenkopf, 2001; Bouras, Kovari, Hof, Riederer, & Giannakopoulos, 2001) in bipolar I disorder. Smaller PFC volume correlates with deficits on sustained attention and inhibition tasks (Sax et al., 1999), and decreased frontal volumes have been observed in adolescents with BD (Chang, Gallelli, & Howe, 2007; Friedman et al., 1999; see also DelBello, Adler, et al., 2004; Lyoo, Lee, Jung, Noam, & Renshaw, 2002).

Neuropsychological studies have also examined attention and working memory functioning of individuals with BD. The continuous performance test (CPT) assesses sustained attention/vigilance. Adults with bipolar I disorder consistently perform worse than normal controls on the CPT in both manic and euthymic states (Clark, Iversen, & Goodwin, 2001; Ferrier, Stanton, Kelly, & Scott, 1999; Fleck, Sax, & Strakowski, 2001; Liu et al., 2002; Sax, Strakowski, McElroy, Keck, & West, 1995; Sax et al., 1998, 1999; Wilder-Willis et al., 2001; but see Swann, Anderson, Dougherty, & Moeller, 2001, for negative findings). Moreover, adults with bipolar I disorder showed decreased activation of medial PFC during performance on a CPT (Strakowski, Adler, Holland, Mills, & DelBello, 2004). Two studies (DelBello, Adler, et al., 2004; Robertson, Kutcher, & Lagace, 2003) did not find CPT differences between youth with BD and normal youth; however, the CPT may not be able to differentiate developmentally normal errors from deficits found in BD, given that attentional control is still developing throughout adolescence (Walshaw et al., in press).

The Stroop color–word naming task (Stroop, 1935) activates the ACC and right orbitofrontal cortex, known to be involved in selective attention and inhibition of interfering stimuli (e.g., Cabeza & Nyberg, 2000). Individuals with bipolar I disorder show impaired Stroop performance regardless of current mood state (Martínez-Arán, Vieta, Reinares, et al., 2004), even when they are euthymic (Cavanagh, van Beck, Muir, & Blackwood, 2002; Gruber, Rogowska, & Yurgelun-Todd, 2004; Thompson et al., 2005; Zalla et al., 2004), and these deficits are stable over a 3-year period (Balanza-Martinez et al., 2005). First-degree relatives of patients with BD also show Stroop impairment (Zalla et al., 2004), suggesting a possible genetic component to the selective attention problems. One study of adolescents with BD found that they showed abnormalities in ventral PFC activation during the Stroop task (Blumberg, Martin, et al., 2003), similar to adults with BD, who display deficits on the task (Benabarre et al., 2005; Blumberg, Leung, et al., 2003).

The Wisconsin Card Sorting Test (WCST; Heaton, 1981) assesses the ability to shift attentional focus or cognitive flexibility and is one of most widely used tests of PFC executive function. In particular, the WCST perseverative errors score measures the extent to which an individual becomes fixated on a dominant rewarded response. Individuals with bipolar I disorder exhibit greater WCST perseverative errors than normal controls (Altshuler et al., 2004; Martínez-Arán, Vieta, Colom, et al., 2004; Morice, 1990; Tien, Ross, Pearlson, & Strauss, 1996; but see Robertson et al., 2003; Verdoux & Liraud, 2000; Zalla et al., 2004, for negative findings), and these deficits occur across mood state (Martínez-Arán, Vieta, Reinares, et al., 2004) and are stable over 3 years (Balanza-Martinez et al., 2005). Moreover, in a prospective study, WCST performance in adolescence predicted bipolar spectrum disorder onset, but not unipolar depression, in young adulthood (Meyer, Carlson, et al., 2004).

Given that the ACC may be centrally involved in selective attention performance (Botvinik et al., 2001; Casey et al., 1997), the possibility that the attentional deficits observed in individuals with BD are associated with differences in ACC activation is worth exploring. Leibenluft and colleagues (2003) reviewed several relevant studies that found an association between mania and increased

ACC activation. Given that attentional control begins to mature in adolescence and that development of attention regulation, in turn, plays a role in the concurrent development of affect regulation (Leibenluft et al., 2003), these studies of attentional function and ACC activation may be relevant to understanding why adolescence is a high-risk period for the onset of BD. Drevets (2001) proposed that the ventral ACC may be involved in mediating the abrupt switches of mood state and arousal seen in BD, which may be relevant to understanding the greater prevalence of rapid cycling observed in adolescent BD as the ACC is maturing.

As noted, normative development of working memory skills, subserved by the dorsolateral PFC (Owen, 2000), should also be an important cognitive capacity underlying efforts at self-regulation and rumination/basking. Relative to controls, adults with bipolar I disorder have consistently shown deficits in verbal working memory (Ferrier et al., 1999; Martínez-Arán, Vieta, Colom, et al., 2004; Thompson et al., 2005) across mood states (Martínez-Arán, Vieta, Reinares, et al., 2004). Also, Chang and colleagues (2004) found that, relative to normal controls, euthymic adolescents with bipolar spectrum disorders showed increased ACC and dorsolateral PFC activation during a visuospatial working memory task. More generally, Chang and colleagues (2007) suggested that PFC overactivation may be a marker of risk for development of BD.

Our hypotheses regarding the dependence of the adolescent onset of BD on the normative development of executive functions served by PFC maturation in adolescence suggest important directions for future research. Specifically, prospective longitudinal studies are needed that track the trajectories of development of executive functions and PFC/ACC activation during the transition to adolescence and relate these trajectories to those of development of maladaptive cognitive styles, self-regulatory attentional processes (e.g., rumination/basking), and hopelessness/hope, and, in turn, the onset of BD.

EMBEDDING THE COGNITIVE VULNERABILITY–STRESS PERSPECTIVE IN A NORMATIVE ADOLESCENT BRAIN AND EMOTIONAL/MOTIVATIONAL DEVELOPMENT CONTEXT

Just as cognitive vulnerability and underlying PFC function are maturing and consolidating in adolescence, the stress half of the cognitive vulnerability–stress model is also undergoing important developments in adolescence. Recall that there is a developmentally normative increase in the number of stressful life events after age 13 for both males and females (Garber et al., 2002; Gest et al., 1999), but especially for adolescent females (Ge et al., 1994), as well as an increase in achievement opportunities, goal striving, and reward seeking (Steinberg, 2008; Steinberg et al., 2006). This developmentally normative adolescent increase in event exposure occurs at the same time as developmental increases in the "stress sensitivity" and "reward sensitivity" of the adolescent brain (Spear, 2007; Steinberg, 2008; Walker et al., 2004). Thus, at the same time that maladaptive cognitive styles and the capacity for rumination are consolidating, adolescents' exposure and reactivity to negative and positive life events are also increasing. This "two-hit" normative augmentation of both vulnerability and stress may help to explain why adolescence is a high-risk period for onset of bipolar spectrum disorders.

The stress response is enhanced during adolescence both at the neural and behavioral levels (Walker, McMillan, & Mittal, 2007; Walker et al., 2004; see Figure 10.2). In response to environmental challenges, the adrenal cortex releases glucocorticoids (cortisol in humans). Cross-sectional and longitudinal studies reveal a gradual rise in salivary and urinary cortisol during middle childhood, with a sharp increase beginning around age 13 and continuing throughout adolescence (see Walker et al., 2004, 2007, for reviews). Longitudinal and prospective studies suggest that excessive cortisol secretion is associated with the onset and persistence of major depression (e.g., Goodyer, Herbert, & Tamplin, 2000, 2003; Goodyer, Herbert, Tamplin, & Altham, 2000).

In addition to the postpubertal increase in cortisol activity, there are other indicators of heightened biobehavioral sensitivity to stress in adolescence. There is a stronger association between stressful events and depression in adolescents than in adults (Gould, Petrie, Kleinman, & Wallenstein, 1994; Pine, Cohen, Johnson, & Brook, 2002; Rice, Harold, & Thapar, 2003). During laboratory exposure to stressful stimuli, adolescents respond with increases in heart rate and cortisol secretion (Buske-Kirschbaum et al., 1997), greater β-adrenergic activation than younger children (Allen & Matthews, 1997), and more persistent skin conductance responding than adults (Miller & Shields, 1980). Dopaminergic function, important in mediating reward behavior, increases in the PFC during adolescence (Spear, 2007). Furthermore, the amygdala, a limbic brain structure involved in emotional reactivity and coordinating responses to stressors with connections to the PFC and ACC, shows continuing maturation well into adolescence (Benes, 2003a, 2003b), which may have particular relevance to BD. Functional imaging studies of adults with bipolar I disorder indicate activation abnormalities of the amygdala (Drevets et al., 2002; Yurgelun-Todd et al., 2000), and children and adolescents with BD show decreased amygdalar volumes compared with normal controls (Blumberg, Kaufman, et al., 2003; Chang et al., 2005; DelBello, Zimmerman, et al., 2004). Thus, adolescence appears to be a period in which individuals are particularly responsive to stressors both behaviorally and biologically.

The augmented stress sensitivity of the adolescent brain may not only help to account for the greater likelihood of onset or exacerbation of BD in adolescence, but it may also contribute to some of the other clinical phenomena associated with adolescent BD. If adolescents overreact to minor events as a result of an increased sensitivity to life events in adolescence, this could contribute to the rapid cycling often observed in adolescent BD. In addition, cortisol secretion has been found to be about 20% higher in postpubertal females than males (Goodyer, Park, Netherton, & Herbert, 2001), and this may contribute to the relatively greater onset of BD in females than males in adolescence. That is, prepubertal-onset cases of BD are overwhelmingly male, whereas there is a more even gender distribution in adolescent-onset BD (Biederman et al., 2005; Geller et al., 1995; Hendrick, Altshuler, Gitlin, Delrahim, & Hammen, 2000).

Individual differences in neural and behavioral stress sensitivity during adolescence may arise as a function of earlier childhood experiences. Earlier we reviewed evidence suggesting that negative parenting and abuse histories may be associated with an earlier age of onset, rapid cycling, and a worse course of BD, the type of phenomenology observed in adolescent-onset BD. Furthermore, maltreatment and parenting involving low care and high criticism are associated with the development of maladaptive cognitive styles that promote vulnerability to unipolar and bipolar mood episodes (Alloy et al., 2004; Alloy, Abramson, Smith, et al., 2006). However, recent evidence indicates that early experiences of poor parental care and maltreatment may promote the development of a hyperreactive stress response system as well (Gunnar, 2007; Meaney, 2007). Gunnar (2007) reviews evidence that children who are exposed to poor caregiving, early adversity, or severe or prolonged abuse are more likely to show increased cortisol stress responsiveness. Thus, the developmentally normative rise in adolescent stress sensitivity may be augmented in adolescents with a history of poor care or abuse. Consequently, childhood abuse and negative parenting experiences may set the stage for the typically observed adolescent onset and features of BD by affecting both the vulnerability and stress components of the cognitive model.

Just as the behavioral and neurobiological stress response is enhanced in adolescence, so too is reward sensitivity (see Figure 10.2; Steinberg, 2008). Normative developmental changes in the dopaminergic system occur at puberty (Chambers, Taylor, & Potenza, 2003; Spear, 2000). In early adolescence, there is a significant increase in functional dopaminergic activity in the PFC (Rosenberg & Lewis, 1995) that, in rodents, is more pronounced in males than females (Sisk & Foster, 2004; Sisk & Zehr, 2005). Given that dopamine plays a crucial role in the brain's reward systems, this increase in circulating PFC dopamine levels may lead to greater sensitivity and efficiency of the reward circuitry and, consequently, to greater behavioral reward seeking and responsiveness (Steinberg, 2008). Consistent with this idea, Steinberg and colleagues (2009) found that behavioral sensation seeking and reward sensitivity increased in youth from age 10 until midadolescence, peaking somewhere between ages 13 and 16. Considered alongside the evidence that hypomanic/manic and depressive episodes are triggered by events involving reward seeking or attainment and loss of rewards, respectively, this normative adolescent increase in reward sensitivity may also contribute to adolescence being a high-risk period for onset of BDs.

EMBEDDING THE COGNITIVE VULNERABILITY–STRESS MODEL IN A GENETIC CONTEXT

BD has a strong genetic predisposition (Kieseppa, Partonen, Haukka, Kaprio, & Lonnqvis, 2004; McGuffin et al., 2003; Merikangas et al., 2002). Among other mechanisms, genetic predisposition may contribute to BD by increasing both stress sensitivity and cognitive vulnerability, particularly during the developmental period of adolescence (see Figure 10.2). Some genetic effects may come "online" during adolescence. On the basis of recent advances showing that hormones affect gene expression (e.g., Kawata, 1995), researchers (e.g., Walker et al., 2004) have suggested that pubertal hormonal changes may trigger the expression of genetic predispositions for various disorders, including mood disorders. This is consistent with the findings that the heritability estimate for depression rises dramatically after puberty (Silberg et al., 1999) and that the risk of affective illness increases as offspring of parents with BD move through adolescence (Egeland et al., 2003; Hillegers et al., 2005; Shaw, 2005). The expression of such genetic vulnerabilities may contribute to adolescents' increased stress responsiveness (e.g., Walker et al., 2004) and, therefore, to the adolescent onset or exacerbation of BD.

Cognitive vulnerability also has a genetic component. Using genetically informative twin designs, two independent studies (Lau, Rijsdijk, & Eley, 2006; Schulman, Keith, & Seligman, 1993) revealed a genetic influence on attributional style. It is plausible that the serotonin transporter genotype (5-HTTLPR), in particular, is related to cognitive vulnerability. The 5-HTTLPR genotype has been related to both unipolar depression (e.g., Caspi et al., 2003) and BD (e.g., Cho et al., 2005; Craddock & Jones, 2001), particularly in interaction with exposure to stressful life events (e.g., Caspi et al., 2003; Eley et al., 2004; Grabe et al., 2004; Kaufman et al., 2004; Kendler, Kuhn, Vittum, Prescott, & Riley, 2005). Both cognitive vulnerability and 5-HTTLPR genotype may participate in vulnerability × stress interactions that moderate the effects of stress on the development of mood episodes. More specifically, recent work (J. H. Meyer et al., 2003, 2004) suggests that serotonin modulates dysfunctional attitudes, one type of cognitive vulnerability for mood disorders. Furthermore, cognitive vulnerability is associated with serotonergic vulnerability as assessed by a strong response to acute tryptophan depletion (Booij & Van der Does, 2007). Finally, individuals with the 5-HTTLPR genetic vulnerability exhibited a stronger attentional bias to emotional word stimuli, another indicator of cognitive vulnerability, than individuals without this genetic predisposition (Beevers, Gibb, McGeary, & Miller, 2007). Thus, cognitive vulnerability may mediate, in part, the effects of genetic predisposition on adolescent-onset BD in response to the rise in adolescent stressors.

Conclusions and Future Directions

In the past decade, major advances occurred in the understanding of adolescent neurodevelopment, with significant maturation of the PFC and concomitant executive functions, as well as augmented activity of the hypothalamic–pituitary–adrenal axis and dopaminergic pathways and increased stress and reward sensitivity, occurring at this time. These normative changes in adolescent brain, cognitive, and emotional/motivational development provide a context for understanding important clinical phenomena of bipolar spectrum disorders from a cognitive vulnerability–stress perspective. Consistent with the cognitive vulnerability–stress model, we reviewed studies indicating that life events may precipitate hypomanic/manic and depressive episodes, perhaps especially when they involve reward gains and losses (BAS relevance), and that individuals with BDs exhibit maladaptive cognitive styles characterized by BAS-relevant features of perfectionism, self-criticism, and excessive goal striving/reward seeking. More-over, several prospective studies found that such cognitive styles combine with relevant life events to predict the depressive and hypomanic/manic symptoms and episodes of individuals with BD. When informed by the normative changes in adolescent brain, cognitive, and emotional/motivational development as well as genetic predisposition, the cognitive vulnerability–stress model may provide important insights into some of the risk factors for the onset or exacerbation, gen-der differences, and symptom presentation of adolescent BD (see Figure 10.2 for a visual representation of these relationships).

In particular, adolescence is a high-risk period for the onset and exacerbation of bipolar spectrum disorders. We suggested that the increased risk for adoles-cent-onset or exacerbation of BD may be explained by the enhanced expression of genetic predispositions and the augmentation of both the cognitive vulnerability and stress components of the cognitive vulnerability–stress model during this developmental period. We presented evidence that maladaptive cognitive styles and self-regulatory attentional processes (rumination/basking) consolidate and come "online" to contribute to mood episodes during adolescence, as a function of normative adolescent PFC maturation and correlated development of executive functions (attentional competence, working memory, hypothetical thinking/deci-sion making, future orientation) that provide "prerequisites" for these cognitive vulnerability processes. We also presented evidence that both exposure to life events and neural and behavioral responsiveness to stress and reward increase during adolescence. Thus, this two-hit normative rise in both cognitive vulner-ability and stress during adolescence may lead to the greater likelihood of BD onset at this time. Moreover, a history of maltreatment and low-care parenting is associated with an earlier age of onset, rapid cycling, and worse course of BD, which may arise, in part, because these early socialization experiences contribute to the development of both maladaptive cognitive styles and a hyperresponsive stress system.

Adolescent (and childhood) BD is characterized by mixed states involving considerable depression and irritability, rapid cycling, and attention problems (e.g., Biederman et al., 2005; Geller et al., 1995, 2004; Leibenluft et al., 2003; Mick et al., 2003; Strober et al., 1988). Females with BD show a predominantly depressive course beginning in adolescence (e.g., Angst, 1978; Leibenluft, 1996; Rasgon et al., 2005; Robb et al., 1998; Roy-Byrne et al., 1985; Viguera et al., 2001). We suggested that in individuals with maladaptive, BAS-relevant cognitive styles that increase vulnerability to both depressive and hypomanic/manic symptoms, certain types of negative life events (e.g., failures that can be overcome, goal obstacles) might precipitate a mixture of hypomanic/manic, depressive, and irritable symptoms. In addition, intra- or interdaily fluctuations in exposure to relevant life events (both independent of and dependent on individuals' behavior) could lead to rapid alternations between depression and hypomania/mania (rapid cycling), particularly during adolescence, when individuals may both be exposed to higher levels of relevant events and be hypersensitive to these stressors. Finally, we speculated that the greater propensity for a depressive course among females starting in adolescence may be related to the findings that females exhibit greater cognitive vulnerability and rumination than males as well as increased cortisol activation beginning in adolescence.

Our hypotheses regarding the basis for the adolescent onset/exacerbation and phenomenology of bipolar spectrum disorders are speculative at present. However, they suggest important directions for future research. First, the trajectories of development of PFC maturation and concomitant executive functioning need to be linked with the developmental trajectories of maladaptive cognitive styles, self-regulatory attentional processes, and hopelessness/hope in prospective studies of adolescents. All of these trajectories, in turn, must be related to the onset and course of bipolar symptoms. Second, longitudinal studies that relate the onset or exacerbation and course of BD to developmental trajectories of exposure to stressful and rewarding events as well as neural and behavioral responsiveness to those stressors and rewards during adolescence are also needed. We hope that the ideas proposed here will inspire researchers to conduct further tests of the cognitive vulnerability–stress model of BDs in an adolescent development context.

ACKNOWLEDGMENTS

Preparation of this chapter was supported by National Institute of Mental Health Grant Nos. MH 52617 and MH 077908 to Lauren B. Alloy and 52662 to Lyn Y. Abramson. This chapter is a revised, expanded, and updated version of Alloy, Abramson, Walshaw, Keyser, and Gerstein (2006) in *Development and Psychopathology, 18*, 1055–1103.

REFERENCES

Abramson, L. Y., Alloy, L. B., Hankin, B. L., Haeffel, G. J., MacCoon, D. G., & Gibb, B. E. (2002). Cognitive vulnerability-stress models of depression in a self-regulatory and psychobiological context. In I. H. Gotlib & C. L. Hammen (Eds.), *Handbook of depression* (3rd ed., pp. 268–294). New York: Guilford Press.

Abramson, L. Y., Alloy, L. B., Hogan, M. E., Whitehouse, W. G., Cornette, M., Akhavan, S., et al. (1998). Suicidality and cognitive vulnerability to depression among college students: A prospective study. *Journal of Adolescence, 21*, 473–487.

Abramson, L. Y., Metalsky, G. I., & Alloy, L. B. (1989). Hopelessness depression: A theory-based subtype of depression. *Psychological Review, 96*, 358–372.

Akiskal, H. S., Djenderedjian, A. H., Rosenthal, R. H., & Khani, M. K. (1977). Cyclothymic disorder: Validating criteria for inclusion in the bipolar affective group. *American Journal of Psychiatry, 134*, 1227–1233.

Akiskal, H. S., Khani, M. K., & Scott-Strauss, A. (1979). Cyclothymic temperamental disorders. *Psychiatric Clinics of North America, 2*, 527–554.

Allen, M. T., & Matthews, K. A. (1997). Hemodynamic responses to laboratory stressors in children and adolescents: The influences of age, race, and gender. *Psychophysiology, 34*, 329–339.

Alloy, L. B., & Abramson, L. Y. (1999). The Temple–Wisconsin Cognitive Vulnerability to Depression (CVD) Project: Conceptual background, design and methods. *Journal of Cognitive Psychotherapy, 13*, 227–262.

Alloy, L. B., & Abramson, L. Y. (2007). The adolescent surge in depression and emergence of gender differences: A biocognitive vulnerability–stress model in developmental context. In E. Walker & D. Romer (Eds.), *Adolescent psychopathology and the developing brain* (pp. 284–312). New York: Oxford University Press.

Alloy, L. B., Abramson, L. Y., Gibb, B. E., Crossfield, A. G., Pieracci, A. M., Spasojevic, J., et al. (2004). Developmental antecedents of cognitive vulnerability to depression: Review of findings from the Cognitive Vulnerability to Depression (CVD) Project. *Journal of Cognitive Psychotherapy, 18*, 115–133.

Alloy, L. B., Abramson, L. Y., Hogan, M. E., Whitehouse, W. G., Rose, D. T., Robinson, M. S., et al. (2000). The Temple–Wisconsin Cognitive Vulnerability to Depression (CVD) Project: Lifetime history of axis I psychopathology in individuals at high and low cognitive risk for depression. *Journal of Abnormal Psychology, 109*, 403–418.

Alloy, L. B., Abramson, L. Y., Neeren, A. M., Walshaw, P. D., Urosevic, S., & Nusslock, R. (2006). Psychosocial risk factors for bipolar disorder: Current and early environment and cognitive styles. In S. Jones & R. Bentall (Eds.), *The psychology of bipolar disorder: New developments and research strategies* (pp. 11–46). Oxford, UK: Oxford University Press.

Alloy, L. B., Abramson, L. Y., Safford, S. M., & Gibb, B. E. (2005). The Cognitive Vulnerability to Depression (CVD) Project: Current findings and future directions. In L. B. Alloy & J. H. Riskind (Eds.), *Cognitive vulnerability to emotional disorders* (pp. 33–61). Mahwah, NJ: Erlbaum.

Alloy, L. B., Abramson, L. Y., Smith, J. B., Gibb, B. E., & Neeren, A. M. (2006). Role of parenting and maltreatment histories in unipolar and bipolar mood disorders: Mediation by cognitive vulnerability to depression. *Clinical Child and Family Psychology Review, 9*, 23–64.

Alloy, L. B., Abramson, L. Y., Tashman, N. A., Berrebbi, D. S., Hogan, M. E., Whitehouse, W. G., et al. (2001). Developmental origins of cognitive vulnerability to depression: Parenting, cognitive, and inferential feedback styles of the parents of individuals at high and low cognitive risk for depression. *Cognitive Therapy and Research, 25*, 397–423.

Alloy, L. B., Abramson, L. Y., Urosevic, S., Bender, R. E., & Wagner, C. A. (2009). Longitudinal predictors of bipolar spectrum disorders: A behavioral approach system (BAS) perspective. *Clinical Psychology: Science and Practice, 16*, 206–226.

Alloy, L. B., Abramson, L. Y., Urosevic, S., Walshaw, P. D., Nusslock, R., & Neeren, A. M. (2005). The psychosocial context of bipolar disorder: Environmental, cognitive, and developmental risk factors. *Clinical Psychology Review, 25*, 1043–1075.

Alloy, L. B., Abramson, L. Y., Walshaw, P. D., Cogswell, A., Grandin, L. D., Hughes, M. E., et al. (2008). Behavioral Approach System (BAS) and Behavioral Inhibition System (BIS) sensitivities and bipolar spectrum disorders: Prospective prediction of bipolar mood episodes. *Bipolar Disorders, 10*, 310–322.

Alloy, L. B., Abramson, L. Y., Walshaw, P. D., Gerstein, R. K., Keyser, J. D., Whitehouse, W. G., et al. (2009). Behavioral Approach System (BAS)-relevant cognitive styles and bipolar spectrum disorders: Concurrent and prospective associations. *Journal of Abnormal Psychology, 118*, 459–471.

Alloy, L. B., Abramson, L. Y., Walshaw, P. D., Keyser, J., & Gerstein, R. K. (2006). A cognitive vulnerability-stress perspective on bipolar spectrum disorders in a normative adolescent brain, cognitive, and emotional development context. *Development and Psychopathology, 18*, 1055–1103.

Alloy, L. B., Abramson, L. Y., Walshaw, P. D., & Neeren, A. M. (2006). Cognitive vulnerability to unipolar and bipolar mood disorders. *Journal of Social and Clinical Psychology, 25*, 726–754.

Alloy, L. B., Abramson, L. Y., Whitehouse, W. G., Hogan, M. E., Panzarella, C., & Rose, D. T. (2006). Prospective incidence of first onsets and recurrences of depression in individuals at high and low cognitive risk for depression. *Journal of Abnormal Psychology, 115*, 145–156.

Alloy, L. B., & Clements, C. M. (1998). Hopelessness theory of depression: Tests of the symptom component. *Cognitive Therapy and Research, 22*, 303–335.

Alloy, L. B., Just, N., & Panzarella, C. (1997). Attributional style, daily life events, and hopelessness depression: Subtype validation by prospective variability and specificity of symptoms. *Cognitive Therapy and Research, 21*, 321–344.

Alloy, L. B., Reilly-Harrington, N. A., Fresco, D. M., & Flannery-Schroeder, E. (2005). Cognitive vulnerability to bipolar spectrum disorders. In L. B. Alloy & J. H. Riskind (Eds.), *Cognitive vulnerability to emotional disorders* (pp. 93–124). Mahwah, NJ: Erlbaum.

Alloy, L. B., Reilly-Harrington, N. A., Fresco, D. M., Whitehouse, W. G., & Zechmeister, J. S. (1999). Cognitive styles and life events in subsyndromal unipolar and bipolar mood disorders: Stability and prospective prediction of depressive and hypomanic mood swings. *Journal of Cognitive Psychotherapy, 13*, 21–40.

Altshuler, L. L., Ventura, J., van Gorp, W. G., Green, M. F., Theberge, D. C., & Mintz, J. (2004). Neurocognitive function in clinically stable men with bipolar I disorder or schizophrenia and normal control subjects. *Biological Psychiatry, 56*, 560–569.

Angst, J. (1978). The course of affective disorders: II. Typology of bipolar manic-depressive illness. *Archives Psychiatrica Nervenkrica, 226*, 65–73.

Ashworth, C. M., Blackburn, I. M., & McPherson, F. M. (1982). The performance of depressed and manic patients on some repertory grid measures: A cross-sectional study. *British Journal of Medical Psychology, 55*, 247–255.

Ashworth, C. M., Blackburn, I. M., & McPherson, F. M. (1985). The performance of depressed and manic patients on some repertory grid measures: A longitudinal study. *British Journal of Medical Psychology, 58*, 337–342.

Balanza-Martinez, V., Tabares-Seisdedos, R., Selva-Vera, G., Martínez-Arán, A., Torrent, C., Salazar-Fraile, J., et al. (2005). Persistent cognitive dysfunctions in bipolar I disorder and schizophrenic patients: A 3-year follow-up study. *Psychotherapy and Psychosomatics, 74*, 113–119.

Bebbington, P., Wilkins, S., Jones, P., Foerster, A., Murray, R., Toone, B., et al. (1993). Life events and psychosis: Initial results from the Camberwell Collaborative Psychosis Study. *British Journal of Psychiatry, 162*, 72–79.

Beck, A. T. (1987). Cognitive models of depression. *Journal of Cognitive Psychotherapy, 1*, 5–37.

Beevers, C. G., Gibb, B. E., McGeary, J. E., & Miller, I. Q. (2007). Serotonin transporter genetic variation and biased attention for emotional word stimuli among psychiatric inpatients. *Journal of Abnormal Psychology, 116*, 208–212.

Bellivier, F., Golmard, J. L., Henry, C., Leboyer, M., & Schurhoff, F. (2001). Admixture analysis of age at onset in bipolar I affective disorder. *Archives of General Psychiatry, 58*, 510–512.

Bellivier, F., Golmard, J. L., Rietschel, M., Schulze, T. G., Malafosse, A., Preisig, M., et al. (2003). Age at onset in bipolar I affective disorder: Further evidence for three subgroups. *American Journal of Psychiatry, 160*, 999–1001.

Benabarre, A., Vieta, E., Martínez-Arán, A., Garcia-Garcia, M., Martin, F., Lomena, F., et al. (2005). Neuropsychological disturbances and cerebral blood flow in bipolar disorder. *Australian and New Zealand Journal of Psychiatry, 39*, 227–234.

Bender, R. E., Alloy, L. B., Sylvia, L. G., Abramson, L. Y., & Urosevic, S. (2009). *Generation of life events in bipolar disorder: A replication and extension of the stress generation theory.* Manuscript submitted for publication.

Benes, F. M. (2003a). Schizophrenia: II. Amygdalar fiber alteration as etiology? *American Journal of Psychiatry, 160*, 1053.

Benes, F. M. (2003b). Why does psychosis develop during adolescence and early adulthood? *Currrent Opinion in Psychiatry, 16*, 317–319.

Benes, F. M., Vincent, S. L., & Todtenkopf, M. (2001). The density of pyramidal and nonpyramidal neurons in anterior cingulate cortex of schizophrenic and bipolar subjects. *Biological Psychiatry, 50*, 395–406.

Bentall, R. P., & Thompson, M. (1990). Emotional Stroop performance and the manic defense. *British Journal of Clinical Psychology, 29*, 235–237.

Biederman, J., Faraone, S. V., Wozniak, J., Mick, E., Kwon, A., Cayton, G., et al. (2005). Clinical correlates of bipolar disorder in a large, referred sample of children and adolescents. *Journal of Psychiatric Research, 39*, 611–622.

Birmaher, B., Axelson, D., Strober, M., Gill, M. K., Valeri, S., Chiappetta, L., et al. (2006). Clinical course of children and adolescents with bipolar spectrum disorders. *Archives of General Psychiatry, 63*, 175–183.

Blumberg, H. P., Kaufman, J., Martin, A., Whiteman, R., Zhang, J. H., Gore, J. C., et al. (2003). Amygdala and hippocampal volumes in adolescents and adults with bipolar disorder. *Archives of General Psychiatry, 60*, 1201–1208.

Blumberg, H. P., Leung, H., Skudlarski, P., Lacadie, C. M., Fredericks, C. A., Harris, B. C., et al. (2003). A functional magnetic resonance imaging study of bipolar disorder. *Archives of General Psychiatry, 60*, 601–609.

Blumberg, H. P., Martin, A., Kaufman, J., Leung, H., Skudlarski, P., Lacadie, C., et al. (2003). Frontostriatal abnormalities in adolescents with bipolar disorder: Preliminary observations from functional MRI. *American Journal of Psychiatry, 160*, 1345–1347.

Booij, L., & Van der Does, A. J. W. (2007). Cognitive and serotonergic vulnerability to depression: Convergent findings. *Journal of Abnormal Psychology, 116*, 86–94.

Botvinik, M., Braver, T. S., Barch, S. M., Carter, C. S., & Cohen, J. D. (2001). Conflict monitoring and cognitive control. *Psychological Review, 108*, 624–652.

Bouras, C., Kovari, E., Hof, P. R., Riederer, B. M., & Giannakopoulos, P. (2001). Anterior cingulate cortex pathology in schizophrenia and bipolar disorder. *Acta Neuropathologica, 102*, 373–379.

Broderick, P. C. (1998). Early adolescent gender differences in the use of ruminative and distracting coping strategies. *Journal of Early Adolescence, 18*, 173–191.

Brown, G. W., & Harris, T. O. (1978). *Social origins of depression: A study of psychiatric disorder in women.* New York: Free Press.

Burke, K. C., Burke, J. D., Regier, D. A., & Rae, D. S. (1990). Age at onset of selected mental disorders in five community populations. *Archives of General Psychiatry, 47*, 511–518.

Buske-Kirschbaum, A., Jobst, S., Wustmans, A., Kirschbaum, C., Rauh, W., & Hellhammer, D. (1997). Attenuated free cortisol response to psychosocial stress in children with atopic dermatitis. *Psychosomatic Medicine, 59*, 419–426.

Cabeza, R., & Nyberg, L. (2000). Imaging cognition: II. An empirical review of 275 PET and fMRI studies. *Journal of Cognitive Neuroscience, 12*, 1–47.

Carter, T. D., Mundo, E., Parikh, S. V., & Kennedy, J. L. (2003). Early age at onset as a risk factor for poor outcome of bipolar disorder. *Journal of Psychiatric Research, 37*, 297–303.

Carver, C. S. (2004). Negative affect deriving from the behavioral approach system. *Emotion*, *4*, 3–22.

Carver, C. S., & Scheier, M. F. (1998). *On the self-regulation of behavior.* Cambridge, UK: Cambridge University Press.

Casey, B. J., Galvan, A., & Hare, T. A. (2005). Changes in cerebral functional organization during cognitive development. *Current Opinion in Neurobiology*, *15*, 239–244.

Casey, B. J., Giedd, J. N., & Thomas, K. M. (2000). Structural and functional brain development and its relation to cognitive development. *Biological Psychology*, *45*, 241–257.

Casey, B. J., Tottenham, N., Liston, C., & Durston, S. (2005). Imaging the developing brain: What have we learned about cognitive development? *Trends in Cognitive Sciences*, *9*, 104–110.

Casey, B. J., Trainor, R., Giedd, J., Vauss, Y., Vaituzis, C. K., Hamburger, S., et al. (1997). The role of the anterior cingulate in automatic and controlled processes: A developmental neuroanatomical study. *Developmental Psychobiology*, *30*, 61–69.

Caspi, A., Sugden, K., Moffitt, T. E., Taylor, A., Craig, I. W., Harrington, H., et al. (2003). Influence of life stress on depression: Moderation by a polymorphism in the 5-HTT gene. *Science*, *301*, 386–389.

Cassano, G. B., Dell'Osso, L., Frank, E., Miniati, M., Fagiolini, A., Shear, K., et al. (1999). The bipolar spectrum: A clinical reality in search of diagnostic criteria and an assessment methodology. *Journal of Affective Disorders*, *54*, 319–328.

Cavanagh, J. T. O., van Beck, M., Muir, W., & Blackwood, D. H. R. (2002). Case-control study of neurocognitive function in euthymic patients with bipolar disorder: An association with mania. *British Journal of Psychiatry*, *180*, 320–326.

Chambers, R., Taylor, J., & Potenza, M. (2003). Developmental neurocircuitry of motivation in adolescence: A critical period of addiction vulnerability. *American Journal of Psychiatry*, *160*, 1041–1052.

Chang, K. D., Adleman, N. E., Dienes, K., Simeonova, D. I., Menon, V., & Reiss, A. (2004). Anomalous prefrontal-subcortical activation in familial pediatric bipolar disorder: A functional magnetic resonance imaging investigation. *Archives of General Psychiatry*, *61*, 781–792.

Chang, K. D., Gallelli, K., & Howe, M. (2007). Early identification and prevention of early-onset bipolar disorder. In D. Romer & E. F. Walker (Eds.), *Adolescent psychopathology and the developing brain: Integrating brain and prevention science* (pp. 315–346). New York: Oxford University Press.

Chang, K. D., Karchemskiy, A., Barnea-Goraly, N., Garrett, A., Simeonova, D. I., & Reiss, A. (2005). Reduced amygdalar gray matter volume in familial pediatric bipolar disorder. *Journal of the American Academy of Child and Adolescent Psychiatry*, *44*, 565–573.

Chang, K. D., Steiner, H., & Ketter, T. A. (2000). Psychiatric phenomenology of child and adolescent bipolar offspring. *Journal of the American Academy of Child and Adolescent Psychiatry*, *39*, 453–460.

Cho, H. J., Meira-Lima, I., Cordeiro, Q., Michelon, L., Sham, P., Vallada, H., et al. (2005). Population-based and family-based studies on the serotonin transporter gene polymorphism and bipolar disorder: A systematic review and meta-analysis. *Molecular Psychiatry*, *10*, 771–781.

Christensen, E. M., Gjerris, A., Larsen, J. K., Bendtsen, B. B., Larsen, B. H., Rolff, H., et al. (2003). Life events and onset of a new phase in bipolar affective disorder. *Bipolar Disorders*, *5*, 356–361.

Chung, R. K., Langeluddecke, P., & Tennant, C. (1986). Threatening life events in the onset of schizophrenia, schizophreniform psychosis, and hypomania. *British Journal of Psychiatry*, *148*, 680–685.

Cicchetti, D., & Rogosch, F. A. (2002). A developmental psychopathology perspective on adolescence. *Journal of Consulting and Clinical Psychology, 70,* 6–20.

Clark, L., Iversen, S. D., & Goodwin, G. M. (2001). A neuropsychological investigation of prefrontal cortex involvement in acute mania. *American Journal of Psychiatry, 158,* 1605–1611.

Cohen, J. D., & Servan-Schreiber, D. (1992). Context, cortex, and dopamine: A connectionist approach to behavior and biology in schizophrenia. *Psychological Review, 99,* 45–77.

Cole, D. A., Ciesla, J. A., Dallaire, D. H., Jacquez, F., Pineda, A. Q., LaGrange, B., et al. (2008). Emergence of attributional style and its relation to depressive symptoms. *Journal of Abnormal Psychology, 117,* 16–31.

Cooke, R. G., Young, L. T., Mohri, L., Blake, P., & Joffe, R. T. (1999). Family-of-origin characteristics in bipolar disorder: A controlled study. *Canadian Journal of Psychiatry, 44,* 379–381.

Coryell, W., Solomon, S., Turvey, C., Keller, M., Leon, A. C., Schettler, P., et al. (2003). The long-term course of rapid-cycling bipolar disorder. *Archives of General Psychiatry, 60,* 914–920.

Cotter, D., Mackay, D., Chana, G., Beasley, C., Landau, S., & Everall, I. P. (2002). Reduced neuronal size and glial cell density in area 9 of the dorsolateral prefrontal cortex in subjects with major depressive disorder. *Cerebral Cortex, 12,* 386–394.

Coverdale, J. H., & Turbott, S. H. (2000). Sexual and physical abuse of chronically ill psychiatric outpatients compared with a matched sample of medical outpatients. *Journal of Nervous and Mental Disease, 188,* 440–445.

Craddock, N., & Jones, I. (2001). Molecular genetics of bipolar disorder. *British Journal of Psychiatry, 178,* S128–133.

Crick, N. R., & Grotpeter, J. K. (1996). Children's treatment by peers: Victims of relational and overt aggression. *Development and Psychopathology, 8,* 367–380.

De Bellis, M. D., Keshavan, M. S., Beers, S. R., Hall, J., Frustaci, K., Masalehdan, A., et al. (2001). Sex differences in brain maturation during childhood and adolescence. *Cerebral Cortex, 11,* 552–557.

DelBello, M. P., Adler, C. M., Amicone, J., Mills, N. P., Shear, P. K., Warner, J., et al. (2004). Parametric neurocognitive task design: A pilot study of sustained attention in adolescents with bipolar disorder. *Journal of Affective Disorders, 82S,* S79–S88.

DelBello, M. P., & Geller, B. (2001). Review of studies of child and adolescent offspring of bipolar parents. *Bipolar Disorders, 3,* 325–334.

DelBello, M. P., Zimmerman, M. E., Mills, N. P., Getz, G. E., & Strakowski, S. M. (2004). Magnetic resonance imaging analysis of amygdala and other subcortical brain regions in adolescents with bipolar disorder. *Bipolar Disorders, 6,* 43–52.

Depue, R. A., & Iacono, W. G. (1989). Neurobehavioral aspects of affective disorders. *Annual Review of Psychology, 40,* 457–492.

Depue, R. A., Krauss, S., & Spoont, M. (1987). A two-dimensional threshold model of seasonal bipolar affective disorder. In D. Magnusson & A. Ohman (Eds.), *Psychopathology: An interactional perspective* (pp. 95–123). New York: Academic Press.

Depue, R. A., Slater, J., Wolfstetter-Kausch, H., Klein, D., Goplerud, E., & Farr, D. (1981). A behavioral paradigm for identifying persons at risk for bipolar depressive disorder: A conceptual framework and five validation studies. *Journal of Abnormal Psychology, 90,* 381–437.

Donnelly, E. F., & Murphy, D. L. (1973). Social desirability and bipolar affective disorder. *Journal of Consulting and Clinical Psychology, 41,* 469.

Drevets, W. C. (2001). Neuroimaging and neuropathological studies of depression: Implications for the cognitive-emotional features of mood disorders. *Current Opinion in Neurobiology, 11*, 240–249.

Drevets, W. C., Price, J. L., Bardgett, M. E., Reich, T., Todd, R. D., & Raichle, M. E. (2002). Glucose metabolism in the amygdala in depression: Relationship to diagnostic subtype and plasma cortisol levels. *Pharmacology, Biochemistry and Behavior, 71*, 431–447.

Drevets, W. C., Price, J. L., Simpson, J. R., Jr., Todd, R. D., Reich, T., Vannier, M., et al. (1997). Subgenual prefrontal cortex abnormalities in mood disorders. *Nature, 386*, 824–827.

Egeland, J. A., Shaw, J. A., Endicott, J., Pauls, D. L., Allen, C. R., Hostetter, A. M., et al. (2003). Prospective study of prodromal features for bipolarity in well Amish children. *Journal of the American Academy of Child and Adolescent Psychiatry, 42*, 786–796.

Ehnvall, A., & Agren, H. (2002). Patterns of sensitization in the course of affective illness: A life-charting study of treatment-refractory depressed patients. *Journal of Affective Disorders, 70*, 67–75.

Eich, E., Macaulay, D., & Lam, R. W. (1997). Mania, depression, and mood-dependent memory. *Cognition and Emotion, 11*, 607–618.

Eley, T. C., Sugden, K., Corsico, A., Gregory, A. M., Sham, P., McGuffin, P., et al. (2004). Gene-environment interaction analysis of serotonin system markers with adolescent depression. *Molecular Psychiatry, 9*, 908–915.

Ellicott, A., Hammen, C., Gitlin, M., Brown, G., & Jamison, K. (1990). Life events and the course of bipolar disorder. *American Journal of Psychiatry, 147*, 1194–1198.

Ernst, C. L., & Goldberg, J. F. (2004). Clinical features related to age at onset in bipolar disorder. *Journal of Affective Disorders, 82*, 21–27.

Feldman, G. C., Joorman, J., & Johnson, S. L. (2008). Responses to positive affect: A self-report measure of rumination and dampening. *Cognitive Therapy and Research, 32*, 507–525.

Ferrier, I. N., Stanton, B. R., Kelly, T. P., & Scott, J. (1999). Neuropsychological function in euthymic patients with bipolar disorder. *British Journal of Psychiatry, 175*, 246–251.

Fleck, D. E., Sax, K. W., & Strakowski, S. M. (2001). Reaction time measures of sustained attention differentiate bipolar disorder from schizophrenia. *Schizophrenia Research, 52*, 251–259.

Floyd, T. D., Alloy, L. B., Smith, J., Neeren, A., & Thorell, G. (2009). *Puberty, ethnicity, and gender differences in depression: Role of cognitive vulnerability and the thin female ideal.* Manuscript in preparation.

Francis-Raniere, E., Alloy, L. B., & Abramson, L. Y. (2006). Depressive personality styles and bipolar spectrum disorders: Prospective tests of the event congruency hypothesis. *Bipolar Disorders, 8*, 1–18.

French, C. C., Richards, A., & Scholfield, E. J. C. (1996). Hypomania, anxiety and the emotional Stroop. *British Journal of Clinical Psychology, 35*, 617–626.

Friedman, L., Findling, R., Kenny, J. T., Swales, T. P., Stuve, T. A., Jesberger, J., et al. (1999). An MRI study of adolescent patients with either schizophrenia or bipolar disorder as compared to healthy control subjects. *Biological Psychiatry, 46*, 78–88.

Garber, J., Keiley, M. K., & Martin, N. C. (2002). Developmental trajectories of adolescents' depressive symptoms: Predictors of change. *Journal of Consulting and Clinical Psychology, 70*, 79–95.

Ge, X., Lorenz, F. O., Conger, R. D., Elder, G. H., & Simons, R. L. (1994). Trajectories of stressful life events and depressive symptoms during adolescence. *Developmental Psychology, 30*, 467–483.

Geller, B., Bolhofner, K., Craney, J. L., Williams, M., DelBello, M. P., & Gundersen, K. (2000). Psychosocial functioning in prepubertal and early adolescent bipolar disorder phenotype. *Journal of the American Academy of Child and Adolescent Psychiatry, 39*, 1543–1548.

Geller, B., Cooper, T. B., Zimerman, B., Frazier, J., Williams, M., Heath, J., et al. (1998). Lithium for prepubertal depressed children with family history predictors of future bipolarity: A double-blind, placebo-controlled study. *Journal of Affective Disorders, 51,* 165–175.

Geller, B., Sun, K., Zimerman, B., Luby, J., Frazier, J., & Williams, M. (1995). Complex and rapid-cycling in bipolar children and adolescents: A preliminary study. *Journal of Affective Disorders, 18,* 259–268.

Geller, B., Tillman, R., Craney, J. L., & Bolhofner, K. (2004). Four-year prospective outcome and natural history of mania in children with a prepubertal and early adolescent bipolar disorder phenotype. *Archives of General Psychiatry, 61,* 459–467.

Gest, S. D., Reed, M. J., & Masten, A. S. (1999). Measuring developmental changes in exposure to adversity: A life chart and rating scale approach. *Development and Psychopathology, 11,* 171–192.

Gibb, B. E., Abramson, L. Y., & Alloy, L. B. (2004). Emotional maltreatment from parents, peer victimization, and cognitive vulnerability to depression. *Cognitive Therapy and Research, 28,* 1–21.

Gibb, B. E., & Alloy, L. B. (2006). A prospective test of the hopelessness theory of depression in children. *Journal of Clinical Child and Adolescent Psychology, 35,* 264–274.

Gibb, B. E., Alloy, L. B., Abramson, L. Y., Rose, D. T., Whitehouse, W. G., Donovan, P., et al. (2001a). History of childhood maltreatment, negative cognitive styles, and episodes of depression in adulthood. *Cognitive Therapy and Research, 25,* 425–446.

Gibb, B. E., Alloy, L. B., Abramson, L. Y., Rose, D. T., Whitehouse, W. G., & Hogan, M. E. (2001b). Childhood maltreatment and college students' current suicidal ideation: A test of the hopelessness theory. *Suicide and Life-Threatening Behavior, 31,* 405–415.

Gibb, B. E., Alloy, L. B., Walshaw, P. D., Comer, J. S., Chang, G. H., & Villari, A. G. (2006). Predictors of negative attributional style change in children. *Journal of Abnormal Child Psychology, 34,* 425–439.

Giedd, J. N. (2004). Structural magnetic resonance imaging of the adolescent brain. *Annals of the New York Academy of Science, 1021,* 77–85.

Giedd, J. N., Blumenthal, J., Jeffries, N. O., Castellanos, F. X., Lui, H., Zijdenbos, A., et al. (1999). Brain development during childhood and adolescence: A longitudinal MRI study. *Nature Neuroscience, 2,* 861–863.

Giedd, J. N., Snell, J. W., Lange, N., Rajapakse, J. C., Casey, B. J., Kozuch, P. L., et al. (1996). Quantitative magnetic resonance imaging of human brain development: Ages 4–18. *Cerebral Cortex, 6,* 551–560.

Glassner, B., & Haldipur, C. V. (1983). Life events and early and late onset of bipolar disorder. *American Journal of Psychiatry, 140,* 215–217.

Glassner, B., Haldipur, C. V., & Dessauersmith, J. (1979). Role loss and working-class manic depression. *Journal of Nervous and Mental Disease, 167,* 530–541.

Gogtay, N., Giedd, J. N., Lusk, L., Hayashi, K. M., Greenstein, D., Vaituzis, A. C., et al. (2004). Dynamic mapping of human cortical development during childhood through early adulthood. *Proceedings of the National Academy of Science, 101,* 8174–8179.

Goldberg, J. F., Gerstein, R. K., Wenze, S. J., Welker, T. M., & Beck, A. T. (2008). Dysfunctional attitudes and cognitive schemas in bipolar manic and unipolar depressed outpatients: Implications for cognitively based psychotherapeutics. *Journal of Nervous and Mental Disease, 196,* 207–210.

Goodwin, F. K., & Jamison, K. R. (2007). *Manic-depressive illness* (2nd ed.). New York: Oxford University Press.

Goodyer, I. M., Herbert, J., & Tamplin, A. (2000a). Recent life events, cortisol, dehydroepiandrosterone, and the onset of major depression in high-risk adolescents. *British Journal of Psychiatry, 177,* 499–504.

Goodyer, I. M., Herbert, J., & Tamplin, A. (2003). Psychoendocrine antecedents of persistent first-episode major depression in adolescents: A community-based longitudinal enquiry. *Psychological Medicine, 33,* 601–610.

Goodyer, I. M., Herbert, J., Tamplin, A., & Altham, P. M. (2000b). First-episode major depression in adolescents: Affective, cognitive and endocrine characteristics of risk status and predictors of onset. *British Journal of Psychiatry, 176,* 142–149.

Goodyer, I. M., Park, R. J., Netherton, C. M., & Herbert, J. (2001). Possible role of cortisol and dehydroepiandrosterone in human development and psychopathology. *British Journal of Psychiatry, 179,* 243–249.

Gould, M. S., Petrie, K., Kleinman, M. H., & Wallenstein, S. (1994). Clustering of attempted suicide: New Zealand national data. *International Journal of Epidemiology, 23,* 1185–1189.

Grabe, H. J., Lange, M., Wolff, B., Votzke, H., Lucht, M., Freyberger, H. J., et al. (2004). Mental and physical distress is modulated by a polymorphism in the 5-HT transporter gene interacting with social stressors and chronic disease burden. *Molecular Psychiatry, 10,* 220–224.

Grandin, L. D., Alloy, L. B., & Abramson, L. Y. (2007). Childhood stressful life events and bipolar spectrum disorders. *Journal of Social and Clinical Psychology, 26,* 460–478.

Gruber, S. A., Rogowska, J., & Yurgelun-Todd, D. A. (2004). Decreased activation of the anterior cingulate in bipolar patients: An fMRI study. *Journal of Affective Disorders, 82,* 191–201.

Gunnar, M. R. (2007). Stress effects on the developing brain. In D. Romer & E. F. Walker (Eds.), *Adolescent psychopathology and the developing brain: Integrating brain and prevention science* (pp. 127–147). New York: Oxford University Press.

Hall, K. S., Dunner, D. L., Zeller, G., & Fieve, R. R. (1977). Bipolar illness: A prospective study of life events. *Comprehensive Psychiatry, 18,* 497–502.

Hammen, C. (1991). Generation of stress in the course of unipolar depression. *Journal of Abnormal Psychology, 100,* 555–561.

Hammen, C., Ellicott, A., & Gitlin, M. (1992). Stressors and sociotropy/autonomy: A longitudinal study of their relationship to the course of bipolar disorder. *Cognitive Therapy and Research, 16,* 409–418.

Hammen, C., Ellicott, A., Gitlin, M., & Jamison, K. (1989). Sociotropy/autonomy and vulnerability to specific life events in patients with unipolar depression and bipolar disorders. *Journal of Abnormal Psychology, 98,* 154–160.

Hammen, C., & Gitlin, M. (1997). Stress reactivity in bipolar patients and its relation to prior history of depression. *American Journal of Psychiatry, 154,* 856–857.

Hammersley, P., Dias, A., Todd, G., Bowen-Jones, K., Reilly, B., & Bentall, R. P. (2003). Childhood trauma and hallucinations in bipolar affective disorder: Preliminary investigation. *British Journal of Psychiatry, 182,* 543–547.

Hankin, B. L., & Abramson, L. Y. (2001). Development of gender differences in depression: An elaborated cognitive vulnerability-transactional stress theory. *Psychological Bulletin, 127,* 773–796.

Hankin, B. L., & Abramson, L. Y. (2002). Measuring cognitive vulnerability to depression in adolescence: Reliability, validity, and gender differences. *Journal of Child and Adolescent Clinical Psychology, 31,* 491–504.

Harmon-Jones, E., Abramson, L. Y., Sigelman, J. D., Bohlig, A., Hogan, M. E., & Harmon-Jones, C. (2002). Proneness to hypomania/mania symptoms or depression symptoms and asymmetrical frontal cortical responses to an anger-evoking event. *Journal of Personality and Social Psychology, 82,* 610–618.

Harmon-Jones, E., & Allen, J. J. B. (1998). Anger and prefrontal brain activity: EEG asymmetry consistent with approach motivation despite negative affect valence. *Journal of Personality and Social Psychology, 74*, 1310–1316.

Harmon-Jones, E., & Sigelman, J. D. (2001). State anger and prefrontal brain activity: Evidence that insult-related relative left prefrontal activity is associated with experienced anger and aggression. *Journal of Personality and Social Psychology, 80*, 797–803.

Harmon-Jones, E., Sigelman, J. D., Bohlig, A., & Harmon-Jones, C. (2003). Anger, coping, and frontal cortical activity: The effect of coping potential on anger-induced left frontal activity. *Cognition and Emotion, 17*, 1–24.

Harris, J. R. (1995). Where is the child's environment?: A group socialization theory of development. *Psychological Review, 102*, 458–489.

Hayward, P., Wong, G., Bright, J. A., & Lam, D. (2002). Stigma and self-esteem in manic depression: An exploratory study. *Journal of Affective Disorders, 69*, 61–67.

Haznedar, M. M., Roversi, F., Pallanti, S., Baldini-Rossi, N., Schnur, D. B., LiCalzi, E. M., et al. (2005). Fronto-thalamo-striatal gray and white matter volumes and anisotropy of their connections in bipolar spectrum illness. *Biological Psychiatry, 57*, 733–742.

Heaton, R. K. (1981). *Wisconsin Card Sorting Test manual.* Odessa, FL: Psychological Assessment Resource.

Hendrick, V., Altshuler, L. L., Gitlin, M. J., Delrahim, S., & Hammen, C. (2000). Gender and bipolar illness. *Journal of Clinical Psychiatry, 61*, 393–396.

Hill, C. V., Oei, T. P., & Hill, M. A. (1989). An empirical investigation of the specificity and sensitivity of the Automatic Thoughts Questionnaire and Dysfunctional Attitudes Scale. *Journal of Psychopathology and Behavioral Assessment, 11*, 291–311.

Hillegers, M. H. J., Reichart, C. G., Wals, M., Verhulst, F. C., Ormel, J., & Nolen, W. A. (2005). Five-year prospective outcome of psychopathology in the adolescent offspring of bipolar parents. *Bipolar Disorders, 7*, 344–350.

Hlastala, S. A., Frank, E., Kowalski, J., Sherrill, J. T., Tu, X. M., Anderson, B., et al. (2000). Stressful life events, bipolar disorder, and the "kindling model." *Journal of Abnormal Psychology, 109*, 777–786.

Hollon, S. D., Kendall, P. C., & Lumry, A. (1986). Specificity of depressogenic cognitions in clinical depression. *Journal of Abnormal Psychology, 95*, 52–59.

Hughes, M. E., Alloy, L. B., Choi, J., Goldstein, K. E., & Black, S. K. (2009). *Responses to positive affect: An examination of positive rumination and dampening.* Manuscript under review.

Hunt, N., Bruce-Jones, W., & Silverstone, T. (1992). Life events and relapse in bipolar affective disorder. *Journal of Affective Disorders, 25*, 13–20.

Hyun, M., Friedman, H. M., & Dunner, D. L. (2000). Relationship of childhood physical and sexual abuse to adult bipolar disorder. *Bipolar Disorders, 2*, 131–135.

Joffe, R. T., MacDonald, C., & Kutcher, S. P. (1989). Life events and mania: A case-controlled study. *Psychiatry Research, 30*, 213–216.

Johnson, L., Andersson-Lundman, G., Aberg-Wistedt, A., & Mathe, A. A. (2000). Age of onset in affective disorder: Its correlation with hereditary and psychosocial factors. *Journal of Affective Disorders, 59*, 139–148.

Johnson, S. L. (2005). Life events in bipolar disorder: Towards more specific models. *Clinical Psychology Review, 25*, 1008–1027.

Johnson, S. L., Cueller, A. K., Ruggero, C., Winett-Perlman, C., Goodnick, P., White, R., et al. (2008). Life events as predictors of mania and depression in bipolar I disorder. *Journal of Abnormal Psychology, 117*, 268–277.

Johnson, S. L., & Fingerhut, R. (2004). Cognitive styles predict the course of bipolar depression, not mania. *Journal of Cognitive Psychotherapy, 18*, 149–162.

Johnson, S. L., McKenzie, G., & McMurrich, S. (2008). Ruminative responses to negative and positive affect among students diagnosed with bipolar disorder and major depressive disorder. *Cognitive Therapy and Research, 32,* 702–713.

Johnson, S. L., Meyer, B., Winett, C., & Small, J. (2000). Social support and self-esteem predict changes in bipolar depression but not mania. *Journal of Affective Disorders, 58,* 79–86.

Johnson, S. L., & Miller, I. (1997). Negative life events and time to recovery from episodes of bipolar disorder. *Journal of Abnormal Psychology, 106,* 449–457.

Johnson, S. L., Sandrow, D., Meyer, B., Winters, R., Miller, I., Solomon, D., et al. (2000). Increases in manic symptoms after life events involving goal attainment. *Journal of Abnormal Psychology, 109,* 721–727.

Joyce, P. R. (1984). Parental bonding in bipolar affective disorder. *Journal of Affective Disorders, 7,* 319–324.

Kaufman, J., Yang, B. Z., Douglas-Palumberi, H., Houshyar, S., Lipschitz, D., Krystal, J. H., et al. (2004). Social supports and serotonin transporter gene moderate depression in maltreated children. *Proceedings of the National Academy of Science, 101,* 17316–17321.

Kawa, I., Carter, J. D., Joyce, P. R., Doughty, C. J., Frampton, C. M., Wells, J. E., et al. (2005). Gender differences in bipolar disorder: Age of onset, course, comorbidity, and symptom presentation. *Bipolar Disorders, 7,* 119–125.

Kawata, M. (1995). Roles of steroid hormones and their receptors in structural organization in the nervous system. *Neuroscience Research, 24,* 1–46.

Keating, D. P. (2005). Cognitive and brain development. In R. J. Lerner & L. D. Steinberg (Eds.), *Handbook of adolescent psychology* (2nd ed.). New York: Wiley.

Kendler, K. S., Kuhn, J. W., Vittum, J., Prescott, C. A., & Riley, B. (2005). The interaction of stressful life events and a serotonin transporter polymorphism in the prediction of episodes of major depression: A replication. *Archives of General Psychiatry, 62,* 529–535.

Kennedy, N., Boydell, J., Kalidindi, S., Fearon, P., Jones, P. B., van Os, J., et al. (2005). Gender differences in incidence and age at onset of mania and bipolar disorder over a 35-year period in Camberwell, England. *American Journal of Psychiatry, 162,* 257–262.

Kennedy, S., Thompson, R., Stancer, H. C., Roy, A., & Persad, E. (1983). Life events precipitating mania. *British Journal of Psychiatry, 142,* 398–403.

Kessler, R. C., Rubinow, D. R., Holmes, C., Abelson, J. M., & Zhao, S. (1997). The epidemiology of DSM-III-R bipolar I disorder in a general population survey. *Psychological Medicine, 27,* 1079–1089.

Kieseppa, T., Partonen, T., Haukka, J., Kaprio, J., & Lonnqvis, J. (2004). High concordance of bipolar I disorder in a nationwide sample of twins. *American Journal of Psychiatry, 161,* 1814–1821.

Kimberg, D. Y., & Farah, M. J. (1993). A unified account of cognitive impairments following frontal lobe damage: The role of working memory in complex, organized behavior. *Journal of Experimental Psychology: General, 112,* 411–428.

Koenig, J. E., Sachs-Ericsson, N., & Miklowitz, D. J. (1997). How do psychiatric patients experience interactions with their relatives? *Journal of Family Psychology, 11,* 251–256.

Kupfer, D. J., Frank, E., Grochocinski, V. J., Cluss, P. A., Houck, P. R., & Stapf, D. A. (2002). Demographic and clinical characteristics of individuals in a bipolar disorder case registry. *Journal of Clinical Psychiatry, 63,* 120–125.

Lam, D., Wright, K., & Smith, N. (2004). Dysfunctional assumptions in bipolar disorder. *Journal of Affective Disorders, 79,* 193–199.

Lau, J. Y. F., Rijsdijk, F., & Eley, T. C. (2006). I think, therefore I am: A twin study of attributional style in adolescents. *Journal of Clinical Psychology and Psychiatry, 47,* 696–703.

Leibenluft, E. (1996). Women with bipolar illness: Clinical and research issues. *American Journal of Psychiatry, 153,* 163–173.

Leibenluft, E., Charney, D. S., & Pine, D. S. (2003). Researching the pathophysiology of pediatric bipolar disorder. *Biological Psychiatry, 53,* 1009–1020.

Leverich, G. S., McElroy, S. L., Suppes, T., Keck, P. E., Jr., Denicoff, K. D., Nolen, W. A., et al. (2002). Early physical or sexual abuse and the course of bipolar illness. *Biological Psychiatry, 51,* 288–297.

Levitan, R. D., Parikh, S. V., Lesage, A. D., Hegadoren, K. M., Adams, M., Kennedy, S. H., et al. (1997). Major depression in individuals with a history of childhood physical or sexual abuse: Relationship to neurovegetative features, mania, and gender. *American Journal of Psychiatry, 155,* 1746–1752.

Liu, R. T., Alloy, L. B., Abramson, L. Y., Iacoviello, B. M., & Whitehouse, W. G. (2009). Emotional maltreatment and depression: Prospective prediction of depressive episodes. *Depression and Anxiety, 26,* 174–181.

Liu, S. K., Chiu, C. H., Chang, C. J., Hwang, T. J., Hwu, H. G., & Chen, W. J. (2002). Deficits in sustained attention in schizophrenia and affective disorders: Stable versus state-dependent markers. *American Journal of Psychiatry, 159,* 975–982.

Liu, X., & Kaplan, H. B. (1999). Explaining gender differences in symptoms of subjective distress in young adolescents. *Stress Medicine, 15,* 41–51.

Lopez-Larson, M. P., DelBello, M. P., Zimmerman, M. E., Schwiers, M. L., & Strakowski, S. M. (2002). Regional prefrontal gray and white matter abnormalities in bipolar disorder. *Biological Psychiatry, 52,* 93–100.

Lovejoy, M. C., & Steuerwald, B. L. (1997). Subsyndromal unipolar and bipolar disorders: II. Comparisons on daily stress levels. *Cognitive Therapy and Research, 21,* 607–618.

Lozano, B. E., & Johnson, S. L. (2001). Can personality traits predict increases in manic and depressive symptoms? *Journal of Affective Disorders, 63,* 103–111.

Lyon, H. M., Startup, M., & Bentall, R. P. (1999). Social cognition and the manic defense: Attributions, selective attention, and self-schema in bipolar affective disorder. *Journal of Abnormal Psychology, 108,* 273–282.

Lyoo, K., Lee, H. K., Jung, J. H., Noam, G. G., & Renshaw, P. F. (2002). White matter hyperintensities on magnetic resonance imaging of the brain in children with psychiatric disorders. *Comprehensive Psychiatry, 43,* 361–368.

MacVane, J. R., Lange, J. D., Brown, W. A., & Zayat, M. (1978). Psychological functioning of bipolar manic-depressives in remission. *Archives of General Psychiatry, 35,* 1351–1354.

Martínez-Arán, A., Vieta, E., Colom, F., Torrent, C., Sánchez-Moreno, J., Reinares, M., et al. (2004). Cognitive impairment in euthymic bipolar patients: Implications for clinical and functional outcome. *Bipolar Disorders, 6,* 224–232.

Martínez-Arán, A., Vieta, E., Reinares, M., Colom, F., Torrent, C., Sánchez-Moreno, J., et al. (2004). Cognitive function across manic or hypomanic, depressed, and euthymic states in bipolar disorder. *American Journal of Psychiatry, 161,* 262–270.

McGuffin, P., Rijsdijk, F., Andrew, M., Sham, P., Katz, R., & Cardno, A. (2003). The heritability of bipolar affective disorder and the genetic relationship to unipolar depression. *Archives of General Psychiatry, 60,* 497–502.

McPherson, H., Herbison, P., & Romans, S. (1993). Life events and relapse in established bipolar affective disorder. *British Journal of Psychiatry, 163,* 381–385.

Meaney, M. J. (2007). Maternal programming of defensive responses through sustained effects on gene expression. In D. Romer & E. F. Walker (Eds.), *Adolescent psychopathology and the developing brain: Integrating brain and prevention science* (pp. 148–172). New York: Oxford University Press.

Merikangas, K. R., Chakravarti, A., Moldin, S. O., Araj, H., Blangero, J. C., Burmeister, M., et al. (2002). Future of genetics of mood disorders research. *Biological Psychiatry, 52,* 457–477.

Meyer, J. H., Houle, S., Sagrati, S., Carella, A., Hussey, D. F., Ginovart, N., et al. (2004). Brain serotonin transporter binding potential measured with carbon 11-labeled DASB positron emission tomography: Effects of major depressive episodes and severity of dysfunctional attitudes. *Archives of General Psychiatry, 61,* 1271–1279.

Meyer, J. H., McMain, S., Kennedy, S., Korman, L., Brown, G., DaSilva, J., et al. (2003). Dysfunctional attitudes and serotonin$_2$ receptors during depression and self-harm. *American Journal of Psychiatry, 160,* 90–99.

Meyer, S. E., Carlson, G. A., Wiggs, E. A., Martinez, P. E., Ronsaville, D. S., Klimes-Dougan, B., et al. (2004). A prospective study of the association among impaired executive functioning, childhood attentional problems, and the development of bipolar disorder. *Development and Psychopathology, 16,* 461–476.

Meyer, T. D., & Krumm-Merabet, C. (2003). Academic performance and expectations for the future in relation to a vulnerability marker for bipolar disorders: The hypomanic temperament. *Personality and Individual Differences, 35,* 785–796.

Mezulis, A. H., Abramson, L. Y., Hyde, J. S., & Hankin, B. L. (2004). Is there a universal positivity bias in attributions?: A meta-analytic review of individual, developmental, and cultural differences in the self-serving attributional bias. *Psychological Bulletin, 130,* 711–747.

Mick, E., Biederman, M. D., Faraone, S. V., Murray, K., & Wozniak, J. (2003). Defining a developmental subtype of bipolar disorder in a sample of nonreferred adults by age of onset. *Journal of Child and Adolescent Psychopharmacology, 13,* 453–462.

Miklowitz, D. J., Goldstein, M. J., & Nuechterlein, K. H. (1995). Verbal interactions in the families of schizophrenic and bipolar affective patients. *Journal of Abnormal Psychology, 104,* 268–276.

Miklowitz, D. J., Goldstein, M. J., Nuechterlein, K. H., Snyder, K. S., & Mintz, J. (1988). Family factors and the course of bipolar affective disorder. *Archives of General Psychiatry, 45,* 225–231.

Miller, E. M., & Shields, S. A. (1980). Skin conductance response as a measure of adolescents' emotional reactivity. *Psychological Reports, 46,* 587–590.

Monroe, S. M., & Harkness, K. L. (2005). Life stress, the "kindling" hypothesis, and the recurrence of depression: Considerations from a life stress perspective. *Psychological Review, 112,* 417–445.

Morice, R. (1990). Cognitive inflexibility and pre-frontal dysfunction in schizophrenia and mania. *British Journal of Psychiatry, 157,* 50–54.

Mueser, K. T., Goodman, L. B., Trumbetta, S. L., Rosenberg, S. D., Osher, F. C., Vidaver, R., et al. (1998). Trauma and posttraumatic stress disorder in severe mental illness. *Journal of Consulting and Clinical Psychology, 66,* 493–499.

Murphy, F. C., Sahakian, B. J., Rubinsztein, J. S., Michael, A., Rogers, R. D., Robbins, T. W., et al. (1999). Emotional bias and inhibitory control processes in mania and depression. *Psychological Medicine, 29,* 1307–1321.

Neeren, A. M., Alloy, L. B., & Abramson, L. Y. (2008). History of parenting and bipolar spectrum disorders. *Journal of Social and Clinical Psychology, 27,* 1021–1044.

Nolen-Hoeksema, A. (1990). *Sex differences in depression.* Stanford, CA: Stanford University Press.

Nolen-Hoeksema, S. (1991). Responses to depression and their effects on the duration of the depressive episode. *Journal of Abnormal Psychology, 100,* 569–582.

Nolen-Hoeksema, S. (2000). The role of rumination in depressive disorders and mixed anxiety/depressive symptoms. *Journal of Abnormal Psychology, 109,* 504–511.

Nolen-Hoeksema, S., Girgus, J. S., & Seligman, M. E. P. (1992). Predictors and consequences of childhood depressive symptoms: A 5-year longitudinal study. *Journal of Abnormal Psychology, 101,* 405–422.

Nolen-Hoeksema, S., & Jackson, B. (2001). Mediators of the gender difference in rumination. *Psychology of Women Quarterly, 25,* 37–47.

Nusslock, C. R., Abramson, L. Y., Harmon-Jones, E., Alloy, L. B., & Hogan, M. E. (2007). A goal-striving life event and the onset of bipolar episodes: Perspective from the behavioral approach system (BAS) dysregulation theory. *Journal of Abnormal Psychology, 116,* 105–115.

O'Connell, R. A., Mayo, J. A., Flatow, L., Cuthbertson, B., & O'Brien, B. E. (1991). Outcome of bipolar disorder on long-term treatment with lithium. *British Journal of Psychiatry, 159,* 123–129.

Ongur, D., Drevets, W. C., & Price, J. L. (1998). Glial reduction in the subgenual prefrontal cortex in mood disorders. *Proceedings of the National Academy of Sciences USA, 95,* 13290–13295.

Owen, A. M. (2000). The role of the lateral frontal cortex in mnemonic processing: The contribution of functional neuroimaging. *Experimental Brain Research, 133,* 33–43.

Panzarella, C., Alloy, L. B., & Whitehouse, W. G. (2006). Expanded hopelessness theory of depression: On the mechanisms by which social support protects against depression. *Cognitive Therapy and Research, 30,* 307–333.

Pardoen, D., Bauwens, F., Dramaix, M., Tracy, A., Genevrois, C., Staner, L., et al. (1996). Life events and primary affective disorders: A one year prospective study. *British Journal of Psychiatry, 169,* 160–166.

Pardoen, D., Bauwens, F., Tracy, A., Martin, F., & Mendlewicz, J. (1993). Self-esteem in recovered bipolar and unipolar out-patients. *British Journal of Psychiatry, 163,* 755–762.

Parker, G. (1979). Parental characteristics in relation to depressive disorders. *British Journal of Psychiatry, 134,* 138–147.

Parker, G. (1983). Parental "affectionless control" as an antecedent to adult depression. *Archives of General Psychiatry, 34,* 138–147.

Paus, T. (2005). Mapping brain maturation and cognitive development during adolescence. *Trends in Cognitive Sciences, 9,* 60–68.

Perris, C., Arrindell, E., Van der Ende, J. V., & Knorr, L. (1986). Perceived depriving parental rearing and depression. *British Journal of Psychiatry, 148,* 170–175.

Perris, H. (1984). Life events and depression: Part 2. Results in diagnostic subgroups, and in relation to the recurrence of depression. *Journal of Affective Disorders, 7,* 25–36.

Pine, D. S., Cohen, P., Johnson, J. G., & Brook, J. S. (2002). Adolescent life events as predictors of adult depression. *Journal of Affective Disorders, 68,* 49–57.

Post, R. (1992). Transduction of psychosocial stress into the neurobiology of recurrent affective disorders. *American Journal of Psychiatry, 149,* 999–1010.

Post, R. M., & Leverich, G. S. (2006). The role of psychosocial stress in the onset and progression of bipolar disorder and its comorbidities: The need for earlier and alternative modes of therapeutic intervention. *Development and Psychopathology, 18,* 1181–1211.

Priebe, S., Wildgrube, C., & Muller-Oerlinghausen, B. (1989). Lithium prophylaxis and expressed emotion. *British Journal of Psychiatry, 154,* 396–399.

Pyszczynski, T., & Greenberg, J. (1987). Self-regulatory perseveration and the depressive self-focusing style: A self-awareness theory of reactive depression. *Psychological Bulletin, 102,* 122–138.

Rajkowska, G., Halaris, A., & Selemon, L. D. (2001). Reductions in neuronal and glial density characterize the dorsolateral prefrontal cortex in bipolar disorder. *Biological Psychiatry, 49,* 741–752.

Rasgon, N., Bauer, M., Grof, P., Gyulai, L., Elman, S., Glenn, T., et al. (2005). Sex-specific self-reported mood changes by patients with bipolar disorder. *Journal of Psychiatric Research, 39,* 77–83.

Reilly-Harrington, N. A., Alloy, L. B., Fresco, D. M., & Whitehouse, W. G. (1999). Cognitive styles and life events interact to predict bipolar and unipolar symptomatology. *Journal of Abnormal Psychology, 108*, 567–578.

Rice, F., Harold, G. T., & Thapar, A. (2003). Negative life events as an account of age-related differences in the genetic aetiology of depression in childhood and adolescence. *Journal of Child Psychology and Psychiatry and Allied Disciplines, 44*, 977–987.

Robb, J. C., Young, L. T., Cooke, R. G., & Joffe, R. T. (1998). Gender differences in patients with bipolar disorder influence outcome in the Medical Outcomes Survey (SF-20) subscale scores. *Journal of Affective Disorders, 49*, 189–193.

Robertson, H. A., Kutcher, S. P., & Lagace, D. C. (2003). No evidence of attentional deficits in stabilized bipolar youth relative to unipolar and control comparators. *Bipolar Disorders, 5*, 330–339.

Robinson, M. S., & Alloy, L. B. (2003). Negative cognitive styles and stress-reactive rumination interact to predict depression: A prospective study. *Cognitive Therapy and Research, 27*, 275–291.

Rose, D. T., & Abramson, L. Y. (1992). Developmental predictors of depressive cognitive style: Research and theory. In D. Cicchetti & S. Toth (Eds.), *Rochester Symposium on Developmental Psychopathology* (Vol. IV, pp. 323–349). Rochester, NY: University of Rochester Press.

Rosenberg, D., & Lewis, D. (1995). Postnatal maturation of the dopaminergic innervation of monkey prefrontal and motor cortices: A tyrosine hydroxylase immunohistochemical analysis. *Journal of Comparative Neurology, 358*, 383–400.

Rosenfarb, I. S., Becker, J., & Khan, A. (1994). Perceptions of parental and peer attachments by women with mood disorders. *Journal of Abnormal Psychology, 103*, 637–644.

Rosenfarb, I. S., Becker, J., Khan, A., & Mintz, J. (1998). Dependency and self-criticism in bipolar and unipolar depressed women. *British Journal of Clinical Psychology, 37*, 409–414.

Rosenfarb, I. S., Miklowitz, D. J., Goldstein, M. J., Harmon, L., Nuechterlein, K. H., & Rea, M. M. (2001). Family transactions and relapse in bipolar disorder. *Family Process, 40*, 5–14.

Roy-Byrne, P., Post, R. M., Uhde, T. W., Porcu, T., & Davis, D. (1985). The longitudinal course of recurrent affective illness: Life chart data from research patients at the NIMH. *Acta Psychiatrica Scandinavica Supplement, 317*, 1–34.

Safford, S. M., Alloy, L. B., Abramson, L. Y., & Crossfield, A. G. (2007). Negative cognitive style as a predictor of negative life events in depression-prone individuals: A test of the stress generation hypothesis. *Journal of Affective Disorders, 99*, 147–154.

Sax, K. W., Strakowski, S. M., Keck, P. E., Jr., McElroy, S. L., West, S. A., & Stanton, S. P. (1998). Symptom correlates of attentional improvement following hospitalization for a first episode of affective psychosis. *Biological Psychiatry, 44*, 784–786.

Sax, K. W., Strakowski, S. M., McElroy, S. L., Keck, P. E., Jr., & West, S. A. (1995). Attention and formal thought disorder in mixed and pure mania. *Biological Psychiatry, 37*, 420–423.

Sax, K. W., Strakowski, S. M., Zimmerman, M. E., DelBello, M. P., Keck, P. E., Jr., & Hawkins, J. M. (1999). Frontosubcortical neuroanatomy and the continuous performance test in mania. *American Journal of Psychiatry, 156*, 139–141.

Schulman, P., Keith, D., & Seligman, M. E. P. (1993). Is optimism heritable: A study of twins. *Behaviour Research and Therapy, 31*, 569–574.

Sclare, P., & Creed, F. (1990). Life events and the onset of mania. *British Journal of Psychiatry, 156*, 508–514.

Scott, J., & Pope, M. (2003). Cognitive styles in individuals with bipolar disorders. *Psychological Medicine, 33*, 1081–1088.

Scott, J., Stanton, B., Garland, A., & Ferrier, I. N. (2000). Cognitive vulnerability in patients with bipolar disorder. *Psychological Medicine, 30,* 467–472.

Segerstrom, S. C., Stanton, A. L., Alden, L. E., & Shortridge, B. E. (2003). A multidimensional structure for repetitive thought: What's on your mind, and how, and how much? *Journal of Personality and Social Psychology, 85,* 909–921.

Shaw, J. A., Egeland, J. A., Endicott, J., Allen, C. R., & Hostetter, A. M. (2005). A 10-year prospective study of prodromal patterns for bipolar disorder among Amish youth. *Journal of the American Academy of Child and Adolescent Psychiatry, 44,* 1104–1111.

Shen, G. C., Alloy, L. B., Abramson, L. Y., & Sylvia, L. G. (2008). Social rhythm regularity and the onset of affective episodes in bipolar spectrum individuals. *Bipolar Disorders, 10,* 520–529.

Silberg, J. L., Pickles, A., Rutter, M., Hewitt, J., Simonoff, E., Maes, H., et al. (1999). The influence of genetic factors and life stress on depression among adolescent girls. *Archives of General Psychiatry, 56,* 225–232.

Simoneau, T. L., Miklowitz, D. J., & Saleem, R. (1998). Expressed emotion and interactional patterns in the families of bipolar patients. *Journal of Abnormal Psychology, 107,* 497–507.

Sisk, C., & Foster, D. (2004). The neural basis of puberty and adolescence. *Nature Neuroscience, 7,* 1040–1047.

Sisk, C., & Zehr, J. (2005). Pubertal hormones organize the adolescent brain and behavior. *Frontiers in Neuroendocrinology, 26,* 163–174.

Smith, J. M., Floyd, T. D., Alloy, L. B., Hughes, M., & Neeren, A. M. (2009). *An integrated model of the gender difference in depression: Pubertal development, response style, and body dissatisfaction.* Manuscript submitted for publication.

Sowell, E. R., Thompson, P. R., & Toga, A. W. (2007). Mapping adolescent brain maturation using structural magnetic resonance imaging. In D. Romer & E. F. Walker (Eds.), *Adolescent psychopathology and the developing brain: Integrating brain and prevention science* (pp. 55–84). New York: Oxford University Press.

Spasojevic, J., & Alloy, L. B. (2001). Rumination as a common mechanism relating depressive risk factors to depression. *Emotion, 1,* 25–37.

Spasojevic, J., & Alloy, L. B. (2002). Who becomes a depressive ruminator?: Developmental antecedents of ruminative response style. *Journal of Cognitive Psychotherapy, 16,* 405–419.

Spear, L. P. (2000). The adolescent brain and age-related behavioral manifestations. *Neuroscience Biobehavioral Review, 24,* 417–463.

Spear, L. P. (2007). The developing brain and adolescent-typical behavior patterns: An evolutionary approach. In D. Romer & E. F. Walker (Eds.), *Adolescent psychopathology and the developing brain: Integrating brain and prevention science* (pp. 9–30). New York: Oxford University Press.

Steinberg, L. (2002). Clinical adolescent psychology: What it is, and what it needs to be. *Journal of Consulting and Clinical Psychology, 70,* 124–128.

Steinberg, L. (2008). A social neuroscience perspective on adolescent risk-taking. *Developmental Review, 28,* 78–106.

Steinberg, L., Dahl, R., Keating, D., Kupfer, D. J., Masten, A. S., & Pine, D. (2006). Psychopathology in adolescence: Integrating affective neuroscience with the study of context. In D. Cicchetti & D. Cohen (Eds.), *Developmental psychopathology: Vol. 2. Developmental neuroscience* (pp. 710–741). New York: Wiley.

Steinberg, L., Graham, S., O'Brien, L., Woolard, J., Cauffman, E., & Banich, M. (2009). Age differences in future orientation and delay discounting. *Child Development, 80,* 28–44.

Strakowski, S. M., Adler, C. M., Holland, S. K., Mills, N., & DelBello, M. P. (2004). A preliminary fMRI study of sustained attention in euthymic, unmedicated bipolar disorder. *Neuropsychopharmacology, 29,* 1734–1740.

Strober, M., Morrell, W., Burroughs, J., Lampert, C., Danforth, H., & Freeman, R. (1988). A family study of bipolar I disorder in adolescence: Early onset of symptoms linked to increased familial loading and lithium resistance. *Journal of Affective Disorders, 15,* 255–268.

Stroop, J. R. (1935). Studies of interference in serial verbal reactions. *Journal of Experimental Psychology, 18,* 643–662.

Swann, A. C., Anderson, J. C., Dougherty, D. M., & Moeller, F. G. (2001). Measurement of inter-episode impulsivity in bipolar disorder. *Psychiatry Research, 101,* 195–197.

Swendsen, J., Hammen, C., Heller, T., & Gitlin, M. (1995). Correlates of stress reactivity in patients with bipolar disorder. *American Journal of Psychiatry, 152,* 795–797.

Thompson, J. M., Gallagher, P., Hughes, J. H., Watson, S., Gray, J. M., Ferrier, I. N., et al. (2005). Neurocognitive impairment in euthymic patients with bipolar affective disorder. *British Journal of Psychiatry, 186,* 32–40.

Thompson, M., & Bentall, R. P. (1990). Hypomanic personality and attributional style. *Personality and Individual Differences, 11,* 867–868.

Tien, A., Ross, D. E., Pearlson, G., & Strauss, M. E. (1996). Eye movements and psychopathology in schizophrenia and bipolar disorder. *Journal of Nervous and Mental Disease, 184,* 331–338.

Tracy, A., Bauwens, F., Martin, F., Pardoen, D., & Mendlewicz, J. (1992). Attributional style and depression: A controlled comparison of remitted unipolar and bipolar patients. *British Journal of Clinical Psychology, 31,* 83–84.

Turner, J. E., Jr., & Cole, D. A. (1994). Developmental differences in cognitive diatheses for child depression. *Journal of Abnormal Child Psychology, 22,* 15–32.

Urosevic, S., Abramson, L. Y., Alloy, L. B., Nusslock, R., Harmon-Jones, E., Bender, R. E., et al. (2009). *Increased rates of behavioral approach system (BAS) activating and deactivating, but not goal-attainment, events in bipolar spectrum disorders.* Manuscript under review.

Urosevic, S., Abramson, L. Y., Harmon-Jones, E., & Alloy, L. B. (2008). Dysregulation of the behavioral approach system (BAS) and bipolar spectrum disorders: Review of theory and evidence. *Clinical Psychology Review, 28,* 1188–1205.

Verdoux, H., & Liraud, F. (2000). Neuropsychological function in subjects with psychotic and affective disorders. Relationship to diagnostic category and duration of illness. *European Psychiatry, 15,* 236–243.

Viguera, A. C., Baldessarini, R. J., & Tondo, L. (2001). Response to lithium maintenance treatment in bipolar disorders: Comparison of women and men. *Bipolar Disorders, 3,* 245–252.

Wagner, C. A., Alloy, L. B., & Abramson, L. Y. (2009). *Parenting, behavioral approach system (BAS)—relevant cognitive styles, and diagnosis and course of bipolar spectrum disorders.* Manuscript under review.

Walker, E. F., McMillan, A., & Mittal, V. (2007). Neurohormones, neurodevelopment and the prodrome of psychosis in adolescence. In D. Romer & E. F. Walker (Eds.), *Adolescent psychopathology and the developing brain: Integrating brain and prevention science* (pp. 264–283). New York: Oxford University Press.

Walker, E. F., Sabuwalla, Z., & Huot, R. (2004). Pubertal neuromaturation, stress sensitivity, and psychopathology. *Development and Psychopathology, 16,* 807–824.

Walshaw, P. D., Alloy, L. B., & Sabb, F. W. (in press). Executive function in bipolar disorder and attention-deficit hyperactivity disorder: In search of distinct phenotypic profiles. Manuscript submitted for publication. *Neuropsychology Review.*

Weissman, M. M., Bland, R. C., Canino, G. J., Faravelli, C., Greenwald, S., Hwu, H. G., et al.

(1996). Cross-national epidemiology of major depression and bipolar disorder. *Journal of the American Medical Association, 276*, 293–299.

Wexler, B. E., Lyons, L., Lyons, H., & Mazure, C. M. (1997). Physical and sexual abuse during childhood and development of psychiatric illnesses during adulthood. *Journal of Nervous and Mental Disease, 185*, 522–534.

Wilder-Willis, K. E., Sax, K. W., Rosenberg, H. L., Fleck, D. E., Shear, P. K., & Strakowski, S. M. (2001). Persistent attentional dysfunction in remitted bipolar disorder. *Bipolar Disorders, 3*, 58–62.

Winters, K. C., & Neale, J. M. (1985). Mania and low self-esteem. *Journal of Abnormal Psychology, 94*, 282–290.

Wozniak, J., Biederman, J., Kiley, K., Ablon, J. S., Faraone, S. V., Mundy, E., et al. (1995). Mania-like symptoms suggestive of childhood-onset bipolar disorder in clinically referred children. *Journal of the American Academy of Child and Adolescent Psychiatry, 34*, 867–877.

Yan, L., Hammen, C., Cohen, A., Daley, S., & Henry, R. (2004). Expressed emotion versus relationship quality variables in the prediction of recurrence in bipolar patients. *Journal of Affective Disorders, 83*, 199–206.

Yurgelun-Todd, D. A., Gruber, S. A., Kanayama, G., Kilgore, W. D., Baird, A. A., & Young, A. D. (2000). fMRI during affect discrimination in bipolar affective disorder. *Bipolar Disorders, 2*, 237–248.

Zalla, T., Joyce, C., Szoke, A., Schurhoff, F., Pillon, B., Komano, O., et al. (2004). Executive dysfunction as potential markers of familial vulnerability to bipolar disorder and schizophrenia. *Psychiatry Research, 121*, 207–217.

CHAPTER 11

Social Cognition and Cognitive Flexibility in Bipolar Disorder

Erin B. McClure-Tone

A rapidly growing literature examines the impact of bipolar disorder (BD) on social cognition, or patterns of thought about interpersonal interaction, and social behavior. Considerable evidence indicates that acquisition and implementation of an array of social cognitive and behavioral skills are disrupted in the context of this psychiatric illness. Furthermore, numerous studies link the social deficits evident in BD with atypical development in brain regions implicated in social and emotional processing. Elucidating the social disruptions evident across the life span in individuals with BD, how these disruptions relate to specific behavioral deficits or endophenotypes, and their underlying neural mechanisms may help inform our understanding not only of psychopathological processes but also of typical social development at the behavioral and neural levels. Additionally, clarification of social deficits and strengths associated with BD, as well as their neural underpinnings, may facilitate the development of effective and explicitly targeted interventions.

Several factors, however, complicate the description and evaluation of social functioning, its component processes, and their typical or atypical development in the context of BD. First and foremost, researchers and clinicians have in recent years classified a diversity of conditions as representative of the BD spectrum, particularly among children and adolescents (Geller et al., 2003; Leibenluft, Charney, Towbin, Bhangoo, & Pine, 2003; Soutullo et al., 2005; Staton, Volness, & Beatty, 2008; Youngstrom, Birmaher, & Findling, 2008). Whether or not symptoms such as grandiosity or elation need to be present in youth and how best to define these symptoms in youth of different ages remain controversial (Staton et al., 2008), as do the boundaries between attention-deficit/hyperactivity disorder

(ADHD) and the BD spectrum (Galanter & Leibenluft, 2008). Furthermore, some researchers have developed criteria for distinguishing strictly diagnosed BD from related conditions; Leibenluft, Charney, and colleagues (2003), for example, make a distinction between narrow and broad phenotypes for mania in pediatric BD. According to this system, individuals with the narrow phenotype meet full *Diagnostic and Statistical Manual of Mental Disorders*, fourth edition (DSM-IV; American Psychiatric Association, 1994) diagnostic criteria for hypomania or mania; those with a related, but broader, phenotype that they term severe mood dysregulation (SMD) exhibit severe irritability and hyperarousal, but do not show the hallmark symptoms of elation or grandiosity (Leibenluft, Charney, et al., 2003). Finally, the role of irritability in BD has been extensively debated (Biederman, Klein, Pine, & Klein, 1998; Leibenluft, Blair, Charney, & Pine, 2003; Leibenluft, Cohen, Gorrindo, Brook, & Pine, 2006). This issue has been complicated to resolve, in part because irritability is normatively common, particularly during some developmental periods, and also frequently reported as characteristic of youth with a range of psychopathology (Leibenluft, Blair, et al., 2003). Thus, not surprisingly, different research groups over the past decade have used varied inclusion criteria to identify participants with pediatric BD, rendering direct comparisons of results across studies difficult. Because of the importance of clarity around fundamental issues of diagnosis and categorization, this chapter will note instances where criteria used to identify youth with BD vary from those listed in the DSM (American Psychiatric Association, 1994).

Second, it remains unclear whether social impairments associated with BD are state dependent (i.e., present only during mood episodes) or reflective of enduring trait-like characteristics that influence cognition and behavior even when individuals are asymptomatic. Commendably, many studies now clearly describe participants' mood states and medications at the time of research participation, and a growing body of research compares medicated and unmedicated and/or euthymic and symptomatic subgroups. Almost no research, however, has looked at whether patterns of social cognition and behavior differ *within* individuals when they are euthymic versus symptomatic or medicated versus unmedicated. This gap in the literature reflects the complexity of conducting such studies. Although within-subject research is of great interest, it is difficult to carry out. Thus, little is known about whether patterns of performance on research tasks reflect stable or transient deficits or strengths within individuals.

Third, the impact of acute BD symptoms and more stable illness-related deficits on social cognition and behavior is likely to vary across development, given differing social demands and expectations that individuals face at different ages. Mood-related behaviors or intensity levels that are considered typical at one developmental stage (e.g., need-related crying among infants, irritability in mid-adolescence) may be considered atypical at other points (Leibenluft et al., 2006; St. James-Roberts & Plewis, 1996). Thus, the developmental context of the affected individual, both at the time of study participation and at illness onset, should ideally be taken into account in evaluating the roles that symp-

---

GOALS OF THIS CHAPTER

- Within a developmental psychopathology context, review the literature regarding affective cue processing, flexible response generation and inhibition, and management of affective states in BD across the life span.
- Identify similarities and differences in social functioning between individuals with and without BD.
- Highlight study, participant, and task characteristics that complicate the interpretation of findings.

---

toms, illness-related deficits, and risk-related deficits play in social success or impairment. Onset before adolescence, for example, may interfere with the successful mastery of basic social cognitive skills (e.g., facial expression decoding or response inhibition) that form the basis of later emerging, more complex skills. In contrast, later onset of illness may result in a markedly different pattern of spared and impaired functions.

The following review of select aspects of social cognitive and behavioral development as they relate to BD is written with an effort to take these complicating factors into account. This review briefly summarizes primary social milestones and their emergence during typical development as well as what we know about their neural underpinnings. It then shifts focus to the literature regarding social functioning in individuals with BD across development and, finally, examines behavioral and neural research regarding component social cognitive and behavioral processes in affected individuals and those who are genetically at risk for BD. There is a particular focus on affective cue processing, flexible response generation and inhibition, and management of affective states that are likely to interfere with effective implementation of these skills.

Typical Social Cognitive Development

Across development, social success depends on the ability to navigate complex, frequently shifting interpersonal and environmental demands. This navigation requires the integration of multiple discrete skills, including accurately perceiving and interpreting social cues, responding flexibly and appropriately to those cues, and regulating one's own emotional reactions throughout (Crick & Dodge, 1994). In typical development, these skills emerge gradually from infancy through adulthood, evolving as the individual negotiates increasingly complex social interactions. In the first years of life, infants learn to use adult cues as reference points, laying a foundation of core social cognitive skills, including joint attention and the capacity for progressively more sophisticated dyadic and triadic interactions with people and objects (Carpenter, Nagell, & Tomasello, 1998). During the preschool years, as their verbal and nonverbal language skills develop, children build on this social cognitive base to become increasingly adept at discriminating among and interpreting social and emotional cues such as facial expressions (McClure, 2000); theorizing about others' states of mind (Milligan, Astington, & Dack, 2007; Wellman, Lopez-Duran, LaBounty, & Hamilton, 2008); and selecting or inhibiting behavioral responses in accordance with situational demands (Lagattuta, 2005).

In the middle childhood period, between approximately 7 and 11 years of age, as peer relationships become increasingly important and focused on mutual trust and assistance (Sullivan, 1953), social cognitive skills refine and expand. Children develop more complex mechanisms for managing their emotions and behaviors in stressful situations (Kliewer, Fearnow, & Miller, 1996), conform more tightly to social rules for displaying emotion (Jones, Abbey, & Cumberland, 1998), become more sophisticated in their understanding of others' mental states (Schwanenflugel, Fabricius, & Alexander, 1994), and learn to implement more flexibly a broad array of tools for and approaches to social problem solving (Crick & Dodge, 1994). These skills continue to develop through adolescence and into adulthood, with successful mastery increasingly important for both personal and occupational success (Fullerton & Ursano, 1994; Reisman, 1985).

Neural Underpinnings of Social Cognitive Development

The acquisition of social cognitive and behavioral skills, a process that begins early in development, appears to depend, at least in part, on the healthy maturation of a core set of interconnected neural structures (Blakemore, 2008; Nelson, Leibenluft, McClure, & Pine, 2005; Paterson, Heim, Friedman, Choudhury, & Benasich, 2006). These brain regions, which undergo structural and functional changes from infancy through adulthood (Giedd, 2004; Gogtay et al., 2004; Sowell, Trauner, Gamst, & Jernigan, 2002), constitute what Nelson and colleagues (2005) have termed the social information processing network (SIPN). This network consists of three reciprocally interactive primary "nodes": the detection node, the affective node, and the cognitive-regulatory node.

The detection node includes the superior temporal sulcus, fusiform face area, and inferior temporal and occipital cortices, all structures that play key roles in the detection and decoding of socially salient environmental features. Available data, which include findings from electrophysiological studies demonstrating distinct neural responses to various classes of social stimuli in human infants, suggest that functional aspects of this node mature as early as the first years of life (Halit, Csibra, Volein, & Johnson, 2004; Halit, de Haan, & Johnson, 2003; Johnson et al., 2005).

The affective node, which comprises regions engaged by reward or punishment cues (e.g., amygdala and ventral striatum), evaluates the emotional significance of salient stimuli and participates in the coordination of appropriate behavioral responses. Available data in nonhuman species suggest that structures within this node contribute to social cognition and behavior in meaningful ways as early as the neonatal period (Bauman, Lavenex, Mason, Capitanio, & Amaral, 2004; Goursaud & Bachevalier, 2007). They continue to evolve across development, undergoing relatively abrupt functional and structural changes during the surge of gonadal hormones that accompanies puberty (Giedd, Castellanos, Rajapakse, Vaituzis, & Rapoport, 1997; Nelson et al., 2005).

The cognitive-regulatory node encompasses several regions within the frontal cortices. Structures within this node, which appear to continue developing well into adolescence and early adulthood (Gogtay et al., 2004), participate in theory-of-mind processes (e.g., attributing mental states to others), inhibition of prepotent responses, and generation of goal-directed behavior (Nelson et al., 2005). Evidence from animal studies indicates that projections between the cognitive-regulatory and affective/detection nodes are consistent with reciprocal feedback loops, such that activity in one node influences or modifies activity in others (Barbas, 2007). Thus, atypical functioning in one node is likely to affect functioning in other nodes, even those that might, in artificial isolation, operate in typical ways.

Interestingly, the different developmental courses for structures in the detection, affective, and cognitive-regulatory nodes might relate to the emergence of dysfunctional behavior patterns at different developmental stages. Many investigators have speculated, for example, about the degree to which adolescent impulsivity and risk taking stem from emotional influences and other processes mediated by the affective node, in the context of limited inhibition or other regulatory influences mediated by the cognitive-regulatory node (Nelson et al., 2005). Such behavioral tendencies may reflect operation of the mature affective node in concert with the immature cognitive-regulatory node. Similarly, atypical development within the early-maturing detection node could have a cascade of effects on functioning in associated brain regions that mature later. It is critical that research articulate more clearly the developmental course of BD at neural as well as phenomenological and functional levels; underlying neural mechanisms may be critically important in determining both concurrent and delayed functional outcomes. Such research needs to focus not only on youth who have been diagnosed with BD but also those at risk, who may show atypical patterns of neural development in the absence of active symptoms.

STUDIES OF SOCIAL FUNCTIONING IN INDIVIDUALS WITH BIPOLAR DISORDER

Social Functioning in Adults with Bipolar Disorder

Social functioning is commonly impaired in adults with BD, which presents obstacles to personal and occupational success during both symptomatic and euthymic periods (Fagiolini et al., 2005; Pope, Dudley, & Scott, 2007; Simon, Bauer, Ludman, Operskalski, & Unutzer, 2007). Indeed, one literature review found that between 30 and 60% of affected adults showed detectable social and occupational impairment during and even after long periods of remission (MacQueen, Young, & Joffe, 2001). Social impairment in adults with BD has typically been measured using self-report scales and has focused on the broad presence or absence of difficulty forming and maintaining close relationships or participating in social leisure activities. A small body of research has examined more specific social skills as well. In one study of adults diagnosed with BD, for example, euthymic individuals generated fewer solutions during a hypothetical social and moral problem-solving task than healthy controls. Furthermore, the more mood episodes experienced by individuals with BD, the less effective their generated solutions were likely to be, by both self- and observer rating (Scott, Stanton, Garland, & Ferrier, 2000).

In adults, social functioning difficulties appear to be pronounced in the presence of active manic or depressive symptoms and, more generally, vary depending on current affective state. For example, hypomania has been particularly strongly associated with elevated friction in relationships (Morriss et al., 2007). Mood states that can be associated with both mania and depression, such as anger, also have the potential to disrupt adult social functioning. For example, adults with BD reported more bursts of sudden, intense, situationally inappropriate anger during depressive episodes than did adults with unipolar depressive disorders (Perlis et al., 2004). Such expressions of unpredictable, inappropriate negative affect are likely to impede effective social interaction under many circumstances (Rydell, Thorell, & Bohlin, 2007; Tamir, Mitchell, & Gross, 2008).

Social Functioning in Youth with Bipolar Disorder

Findings regarding social functioning among youth diagnosed with BD are less consistent than those in the adult literature. This reflects several factors: first, the heterogeneity of conditions labeled as BD among children and adolescents; second, the differing social demands that youth face at different ages; third, variability in study designs, which include retrospective, cross-sectional, and longitudinal approaches; and fourth, the need to obtain reports regarding social behavior from multiple sources, such as parents and their affected children. Although data from both sources are valuable, parent reports need to be evaluated carefully because parent mood symptoms/disorders, which are likely to be common given the familial nature of BD, may influence parents' perceptions of and interactions with their children (Brotman et al., 2007; De Los Reyes & Kazdin, 2006; Edvardsen et al., 2008). In light of this caveat, some research has found that youth with BD have impaired relationships with family members and peers. Most of this research has focused on older children and adolescents (Geller et al., 2000; Robertson, Kutcher, Bird, & Grasswick, 2001; Schenkel, West, Harral, Patel, & Pavuluri, 2008); published research that characterizes patterns of social behavior in preschool and early elementary–age children with BD spectrum disorders or symptoms is notably lacking.

A few studies focused on middle childhood through late adolescence have yielded evidence of elevated conflict between individuals with BD and their parents, regardless of the child's current mood state (Table 11.1). In one of the first studies of psychosocial functioning in pediatric BD, Geller and colleagues found that affected youth (some of whom also had comorbid ADHD) and their mothers reported less maternal–child warmth, more maternal–child and paternal–child tension, and more problematic peer relationships than did both ADHD and nonpsychiatric control groups (Geller et al., 2000). Further research on this sample, which the authors followed longitudinally for 2 years, yielded evidence of additional differences in social behavior among groups. By parent report, youth with BD were less cooperative than both youth with ADHD and controls. Furthermore, compared with controls, members of the BD and ADHD groups were more novelty seeking, more reward dependent, and less persistent or self-directed. Youth with BD described themselves as less persistent and self-directed as well as more novelty seeking than controls but did not differ in self-report from peers with ADHD (Tillman et al., 2003).

Schenkel, West, and colleagues (2008) replicated and extended Geller and colleagues' findings regarding family interaction patterns by asking mothers to evaluate their relationships with their 8- to 17-year-old (mean, 11.27 years) children with or without BD. In this study, mothers of healthy controls (n = 30) reported feeling more warmly toward and having better relationships and less conflict with their children than did mothers of medicated, euthymic BD youth (n = 30). Mothers with younger children with BD, as well as those whose children had earlier symptom onset, reported the most conflictual relationships with their offspring (Schenkel, West, et al., 2008). Notably, the presence of both mother and father mood disorder diagnoses predicted significantly lower maternal ratings of warm and intimate relationships with their children, underscoring the importance of taking parent, as well as child, mental health into account when evaluating social and relational characteristics of youth with BD.

A few studies have examined self-perceived social and family functioning in adolescents with BD, yielding findings similar to those obtained from affected adults. In research focused on family interaction, for example, older adolescents (18–19 years old) with bipolar I disorder who were mildly symptomatic but not in depressive or manic episodes reported significantly more problems with their parents than did peers with unipolar major depressive disorder (MDD) or community controls. For all groups, however, problematic interactions between adolescents and parents were minor and infrequent. Youth with BD, relative to controls, reported less positive relationships with siblings and described their families as less cohesive (Robertson et al., 2001).

A study focused more explicitly on individual social coping skills also yielded findings consistent with those from adult-focused research. Specifically, 13- to 17-year-old adolescents with postpubertal-onset BD (n = 24) reported more external loci of control and greater difficulties regulating emotion in anger-provoking situations than healthy comparison youth (n = 39). Participants with BD also

TABLE 11.1. Summary of Studies of Social Functioning in Bipolar Disorder from Childhood through Adulthood

Study	BD group (n)	Mood state at time of study	Mean age, years (SD)	Comparison group (n)	Mean age, years (SD)	Method	Findings
Child/adolescent cross-sectional studies							
Geller et al. (2000)	BDI: 93	Manic	10.9 (2.7)	ADHD: 81 HC: 94	9.7 (2.0) 11.1 (2.6)	Mother report	Mother–child warmth: BD < ADHD, HC
							Parent–child tension: BD > ADHD, HC
							Peer relationship quality: BD < ADHD, HC
Tillman et al. (2003)	BDI: 101	Not reported	~12.8[a]	ADHD: 68 HC: 94	~11.6[a] ~13.1[a]	Mother report	Cooperativeness (mother): BD < ADHD, HC
						Self-report	Persistence/self-direction (mother): BD < HC
							Persistence/self-direction (self): BD < HC
							Novelty seeking (mother/self): BD < HC
							Reward dependence (mother): BD < HC
Schenkel, West, et al. (2008)	BD: 30	Euthymic	11.6 (2.7)	HC: 30	10.9 (2.7)	Mother report	Mother–child warmth: BD < HC
							Mother–child conflict: BD > HC

(cont.)

Study	Sample	Mood state	Age	Comparison group	Comparison age	Measure	Findings
Robertson et al. (2001)	BDI: 44	Euthymic	19.9 (2.9)	UD: 30 HC: 45	18.5 (2.8) 18.2 (1.6)	Self-report	Parent relationship quality: BD < UD, HC Sibling relationship quality: BD < UD, HC Family cohesion: BD < UD, HC
Rucklidge (2006)	BDI/II/NOS: 24	Not reported	13–17[b]	HC: 39	13–17[b]	Self-report	External locus of control: BD > HC Anger regulation: BD < HC Effective coping: BD < HC
Retrospective studies							
Kutcher et al. (1998)	BDI: 28	Euthymic	13–19 years at time of first mood episode	—	—	Retrospective parent report re premorbid functioning, school records	Peer relations: rated "excellent" in 30%, "as expected" in 60%, "problematic" in 10%
Cannon et al. (1997)	BD: 28	n/a	32 (9.3) 23.4 (5.4) at first hospital admission	SZ: 70 HC: 100	26.8 (6.7) 23.3 (5.7) at first hospital admission 27.5 (7.1)	Retrospective maternal report re premorbid functioning	Social adjustment: HC > BD > SZ

339

TABLE 11.1. (*cont.*)

Study	BD group (n)	Mood state at time of study	Mean age, years (SD)	Comparison Group (n)	Mean age, years (SD)	Method	Findings
High-risk studies							
Reichart et al. (2007)	High risk (parent with BD): 11–17 years old, 102; 18–26 years old, 106	n/a	11–17 years, 18–26 years (means not reported)	Low risk (no parent with BD): 11–17 years old, 1,122; 18–26 years old, 1,175	11–17 years, 18–26 years (means not reported)	Parent, teacher, and child report	11–17 years: no differences 18–26 years: adaptive functioning, family relationships: high risk < low risk
Petti et al. (2004)	High risk (parent with BD): 23 (9 had an affective disorder diagnosis)	n/a	7–16 years (mean age by risk group not reported)	Low risk (no parent with BD): 27 (three had an affective disorder diagnosis)	7–16 years (mean age by risk group not reported)	Parent and self-report	Social dysfunction associated with child diagnosis but not with risk group status
Anderson & Hammen (1993)	High risk (parent with BD): 18		13.7 (2.8)	High risk (parent with MDD): 22 Low risk (no parent disorder): 38	12.4 (2.6) 11.7 (2.3)	Mother and teacher report	Social functioning: high MDD risk < high BD risk, low risk

Adult cross-sectional studies

Study	Sample	Mood state	Age	Comparison	Age	Assessment	Findings
Fagiolini et al. (2005)	BDI/II/NOS: 103	Euthymic	42.6 (11.2)	—		Self-report	General functional and social impairment relative to normative data
Pope et al. (2007)	BDI/II: 77	Euthymic, mildly depressed, hypomanic	42.1 (11.1)	—		Self-report	Moderately impaired interpersonal functioning
Scott et al. (2000)	BDI: 41	Euthymic	44.7 (10.5)	HC: 20	42 (14.6)	Self- and observer ratings on Means Ends Problem-Solving Scale	Number of solutions generated: BD < HC
Morriss et al. (2007)	BDI/II: 253	Euthymic (n = 171) MDD (n = 60) Hypomanic (n = 22)	41.2 (10.9)	—		Interviewer rating (Social Adjustment Scale)	Full sample: moderately impaired social functioning. Social performance: H, MDD < E. Interpersonal behavior: H, MDD < E. Interpersonal friction: H > MDD, H > E
Perlis et al. (2004)	BDI/II: 29	Depressed	42.9 (11.9)	MDD: 50	38.2 (13.8)	Self-report (Anger Attacks Questionnaire)	Anger attacks: BD > MDD

Note. BD, bipolar disorder (BDI, bipolar disorder type I; BDII, bipolar disorder type II; BD NOS, bipolar disorder not otherwise specified); ADHD, attention-deficit/hyperactivity disorder; HC, healthy control; UD, unipolar depression; MDD, major depressive disorder; SZ, schizophrenia; E, euthymia.
[a]Tillman et al. (2003) gathered 2-year follow-up data on the sample recruited for Geller et al. (2000). Ages at follow-up were not reported (ages at baseline were), so ages presented are estimates based on the baseline data.
[b]Means and standard deviations were not reported.

endorsed less effective coping strategies than control participants; for example, in coping with difficult situations, they described themselves as less capable, more likely to reduce tension using maladaptive methods (e.g., screaming, substance use, taking frustration out on others), and more likely to blame themselves for their problems. Furthermore, adolescents with BD perceived themselves as less solution focused than controls (Rucklidge, 2006).

Social Impairment in Bipolar Disorder:
Marker of Illness or Vulnerability to Illness?

The studies described previously provide important snapshots of perceived social functioning in youth with BD, from both their own and their parents' perspectives. They are limited, however, on several fronts, leaving many questions open. First, they provide limited insight into the timing of social impairments in pediatric BD. Are such deficits "episode indicators" evident during active periods of illness but not remission (Nuechterlein & Dawson, 1984)? Alternatively, do they constitute "mediating vulnerability indicators" or chronic characteristics of affected youth, which become particularly severe during episodes? Given findings regarding state-related cognitive deficits in adults with active or remitted BD (Bozikas et al., 2005; Iacono, Peloquin, Lumry, Valentine, & Tuason, 1982; Liu et al., 2002), this question merits closer examination.

One approach is to examine functioning before illness onset in youth who eventually develop BD, either retrospectively in affected populations or prospectively in high-risk groups. The first studies to take this approach examined school records or asked parents to evaluate retrospectively whether affected children had displayed social impairment before their symptoms became evident. Kutcher, Robertson, and Bird (1998) found that parent recollections and school records regarding a sample of individuals with adolescent-onset BD (mean age at first depressive episode, 15.8 years; mean age at first manic episode, 16.7 years) yielded little evidence of premorbid social impairment. Indeed, their data indicated that 90% of the sample had average to excellent peer relationships before illness onset (Kutcher et al., 1998). In a second retrospective study, mothers of older adolescents and adults with BD, schizophrenia, or no impairment (aged 16–50 years) were asked to evaluate childhood and adolescent social functioning in their offspring. In contrast to Kutcher and colleagues' findings, individuals who had developed BD were rated as less socially adept during youth than controls, although impairment was less severe and long standing in the BD group than in those who later developed schizophrenia (Cannon et al., 1997).

These findings must be interpreted cautiously because of their retrospective nature. First, awareness of their children's diagnoses and, later, diagnosis-associated behaviors may have biased parents' recollections of earlier behavior either positively or negatively. Second, because no data were provided regarding family history of psychopathology in either study, it is unclear whether and how current or past symptoms in the maternal reporters influenced their descriptions of their children. Such confounds are difficult to avoid in retrospective studies, although use of additional sources, such as the school records that Kutcher and colleagues (1998) reviewed, mitigates the potential impact of parent biases. Therefore, researchers have shifted to studies focused on current behavior or, when possible, prospective longitudinal designs, typically targeting the offspring of adults with BD.

Using cross-sectional data from a longitudinal study, researchers compared social functioning between high- and low-risk youth in both younger (11–18 years) and older (18–26 years) age ranges (Reichart et al., 2007). Participants in the high-risk group each had a parent with BD; low-risk peers were drawn from large samples of the Dutch general population. Within both age ranges, the two risk groups differed minimally on well-normed, standardized parent-, teacher-, and child-report measures of social functioning, but adaptive functioning and family relationships were poorer in older high-risk participants than in their low-risk peers, particularly those who had been diagnosed with a lifetime mood or other disorder. Findings from this study are complicated by the fact that over half of the high-risk sample had been diagnosed with either a mood disorder or another psychiatric illness by the end of the study. Thus, current symptoms at the time of evaluation may have affected their social behavior independently of familial risk.

Petti and colleagues (2004) used a within-family design to contrast an array of psychosocial variables between 7- to 16-year-old offspring with parents who either did (n = 23) or did not (n = 27) have BD. Of the youth with affected parents, nine had affective disorders of their own; three of the offspring of nonaffected parents received affective disorder diagnoses. Children with affective disorders, regardless of parent diagnosis, reported receiving more social support in the form of positive regard from classmates, teachers, and parents than did healthy youth. Neither child nor parent diagnostic status differentiated participants with regard to perceptions of family closeness, although parents of diagnosed children reported more disciplinary issues than parents of healthy children (Petti et al., 2004).

Although several prospective longitudinal studies of offspring at risk for BD have been conducted or are underway (Alloy, Abramson, Walshaw, Keyser, & Gerstein, 2006; Anderson & Hammen, 1993; Hillegers et al., 2004), surprisingly few have published data regarding social functioning in their participants. In one such study, Anderson and Hammen (1993) followed four groups of 8- to 16-year-old children (offspring of unipolar depressed, bipolar, medically ill, and psychiatrically typical women; n = 96) for 2 years. During the course of the study, mothers evaluated the social competence, academic performance, and behavior problems of their children at 6-month intervals. Teachers also completed standard measures, whenever possible, regarding each child's behavior and social functioning at school. Results yielded little evidence of social or behavioral impairment among children of mothers with BD, who differed minimally from the children of control mothers. In contrast, children of mothers with unipolar depression showed chronically and significantly poorer social functioning on all measures compared with the other three groups, including the offspring of BD (Anderson & Hammen, 1993). This finding could reflect a number of factors, including differences between mothers with unipolar depression and BD in symptom severity or chronicity, treatment history (e.g., mothers with BD may have received treatment earlier or more consistently than those with unipolar depression), or social support. Furthermore, although the researchers gathered data regarding child diagnoses, these data were not presented in the Anderson and Hammen study; it is thus difficult to evaluate the impact, if any, of active child symptoms on social functioning.

Social Functioning in Bipolar Disorder: Summary and Future Directions

Taken together, these findings suggest that once children have begun to exhibit BD symptoms, they are likely to lag behind their peers in terms of social functioning regardless of whether they are observed in an active mood episode. The research base with regard to this example of equifinality is strikingly incomplete, and further study is clearly warranted, with attention to several factors. First, although researchers have begun to conduct prospective, longitudinal studies focused on outcomes in children who are at risk for BD or show early symptoms of the disorder, few characterize social functioning in these youth across different developmental phases.

Second, almost no research has targeted participants in infancy or early childhood and followed their development through adolescence or adulthood. Indeed, most prospective studies focused on pediatric BD or risk for BD have enrolled participants in middle childhood or early adolescence and followed them for 2 to 5 years (Anderson & Hammen, 1993; Geller et al., 2002; Hillegers et al., 2004). Research over longer periods of time is expensive and difficult to conduct but absolutely essential to answer questions about the onset of social deficits associated with BD. Notably, several groups have prospective studies underway that are aimed at identifying and following young children with mood symptoms and/or family histories of BD.

Third, as noted earlier, extant studies differ according to whether they take into account child and parent symptoms and medication status at the time of data collection and the impact of these variables on reports regarding child behavior and functioning. Given the risk that current mood state may bias responses, future research, in keeping with recent trends in work on pediatric BD, must evaluate the impact of mood on reports regarding social behavior. More routine inclusion of reports from nonfamilial sources (teachers, peers, research observers) would not only provide useful information regarding potential biases in parent or child reporters but would also help clarify how social functioning in affected or at-risk youth varies across different settings (e.g., school, home).

Fourth, even if social functioning is typically healthy before the onset of BD, trajectories of social functioning may, in keeping with the concept of multifinality, vary across youth who become symptomatic at different ages, who express the disorder in different ways (e.g., rapid cycling, predominantly depressed, predominantly manic), who have varying comorbid diagnoses, or who experience different levels of environmental support or adversity. For example, symptoms that manifest early may, in keeping with the "scar hypothesis" (Lewinsohn, Steinmetz, Larson, & Franklin, 1981), affect children in enduring ways that influence their later social functioning. Children whose symptoms cycle more unpredictably or rapidly may elicit different responses from those in their environments (e.g., increased frustration) than do children whose symptoms appear in the context of circumscribed episodes, leading the two groups to develop different styles of interpersonal interaction and different types of social strengths and weaknesses. No research has examined individual difference variables such as sex and age in relation to psychosocial outcomes in BD.

Environmental factors that may serve as protective or risk factors and thus diminish or amplify the social consequences of BD also merit attention. In particular, what do families, teachers, peers, and others in the environment do that helps some children avoid negative social outcomes or that increases risk for such outcomes in others? Additionally, where do youth with BD resemble typical peers? Findings from at least one study, for example, suggest that adolescents with BD show social *performance* deficits by their own and their parents' reports. Specifically, adolescents with BD rate themselves as more inappropriately assertive, impulsive, jealous, withdrawn, and overconfident than do healthy controls, and their parents rate them as more likely to behave inappropriately in social situations. However, they do not differ from healthy controls in their social *knowledge* (Goldstein, Miklowitz, & Mullen, 2006). Notably, social skills evaluations in this study took place when participants' BD symptoms were well controlled, decreasing the possibility of mood/state-related biases in self-ratings.

Finally, there is a need to elucidate the specific deficits that underlie social dysfunction in BD. Difficulties in encoding facial emotions, for example, may be more likely than global patterns of social behavior or cognition to represent stable endophenotypes (enduring vulnerability characteristics) of the disorder. By isolating component skills, in addition to global patterns of social success or failure, research may facilitate the development of targeted prevention or intervention approaches that will decrease the effects of BD on social development and functioning. In the next sections, research on specific social deficits associated with BD, as well as their neural correlates, is reviewed.

SPECIFIC SOCIAL DEFICITS ASSOCIATED WITH BIPOLAR DISORDER

Clinicians and researchers have long recognized that individuals with BD show not only evidence of general social dysfunction but also broad symptomatic patterns (e.g., irritability, impulsivity, withdrawal) that are likely to interfere with relationships. Only recently has research begun to characterize more precisely the nature of behavioral and social cognitive deficits associated with the disorder. Studies over the past several years have compared individuals with and without BD on a wide array of social and social cognitive variables that reflect multiple social information processing stages, such as those that Crick and Dodge (1994) described in a seminal theoretical report (Crick & Dodge, 1994). In keeping with Crick and Dodge's model, the present chapter focuses specifically on work regarding the accurate perception and interpretation of social cues, the formulation of flexible and appropriate responses to those cues, and the regulation of emotional reactions in individuals, predominantly youth, with and without BD.

Perception and Interpretation of Social Cues

Several studies in recent years have targeted the recognition and interpretation of social cues as potentially deficient skills in individuals with BD. Much of this research has found that BD is associated with deficits in the labeling of emotional facial expressions, in samples of both adults (Getz, Shear, & Strakowski, 2003; Lembke & Ketter, 2002) and children (Guyer et al., 2007; McClure, Pope, Hoberman, Pine, & Leibenluft, 2003; McClure et al., 2005; Rich, Grimley, et al., 2008; Schenkel, Pavuluri, Herbener, Harral, & Sweeney, 2007), although specific patterns of performance vary across studies. Studies have focused predominantly on adults or adolescents; relatively little is known about facial expression processing in younger children with BD or individuals who are at risk for the disorder. Furthermore, whether documented deficits are trait based or state based (i.e., related to current mood state) remains unclear, although some studies have made efforts to address this issue. A growing body of evidence indicates that at least some aspects of facial expression processing are impaired regardless of current mood.

In the most comprehensive study to date of youth with different psychological disorders, Guyer and colleagues (2007) compared performance on a facial emotion labeling task among adolescents (mean ages by group ranged from approximately 12–15 years) with BD ($n = 42$), severe mood dysregulation (SMD; $n = 39$) (Leibenluft, Charney, et al., 2003), anxiety or MDD ($n = 44$), ADHD/conduct disorder ($n = 35$), and controls ($n = 92$). Consistent with earlier, smaller studies (e.g., McClure et al., 2003, 2005), results indicated expression labeling deficits across an array of facial emotions (happy, sad, angry, fearful) in the BD and SMD groups relative to controls and other clinical groups. Errors did not differ based on the ages of the face stimuli or the emotions (happy, sad, angry, or fearful) displayed; however, the authors note that power limitations may have obscured such specific group differences (Guyer et al., 2007). Interpretation of study findings is complicated by the facts that current mood state (euthymic, manic, depressed) varied within the BD group, and that many participants within the BD and SMD groups were medicated at the time of evaluation, unlike members of the other groups. Post hoc analyses, however, comparing euthymic participants with BD ($n = 25$) and control ($n = 92$) groups indicated comparable deficits to those seen in the combined euthymic/symptomatic BD group. Indeed, McClure and colleagues

(2005) obtained similar results in a smaller sample. Furthermore, unmedicated BD/SMD youth differed from controls in their overall task performance, with consistently lower scores.

Whereas Guyer and colleagues (2007) examined skill at classifying emotions into discrete categories, Rich, Grimley, and colleagues (2008) evaluated capacity to correctly identify facial expressions presented at gradually increasing emotional intensity in adolescents with narrow-phenotype BD, SMD, and no diagnosis. Each stimulus began as a neutral face and was morphed gradually into an emotional (happy, surprised, sad, angry, fearful, disgusted) face; participants pressed a button as soon as they believed they had accurately identified the depicted expression. Regardless of the emotion presented, youth with BD and SMD required more intensity to be apparent before they responded at all; they also correctly identified disgusted, surprised, happy, and fearful faces at later points than did controls.

Another recent study focused more explicitly on associations between facial expression processing deficits and both medication and current mood state in youth with DSM-IV BD (Schenkel et al., 2007). This study compared performance on two facial expression processing tasks in young adolescents (mean age, 11–12 years) who were either healthy (*n* = 28), diagnosed with BD and euthymic (*n* = 29), or diagnosed with BD and acutely symptomatic (*n* = 29). On the first task, which required participants to identify which of two faces displayed a single emotion more intensely, only symptomatic youth with BD performed more poorly than controls. On the second task, which involved rating emotional expressions along a 7-point continuum ranging from *very happy* to *neutral* to *very sad*, both euthymic and symptomatic youth with BD underestimated the intensity of emotional faces compared with healthy controls. Results suggest that some emotion processing impairments may be associated with acute symptomatology, whereas other kinds of impairment may constitute trait or risk markers.

Consistent with the possibility that impairment in particular aspects of emotion processing may be related to risk for BD, Brotman and colleagues (2008) found that 4- to 18-year-olds without BD diagnoses but with an affected parent or sibling performed more poorly than controls on a facial expression labeling task. Their peers diagnosed with BD also performed more poorly than controls (Brotman et al., 2008).

Thus, on tasks that involve different kinds of facial expression processing (e.g., discrimination, labeling, evaluation of intensity), children and adolescents with BD appear to show fairly consistent deficits, some of which are apparent regardless of current mood state (e.g., expression labeling and intensity rating) and thus may represent endophenotypes for the disorder and others of which relate more specifically to the presence of active symptoms (e.g., discrimination between expressions that differ subtly in intensity). More research is needed to delineate the impact that such facial expression processing deficits have on day-to-day social behavior; the first study to examine this question in youth with BD indicates that they may correlate meaningfully with impaired social reciprocity skills (Rich, Grimley, et al., 2008). In notable contrast, in this study, facial expres-

---

PERCEPTION AND INTERPRETATION OF SOCIAL CUES

- Both adults and youth with BD, as well as youth at risk for BD, perform more poorly than controls on facial expression recognition tasks.

- Although some deficits appear consistent across euthymic and manic/depressed mood states (e.g., facial expression labeling), others appear to emerge only during mood episodes (e.g., discrimination among subtly differing expressions).

- Deficits in processing more complex social cues, such as those associated with inferences regarding others' mental states, are also evident in adolescents and adults with BD.

---

sion processing deficits correlated significantly with family dysfunction in youth with SMD, but not with BD, which suggests that the effects of emotion processing deficits may vary markedly depending on the nature and severity of a child's dysfunction.

At least two studies on perception of social cues in individuals with BD focused more broadly on performance on theory-of-mind or social inference tasks. Like most of the research on facial expression processing in BD, this body of work has been limited to studies of adolescents and adults (Kerr, Dunbar, & Bentall, 2003; Schenkel, Marlow-O'Connor, Moss, Sweeney, & Pavuluri, 2008), with little to no attention yet to preadolescent children or asymptomatic individuals at risk for BD. This small literature suggests that BD may be associated not only with deficits in basic emotion processing but also with impairment in more complex social cognitive domains. Schenkel, Marlow-O'Connor, and colleagues (2008) examined performance on two theory-of-mind tasks, one designed to measure ability to infer others' intents and the other developed to tap false-belief understanding in emotional contexts. Adolescents with BD who showed at least two hallmark symptoms (elation, irritability, grandiosity; $n = 26$) performed significantly more poorly than healthy controls ($n = 20$) on both tasks (Schenkel, Marlow-O'Connor, et al., 2008). Findings were comparable to those obtained in studies of adults with BD, in which symptomatic individuals (Kerr et al., 2003) and, in some studies, euthymic patients with BD (Bora et al., 2005; Pollak & Tolley-Schell, 2003) showed theory-of-mind deficits.

Formulation of Appropriate Responses to Social Cues

Surprisingly little research has examined whether BD is associated with aberrant responses in social situations, particularly early in development. Such a pattern of deficits seems plausible, given the evidence that affected individuals appear to misread or misinterpret others' cues and thus may generate responses that are incongruent or inappropriate. Towbin, Pradella, Gorrindo, Pine, and Leibenluft (2005) compared patterns of social behavior among 8- to 18-year-old youth with

BD, SMD, or major depression and/or anxiety disorders using a series of parent-report measures developed to identify children with characteristics of pervasive developmental disorders (e.g., autism, Asperger) and describe their social functioning. Results indicated marked social interaction deficits in the BD and SMD groups compared with the MDD/anxiety group. Furthermore, when scores were compared with normative data, 62% of youth with bipolar type I disorder, 67% of youth with bipolar type II disorder, and 72% of youth with SMD scored in the autism spectrum range on at least one measure (Towbin et al., 2005). Although these findings are striking, they also raise questions about the discriminant validity of the instruments. In a recent follow-up to this study, Pine, Guyer, Goldwin, Towbin, and Leibenluft (2008) administered the same three measures to a larger sample of youth with BD, SMD, MDD, an anxiety disorder, or no diagnosis. Consistent with their earlier findings, scores on all three measures were higher in participants with mood disorders (BD, SMD, MDD) than in those with anxiety disorders or no diagnosis, reflecting more impairment in social reciprocity and language as well as elevated levels of behavioral rigidity and stereotypy in the mood-disordered groups.

The measures that Towbin and colleagues (2005) and Pine and colleagues (2008) administered tapped a broad array of expressive language and interpersonal interaction skills as rated by parents. Although informative about general social behavior as observed by adults who interact frequently with the child, global scores from these measures provide limited information about specific response formulation skills that might be impaired in youth with BD. As a first step toward addressing this question, McClure and colleagues (2005) administered to adolescents with BD (*n* = 40) and healthy controls (*n* = 22) a more focused measure of pragmatic language skill or the ability to use language effectively to achieve social goals. Comparison of BD and control groups showed that even when global oral expression skill was covaried, the BD group obtained lower scores on the pragmatic language measure, as well as on measures of facial expression labeling, than controls (McClure et al., 2005).

FORMULATION OF RESPONSES TO SOCIAL CUES

- Limited research has examined patterns of response to social stimuli in individuals with BD.
- There is some evidence that youth with BD and other mood disturbances perform atypically on measures of social reciprocity and language and show elevated levels of behavioral rigidity and stereotypy.
- Pragmatic language deficits have also been observed in youth with BD.
- Questions remain, however, regarding specificity of these deficits to BD, associations with mood state, and associations with medication status.

Further research is clearly needed examining social communication skills, at both macro- and microlevels, in individuals with BD across development. The small number of existing studies provides suggestive evidence that impairment in these domains may be associated with the disorder. However, these studies provide little information about whether and how mood state, age, or medication status may relate to patterns of spared and impaired function. Further research exploring links between social perceptual deficits in domains such as facial expression processing and social communication deficits would also be informative.

Regulation of Behavioral and Emotional Reactions

Social situations require not only that individuals generate appropriate responses, but also that they implement these responses in ways that are consistent with continually changing environmental demands. Such cognitive and behavioral flexibility (Cools, Clark, & Robbins, 2004) must further be combined with effective regulation of one's own emotional reactions to an unfolding interaction, which may not proceed in expected ways and may provoke frustration or anger. A number of studies have examined cognitive flexibility and emotional regulation in individuals with BD. Research on adults consistently suggests the presence of at least subtle and enduring deficits regardless of mood state (Fleck et al., 2003; Martínez-Arán et al., 2004; Mur, Portella, Martínez-Arán, Pifarré, & Vieta, 2007).

In adolescent samples, researchers have typically examined cognitive flexibility outside of social contexts, using neuropsychological tasks designed to measure aspects of executive functioning, such as the ability to shift attention between the perceptual features of complex stimuli in response to contingency cues. Such tasks include the classic Trails B measure (Lezak, 2004) and Wisconsin Card Sorting Test (WCST; Heaton, Chelune, Talley, Kay, & Curtiss, 1993), as well as the intra-extra dimensional (IED) shift task (Robbins et al., 1998). The IED shift task, which incorporates simple and compound reversal trials of varying difficulty, was originally designed as an analogue to the WCST for use with nonhuman primates but has been adapted for use with humans as well. Additionally, the change task, which measures the ability to inhibit a prepotent response and substitute an alternate one, provides another approach to examining response flexibility (Logan, Schachar, & Tannock, 1997). This task has the advantage that difficulty can be adjusted with a tracking algorithm to ensure that subjects execute correct responses approximately 50% of the time on trials requiring response substitution.

Dickstein, Nelson, and colleagues (2007) administered the IED shift task and the change task to youth with BD (n = 50; mean age, 13.1 years) and SMD (n = 44; mean age, 12.2 years) and to controls (n = 43; mean age, 13.6 years). On the IED shift task, adolescents with BD were impaired on simple reversal learning trials compared with control and SMD groups. Furthermore, on the change task, the BD group members were also impaired on change trials that involved substituting novel responses for prepotent responses relative to adolescents with SMD. These deficits appeared to be independent of current mood state, comorbid anxiety, and comorbid ADHD and could, according to the authors, reflect impaired capacity to adapt to altered stimulus–reward associations. Participants with SMD only showed impaired performance relative to controls on compound reversal trials, which the authors speculated may represent deficits in selective attention (Dickstein, Nelson, et al., 2007).

Meyer and colleagues (2004) conducted a prospective study of cognitive flexibility in offspring of mothers with mood disorders (unipolar or bipolar) or no history of psychiatric illness. Offspring, who had been administered the WCST and Trails B during adolescence, were grouped according to their own diagnoses in young adulthood and compared with regard to their performance on both measures. Of the offspring of mothers with mood disorders who had developed BD themselves by their late teens or 20s, 67% showed impairment on the WCST, making perseverative errors and generating fewer conceptual-level responses. Impairment rates were much lower among offspring who remained free of psychopathology (17%) or who developed major depression (19%). The presence of this impaired pattern of performance before the onset of BD symptoms is consistent with the possibility that cognitive flexibility deficits represent a risk marker for the disorder (Meyer et al., 2004). Additional data, however, indicate that the associations between cognitive inflexibility and risk for BD are more complex. In a subsequent study of the same sample, Meyer and colleagues (2006) found that WCST performance mediated associations between maternal negativity when their offspring were toddlers and the later development of BD in their children. This pattern of findings suggests a dynamic pattern of interactions among genetic risk, parent behavior, child cognition, and child outcome and points to the need for further longitudinal work that examines reciprocal influences among these and other relevant variables.

One recent study of youth with BD focused on emotion regulation in response to changing contingencies, in addition to regulation of cognitive and behavioral responses to such environmental demands (Rich et al., 2007). Children and adolescents (ages 7–17 years) with BD (most were euthymic; four had hypomania or mixed hypomania; 88.6% were medicated), SMD (all were euthymic, 9.5% were medicated), or no diagnosis completed the Affective Posner Task, which assesses attention under a variety of emotional circumstances and contingencies. In the first (nonemotional) condition, participants received verbal feedback about their accuracy and speed on an attentional measure; in the second condition, they won or lost money based on their performance on the same task; and in the third (frustration) condition, they won or lost money based on a rigged algorithm that caused them to lose money on most trials on which they performed accurately as well as those on which they made errors or responded too slowly. Groups showed significant differences in self-reported arousal during the frustration condition, with the patient groups reporting more arousal than controls. In the two conditions that linked speed and accuracy to monetary gain or loss, the patient groups also responded more quickly than controls when they lost money. The similarities

---

REGULATION OF BEHAVIORAL AND EMOTIONAL REACTIONS

- Adults and adolescents with BD show deficits on measures of cognitive flexibility.
- Some prospective longitudinal research suggests that cognitive flexibility deficits may be a risk marker for BD.
- Youth with BD and other mood pathology show heightened emotional reactions to frustration relative to healthy peers.

---

in response between the BD and SMD groups suggest that heightened emotional reactions to frustration may be broadly associated with mood pathology rather than specifically linked to BD. Further research that includes additional clinical samples, such as youth with pervasive developmental disorder or schizophrenia, would help clarify this issue.

NEURAL CORRELATES OF SOCIAL COGNITIVE DEFICITS IN BIPOLAR DISORDER

Recent models of BD conceptualize the condition in terms of dysfunction in two primary neural systems that, as described in Nelson and colleagues' (2005) SIPN framework, are thought to mediate mood regulation/emotion processing and cognitive control functions (Phillips & Vieta, 2007). Indeed, considerable evidence suggests that individuals with BD across the life span show atypically elevated activity in a system that encompasses the amygdala and subcortical structures, combined with abnormally decreased activity in a prefrontal cortical neural system that subserves control processes such as cognitive flexibility (Bearden, Hoffman, & Cannon, 2001; Phillips & Vieta, 2007). The next section presents a review of the literature regarding these two systems as they relate to BD across development, with a focus on studies that have examined neural correlates of social cue perception, specifically facial expression processing, and cognitive or response flexibility.

Neural Differences Associated with Facial Expression Processing in Bipolar Disorder

Given the evidence that impaired processing of social cues such as facial expressions may represent an endophenotype for BD, as well as the importance of accurate and efficient perception and interpretation of such cues for successful social interaction, it is not surprising that a growing body of research has examined neural correlates of this skill in BD. In adults, several studies comparing neural activation during different facial expression processing tasks among healthy controls, actively manic patients with BD (Altshuler et al., 2005), and individuals with medication-stabilized BD in varying current mood states (Yurgelun-Todd et al., 2000) have yielded a fairly consistent pattern of increased activation in the amygdala and other subcortical regions and decreased prefrontal activation in participants with BD.

Findings have varied across studies, possibly reflecting differences in tasks, facial expressions displayed, and participant characteristics, including clinical state. One study, for example, indicated elevated activity in subcortical structures and prefrontal regions in euthymic and depressed patients with BD relative to both controls and patients with MDD during passive viewing of emotional faces (Lawrence et al., 2004), and another study demonstrated decreased amygdala and subgenual cingulate cortex and increased posterior cingulate cortex and posterior insula activation in manic patients with BD when they rated the intensity of sad faces (Lennox, Jacob, Calder, Lupson, & Bullmore, 2004). Indeed, findings from one study that compared manic BD, depressed BD, and control groups during both implicit and explicit recognition of facial expressions suggest that, although atypical activation is present regardless of mood state in BD, it varies in pattern depending on the task and stimulus used (Chen et al., 2006). Few data are available regarding neural responses to facial expressions in euthymic adults with BD. One study found more hippocampal activation rather than amygdala activation to fearful faces in euthymic adults with BD versus controls (Malhi et al., 2007).

Thus, in adults with BD, the literature points to a pattern of atypical subcortical, typically amygdala or hippocampal, activation in combination with atypical prefrontal activation, with differences across studies and participant mood states in the structures that show hyper- or hypoactivation. More recent research has focused on interactions among different neural systems during facial expression viewing tasks. In manic adults with BD, the ventrolateral prefrontal cortex shows reduced regulation of the amygdala during expression labeling (Foland et al., 2008). Findings from several recent studies suggest that these functional neural anomalies may be ameliorated by medication: Patterns of activation in response to facial expressions during a recognition task changed after treatment with lamotrigine so that patterns among patients with BD more closely resembled those in healthy controls (Haldane et al., 2008; Jogia, Haldane, Cobb, Kumari, & Frangou, 2008). Blumberg and colleagues (2005) obtained similar findings following treatment with varied medications in a sample of 17 adults with BD. A recent review of the literature on medication effects on functional neuroimaging findings in BD, however, suggests that it may be premature to draw conclusions on this front (Phillips, Travis, Fagiolini, & Kupfer, 2008).

Studies examining neural correlates of facial expression processing in youth with BD have focused primarily on older children and adolescents. Neuroimaging studies of younger children are rare, particularly in clinical populations that are likely to find the imaging context stressful and have difficulty lying still in the magnetic resonance imaging (MRI) scanner for long periods of time. Furthermore, although several studies include at least some participants as young as 7 to 8 years, few samples have yet been large enough to permit examination of age or pubertal status effects. As in the adult literature, sample composition has varied across studies in terms of current mood state, and tasks and target facial expressions have also differed from study to study, rendering direct comparisons of findings difficult. Broadly, however, results have resembled those obtained in research on adults, with atypical activity to emotional faces apparent in subcortical limbic regions and in prefrontal structures.

One study compared patterns of neural activation during passive viewing of emotionally expressive (happy, angry, neutral) faces between euthymic, unmedicated adolescents with BD (mean age, 14.3 years) and healthy comparison participants (mean age, 14.9 years). Relative to the comparison group, adolescents with BD showed decreased activation to angry and happy faces in orbitofrontal and dorsolateral prefrontal regions as well as in the occipital visual cortex. In response to happy faces alone, the BD group showed decreased medial prefrontal activation and greater activation in the right amygdala and bilateral pregenual anterior cingulate cortex (Pavuluri, O'Connor, Harral, & Sweeney, 2007). Another study required participants to rate different characteristics of emotional faces that they then had to identify during a surprise recognition task (Dickstein, Rich, et al., 2007). In this study, adolescents with BD (mean age, 14.2 years) who were either euthymic, depressed, or hypomanic showed increased neural activation relative to controls (mean age, 14.7 years) in the striatum and anterior cingulate cortex in response to happy faces that they recognized later during a memory task and in the orbitofrontal cortex in response to successfully encoded angry faces.

Interestingly, neutral as well as emotional faces appear to elicit differential responses from youth with BD (Rich et al., 2006). In a mixed sample of euthymic, depressed, and hypomanic adolescents with BD, Rich and colleagues (2006) found evidence of greater activation in patients, compared with controls, in the left amygdala, accumbens, putamen, and ventral prefrontal cortex when rating the hostility conveyed by neutral faces. Furthermore, when participants rated their own fear of neutral faces, the BD group showed greater activation in the left amygdala and bilateral accumbens. Participants with BD appeared to perceive the faces more negatively than did controls; they rated neutral faces as more hostile and reported more fear when viewing them. Taken together with Rich, Grimley, and colleagues' (2008) finding that youth with BD were slower than healthy controls to identify emotions depicted on faces as they morphed from neutral to intensely emotional, these results could suggest that, although youth with BD may be biased to perceive ambiguous cues as negative, they have difficulty making finer discriminations among the negative emotions that the cue might convey. Alternatively, this set of findings could indicate that youth with BD are overly sensitive to negative facial expressions across the board.

As in the adult literature, research has started moving away from examination of activation in specific structures in isolation and toward a focus on patterns of connectivity or interaction among brain regions. In one such study, Rich, Fromm, and colleagues (2008) examined functional connectivity between the left amygdala and other neural structures during a task that directed attention toward emotional and nonemotional aspects of expressive faces in adolescents with BD and controls. Results, which resembled Foland and colleagues' (2008) findings in adults, indicated less functional connectivity between the left amygdala and the right posterior/precuneus region, as well as the right fusiform/parahippocampal gyri, in youth with BD than in controls (Rich, Fromm, et al., 2008).

Findings from research that used emotionally valenced pictures (scenes rather than faces) as stimuli (Eaton et al., 2008) provide preliminary evidence that treatment may alter these patterns of activation in adolescents, as it appears to do in adults. In this study, a small sample ($n = 8$) of adolescents with BD who were currently in depressive episodes were treated with lamotrigine for 8 weeks, and patterns of neural activation in response to positive and negative pictures before and after treatment were compared. Results indicated that amygdala activation in response to negative images declined from pre- to posttreatment scans in association with clinical improvement. As the authors point out, replication in a controlled sample is needed to evaluate whether other factors, such as habituation, might have influenced changes in activation patterns; however, this study provides an important first step toward more precisely characterizing the effects of successful treatment.

Taken together, the adult and adolescent literatures on neural correlates of facial expression processing in BD provide compelling evidence that subcortical, primarily limbic, and prefrontal systems interact atypically in response to social cues such as expressive faces in the context of the disorder. Although few studies have compared participants across mood states, findings suggest that atypical patterns of activation are present in the context of euthymia as well as mania and depression, but that euthymia achieved via successful treatment may dampen the effects of the disorder. Further research is needed that replicates existing studies in samples of participants in different developmental stages (e.g., comparisons of adults and adolescents with BD) and mood states (e.g., comparisons of manic vs. euthymic participants or within-participant longitudinal research with scans obtained during different mood episodes). Additionally, consistent use of stan-

---

NEURAL CORRELATES OF FACIAL EXPRESSION PROCESSING

- Both adults and youth with BD show atypical activity to emotional faces in subcortical limbic regions and in prefrontal structures.

- Atypical patterns of activation are present in euthymic as well as manic and depressed individuals.

- Euthymia achieved through successful treatment has been linked to normalization of activation patterns to emotional faces.

- Direct comparisons of activation patterns between individuals with BD in different age groups and mood states as well as standard task procedures across studies are needed to clarify the literature.

dard tasks may help clarify the literature. The diverse array of facial expression processing tasks used in neuroimaging research makes it more difficult to elicit subtly different patterns of neural response than would comparable stimuli.

Neural Differences Associated with Cognitive Flexibility and Related Functions in Bipolar Disorder

The literature on neural correlates of cognitive flexibility and related functions in BD, such as response inhibition and regulation, is less explicitly socioemotional in focus than the facial expressing processing literature. However, in at least a few studies of adults and adolescents, researchers have used tasks that combine cognitive and emotional demands and thus tap underlying skills comparable to those required by effective social interactions. Like studies regarding facial expression processing, research on cognitive flexibility and response inhibition in the context of BD consistently points to the presence of atypical activation in prefrontal and subcortical networks that include limbic and striatal structures, although patterns of anomaly differ among the samples under study.

Studies of cognitive flexibility and response inhibition in adults with BD have typically used modifications of the classic Stroop and go/no-go tasks, which require selective attention, inhibition of prepotent responses, and substitution of alternate responses that demand more effort to generate. In samples of adults with BD who were euthymic (Kronhaus et al., 2006; Lagopoulos & Malhi, 2007; Malhi, Lagopoulos, Sachdev, Ivanovski, & Shnier, 2005) or in varied mood states (Roth et al., 2006; Yurgelun-Todd et al., 2000), activation during emotional and non-emotional variants of the Stroop task differed significantly from that observed in healthy controls. Specifically, across most studies, researchers found evidence of decreased prefrontal activation in patients compared with controls, regardless of the task variant used. The precise location of reduced prefrontal activation varied from study to study; however, findings of attenuated activity in ventral and medial prefrontal regions emerged with some consistency. Notably, one study found evidence of increased dorsolateral prefrontal activation, combined with decreased anterior cingulate activity, in adults with BD versus controls (Yurgelun-Todd et al., 2000), and two studies that focused on depressed adults with BD found no differences from controls in frontal regions during a Stroop measure (Marchand, Lee, Thatcher, Jensen, et al., 2007; Marchand, Lee, Thatcher, Thatcher, et al., 2007). Thus, the literature in adults is not entirely consistent. Task variations, as well as sample differences, may have influenced study outcomes, underscoring the need for consistent use of tasks across studies.

In research that has used go/no-go tasks, findings have varied depending on participants' mood states. In a study of neural activity during emotional versus nonemotional go/no-go tasks, euthymic adults with BD showed increased activation in the orbitofrontal cortex, temporal regions, insula, and both anterior and posterior cingulate cortices relative to healthy controls (Wessa et al., 2007). In contrast, Altshuler and colleagues (2005) found evidence of decreased right orbitofrontal cortex, hippocampus, and left cingulate cortex activation in actively manic adults with BD during a nonemotional go/no-go variant. Differences in both tasks and conditions used to construct contrasts, as well as sample differences, probably influenced study findings, which again highlights the need for replication using identical tasks in different samples and task variants in samples that differ according to mood state. Furthermore, explicit incorporation of emotional versus nonemotional stimuli into go/no-go tasks elicits different patterns of neural engagement (Shafritz, Collins, & Blumberg, 2006), which underscores the need for caution in directly comparing findings across studies that use different measures.

In adolescents, research using Stroop tasks has also yielded evidence of atypical neural activation. Patterns of activation difference, however, have been only partially consistent with those observed in most studies of adults. In one study, Blumberg and colleagues (2003) replicated adult findings of increased ventral prefrontal cortical activation in samples of depressed and euthymic adolescents with BD during a Stroop color-naming task; manic participants with BD, in contrast, showed attenuated activation in this region (Blumberg, Leung, et al., 2003). In a second study, the same research group found increased putamen and thalamus activation in adolescents with BD relative to controls during a Stroop color-naming task but no evidence of group differences in prefrontal activation (Blumberg, Martin, et al., 2003). Given that prefrontal regions continue to develop during adolescence and into early adulthood (Gogtay et al., 2004), these findings, in conjunction with those in adults, raise questions about whether developmental factors may influence patterns of atypical neural development in the context of BD.

A series of neuroimaging studies has used the stop signal task, a go/no-go task variant that permits separate examination of successful and unsuccessful response inhibitions and substitutions, to compare neural activation between adolescents with BD and healthy controls (Leibenluft et al., 2007; Nelson et al., 2007). Nelson and colleagues (2007) focused on trials tapping response flexibility, or the successful substitution of an effortful response for a prepotent response. They found that, in the context of comparable task performance, participants with BD showed more activation in the dorsolateral prefrontal cortex and primary motor cortex than did matched controls. In the Leibenluft and colleagues (2007) study, analyses focused instead on failure to correctly inhibit responses and yielded evidence of attenuated striatal and right ventral prefrontal cortex activation in BD patients compared with controls. Taken together, these findings suggest that dysfunction in frontostriatal circuits disrupts regulation of cognitive and motor responses in BD during adolescence.

Little functional neuroimaging research in adolescents with BD has incorporated socioemotional components into cognitive and behavioral flexibility measures. In their 2007 study, however, during which they administered the Affective Posner Task to adolescents with BD, adolescents with SMD, and healthy controls, Rich and colleagues gathered data regarding event-related potentials (ERPs) along

---

NEURAL CORRELATES OF COGNITIVE FLEXIBILITY

- Results indicate dysfunction of frontostriatal regions in the pathophysiology of BD across development.

- Frontostriatal circuitry may be involved in cognitive, affective, and motor responses: response inhibition, flexibility, planning, or modulating emotions when making choices.

- These pathophysiological findings are not unique to BD but have also been observed in ADHD or obsessive–compulsive disorder.

- Findings are not exclusive to BD, but studies are limited by use of different procedures, lack of control over mood states, and sampling differences.

---

with the behavioral data discussed earlier. ERP activation patterns differed significantly between youth with BD and members of the other two groups in the frustration condition, with the BD group showing decreases in parietal P3 amplitude. The authors interpreted this finding as suggestive of attentional deficits in the context of frustration in the participants with BD (Rich et al., 2007).

Taken together, the adolescent and adult literatures regarding neural correlates of cognitive flexibility and response inhibition in BD implicate dysfunction in frontostriatal regions in the pathophysiology of the disorder across development. As Blumberg and colleagues (2004) have asserted, however, the manifestations of this dysfunction may vary depending on the timing of disorder onset because of variability in the maturation rates of different structures within frontostriatal circuits. Thus, disorder onset during early adolescence may affect neural activity and behavior differently than does disorder onset in early adulthood (Blumberg et al., 2004).

Notably, comparable findings of atypical activation during cognitive flexibility and response inhibition tasks have been obtained in studies focused on varied clinical groups, such as individuals with ADHD (Smith, Taylor, Brammer, Toone, & Rubia, 2006) and obsessive–compulsive disorder (Gu et al., 2008). This suggests that frontostriatal anomalies may be markers associated broadly with psychopathology rather than with specific disorders. Research comparing patterns of activation between different clinical groups during cognitive flexibility and response inhibition tasks would help to clarify this issue.

SUMMARY, CONCLUSIONS, AND FURTHER QUESTIONS

The preponderance of evidence is consistent with the presence of neurally mediated social cognitive deficits associated with BD. These deficits appear consistently in affected individuals regardless of whether their symptoms emerge early or later in development. Atypical patterns of emotional cue (particularly facial expression) processing, which have been identified fairly consistently in both euthy-mic individuals with BD and those at risk for the disorder, are of great interest as potential endophenotypes mediated by functional anomalies in frontolimbic neural circuits. Similarly, cognitive and behavioral inflexibility in social and non-social contexts holds promise as a risk-related marker, although more research is needed on this topic in at-risk and euthymic samples. Focus on such discrete and specific aspects of social cognition and behavior is likely to be more fruitful for researchers than examination of broader measures of social function, particularly if the aim is to identify correlates of risk rather than active symptoms. It may also enhance development of specific interventions that target these dysfunctions.

A number of questions remain to be answered if we are to understand and address the functional impact of BD on social behavior and cognition. First, most published research, particularly with regard to neural mechanisms, still focuses on actively ill participants (either those who are currently in mood episodes or remission from such episodes) rather than those at risk for BD. Studies that test the same individuals with BD in different mood states, although difficult to con-duct, are critically important for the elucidation of risk and prodromal mark-ers that might inform prevention and early treatment efforts. Numerous research groups are working to fill this gap.

In a groundbreaking study of neural markers of risk, Gogtay and colleagues (2007) gathered longitudinal data regarding brain structure in youth who were undiagnosed but were suspected to have childhood onset schizophrenia. All 32 participants, who underwent repeated structural MRI scans over a 4- to 8-year period, showed diffuse impairment in multiple domains, including emotional and attentional dysregulation at study onset. In a subsample ($n = 9$) who developed manic episodes in the course of the study, the authors examined patterns of neu-ral change. Results indicated subtle differences from controls, including bilateral decreases in anterior cingulate regions and increases in left temporal structures over time in the youth who developed mania, as well as the nonmanic but impaired participants, who met DSM-IV criteria for psychosis not otherwise specified and ADHD as well as other comorbid disorders (Gogtay et al., 2007). Such research, with a focus on functional and structural changes over time in high-risk youth, is critical if we are to clarify the antecedents of BD and identify markers of risk.

Given the mixed findings regarding broad patterns of social function before illness onset, premorbid neural markers have the potential to be more reliable early indicators of risk for BD. The specificity of such neural markers, however, remains in question: Gogtay and colleagues (2007) obtained similar atypical find-ings both in youth who developed mania and in those who did not, which could indicate that neural anomalies are generic markers of risk for later impairment.

Second, consistency among researchers in their definitions of BD, particu-larly pediatric BD, is needed. Although experts in the field increasingly recognize that children and adolescents can show episodic patterns of mood dysfunction that parallel those documented in adults, studies vary in the breadth of their inclusion criteria and the symptoms that they identify as cardinal. Until there is consensus about a clear, empirically validated phenotype or set of phenotypes for the disorder across development, investigators should articulate the precise criteria according to which participants were identified as having BD. Given the many variations in manifestations of mood dysregulation, particularly among youth (e.g., rapid cycling, predominantly irritable), it is important that research participants be as carefully characterized as possible so that the same diagnostic label is not applied to individuals with related, but diverse, conditions. One framework that has proved useful is Leibenluft, Charney, and colleagues' (2003) distinction between narrow-phenotype BD and severe mood dysregulation, which resembles BD but does not follow the episodic pattern observed in adults. Similarly, Geller and colleagues have defined an ultrarapid cycling phenotype in youth that merits continued study (Tillman & Geller, 2007). Careful attention to different expressions of bipolar spectrum conditions will only advance the field and facilitate the effective treatment of and provision of social support for affected individuals.

Third, it will be important to consider the impact of development on the socioemotional impact of BD. Mixed findings regarding the interpersonal correlates and consequences of actively symptomatic and remitted BD, particularly among youth, may reflect at least in part the different effects that the disorder may have at different ages or during different developmental periods. Symptoms that emerge in early childhood are likely to disrupt different social learning processes compared with those that do not emerge until adolescence or later. Furthermore, the varying social demands that individuals face at different ages as well as the varying amounts of control that they have over their social environments (e.g., whereas children are required to attend school, older adolescents and adults can opt to avoid structured social settings) are likely to interact with BD manifestations to influence the impact of the disorder. Consideration of such developmental differences will be useful as researchers continue to elucidate the social cognitive and behavioral effects of BD across development.

A fourth question that relates closely to the third revolves around the interaction of neural and environmental factors to influence social outcomes in youth and adults with BD. In particular, are there family or community characteristics that might ameliorate or prevent negative outcomes or, conversely, promote them? Not surprisingly, given the difficulty of recruiting sizable samples of youth with or at risk for BD, only recently has research begun to target interactions of environmental and neural factors as predictors of social and functional outcomes, particularly at different points in development. Such work will be critically important not only for the development of preventive approaches (Chang, Howe, Gallelli, & Miklowitz, 2006) but also for the refinement and targeting of existing pharmacological (DelBello & Kowatch, 2006) and empirically based psychosocial treatments (Miklowitz & Otto, 2007). Research regarding outcomes associated with various combinations of neural vulnerabilities and environmental stressors may be especially helpful for clinicians and community support agencies as they develop and implement preventive and remedial measures aimed at helping families and schools support affected or high-risk youth.

In particular, multisystemic interventions designed to promote resilience, such as those that have been successfully implemented to treat aggressive or conduct-disordered youth (Bierman et al., 2004; Henggeler, Schoenwald, Borduin, Rowland, & Cunningham, 1998) may be able to make effective use of research that integrates environmental and biological perspectives. Multisystemic interventions are family- and community-based approaches to treatment that target factors in the social ecology (family, peers, school, neighborhood, and community) that contribute to problem behavior (Henggeler et al., 1998). Not only do they treat psychological problems as multiply determined and maintained, but they also have demonstrated at least modest long-term success at changing patterns of social behavior and cognition in both peer (Bierman et al., 2004) and family contexts (Curtis, Ronan, & Borduin, 2004). Comparable intervention at multiple levels (pharmacological, psychotherapeutic, family, school, community) in youth with BD, particularly if implemented early in the course of the disorder, might help affected individuals compensate for or remediate the socioemotional problems that commonly accompany their psychiatric symptoms.

ACKNOWLEDGMENTS

I would like to thank the editors and Dr. Ellen Leibenluft for helpful feedback on earlier versions of this chapter.

REFERENCES

Alloy, L. B., Abramson, L. Y., Walshaw, P. D., Keyser, J., & Gerstein, R. K. (2006). A cognitive vulnerability-stress perspective on bipolar spectrum disorders in a normative adolescent brain, cognitive, and emotional development context. *Development and Psychopathology*, *18*(4), 1055–1103.

Altshuler, L. L., Bookheimer, S., Proenza, M. A., Townsend, J., Sabb, F., Firestine, A., et al. (2005). Increased amygdala activation during mania: A functional magnetic resonance imaging study. *American Journal of Psychiatry*, *162*(6), 1211–1213.

American Psychiatric Association. (1994). *Diagnostic and statistical manual of mental disorders* (4th ed.). Washington, DC: Author.

Anderson, C. A., & Hammen, C. L. (1993). Psychosocial outcomes of children of unipolar depressed, bipolar, medically ill, and normal women: A longitudinal study. *Journal of Consulting and Clinical Psychology*, *61*(3), 448–454.

Barbas, H. (2007). Flow of information for emotions through temporal and orbitofrontal pathways. *Journal of Anatomy*, *211*(2), 237–249.

Bauman, M. D., Lavenex, P., Mason, W. A., Capitanio, J. P., & Amaral, D. G. (2004). The development of mother–infant interactions after neonatal amygdala lesions in rhesus monkeys. *Journal of Neuroscience*, *24*(3), 711–721.

Bearden, C. E., Hoffman, K. M., & Cannon, T. D. (2001). The neuropsychology and neuroanatomy of bipolar affective disorder: A critical review. *Bipolar Disorders, 3*(3), 106–150; discussion 151–103.

Biederman, J., Klein, R. G., Pine, D. S., & Klein, D. F. (1998). Resolved: Mania is mistaken for ADHD in prepubertal children. *Journal of the American Academy of Child and Adolescent Psychiatry, 37,* 1091–1096; discussion, 1096–1099.

Bierman, K. L., Coie, J. D., Dodge, K. A., Foster, E. M., Greenberg, M. T., Lochman, J. E., et al. (2004). The effects of the fast track program on serious problem outcomes at the end of elementary school. *Journal of Clinical Child and Adolescent Psychology, 33*(4), 650–661.

Blakemore, S.-J. (2008). Development of the social brain during adolescence. *Quarterly Journal of Experimental Psychology, 61*(1), 40–49.

Blumberg, H., Donegan, N., Sanislow, C., Collins, S., Lacadie, C., Skudlarski, P., et al. (2005). Preliminary evidence for medication effects on functional abnormalities in the amygdala and anterior cingulate in bipolar disorder. *Psychopharmacology, 183*(3), 308–313.

Blumberg, H. P., Kaufman, J., Martin, A., Charney, D. S., Krystal, J. H., & Peterson, B. S. (2004). Significance of adolescent neurodevelopment for the neural circuitry of bipolar disorder. *Annals of the New York Academy of Sciences, 1021*(1), 376–383.

Blumberg, H. P., Leung, H.-C., Skudlarski, P., Lacadie, C. M., Fredericks, C. A., Harris, B. C., et al. (2003). A functional magnetic resonance imaging study of bipolar disorder: State- and trait-related dysfunction in ventral prefrontal cortices. *Archives of General Psychiatry, 60*(6), 601–609.

Blumberg, H. P., Martin, A., Kaufman, J., Leung, H.-C., Skudlarski, P., Lacadie, C., et al. (2003). Frontostriatal abnormalities in adolescents with bipolar disorder: Preliminary observations from functional MRI. *American Journal of Psychiatry, 160*(7), 1345–1347.

Bora, E., Vahip, S., Gonul, A. S., Akdeniz, F., Alkan, M., Ogut, M., et al. (2005). Evidence for theory of mind deficits in euthymic patients with bipolar disorder. *Acta Psychiatrica Scandinavica, 112*(2), 110–116.

Bozikas, V. P., Andreou, C., Giannakou, M., Tonia, T., Anezoulaki, D., Karavatos, A., et al. (2005). Deficits in sustained attention in schizophrenia but not in bipolar disorder. *Schizophrenia Research, 78*(2–3), 225–233.

Brotman, M. A., Guyer, A. E., Lawson, E. S., Horsey, S. E., Rich, B. A., Dickstein, D. P., et al. (2008). Facial emotion labeling deficits in children and adolescents at risk for bipolar disorder. *American Journal of Psychiatry, 165*(3), 385–389.

Brotman, M. A., Kassem, L., Reising, M. M., Guyer, A. E., Dickstein, D. P., Rich, B. A., et al. (2007). Parental diagnoses in youth with narrow phenotype bipolar disorder or severe mood dysregulation. *American Journal of Psychiatry, 164*(8), 1238–1241.

Cannon, M., Jones, P., Gilvarry, C., Rifkin, L., McKenzie, K., Foerster, A., et al. (1997). Premorbid social functioning in schizophrenia and bipolar disorder: Similarities and differences. *American Journal of Psychiatry, 154*(11), 1544–1550.

Carpenter, M., Nagell, K., & Tomasello, M. (1998). Social cognition, joint attention, and communicative competence from 9 to 15 months of age. *Monographs of the Society for Research in Child Development, 63*(4), 1–143.

Chang, K., Howe, M., Gallelli, K. I. M., & Miklowitz, D. (2006). Prevention of pediatric bipolar disorder: Integration of neurobiological and psychosocial processes. *Annals of the New York Academy of Sciences, 1094*(1), 235–247.

Chen, C.-H., Lennox, B., Jacob, R., Calder, A., Lupson, V., Bisbrown-Chippendale, R., et al. (2006). Explicit and implicit facial affect recognition in manic and depressed states of bipolar disorder: A functional magnetic resonance imaging study. *Biological Psychiatry, 59*(1), 31–39.

Cools, R., Clark, L., & Robbins, T. W. (2004). Differential responses in human striatum and prefrontal cortex to changes in object and rule relevance. *Journal of Neuroscience*, 24(5), 1129–1135.

Crick, N. R., & Dodge, K. A. (1994). A review and reformulation of social information-processing mechanisms in children's social adjustment. *Psychological Bulletin*, 115(1), 74–101.

Curtis, N. M., Ronan, K. R., & Borduin, C. M. (2004). Multisystemic treatment: A meta-analysis of outcome studies. *Journal of Family Psychology*, 18(3), 411–419.

De Los Reyes, A., & Kazdin, A. E. (2006). Informant discrepancies in assessing child dysfunction relate to dysfunction within mother–child interactions. *Journal of Child and Family Studies*, 15(5), 645–663.

DelBello, M. P., & Kowatch, R. A. (2006). Pharmacological interventions for bipolar youth: Developmental considerations. *Development and Psychopathology*, 18, 1231–1246.

Dickstein, D. P., Nelson, E. E., McClure, E. B., Grimley, M. E., Knopf, L., Brotman, M. A., et al. (2007). Cognitive flexibility in phenotypes of pediatric bipolar disorder. *Journal of the American Academy of Child and Adolescent Psychiatry*, 46(3), 341–355.

Dickstein, D. P., Rich, B. A., Roberson-Nay, R., Berghorst, L., Vinton, D., Pine, D. S., et al. (2007). Neural activation during encoding of emotional faces in pediatric bipolar disorder. *Bipolar Disorders*, 9(7), 679–692.

Eaton, W. W., Shao, H., Nestadt, G., Lee, B. H., Bienvenu, O. J., & Zandi, P. (2008). Population-based study of first onset and chronicity in major depressive disorder. *Archives of General Psychiatry*, 65(5), 513–520.

Edvardsen, J., Torgersen, S., Roysamb, E., Lygren, S., Skre, I., Onstad, S., et al. (2008). Heritability of bipolar spectrum disorders. Unity or heterogeneity? *Journal of Affective Disorders*, 106(3), 229–240.

Fagiolini, A., Kupfer, D. J., Masalehdan, A., Scott, J. A., Houck, P. R., & Frank, E. (2005). Functional impairment in the remission phase of bipolar disorder. *Bipolar Disorders*, 7(3), 281–285.

Fleck, D. E., Shear, P. K., Zimmerman, M. E., Getz, G. E., Corey, K. B., Jak, A., et al. (2003). Verbal memory in mania: Effects of clinical state and task requirements. *Bipolar Disorders*, 5(5), 375–380.

Foland, L. C., Altshuler, L. L., Bookheimer, S. Y., Eisenberger, N., Townsend, J., & Thompson, P. M. (2008). Evidence for deficient modulation of amygdala response by prefrontal cortex in bipolar mania. *Psychiatry Research: Neuroimaging*, 162(1), 27–37.

Fullerton, C. S., & Ursano, R. J. (1994). Preadolescent peer friendships: A critical contribution to adult social relatedness? *Journal of Youth and Adolescence*, 23(1), 43–63.

Galanter, C. A., & Leibenluft, E. (2008). Frontiers between attention deficit hyperactivity disorder and bipolar disorder. *Child and Adolescent Psychiatric Clinics of North America*, 17(2), 325–346.

Geller, B., Bolhofner, K., Craney, J. L., Williams, M., DelBello, M. P., & Gundersen, K. (2000). Psychosocial functioning in a prepubertal and early adolescent bipolar disorder phenotype. *Journal of the American Academy of Child and Adolescent Psychiatry*, 39(12), 1543–1548.

Geller, B., Craney, J. L., Bolhofner, K., DelBello, M. P., Axelson, D., Luby, J., et al. (2003). Phenomenology and longitudinal course of children with a prepubertal and early adolescent bipolar disorder phenotype. In B. Geller & M. P. DelBello (Eds.), *Bipolar disorder in childhood and early adolescence* (pp. 25–50). New York: Guilford Press.

Geller, B., Craney, J. L., Bolhofner, K., Nickelsburg, M. J., Williams, M., & Zimerman, B. (2002). Two-year prospective follow-up of children with a prepubertal and early adolescent bipolar disorder phenotype. *American Journal of Psychiatry*, 159(6), 927–933.

Getz, G. E., Shear, P. K., & Strakowski, S. M. (2003). Facial affect recognition deficits in bipolar disorder. *Journal of the International Neuropsychological Society, 9*(4), 623–632.

Giedd, J. N. (2004). Structural magnetic resonance imaging of the adolescent brain. *Annals of the New York Academy of Sciences, 1021*(1), 77–85.

Giedd, J. N., Castellanos, F. X., Rajapakse, J. C., Vaituzis, A. C., & Rapoport, J. L. (1997). Sexual dimorphism of the developing human brain. *Progress in Neuro-Psychopharmacology and Biological Psychiatry, 21*(8), 1185–1201.

Gogtay, N., Giedd, J. N., Lusk, L., Hayashi, K. M., Greenstein, D., Vaituzis, A. C., et al. (2004). Dynamic mapping of human cortical development during childhood through early adulthood. *Proceedings of the National Academy of Sciences USA, 101*(21), 8174–8179.

Gogtay, N., Ordonez, A., Herman, D. H., Hayashi, K. M., Greenstein, D., Vaituzis, C., et al. (2007). Dynamic mapping of cortical development before and after the onset of pediatric bipolar illness. *Journal of Child Psychology and Psychiatry, 48*(9), 852–862.

Goldstein, T. R., Miklowitz, D. J., & Mullen, K. L. (2006). Social skills knowledge and performance among adolescents with bipolar disorder. *Bipolar Disorders, 8*(4), 350–361.

Goursaud, A.-P. S., & Bachevalier, J. (2007). Social attachment in juvenile monkeys with neonatal lesion of the hippocampus, amygdala and orbital frontal cortex. *Behavioural Brain Research, 176*(1), 75–93.

Gu, B.-M., Park, J.-Y., Kang, D.-H., Lee, S. J., Yoo, S. Y., Jo, H. J., et al. (2008). Neural correlates of cognitive inflexibility during task-switching in obsessive–compulsive disorder. *Brain, 131*(1), 155–164.

Guyer, A. E., McClure, E. B., Adler, A. D., Brotman, M. A., Rich, B. A., Kimes, A. S., et al. (2007). Specificity of facial expression labeling deficits in childhood psychopathology. *Journal of Child Psychology and Psychiatry, 48*(9), 863–871.

Haldane, M., Jogia, J., Cobb, A., Kozuch, E., Kumari, V., & Frangou, S. (2008). Changes in brain activation during working memory and facial recognition tasks in patients with bipolar disorder with lamotrigine monotherapy. *European Neuropsychopharmacology, 18*(1), 48–54.

Halit, H., Csibra, G., Volein, A., & Johnson, M. H. (2004). Face-sensitive cortical processing in early infancy. *Journal of Child Psychology and Psychiatry, 45*(7), 1228–1234.

Halit, H., de Haan, M., & Johnson, M. H. (2003). Cortical specialisation for face processing: Face-sensitive event-related potential components in 3- and 12-month-old infants. *NeuroImage, 19*(3), 1180–1193.

Heaton, R. K., Chelune, G. J., Talley, J., Kay, K. K., & Curtiss, G. (1993). *Wisconsin Card Sorting Test manual.* Odessa, FL: Psychological Assessment Resources.

Henggeler, S. W., Schoenwald, S. K., Borduin, C. M., Rowland, M. D., & Cunningham, P. B. (1998). *Multisystemic treatment of antisocial behavior in children and adolescents.* New York: Guilford Press.

Hillegers, M. H. J., Burger, H., Wals, M., Reichart, C. G., Verhulst, F. C., Nolen, W. A., et al. (2004). Impact of stressful life events, familial loading and their interaction on the onset of mood disorders: Study in a high-risk cohort of adolescent offspring of parents with bipolar disorder. *British Journal of Psychiatry, 185*(2), 97–101.

Iacono, W. G., Peloquin, L. J., Lumry, A. E., Valentine, R. H., & Tuason, V. B. (1982). Eye tracking in patients with unipolar and bipolar affective disorders in remission. *Journal of Abnormal Psychology, 91*(1), 35–44.

Jogia, J., Haldane, M., Cobb, A., Kumari, V., & Frangou, S. (2008). Pilot investigation of the changes in cortical activation during facial affect recognition with lamotrigine monotherapy in bipolar disorder. *British Journal of Psychiatry, 192*(3), 197–201.

Johnson, M. H., Griffin, R., Csibra, G., Halit, H., Farroni, de Haan, M., et al. (2005). The emergence of the social brain network: Evidence from typical and atypical development. *Development and Psychopathology, 17*(3), 599–619.

Jones, D. C., Abbey, B. B., & Cumberland, A. (1998). The development of display rule knowledge: Linkages with family expressiveness and social competence. *Child Development, 69*(4), 1209–1222.

Kerr, N., Dunbar, R. I. M., & Bentall, R. P. (2003). Theory of mind deficits in bipolar affective disorder. *Journal of Affective Disorders, 73*(3), 253–259.

Kliewer, W., Fearnow, M. D., & Miller, P. A. (1996). Coping socialization in middle childhood: Tests of maternal and paternal influences. *Child Development, 67*(5), 2339–2357.

Kronhaus, D. M., Lawrence, N. S., Williams, A. M., Frangou, S., Brammer, M. J., Williams, S. C. R., et al. (2006). Stroop performance in bipolar disorder: Further evidence for abnormalities in the ventral prefrontal cortex. *Bipolar Disorders, 8*(1), 28–39.

Kutcher, S., Robertson, H. A., & Bird, D. (1998). Premorbid functioning in adolescent onset bipolar I disorder: A preliminary report from an ongoing study. *Journal of Affective Disorders, 51*(2), 137–144.

Lagattuta, K. H. (2005). When you shouldn't do what you want to do: Young children's understanding of desires, rules, and emotions. *Child Development, 76*(3), 713–733.

Lagopoulos, J., & Malhi, G. S. (2007). A functional magnetic resonance imaging study of emotional Stroop in euthymic bipolar disorder. *NeuroReport, 18*(15), 1583–1587.

Lawrence, N. S., Williams, A. M., Surguladze, S., Giampietro, V., Brammer, M. J., Andrew, C., et al. (2004). Subcortical and ventral prefrontal cortical neural responses to facial expressions distinguish patients with bipolar disorder and major depression. *Biological Psychiatry, 55*(6), 578–587.

Leibenluft, E., Blair, R. J., Charney, D. S., & Pine, D. S. (2003). Irritability in pediatric mania and other childhood psychopathology. *Annals of the New York Academy of Sciences, 1008*, 201–218.

Leibenluft, E., Charney, D. S., Towbin, K. E., Bhangoo, R. K., & Pine, D. S. (2003). Defining clinical phenotypes of juvenile mania. *American Journal of Psychiatry, 160*(3), 430–437.

Leibenluft, E., Cohen, P., Gorrindo, T., Brook, J. S., & Pine, D. S. (2006). Chronic versus episodic irritability in youth: A community-based, longitudinal study of clinical and diagnostic associations. *Journal of Child and Adolescent Psychopharmacology, 16*(4), 456–466.

Leibenluft, E., Rich, B. A., Vinton, D. T., Nelson, E. E., Fromm, S. J., Berghorst, L. H., et al. (2007). Neural circuitry engaged during unsuccessful motor inhibition in pediatric bipolar disorder. *American Journal of Psychiatry, 164*(1), 52–60.

Lembke, A., & Ketter, T. A. (2002). Impaired recognition of facial emotion in mania. *American Journal of Psychiatry, 159*(2), 302–304.

Lennox, B. R., Jacob, R., Calder, A. J., Lupson, V., & Bullmore, E. T. (2004). Behavioural and neurocognitive responses to sad facial affect are attenuated in patients with mania. *Psychological Medicine, 34*(5), 795–802.

Lewinsohn, P. M., Steinmetz, J. L., Larson, D. W., & Franklin, J. (1981). Depression-related cognitions: Antecedent or consequence? *Journal of Abnormal Psychology, 90*, 213–219.

Lezak, M. D. (2004). *Neuropsychological assessment* (4th ed.). New York: Oxford University Press.

Liu, S. K., Chiu, C.-H., Chang, C.-J., Hwang, T.-J., Hwu, H.-G., & Chen, W. J. (2002). Deficits in sustained attention in schizophrenia and affective disorders: Stable versus state-dependent markers. *American Journal of Psychiatry, 159*(6), 975–982.

Logan, G. D., Schachar, R. J., & Tannock, R. (1997). Impulsivity and inhibitory control. *Psychological Science, 8*(1), 60–64.

MacQueen, G. M., Young, L. T., & Joffe, R. T. (2001). A review of psychosocial outcome in patients with bipolar disorder. *Acta Psychiatrica Scandinavica, 103*(3), 163–170.

Malhi, G. S., Lagopoulos, J., Sachdev, P. S., Ivanovski, B., & Shnier, R. (2005). An emotional Stroop functional MRI study of euthymic bipolar disorder. *Bipolar Disorders, 7*(Suppl. 5), 58–69.

Malhi, G. S., Lagopoulos, J., Sachdev, P. S., Ivanovski, B., Shnier, R., & Ketter, T. (2007). Is a lack of disgust something to fear? A functional magnetic resonance imaging facial emotion recognition study in euthymic bipolar disorder patients. *Bipolar Disorders, 9*(4), 345–357.

Marchand, W. R., Lee, J. N., Thatcher, G. W., Jensen, C., Stewart, D., Dilda, V., et al. (2007). A functional MRI study of a paced motor activation task to evaluate frontal-subcortical circuit function in bipolar depression. *Psychiatry Research: Neuroimaging, 155*(3), 221–230.

Marchand, W. R., Lee, J. N., Thatcher, J., Thatcher, G. W., Jensen, C., & Starr, J. (2007). A preliminary longitudinal fMRI study of frontal-subcortical circuits in bipolar disorder using a paced motor activation paradigm. *Journal of Affective Disorders, 103*(1–3), 237–241.

Martínez-Arán, A., Vieta, E., Reinares, M., Colom, F., Torrent, C., Sánchez-Moreno, J., et al. (2004). Cognitive function across manic or hypomanic, depressed, and euthymic states in bipolar disorder. *American Journal of Psychiatry, 161*(2), 262–270.

McClure, E. B. (2000). A meta-analytic review of sex differences in facial expression processing and their development in infants, children, and adolescents. *Psychological Bulletin, 126*(3), 424–453.

McClure, E. B., Pope, K., Hoberman, A. J., Pine, D. S., & Leibenluft, E. (2003). Facial expression recognition in adolescents with mood and anxiety disorders. *American Journal of Psychiatry, 160*(6), 1172–1174.

McClure, E. B., Treland, J. E., Snow, J., Schmajuk, M., Dickstein, D. P., Towbin, K. E., et al. (2005). Deficits in social cognition and response flexibility in pediatric bipolar disorder. *American Journal of Psychiatry, 162*(9), 1644–1651.

Meyer, S. E., Carlson, G. A., Wiggs, E. A., Martinez, P. E., Ronsaville, D. S., Klimes-Dougan, B., et al. (2004). A prospective study of the association among impaired executive functioning, childhood attentional problems, and the development of bipolar disorder. *Development and Psychopathology, 16*(2), 461–476.

Meyer, S. E., Carlson, G. A., Wiggs, E. A., Ronsaville, D. S., Martinez, P. E., Klimes-Dougan, B., et al. (2006). A prospective high-risk study of the association among maternal negativity, apparent frontal lobe dysfunction, and the development of bipolar disorder. *Development and Psychopathology, 18*(2), 573–589.

Miklowitz, D. J., & Otto, M. W. (2007). Psychosocial interventions for bipolar disorder: A review of literature and introduction of the systematic treatment enhancement program. *Psychopharmacology Bulletin, 40*(4), 116–131.

Milligan, K., Astington, J. W., & Dack, L. A. (2007). Language and theory of mind: Meta-analysis of the relation between language ability and false-belief understanding. *Child Development, 78*(2), 622–646.

Morriss, R., Scott, J., Paykel, E., Bentall, R., Hayhurst, H., & Johnson, T. (2007). Social adjustment based on reported behaviour in bipolar affective disorder. *Bipolar Disorders, 9*(1–2), 53–62.

Mur, M., Portella, M. J., Martínez-Arán, A., Pifarré, J., & Vieta, E. (2007). Persistent neuropsychological deficit in euthymic bipolar patients: Executive function as a core deficit. *Journal of Clinical Psychiatry, 68*(7), 1078–1086.

Nelson, E. E., Leibenluft, E., McClure, E. B., & Pine, D. S. (2005). The social re-orientation of adolescence: A neuroscience perspective on the process and its relation to psychopathology. *Psychological Medicine, 35*(2), 163–174.

Nelson, E. E., Vinton, D. T., Berghorst, L., Towbin, K. E., Hommer, R. E., Dickstein, D. P., et al. (2007). Brain systems underlying response flexibility in healthy and bipolar adolescents: An event-related fMRI study. *Bipolar Disorders, 9*(8), 810–819.

Nuechterlein, K. H., & Dawson, M. E. (1984). A heuristic vulnerability/stress model of schizophrenic episodes. *Schizophrenia Bulletin, 10*(2), 300–312.

Paterson, S. J., Heim, S., Friedman, J. T., Choudhury, N., & Benasich, A. A. (2006). Development of structure and function in the infant brain: Implications for cognition, language and social behaviour. *Neuroscience and Biobehavioral Reviews, 30*(8), 1087–1105.

Pavuluri, M. N., O'Connor, M. M., Harral, E., & Sweeney, J. A. (2007). Affective neural circuitry during facial emotion processing in pediatric bipolar disorder. *Biological Psychiatry, 62*(2), 158–167.

Perlis, R. H., Smoller, J. W., Fava, M., Rosenbaum, J. F., Nierenberg, A. A., & Sachs, G. S. (2004). The prevalence and clinical correlates of anger attacks during depressive episodes in bipolar disorder. *Journal of Affective Disorders, 79*(1–3), 291–295.

Petti, T., Reich, W., Todd, R. D., Joshi, P., Galvin, M., Reich, T., et al. (2004). Psychosocial variables in children and teens of extended families identified through bipolar affective disorder probands. *Bipolar Disorders, 6*(2), 106–114.

Phillips, M. L., Travis, M. J., Fagiolini, A., & Kupfer, D. J. (2008). Medication effects in neuroimaging studies of bipolar disorder. *American Journal of Psychiatry, 165*(3), 313–320.

Phillips, M. L., & Vieta, E. (2007). Identifying functional neuroimaging biomarkers of bipolar disorder: Toward DSM-V. *Schizophrenia Bulletin, 33*(4), 893–904.

Pine, D. S., Guyer, A. E., Goldwin, M., Towbin, K. A., & Leibenluft, E. (2008). Autism spectrum disorder scale scores in pediatric mood and anxiety disorders. *Journal of the American Academy of Child and Adolescent Psychiatry, 47*(6), 652–661.

Pollak, S. D., & Tolley-Schell, S. A. (2003). Selective attention to facial emotion in physically abused children. *Journal of Abnormal Psychology, 112*(3), 323–338.

Pope, M., Dudley, R., & Scott, J. (2007). Determinants of social functioning in bipolar disorder. *Bipolar Disorders, 9*(1), 38–44.

Reichart, C. G., van der Ende, J., Wals, M., Hillegers, M. H. J., Nolen, W. A., Ormel, J., et al. (2007). Social functioning of bipolar offspring. *Journal of Affective Disorders, 98*(3), 207–213.

Reisman, J. M. (1985). Friendship and its implications for mental health or social competence. *Journal of Early Adolescence, 5*(3), 383–391.

Rich, B. A., Fromm, S. J., Berghorst, L. H., Dickstein, D. P., Brotman, M. A., Pine, D. S., et al. (2008). Neural connectivity in children with bipolar disorder: Impairment in the face emotion processing circuit. *Journal of Child Psychology and Psychiatry, 49*(1), 88–96.

Rich, B. A., Grimley, M. E., Schmajuk, M., Blair, K. S., Blair, R. J., & Leibenluft, E. (2008). Face emotion labeling deficits in children with bipolar disorder and severe mood dysregulation. *Development and Psychopathology, 20*(2), 529–546.

Rich, B. A., Schmajuk, M., Perez-Edgar, K. E., Fox, N. A., Pine, D. S., & Leibenluft, E. (2007). Different psychophysiological and behavioral responses elicited by frustration in pediatric bipolar disorder and severe mood dysregulation. *American Journal of Psychiatry, 164*(2), 309–317.

Rich, B. A., Vinton, D. T., Roberson-Nay, R., Hommer, R. E., Berghorst, L. H., McClure, E. B., et al. (2006). Limbic hyperactivation during processing of neutral facial expressions in children with bipolar disorder. *Proceedings of the National Academy of Sciences USA, 103*(23), 8900–8905.

Robbins, T. W., James, M., Owen, A. M., Sahakian, B. J., Lawrence, A. D., McInnes, L., et al. (1998). A study of performance on tests from the CANTAB battery sensitive to frontal lobe dysfunction in a large sample of normal volunteers: Implications for theories of executive functioning and cognitive aging. *Journal of the International Neuropsychological Society, 4*(5), 474–490.

Robertson, H. A., Kutcher, S. P., Bird, D., & Grasswick, L. (2001). Impact of early onset bipolar disorder on family functioning: Adolescents' perceptions of family dynamics, communication, and problems. *Journal of Affective Disorders, 66*(1), 25–37.

Roth, R. M., Koven, N. S., Randolph, J. J., Flashman, L. A., Pixley, H. S., Ricketts, S. M., et al. (2006). Functional magnetic resonance imaging of executive control in bipolar disorder. *NeuroReport, 17*(11), 1085–1089.

Rucklidge, J. J. (2006). Psychosocial functioning of adolescents with and without paediatric bipolar disorder. *Journal of Affective Disorders, 91*(2), 181–188.

Rydell, A.-M., Thorell, L. B., & Bohlin, G. (2007). Emotion regulation in relation to social functioning: An investigation of child self-reports. *European Journal of Developmental Psychology, 4*(3), 293–313.

Schenkel, L. S., Marlow-O'Connor, M., Moss, M., Sweeney, J. A., & Pavuluri, M. N. (2008). Theory of mind and social inference in children and adolescents with bipolar disorder. *Psychological Medicine, 38*, 791–800.

Schenkel, L. S., Pavuluri, M. N., Herbener, E. S., Harral, E. M., & Sweeney, J. A. (2007). Facial emotion processing in acutely ill and euthymic patients with pediatric bipolar disorder. *Journal of the American Academy of Child and Adolescent Psychiatry, 46*(8), 1070–1079.

Schenkel, L. S., West, A. E., Harral, E. M., Patel, N. B., & Pavuluri, M. N. (2008). Parent–child interactions in pediatric bipolar disorder. *Journal of Clinical Psychology, 64*(4), 422–437.

Schwanenflugel, P. J., Fabricius, W. V., & Alexander, J. (1994). Developing theories of mind: Understanding concepts and relations between mental activities. *Child Development, 65*(6), 1546–1563.

Scott, J., Stanton, B., Garland, A., & Ferrier, I. N. (2000). Cognitive vulnerability in patients with bipolar disorder. *Psychological Medicine, 30*(2), 467–472.

Shafritz, K. M., Collins, S. H., & Blumberg, H. P. (2006). The interaction of emotional and cognitive neural systems in emotionally guided response inhibition. *NeuroImage, 31*(1), 468–475.

Simon, G. E., Bauer, M. S., Ludman, E. J., Operskalski, B. H., & Unutzer, J. (2007). Mood symptoms, functional impairment, and disability in people with bipolar disorder: Specific effects of mania and depression. *Journal of Clinical Psychiatry, 68*(8), 1237–1245.

Smith, A. B., Taylor, E., Brammer, M., Toone, B., & Rubia, K. (2006). Task-specific hypoactivation in prefrontal and temporoparietal brain regions during motor inhibition and task switching in medication-naive children and adolescents with attention deficit hyperactivity disorder. *American Journal of Psychiatry, 163*(6), 1044–1051.

Soutullo, C. A., Chang, K. D., Díez-Suárez, A., Figueroa-Quintana, A., Escamilla-Canales, I., Rapado-Castro, M., et al. (2005). Bipolar disorder in children and adolescents: International perspective on epidemiology and phenomenology. *Bipolar Disorders, 7*(6), 497–506.

Sowell, E. R., Trauner, D. A., Gamst, A., & Jernigan, T. L. (2002). Development of cortical and subcortical brain structures in childhood and adolescence: A structural MRI study. *Developmental Medicine and Child Neurology, 44*(1), 4–16.

St. James-Roberts, I., & Plewis, I. (1996). Individual differences, daily fluctuations, and developmental changes in amounts of infant waking, fussing, crying, feeding, and sleeping. *Child Development, 67*(5), 2527–2540.

Staton, D., Volness, L. J., & Beatty, W. W. (2008). Diagnosis and classification of pediatric bipolar disorder. *Journal of Affective Disorders, 105*(1), 205–212.

Sullivan, H. S. (1953). *The interpersonal theory of psychiatry.* New York: Norton.

Tamir, M., Mitchell, C., & Gross, J. J. (2008). Hedonic and instrumental motives in anger regulation. *Psychological Science, 19*(4), 324–328.

Tillman, R., & Geller, B. (2007). Diagnostic characteristics of child bipolar I disorder: Does the "treatment of early age mania (team)" sample generalize? *Journal of Clinical Psychiatry, 68*(2), 307–314.

Tillman, R., Geller, B., Craney, J. L., Bolhofner, K., Williams, M., Zimerman, B., et al. (2003). Temperament and character factors in a prepubertal and early adolescent bipolar disorder phenotype compared to attention deficit hyperactive and normal controls. *Journal of Child and Adolescent Psychopharmacology, 13*(4), 531–543.

Towbin, K. E., Pradella, A., Gorrindo, T., Pine, D. S., & Leibenluft, E. (2005). Autism spectrum traits in children with mood and anxiety disorders. *Journal of Child and Adolescent Psychopharmacology, 15*(3), 452–464.

Wellman, H. M., Lopez-Duran, S., LaBounty, J., & Hamilton, B. (2008). Infant attention to intentional action predicts preschool theory of mind. *Developmental Psychology, 44*(2), 618–623.

Wessa, M., Houenou, J., Paillere-Martinot, M.-L., Berthoz, S., Artiges, E., Leboyer, M., et al. (2007). Fronto-striatal overactivation in euthymic bipolar patients during an emotional go/nogo task. *American Journal of Psychiatry, 164*(4), 638–646.

Youngstrom, E. A., Birmaher, B., & Findling, R. L. (2008). Pediatric bipolar disorder: Validity, phenomenology, and recommendations for diagnosis. *Bipolar Disorders, 10*, 194–214.

Yurgelun-Todd, D. A., Gruber, S. A., Kanayama, G., Killgore, W. D., Baird, A. A., & Young, A. D. (2000). fMRI during affect discrimination in bipolar affective disorder. *Bipolar Disorders, 2*(3, Pt. 2), 237–248.

CHAPTER 12

The Role of Stress in the Onset, Course, and Progression of Bipolar Illness and Its Comorbidities

Implications for Therapeutics

Robert M. Post and David J. Miklowitz

A lthough bipolar disorder (BD) has among the highest heritability of the major psychiatric illnesses, a substantial portion of identical twins remain discordant for the illness. Additionally, some 50% of patients with bipolar illness do not have a positive family history of BD in first-degree relatives, indicating that environmental mechanisms as well as genetic vulnerability are at play. The data suggest the likelihood that gene × environment interactions play an important role in the onset and evolution of BD. Moreover, gene × environment interactions are an extremely important guide for therapeutics because environmental stressors can be anticipated and modulated; in many instances, the detrimental clinical and neurobiological effects of stress can either be blunted or prevented altogether.

A modicum of evidence suggests that environmental stressors play a role in (1) vulnerability to onset (and to earlier onset) of BD compared with those without such early adversity; (2) the precipitation of depressive and manic episodes; (3) the adoption of substance abuse comorbidity and reinstatement of such substance abuse in those who had been abstinent; and (4) the relapse and recrudescence of episodes of affective illness in a stabilized patient during pharmacotherapy. In each of these instances, a neuroprotective factor (brain-derived neurotrophic factor [BDNF]) that is stress sensitive is involved (see Figure 12.1). These findings

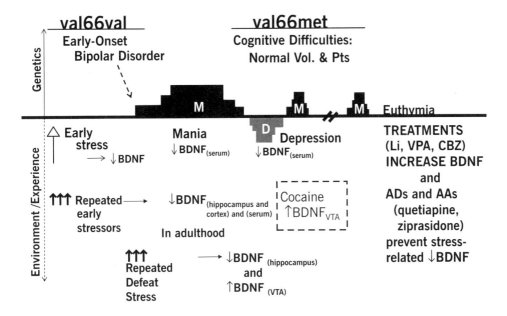

FIGURE 12.1. Brain-derived neurotrophic factor (BDNF) is involved in the onset, course, and treatment of bipolar disorder. (AAs, atypical antipsychotics; ADs, antidepressants; CBZ, carbamazepine; Li, lithium; VPA, valproate; VTA, ventral tegmental area)

suggest the importance of psychotherapeutic approaches not only to stress modulation but also to pharmacotherapy.

In this chapter, we examine the role of psychosocial stress across the different phases of BD. We also examine the mutual interactions of stress and biological (e.g., BDNF) or genetic vulnerability in the onset and course of the disorder. We discuss the role of stressors before illness onset, during the earliest phases of the disorder, and after multiple episodes as revealed in the kindling and stress sensitization models. After a review of stress mechanisms, we conclude with recommendations for psychosocial treatment approaches based on these mechanisms.

BRAIN-DERIVED NEUROTROPHIC FACTOR

There is now excellent evidence that the major mood stabilizers (lithium, carbamazepine, and valproate) can increase BDNF, and some of the atypical antipsychotics (quetiapine and ziprasidone), like unimodal antidepressants, can prevent stress from lowering BDNF in the hippocampus (Duman & Monteggia, 2006; Post, 2007). Several psychopharmacological approaches not only are effective in preventing episodes but may have direct and secondary consequences in mitigating and preventing the effects of stress on a variety of neurochemical systems, including BDNF. Evidence suggests that each episode of either mania or depression is associated with decrements in BDNF in the serum of patients in proportion to the severity of the depressive (Cunha et al., 2006; Karege et al., 2002; Shimizu et al., 2003) or manic (Cunha et al., 2006) episode. Moreover, there are episode-related increases in oxidative stress and the production of free radicals and other toxic substances that can endanger cell function or survivability. Thus, affective episodes bring with them the dual liability of (1) a decrement in neuroprotective factors at a time when these factors are needed to counter other effects of stress involved in the precipitation and maintenance of episodes; and (2) the increase in oxidative stress associated with each affective episode itself.

The effect of stress in affective episodes has a passive role in the general endangerment of cell function and viability. In addition, there appears to be a much more active and selective process of stress-mediated effects through specific enhancement and alterations of neurochemical pathways in the ventral striatum (nucleus accumbens), a key area of mood, motivation, activity, and reward modulation. Animals subjected to repeated bouts of defeat stress (i.e., stressors involving uncontrollable negative outcomes) show increases in BDNF in the dopaminergic ventral tegmental area/nucleus accumbens pathway in contrast to the decrements in BDNF in the hippocampus (Berton et al., 2006; Eisch et al., 2003; Tsankova et al., 2006). If either of these alterations in BDNF is prevented, the depressive-like consequences of repeated defeat stress experiences do not manifest themselves (Berton et al., 2006; Tsankova et al., 2006).

Thus, it appears that an active or conditioned component of defeat stress or helplessness/hopelessness behaviors may be mediated through an overactivated or overlearned dopaminergic pathway. This same pathway has been intimately implicated in the manifestation of drug abuse behaviors such as cocaine-induced hyperactivity and behavioral sensitization. In this form of sensitization, the increased behavioral responsivity to the same dose of cocaine over time is environmental context dependent and thus appears to have important conditioned components similar to the defeat stress paradigm (Post, 1992). Likewise, if BDNF increases are prevented, cocaine sensitization is prevented as well. These data give us potentially converging neural substrates that might account for several related processes in the developmental course of BD: the increased reactivity to stressors on repetition (stress sensitization), increased vulnerability to episode occurrence upon repetition (episode sensitization), and increased motoric responsivity to repeated cocaine administration (psychomotor stimulant-induced behavioral sensitization; Figure 12.2).

Although multiple neurobiological mechanisms are involved in each of these processes, we highlight the data suggesting a convergence of the role of BDNF in each of these sensitization phenomena as well as in the cross-sensitization of each to the other. The potential role of BDNF in these aspects of the progression of the illness becomes even more cogent as one then considers the role of psychopharmacological agents and psychosocial treatments in altering BDNF and related neurobiological mechanisms (Post, 2007).

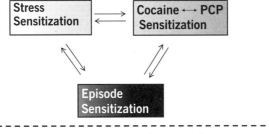

FIGURE 12.2. Cross-sensitization among stressors, drugs of abuse, and episodes. (PCP, phencyclidine)

STRESSORS AS VULNERABILITY FACTORS
FOR EARLY ONSET OF ILLNESS

Extreme life stressors in early childhood, such as physical or sexual abuse, appear to be associated with an earlier age of onset of BD compared with those without these environmental adversities (Brown, McBride, Bauer, & Williford, 2005; Garno, Goldberg, Ramirez, & Ritzler, 2005; Leverich, McElroy, et al., 2002; Leverich et al., 2003; Leverich & Post, 2006; Post & Leverich, 2006, 2008). Moreover, their occurrence is associated with a more complicated and adverse unfolding of the course of bipolar illness, more episodes, more substance abuse comorbidity, and an increased incidence of medically serious suicide attempts (Leverich et al., 2003, 2007).

Although not quite as well delineated as recent data in unipolar disorder, there appear to be gene × environment interactions in the onset of BD. Caspi and colleagues (2003) reported that individuals with greater amounts of early life adversity were more likely to have the onset of a stress-induced major depressive episode later in life if they had one or, even more so, two of the short forms of the serotonin transporter as opposed to the more effective long form of the transporter ($5HT-T_{LL}$). These findings in unipolar depression have been partially replicated in childhood (Taylor et al., 2006) and in adolescence (Cicchetti, Rogosch, & Sturge-Apple 2007; Eley et al., 2004), suggesting the kinds of gene × environment interactions that are likely to further emerge with increasing intensity of study. They also give neurobiological credence to the clinical view that some individuals appear to be relatively immune to stressor-related precipitation of a depressive episode, whereas others are extremely vulnerable. While it appeared that common variations in the serotonin transporter, as well as in BDNF and other substances implicated in stress reactivity and the affective disorders, played an important modulatory role (Kim et al., 2007) in the development of affective disorder, a recent meta-analysis has not confirmed these findings (Nierenberg, 2009). What did prove statistically significant, however, was the relationship of the numbers of psychosocial stressors in childhood with the likelihood of developing depression in adulthood.

In the case of precipitation of the onset of bipolar illness, the data have not yet been closely linked to common gene variants in the population called single nucleotide polymorphisms (SNPs). However, in those with a positive family history of affective disorders in the parental generation, there is an earlier onset of bipolar illness compared with those without this familial vulnerability, which, of course, could be mediated through either genetic or environmental factors (Figure 12.3). As noted, severe early childhood adversity is also associated with an earlier age of onset of bipolar illness. Moreover, if both occur, there appears to be an additive effect such that onset is earliest if there is a childhood psychosocial stressor and a positive family history of affective illness in the parents.

There also appears to be a "dose" effect of the occurrence of stressors on subsequent course of illness variables, such as whether a patient makes a medically serious suicide attempt later in life. With more frequent instances of physical abuse, the incidence of suicide increases from about 25% in its absence to about 50% in its repeated occurrence. The occurrence of even one episode of sexual abuse appears to increase risk of suicide, and if both physical and sexual abuse occurs, the rate of suicide attempts is the highest, with some 55% of patients making a serious suicide attempt.

Findings at the level of BDNF in the serum of patients mirror those seen in preclinical studies in which chronic neonatal stressors can lead to persistent

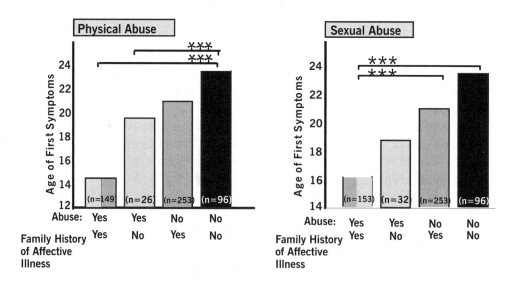

FIGURE 12.3. Additive effect of a positive family history of affective illness and history of early psychosocial trauma on age of onset of bipolar illness.

GENES AND PSYCHIATRIC DISORDER

Looking for single genes that cause psychiatric illness has been unproductive and is now a largely disreputable pursuit. Studies of multiple genes as vulnerability factors that interact with environmental circumstances may have greater merit. The argument about nature versus nurture is passé; development is a continuous interaction of nature and nurture.

---

decreases in BDNF in the brains of adult animals. Kauer Sant'Anna and colleagues (2007) report that those patients with BD with a history of childhood adversity (physical or sexual abuse) had persistently lower BDNF in serum as adults compared with those without such a history. How these findings might relate to the earlier age of onset of bipolar illness in those with childhood adversities remains for further exploration.

Recent studies (Lang, Hellweg, Seifert, Schubert, & Gallinat, 2007) indicate a correlation of BDNF and measures of neuronal integrity (i.e., N-acetyl aspartate measured by magnetic resonance spectroscopy). These correlations further support the likely association of low serum BDNF and neural vulnerability.

PRECLINICAL CORRELATES OF LASTING EFFECTS OF EARLY ADVERSITY

Rat pups subjected to a variety of stressors early in life can subsequently have lifelong alterations in their anxiety behavior, hypercorticosteronemia (excessive corticosterone production), and changes in the set point in the brain for producing corticotrophin-releasing factor, BDNF, and even neurogenesis (Coe et al., 2003; Francis, Caldji, Champagne, Plotsky, & Meaney, 1999; Francis, Diorio, Liu, & Meaney, 1999; Plotsky et al., 2005; Roth, Lubin, Funk, & Sweatt, 2009). Repeated 15-minute periods of maternal separation stress in the first week of life yield less anxious animals with better hippocampal functioning late in life. This is because the mother appears overjoyed with the reunion and engages in increased attention (licking and grooming) of that pup. In contrast, pups subjected to repeated 3 hours of maternal deprivation stress show a high level of stress hormones, anxious behavior, and learning and memory deficits in late life.

After 3 hours of separation, the frantic mother no longer recognizes the smell of the returned pup, which is not attended to and may even by trampled on in the mother's agitation. If another pup is substituted during the separation, the mother does not realize the loss and is not agitated, and the separated pup never develops the anxious phenotype. Other stressors, if repeated, can be associated with decreased levels of BDNF seen acutely not only in the hippocampus (Smith, Makino, Kvetnansky, & Post, 1995; Zhang et al., 2002) but also in the prefrontal cortex of the animal as an adult (Roceri et al., 2004). As noted, the set point for neurogenesis can be permanently altered for the rest of the animal's life. Even the prenatal environment can have an impact on cognitive function in adults, in part mediated by structural and BDNF changes in the hippocampus (Gomez-Pinilla & Vaynman, 2005).

This array of changes has been linked to long-term alterations in gene expression and, most recently, has been traced further into the inner workings of cell at the level of DNA itself. The induction of proteins known as transcription factors bind to DNA promotor regions to turn on or off transcription of specific genes, giving rise to an infinite array of changes in synaptic efficacy and plasticity. Now we know another way that DNA (whose sequence structure remains invariant) can be further modified based on input from the environment. The histones (around which DNA is wrapped) and DNA itself can become methylated, usually making DNA more tightly coiled and less available for the initiation of transcription. These "epigenetic" modifications of DNA and histories (methylation and acetylation) are induced by environmental events and can change how readily a large number of genes are transcribed for the remainder of the animal's life (Bredy et al., 2007). This could explain why some stressors during critical periods of development can change biochemistry and behavior for an animal's whole life span (Roth et al., 2009).

If animals have repeated neonatal stresses that render them highly anxious and hypercorticosteronemic for life, antidepressants such as the serotonin selective reuptake inhibitors are able to reverse this process, yielding normal levels of anxiety and corticosterone secretion. However, if the antidepressants are stopped, the animals immediately revert to the former (epigenetic) signature of high anxiety and high corticosterone. This appears to carry a pessimistic view for the long-term reversal of some of these environmentally mediated altered biochemical and behavioral set points. New data, however, suggest that histone and DNA methylation and acetylation are also modifiable by selective drugs. For example, valproate is a histone deacetylase inhibitor that can reverse or modify some environmentally induced changes that might otherwise be permanent (Bredy et al., 2007). DNA methylation is important for activity-dependent BDNF gene regulation, which is also critical to persistence of long-term memory (Bekinschtein et al., 2007). Traumatic memories can last a lifetime and are difficult to extinguish. The rate of extinction learning can be modified by some drugs acting on DNA methylation as well (Martinowich et al., 2003).

Another potentially optimistic view is drawn from the data of Champagne and Meaney (2001, 2006). They demonstrated that some rodent mothers were naturally high lickers of their infants, and others were low lickers. The offspring of the low lickers were more anxious and hypercorticosteronemic compared with the offspring of the high-licking mothers. However, if the animals were cross-fostered, what had been thought to be an inherent genetic transmission of these behavioral and biochemical traits was, in fact, reversed by the altered cross-fostered maternal behavior. Moreover, when these rodents themselves had offspring, the offspring continued to maintain the cross-fostered phenotype. This

---

EARLY LIFE STRESS AND BDNF

Repeated early life stressors in rodents can permanently change brain levels of brain-derived neurotrophic factor (BDNF) in adulthood, lower the level of neurogenesis, decrease the size of the hippocampus, increase the size of amygdala, and render the animal more anxious with higher levels of secretion of the stress hormone, corticosterone.

---

suggests that transgenerationally altered behavior can potentially occur even with an initial single generational environmental manipulation (Francis, Caldji, et al., 1999; Francis, Diorio, et al., 1999).

Data from McEwen (2003) suggest that early adversity can alter different regions of the brain and their functioning in a differential pattern. That is, repeated stressors lead to decrements in hippocampal volume in adults and associated deficits in hippocampal-dependent spatial learning. Intriguingly, the same animals show increased size of the amygdala and increased amygdala responsiveness in fear-dependent behaviors. These data become of special interest in relationship to the emerging neurobiology of bipolar illness, suggesting cortical and hippocampal deficits in structure and function. At the same time, there is evidence for amygdala increases in volume and hyperreactivity in a variety of amygdala-dependent paradigms (such as facial emotion recognition, especially for fear) in both childhood and adult bipolar illness (e.g., Rich et al., 2006).

A particularly interesting set of observations comes from multiple authors who have found that the amygdala volume is small in those with childhood- and adolescent-onset BD (Blumberg et al., 2003; Chang, Steiner, Dienes, Adleman, & Ketter, 2003; Rich et al., 2006, 2008), whereas many studies indicate that the amygdala is increased in volume in adults with bipolar illness compared with normal volunteers (Altshuler et al., 2000; Strakowski et al., 1999). This pattern may suggest the altered developmental trajectory of amygdala functioning, with the possibility of use- or overuse-dependent neuroplasticity contributing to increased amygdala volume. In much the same way, taxi drivers in England have been shown to have increased hippocampal volume on magnetic resonance imaging scans, presumably because of increased use of this structure on a daily basis in their normal occupational pursuits (Maguire et al., 2003). Alternatively, it is possible that those with larger hippocampi to begin with are more likely to feel comfortable with spatial navigation and may adopt taxi driving as a livelihood, and the direction of causality remains to be demonstrated.

It is unclear why there should be this altered trajectory of amygdala development in children, which then not only reverses itself in adulthood but also proceeds in the opposite direction of larger size. Altshuler and colleagues (2000) reported that the increased size of the amygdala is directly proportional to the number of hospitalizations for mania, although subsequent investigations have not directly linked these two variables. What is clear in both children and adults is that there are deficits in facial emotion recognition that are highly dependent on amygdala functioning. In a variety of facial recognition paradigms, the amygdala appears overreactive in both adults and children with BD (Rich et al., 2006). Thus, these findings in the clinic take on particular interest in relationship to the animal data in suggesting not only the possibility of genetic vulnerability mediating these differential alterations in brain and behavior, but also that some may be driven by early life experience and also, potentially, in the interaction of genes and environment.

To the extent that there are stressor-induced changes that occur early in life and that lead to these long-lasting alterations in brain structure and function, these changes may be amenable to moderation, prevention altogether, or remediation with appropriate pharmacology. The new data on the ability to alter histones and DNA methylation even raise the potential that some of these alterations, which one might have thought were lifelong and immutable, could be reversed in a sustained fashion even in the absence of the need for continued treatment. Today's speculations may seem entirely implausible and fantastic, but the explosive developments in understanding normal developmental neurobiology and its modulation repeatedly suggest that we are in for very major surprises in the future.

THE BRAIN-DERIVED NEUROTROPHIC FACTOR THE LINK TO ILLNESS-ONSET VULNERABILITY

In the general population, there are several very common variants in the gene coding for the proBDNF molecule, which then gets released into the synapses and broken down by enzymes to form BDNF itself. This conversion of released proBDNF to BDNF in the synapse may have important physiological implications because proBDNF binds tightly to a general low-affinity receptor for many neurotrophic factors (p75), which has been implicated in preprogrammed cell death (apoptosis). BDNF itself acts at its own specific high-affinity receptor (TrkB), which is necessary for the variety of neurotrophic and neuroprotective effects of BDNF.

BDNF is also necessary for long-term learning and memory. Rodents whose BDNF levels are "knocked down" to those of half the usual amount are unable to learn a Morris water maze and have deficient hippocampal long-term potentiation, one of the more robust in vitro models of learning and memory in the hippocampal slice (Korte et al., 1995). Early in development, BDNF also appears critical for normal neurogenesis and synaptogenesis in addition to mediating these long-term changes in learning and memory in the adult animal (Alonso et al., 2005).

BDNF has two common variants in the general population based on a single nucleotide substitution or polymorphism (SNP). The most common form of BDNF in humans has two valines at the 66 position of proBDNF, and this form is the most active (Egan et al., 2003). A slightly less common variant in the general population involves the substitution of the single methionine for one of the valines, or what is called val-66-met proBDNF. This SNP, when induced in animals, is associated with deficient BDNF transport throughout the cell and dendrites and a lesser magnitude of long-term potentiation.

In a variety of normal volunteer control groups and patients with BD or with schizophrenia, those with a val-66-met allele have minor cognitive deficits in tests that tap into working or episodic memory. If two methionines occur at the 66 position (met-66-met proBDNF), the deficits are still mild but more striking than those observed with a single methionine substitution at this position. Normal volunteers with the val-66-met allele not only have these minor cognitive difficulties, but they also have significantly smaller hippocampal and prefrontal cortical volumes compared with volunteers with the val-66-val allele.

Given the fact that many patients with bipolar illness experience minor to substantial cognitive deficits even while euthymic between episodes of illness, one might have expected bipolar illness to be associated with the poorer functioning met alleles. However, the opposite appears to be the case, and more than five studies indicate that the better functioning val-66-val allele of proBDNF is associated with an increased incidence of bipolar illness (Post, 2007). In several studies, better functioning val-66-val allele of proBDNF is also associated with early onset or a more rapid cycling course (Post, 2007).

To what differential characteristics of bipolar illness these two common BDNF variants relate remains to be further delineated. However, it is intriguing to speculate that the well-documented and replicated findings of increased creativity in patients with bipolar illness could be linked to the presence of the better functioning val-66-val allele, while, hypothetically, those with the more severe cognitive deficits could be among those with one or more met alleles. Given the ease of measurement of this single nucleotide polymorphism, both of these hypotheses are readily testable and likely to be confirmed or disconfirmed in the very near future.

Whereas we have focused rather selectively on the BDNF story, we must reemphasize that the BDNF gene vulnerability findings are likely to be one of a multitude of SNPs, perhaps including those in the serotonin transporter (Caspi et al., 2003). Current estimates suggest that somewhere between eight and 12 SNPs may be necessary for the manifestation of illnesses such as BD or schizophrenia, with each SNP gene variant conveying a very small effect that, in combination with many others, perhaps exceeds the threshold for illness emergence. Thus, potentially having the val-66-val allele of BDNF may confer a small, statistically significant increased risk of bipolar illness onset, but without a multitude of other genetic and environmental factors this would not be a very robust predictor of illness onset. Thus, the presence of a val-66-val allele cannot inform the utility of primary prevention strategies in those at high risk by virtue of a positive family history of bipolar illness in first-degree relatives. However, we hope in the very near future not only that measurement of an array of SNPs will be able to help in the prediction of such vulnerability but also may be useful in helping clinicians to predict individual clinical responsiveness or adverse side effects to a given therapeutic agent.

SINGLE-NUCLEOTIDE POLYMORPHISMS (SNPs)

SNPs are common inherited variations in genes in the general population, as opposed to mutations, which are by definition rare (i.e., about one per million individuals). It is thought that the co-occurrence of some eight to 10 different SNPs might be needed for the manifestation of a complex illness like BD.

This contribution to the field of prediction of drug responsiveness would be of immense importance to those with adult-onset BD wherein often a series of long-term clinical trials are required in order to find an adequate prophylactic regimen with one or more agents. The issue is even more pressing in children for whom there are, as yet, no U.S. Food and Drug Administration (FDA)–approved medications for those with childhood-onset bipolar illness younger than 10 years, and a number of the drugs widely used for this purpose carry mild to very substantial risks of side effects. (Most of the atypical antipsychotics are now FDA approved for children older than 10, however.) Thus, delineating the most appropriate treatment for these children early in the course of the illness by means of their SNP profile and other clinical and biological variables could contribute markedly to their well-being and even long-term survival. As discussed in more detail in the following sections, the treatment of childhood-onset bipolar illness is often delayed by a decade or more (Leverich et al., 2003, 2007), and the ability to assign the appropriate treatment early in the course of the illness may have a great moderating effect on its morbidity, comorbidity, and ultimate increased risk of death by suicide or other medical illnesses in adulthood.

Childhood-Onset Bipolar Illness: Cohort and Anticipation Effects

There has been an explosion in the recognition of childhood bipolar-like illness in youngsters over the past 10 years. One study reported 20,000 registered visits to clinicians of children and adolescents with a bipolar diagnosis in the mid to late 1990s, but this increased 40-fold to 800,000 visits a decade later (Moreno et al., 2007). Much of the speculation and controversy have revolved around two

---

NUMBER OF EARLY LIFE STRESSORS AND DEPRESSION IN ADULTS

Early life stressors in humans sensitize an individual to the precipitation of a depressive episode after the occurrence of a stressor in adulthood. The greater the number of childhood adversities, the more likely is depression in adulthood.

---

hypotheses: (1) that the illness was always highly prevalent but little recognized and (2) that with the controversies about the current boundaries of bipolar illness in children, particularly those with the BD not otherwise specified (NOS) variant, the disorder is being markedly overdiagnosed, and these children do not have the bona fide disorder (Carlson & Meyer, 2006).

Surprisingly, few have dealt with an alternative third possibility: that much of the increase is real and that the first two suggested explanations are only contributors to the markedly increased prevalence of the diagnosis. In fact, considerable data support the belief that not only is the incidence of bipolar and unipolar disorder increasing in children and in the general population, but also disorder onset is occurring earlier. Lange and McInnis (2002) have reviewed the substantial literature and found that there are two likely contributors: (1) a cohort or year of birth effect and (2) an anticipation or generational effect.

In the cohort effect, multiple investigators have found that there is an increased incidence and an earlier age of onset of both unipolar and bipolar depression in children in essentially every birth cohort (20 years or so) since World War I. Gershon, Hamovit, Guroff, and Nurnberger (1987), Weissman and colleagues (1993), and many other investigators have noted the earlier age of onset and increased incidence using the same criteria, so that the observations do not appear to be an artifact of altered definition of these syndromes or the thresholds for diagnosis.

At the same time, multiple studies have seen an anticipation effect of rather striking proportions such that if a parent had bipolar illness with an onset at age 25 and his or her offspring did acquire the illness, it would occur, on average, 10 years earlier than the parental generation, or at age 15 (Lange & McGinnis, 2002). There are both genetic and environmental potential mechanisms for such an anticipation effect. Huntington's chorea and fragile X are among two of the more well-known neurological disorders showing such an anticipation effect by virtue of parents with the Huntington's chorea vulnerability passing on a greater number of DNA triple repeats coding for the amino acid glutamine in huntington protein than they themselves had. The number of triple repeats one inherits is inversely proportional to an earlier age of onset of the illness. There are mixed data as to whether such a triple-repeat process is occurring in bipolar illness, and, obviously, a variety of environmental mechanisms remain candidates for both the anticipation and cohort effects.

Many investigators have their favorite candidate mechanisms to explain the cohort effect, with possibilities ranging from the increased divorce rate and breakup of the nuclear family; increased prevalence of alcohol and substance abuse in the population; and the near-epidemic proportions of childhood physical and sexual abuse that have been documented by public health authorities and the unreported incidence that is estimated in the United States and Canada to involve some 20% of the general population. Others think about TV, video games, stressors, pollution, population expansion, and a variety of others as possibilities.

The cohort effect seems to have occurred in many countries throughout the world, with one locale being an exception: the territory of Puerto Rico. This makes

---

INCREASED DIAGNOSIS OF CHILDHOOD BIPOLAR ILLNESS

The number of visits for a diagnosis of childhood-onset bipolar illness has increased 40-fold from 20,000 visits about 10 years ago to 800,000 more recently (Moreno et al., 2007). A variety of mechanisms have been proposed: increased recognition; diagnostic criteria changes and overinclusiveness; as well as real cohort and anticipation effects potentially driven by environmental alterations.

---

one consider the possibility that the maintenance of the extended family structure and other related factors may serve as protective mechanisms deserving further exploration. Delineation of the particular mechanisms involved in the cohort and anticipation effects would be of some import because, in many instances, they could lead to public health efforts and attempts at amelioration of some of these factors.

A Higher Incidence of Childhood-Onset Bipolar Illness in the United States Than in the Netherlands or Germany?

Clinicians, academic centers, and advocacy groups in the United States have been besieged with children and family members requesting better information and treatment of childhood-onset BD. This trend has been less readily apparent in a number of European countries. For example, Chang and collaborators (2003) had observed a high incidence of BDs in offspring of adults with BD in their clinic in Stanford, California, compared with the expected low rate in the general population. Conversely, few children with BD have been seen in a similar high-risk study conducted in Utrecht, the Netherlands by Reichart and colleagues (2004).

Many of the speculations about these findings have centered around diagnostic differences among countries or even differential rates of treatment of young children with psychomotor stimulants for attention-deficit/hyperactivity disorder (ADHD). However, recent data collected in our Bipolar Collaborative Network (BCN) suggest that these differences are real and not just an artifact of differential diagnostic criteria or different levels of care and vigilance in observation. We enrolled adults (mean age, 42 years) with clear-cut diagnoses of BD into a treatment outcome network and included four sites in the United States (Los Angeles, Dallas, Cincinnati, and Bethesda) and three in Europe (Utrecht, the Netherlands, and Freiburg and Munich, Germany).

On both patient self-reported questionnaires and the formal Structured Clinical Interview for DSM Disorders administered by trained clinicians, we found that patients in the United States reported double the incidence of childhood and adolescent onsets of the illness compared with those in the Netherlands or Germany (Post et al., 2008). The data were particularly striking in those with preteen childhood onsets (i.e., up to age 12). Twenty-two percent of those in the United States reported onsets of either depression or mania before age 13 compared with only 2% of the adults in both the Netherlands and Germany. These strikingly high rates of childhood-onset bipolar illness in the United States were also mirrored by the 28% of United States adults in the Systematic Treatment Enhancement Program for Bipolar Disorder (STEP-BD) cohort reporting age of onset before 13 years (Perlis et al., 2004).

Given the possibility that this differential incidence was real, which needs to be further documented by using the same epidemiological instruments in a number of countries throughout the world, we immediately looked for different vulnerability factors in the two patient populations. Surprisingly, we found double the incidence of positive family histories of affective disorders (unipolar or bipolar) in the United States compared with those in the Netherlands and Germany. Because we had previously identified childhood-onset adversity as a risk factor for early onset, we examined the incidence of childhood physical or sexual abuse in the two transcontinental locales. The incidence again was approximately double in the United States (22%) compared with about 11% in the two European countries, depending on the exact measure (Post et al., 2008).

Thus, the differential incidence of the two most robust correlates of early-onset bipolar illness, genetic or familial vulnerability and extreme psychosocial adversities, were both consistent with the doubling of the incidence of childhood and adolescent-onset bipolar illness in the United States compared with these two locales in Europe. Together, these findings suggest that there is more to the story than differences in recall or diagnostic criteria.

Although the increased incidence of childhood adversity in the United States has a variety of speculative explanations, it is not at all clear why there could be an increased familial loading for affective illness in the United States compared with these two European countries. A number of candidate mechanisms remain plausible but have yet to be adequately investigated. One is the possibility that those with "more adventuresome genes" and greater proneness to BD were among those who left Europe and migrated to the United States in greater numbers than those with lesser vulnerability genes. Another possibility is that of increased assortative mating in the United States, which is actually supported by our data. That is, with greater mobility of residents in the United States, persons with bipolar illness may be more likely to marry other individuals with either bipolar or unipolar disorder and thus add bilineal genetic risk for onset of illness. This would converge with multiple studies of childhood-onset bipolar illness, which have found that those with the earliest onsets of illness do, in fact, have a higher positive family history of bipolar illness than those with later, or adult, onsets.

Another possibility is that explicated by David Comings in his book *The Gene Bomb* (1995). He postulated that in the United States there is a faster generation time of those carrying genes for affective disorders, sociopathy, substance abuse, and the like compared with individuals who carry fewer of these genes and tend to stay in college or graduate school and not have children until much later in life.

He demonstrates that over a very few generations such rapidity of reproduction would have a very major effect on the gene pool, particularly if multiple genes of small effect were playing a role in multiple illnesses, many of which could also contribute to the risk of BD. Gotlib, Lewinsohn, and Seeley (1998) also found that females with major depression married earlier than those without MDD; those with early-life sexual trauma with or without posttraumatic stress disorder (PTSD) also tend to have intercourse, drop out of school, and bear children earlier than those without these adversities.

A panoply of psychosocial differences across the Atlantic could also contribute to the increased incidence of childhood-onset BD. Further speculation and discussion of these is outside the realm of this chapter other than to note two interesting candidates: an increase in a variety of stressors and decrease in amount of vacation time taken by families. Nonetheless, we would note that identification of some of the environmental and familial factors that contribute to this differential incidence in the United States could lead to attempts for their amelioration, and, conversely, the potential protective effects at play in Europe might be more widely emulated. However, recent data from Norway, Italy, Turkey, and Spain also suggest a considerable incidence of childhood-onset BD, and variations within different countries in Europe, if replicated, could also provide further hints as to the possible mechanisms (Diler, Uguz, Seydaoglu, & Avci, 2008; Soutullo et al., 2005).

CHILDHOOD-ONSET BIPOLAR ILLNESS CARRIES A DIFFICULT PROGNOSIS THROUGHOUT YOUTH AND INTO ADULTHOOD

The data reviewed previously are based on highly convergent observations from our BCN and STEP-BD bipolar outpatient networks in which those with the earliest age of onset had more rapid-cycling illness, more substance abuse, more suicide attempts, and a variety of other measures of a difficult course of illness. In the BCN, these outcomes were validated with prospective observations during a year or more of naturalistic treatment by experts. Those with the earliest age of onset had more depression, more severe depression, and less time euthymic compared with those with adult onsets.

These data are also consistent with the difficult courses of illness reported in current clinical cohorts of children followed by Geller and colleagues (2002); Geller, Tillman, Craney, and Bolhofner (2004); DelBello, Adler, Whitsel, Standford, and Strakowski (2007); and Birmaher and associates (2006). Birmaher and colleagues found that it took some 9 months to stabilize those with bipolar I and bipolar II illness, and with the more controversial BD NOS children it took more than 2½ years to achieve this acute stabilization. A very substantial portion of all of these children relapsed upon further observation (although less so in the BD NOS category). Similarly, Geller and colleagues and DelBello and colleagues found that, although a moderate incidence of children acutely stabilized, there was an extremely high relapse rate, and the children spent a large proportion of their young lives during these follow-up observations affectively ill rather than euthymic.

One caveat here is the nature of the treatment these children received in the community. For example, in Geller and colleagues' follow-up study, the majority were not treated with the recommended consensus guidelines (Kowatch et al., 2005; Post & Wozniak, 2009), that is, with mood stabilizers or atypical antipsychotics. Moreover, in our BCN outpatient clinic, as previously mentioned, those with the earliest onsets had the longest times to first treatment for either depression or their mania. In a new analysis, we found that the duration of the delay to first treatment was independently related to a more adverse outcome in prospectively rated adults; this included more time and severity of depression, less time euthymic, and more episodes and days of ultradian cycling (Post et al., in press).

These observations raise the possibility that long periods of untreated affective disorder not only lead to recurrent episodes, but also increase the likelihood of becoming involved in substance abuse and other high-risk behaviors (Wilens et al., 2004). These results could mirror those in schizophrenia, in which the duration of untreated psychosis is a predictor of poor outcome (Emsley, Chiliza, & Schoeman, 2008). If one had early concerted effective treatment, the question remains as to whether this would yield a more benign course of illness. Such clinical efforts are obviously worthwhile in their own right, independent of any fundamental change in illness progression.

Another possibility is that childhood-onset illness, with its greater loading of genetic vulnerability, is a more difficult and aggressive form of the illness in its own right. This would be akin to the observations in, for example, Huntington's chorea, wherein the number of triple repeats is inversely proportional to the age of onset, and the greater number of triple repeats yields a more rapidly progressive illness in younger individuals. Such an aggressive form may or may not be the case in childhood-onset bipolar illness, and a modicum of data suggest that the childhood-onset variety of illness may be as amenable to treatment (or more so) than the adult variety.

This view is based on clinical vignettes and inferences from the studies of Calabrese and colleagues (2006) in adults and Findling and colleagues (2005, 2006) in children, in which acute stabilization was attempted with the combination of lithium and valproate. In adult outpatients with rapid-cycling BD, only 25% of the observed cases and 17% of the intent-to-treat cases stabilized acutely enough to be randomized to either monotherapy, and 50% of the patients so randomized relapsed on either monotherapy. In partial contrast, Findling and colleagues (2005) showed that 43% of children stabilized on the combination of lithium and valproate, but here too, disappointingly, two-thirds of the children relapsed on randomization to either monotherapy. The vast majority, however, re-responded once the combination was reinstituted. In addition, the majority of patients were

> ### BIPOLAR DISORDER NOT OTHERWISE SPECIFIED
>
> Children with the most controversial BD NOS diagnosis are equally ill and dysfunctional and even take much longer to stabilize than those with bipolar type II and I disorders. The focus should change to finding the best treatment options for all of the bipolar spectrum presentations as well as the nonbipolar variants.

also treated with psychomotor stimulants for their residual ADHD. These investigators interpreted the two studies to suggest that the childhood-onset variety of illness might, at least initially, be more amenable to acute stabilization with the same drugs that are widely used for adults with rapid-cycling BD.

A slightly different perspective on this study suggests that, although the childhood-onset patients may be as or more amenable to treatment with some of the same agents as adults, the vast majority of children require complex combination therapy with these two mood stabilizers, adjunctive psychomotor stimulants, and, in a number of cases, other adjunctive treatments as well, reflecting a high level of general treatment difficulty and a very low level of adequate response to monotherapy (Birmaher et al., 2006).

Another possibility, of course, is that we have yet to define optimal treatments for childhood-onset BD, and with more appropriate choice of medicines and convergence with the best psychotherapeutic approaches, it might have a more benign course. What effectively inhibits the development of the initial phases of the illness may not be exactly the same treatments that are effective against the full-blown variety. Moreover, the early developmental nature of the central nervous system may require differential therapeutics. A particularly cogent clinical example of this phenomenon is the observation that the gamma-aminobutyric acid-B agonist baclofen is a highly effective anticonvulsant against amygdala-kindled seizures in young rodents (Mares, Lindovsky, Slamberová, & Kubová, 2007) but is completely without effect in adult rodents.

From an entirely different perspective, it is possible that the bipolar process, interacting with stages of neurobiological and psychosocial development in children, could exert more damaging long-term effects than the same type of illness in early adulthood when many of the psychosocial and neurodevelopmental tasks of childhood and adolescence have been completed. Whatever turns out to be the explanation, it is clear that the childhood-onset variety of bipolar illness is often inadequately recognized, and treatment is too often either delayed, inadequate, or inappropriate (Post, 2009).

As illustrated in Figure 12.4, the severity of bipolar illness in children and adults tends to increase progressively over the various stages of illness evolution from (1) symptom-free vulnerability to (7) treatment resistance. All too often the illness is treated prophylactically in a late stage of illness after (5) recurrence or (6) progression, when considerable disability and treatment resistance have already been acquired. Earlier recognition and consistent long-term treatment of the (3) prodrome and (4) full syndrome may lessen the severity of the later stages or prevent them from occurring altogether.

Eventually as clinical and biological (genetic and environmental) markers of vulnerability to illness onset become better defined, one could even hope to move treatment back into the (2) presymptomatic phase in hopes of achieving primary prevention. Treating the (3) prodromal phase and the associated comorbidities of anxiety and externalizing disorders would be considered secondary prevention or intervention before the onset of (5) full-blown episodes. Even sustained effective treatment of the first full-blown symptoms meeting criteria for the diagnosis of a manic or depressive episode—that is, (5) syndrome—and its comorbidities, in order to prevent recurrences and achieve tertiary prevention, would be highly preferable to many current treatment practices, which all too often involve only short-term treatment (Rx: picket-fence symbols in Figure 12.4) which is discontinued and results in recurrences of episodes of equal or greater severity/disability as schematized on the y-axis.

Episode recurrences may result in the development of sustained baseline dysthymia, cognitive dysfunction, or other disabilities and psychosocial losses illustrated in the recurrence (5) and progression (6) phases. During the progression phase, patients fail to return to baseline euthymia and premorbid functioning between episodes. Finally, in the latest phase of treatment resistance (7), there is a failure to prevent episodes altogether with medications that had previously been effective (i.e., loss of responsiveness based on repeated drug holidays [discontinuation-induced refractoriness] or based on continued treatment [the development of tolerance]).

COURSE OF ILLNESS IN EARLY-ONSET BIPOLAR DISORDER

1. Early onset bipolar illness is common.

2. Early onset is a predictor of a poorer, more treatment-refractory course of illness.

3. First treatment for mania or depression can be delayed an average of 10–15 years in those with adolescent (before age 19) and childhood (before age 13) onsets, respectively.

4. Years delay to first treatment is an independent risk factor for a poor outcome in adulthood.

5. Treatments for the earliest phases of the disorder may not be the same as those relevant to relapse prevention after the full-blown development of illness.

6. Treatments for early-onset BD in the community often do not follow practice guidelines.

7. Early recognition and treatment of childhood-onset bipolar illness may help convert it to a more benign condition.

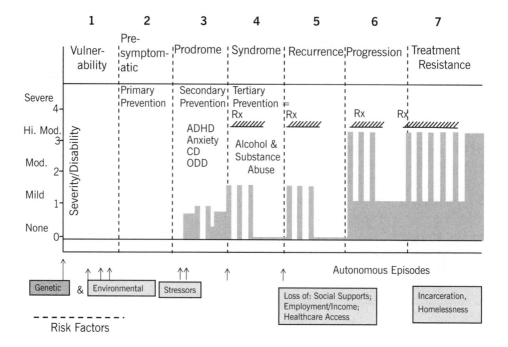

FIGURE 12.4. Stages of bipolar illness evolution. (ADHD, attention-deficit/hyperactivity disorder; CD, conduct disorder; ODD, oppositional defiant disorder)

STRESS SENSITIZATION

As Kraepelin (1921) observed, and of which the literature is generally supportive, initial episodes of unipolar or bipolar disorder are often precipitated by psychosocial stressors, but with sufficient recurrences episodes can begin to occur more autonomously (Post, 1992, 2004, 2007). One postulates an increased sensitivity to stressors inducing affective episodes to the point where they occur without provocation, but not the opposite perspective, which is often mistaken in the literature, that stressors later in the course of illness no longer are able to precipitate episodes. Kendler, Thornton, and Gardner (2000, 2001) elegantly validated the stress-sensitization notion over the first five to seven episodes of recurrent unipolar illness wherein stress has appeared important to episode occurrence and thereafter episodes emerged more spontaneously.

Stress sensitization is also apparent in the work of Caspi and colleagues (2003) whereby severe childhood adversities are associated with increased reactivity to stress-induced depressive episodes in late life, albeit in a genetically defined subgroup. As we have previously noted, early stressful life events in patients in our bipolar network were associated with an earlier age of onset of bipolar illness and an increased number of suicide attempts (Leverich, McElroy, et al., 2002;

Leverich, Perez, & Luckenbaugh, 2002). However, what we observed is that, over a subsequent course of illness, those individuals who had these initial stressors continued to have significantly more stressors of the negative variety, both at their first onset of illness and then over the course of subsequent episodes, including the most recent episode (Table 12.1). This suggests that there may be a component of increased exposure to stressful life events in those with early adversities, and these two factors may interact in predicting the occurrence of subsequent episodes (see also Dienes et al., 2006).

TABLE 12.1. Reported Negative Events/Stressors and Type of Abuse in Childhood

	Abuse	No abuse	p-value
Physical			
Mean number of reported stressors prior to illness onset	4.61	2.33	p = .0000002***
Mean number of reported stressors prior to *most recent episode*	4.61	2.38	p = .0000008***
Sexual			
Mean number of reported stressors prior to illness onset	3.99	2.57	p = .0002***
Mean number of reported stressors prior to *most recent episodes*	3.53	2.68	p = .024*

Negative events include:		Physical	Sexual
Unemployment problems/problems with housing/ financial problems	[onset]	***	*
	[most recent episode]	**	*
Problems with spouse or significant other/lack of family support/lack of person you can trust, confide in	[onset]	***	***
	[most recent episode]	***	**
Loss of social support/loss of important other by death	[onset]	***	***
	[most recent episode]	**	*
Problems with access to health care services/ inadequate coverage	[onset]	**	
	[most recent episode]	***	
Problems meeting demands of social/occupational roles	[onset]	**	*
	[most recent episode]	***	
Legal problems	[onset]		**
	[most recent episode]	**	
Medical illness problems	[onset]	***	
	[most recent episode]	***	

Note. Data from Leverich, Perez, Luckenbaugh, and Post (2002); Post and Leverich (2006).

EPISODE SENSITIZATION

Kraepelin described the huge variation in course of illness within and among individuals with BD, but was among the first to observe a tendency for initial episodes to be more widely separated by longer well-intervals but with successive recurrences the well-intervals shortened and patients began to cycle faster. This is not an invariant property because some patients begin to cycle quite rapidly at the very onset of their illness, but it does appear to be a modal type of presentation in many individuals despite attempts at acute or prophylactic treatment. It should be emphasized, however, that when adequate prophylactic treatment is given, the episode sensitization hypothesis does not suggest that cycle acceleration is relentless and long-term remissions cannot be achieved.

Using the Danish case registry of more than 20,000 individuals, Kessing, Andersen, Mortensen, and Bolwig (1998) demonstrated that in both unipolar and bipolar depression the number of previous hospitalizations for depression was highly predictive of the incidence and rapidity of onset of the next depressive episode/hospitalization. These are among the clearest data documenting the phenomenon of episode sensitization: that each recurrence appears to propel one toward the next episode and increase vulnerability to recurrence.

CROSS-SENSITIZATION AMONG STRESSORS, EPISODES, AND SUBSTANCES OF ABUSE

Stressors can not only increase reactivity to subsequent stressors and be involved in the precipitation of affective episodes, but can also predispose to the onset, maintenance, and relapse of substance abuse (Figure 12.2). Stressed animals show increased reactivity to stimulants, and stimulant-sensitized animals show increased reactivity to stressors. Behavioral sensitization to the psychomotor stimulants involves increased reactivity to the repetition of the same dose of a drug, particularly when it is administered in the same environmental context, suggesting an important conditioned component of the sensitization. There is some evidence that behavioral sensitization can occur in clinical populations because those using cocaine repeatedly show more dysphoric activation, and increasing amounts of paranoia and psychosis may also begin to emerge.

Thus, the patient with stressful life events, recurrent episodes of affective illness, and substance abuse comorbidity is in the unfortunate position of having each of these components individually carry the liability of increasing severity with repetition or recurrence. In addition, although each of these processes can be associated with progressive increases in vulnerability and reactivity, it is even more problematic that each can show cross-sensitization to the other. This can vastly complicate the course of bipolar illness. Thus, whereas stressors are involved in the precipitation of episodes, they can also be involved in the increased incidence, initiation, and reinstatement of cocaine abuse (Covington

& Miczek, 2001; see review in Kalivas & Volkow, 2005; Post & Post, 2004). Conversely, cocaine-sensitized animals are hyperresponsive to many stressors as well (Kalivas & Stewart, 1991). Patients with unipolar and bipolar recurrent affective disorder are at a much higher risk of becoming involved in substance abuse (McElroy et al., 2001), and substance use can also adversely exacerbate affective episodes (Fleck, Arndt, DelBello, & Strakowski, 2006; Sonne, Brady, & Morton, 1994; Strakowski, DelBello, Fleck, & Arndt, 2000). As noted early in this chapter, there is now convergent evidence that BDNF can play a role in each type of sensitization and thus potentially be involved in some of the mechanisms of cross-sensitization among stressors, episodes, and substances of abuse (see Figure 12.2).

CLINICAL AND PRECLINICAL MECHANISMS OF SENSITIZATION AND CROSS-SENSITIZATION

Brain-Derived Neurotrophic Factor, Oxidative Stress, and Episode Recurrence

The mechanisms underlying episode sensitization have remained relatively obscure until recently. There is now a fund of evidence from multiple studies in unipolar and bipolar patient populations that each episode of depression and of mania is associated with decrements in patients' BDNF in serum in proportion to the severity of the symptoms of that episode. Although it is not yet definitive, it is highly likely that some of the serum BDNF is either coming from or reflective of similar alterations in the brain. Thus, to the extent that BDNF drops and oxidative stress (generation of free radicals and other intracellular toxins) increases with every episode (Andreazza et al., 2008), we can begin to understand how recurrent episodes could have increasingly adverse effects on the brain and other organ systems (Kapczinski, Frey, Kauer-Sant'Anna, & Grassi-Oliveira, 2008).

The work of Kessing and Andersen (2003) indicates that those with a history of two prior unipolar or bipolar depressive episodes are at equal risk as the general population for developing dementia in late life. However, once one has four unipolar or bipolar depressive episodes, this doubles the risk of late-life dementia, and every episode thereafter conveys a small added increased risk. The data on low levels of neuroprotective factors like BDNF and increases in oxidative stress offer very plausible mechanisms for how affective episodes could endanger brain functioning and lead to increasing amounts of cognitive decline.

There is also a very robust neuropsychological literature that indicates that many measures of cognitive dysfunction that continue to be manifest, even in patients during euthymic intervals, occur as a function of number of prior episodes (Schretlen et al., 2007; Torres, Boudreau, & Yatham, 2007). Thus, minor cognitive alterations, as well as the incidence of late-life dementia, appear to be at least correlated with numbers of episodes. Although the direction or causality cannot be unequivocally demonstrated, the data would certainly reemphasize the importance of reducing numbers of episodes in the hope of avoiding cognitive disabilities.

Repeated Defeat Stress and Depression

A preclinical model for the induction of depressive behaviors has parallels to human stressful experiences that are depressogenic. In this model an intruder animal is introduced to the home cage of another rodent, who furiously defends its own territory and violently defeats the intruder animal (Berton et al., 2006; Tsankova et al., 2006). If the animal is not rescued, it may even be killed. The intruder can be protected by a glass barrier, but it can still see and smell the aggressor. Repeated occurrences of this defeat stress are associated with reductions of BDNF in the hippocampus and, remarkably, with increases in BDNF in the dopaminergic pathway from the ventral tegmental area (VTA) to the nucleus accumbens. The seminal studies from the laboratory of Eric Nestler (e.g., Berton et al., 2007; Nestler & Carlezon, 2006; Tsankova et al., 2006) have demonstrated that blocking either the hippocampal BDNF decreases or the increases in BDNF in the VTA–accumbens pathway prevents the manifestation of defeat stress behaviors. These data strongly support the view that the BDNF alterations are crucial to the development of depressive-like behaviors.

It is particularly noteworthy that repeated cocaine administration is also associated with increases in BDNF in this same VTA–nucleus accumbens pathway, and the prevention of these BDNF increases by a variety of genetic manipulations also prevent the occurrence of cocaine-induced behavioral sensitization (Nestler & Carlezon, 2006). Thus, differential alterations in BDNF in the brain—reductions in hippocampus and increases in the dopaminergic pathway—are likely to be critically involved in the stress sensitization phenomena leading to depressive-like behavior and cocaine-induced behavioral sensitization. This convergence of common mechanisms involving BDNF also represents a potential mechanistic explanation for the observations of cross-sensitization among stressors, episodes, and cocaine, wherein each can exacerbate the others.

At the same time, this convergence offers unique opportunities for potential therapeutic intervention whereby amelioration of the BDNF decrements in the glutamatergic neurons in the hippocampus or the increases in the dopamine pathway could, in part, moderate each type of sensitization and their cross-sensitization. In

---

DEFEAT STRESS

Repeated defeat stress decreases BDNF in the hippocampus and increases BDNF in the ventral tegmental area–nucleus accumbens dopamine pathway. If either change in BDNF is prevented, depressive-like symptoms and behaviors do not occur.

particular, it appears that the conditioned or context-dependent behaviors (based on habit memory as opposed to conscious representational memory-dependent hippocampal mechanisms) may be mediated in part through the VTA–nucleus accumbens–dopaminergic pathway, as evidenced in repeated defeat stress experiences or cocaine-induced behavioral sensitization. Targeting this overreactivity could theoretically help reduce or prevent the increased vulnerability to stressors, affective episodes, and cocaine self-administration as well as reinstatement of cocaine-seeking behavior once it has been extinguished.

This commonality could prove to be a single target of therapeutics with potential positive effects in the affective disorders and substance abuse disorders. Kalivas and Volkow (2005) reviewed findings that animals trained to press a lever for cocaine and then extinguished from this habit (because pushing the lever no longer delivers cocaine) will rapidly reinstitute bar-pressing and cocaine-seeking behaviors when faced with stressful experiences, appropriate environmental context cues, or a priming dose of cocaine itself. Kalivas, Lalumiere, Knackstedt, and Shen (2008) found that such induced reinstatement behavior was associated with marked increased secretion of glutamate in the nucleus accumbens, and administering the compound N-acetylcysteine (NAC) would normalize the overactive glutamate release and be associated with decreased cocaine-reinstatement behaviors. Zhou and Kalivas (2008) took these preclinical observations into the clinic and found that cocaine addicts had decreased cocaine craving when administered NAC, and heroin addicts also experienced the same phenomenon. Others have reported that NAC also inhibits gambling addiction, alcohol and cigarette cravings, and trichtillomania, each of which appears to involve an overactive habit memory system.

Quite independently, Michael Berk in Australia found that NAC administered to inadequately responsive patients with BD resulted in dramatic improvements in most measures of outcome relative to placebo after 3 and 6 months, with particularly impressive effects in the reduction of depression (Berk et al., 2008). NAC is a glutathione precursor and has potential antioxidant properties, and it is unclear whether this component of NAC or its ability to increase cystine–glutamate exchange in the nucleus accumbens and subsequently downregulate glutamate release (by actions on metabotrophic receptors) is the critical element in its positive clinical effects. Nonetheless, these data, and the findings with BDNF, raise the possibility that common manipulations in these convergent pathways could

---

TREATMENT AND BDNF

Treating bipolar illness effectively with medications would likely (1) increase BDNF in the brain and help protect neurons and glia; (2) prevent episodes and their associated drops in BDNF; and (3) help prevent stress-induced decreases in hippocampal BDNF.

have benefits in multiple domains of the triad of stress sensitization, episode sensitization, and cocaine-induced behavioral sensitization, each of which is all too common in patients with BD.

SOME PSYCHOPHARMACOLOGICAL TREATMENTS INCREASE BRAIN-DERIVED NEUROTROPHIC FACTOR AND PREVENT ITS DECREASE BY STRESS

The effects of pharmacological agents on BDNF form the linchpin of a new view of affective disorders. The fact that a number of drugs increase BDNF, or prevent stress from decreasing it, suggests that these agents may play multiple roles in clinical therapeutics. Not only when they are used appropriately in pharmaco-prophylaxis do they prevent episodes, but they may, in their own right, increase BDNF, as seen with the mood stabilizers lithium, carbamazepine, and valproate; the atypical quetiapine; and all antidepressants (Duman & Monteggia, 2006; Post, 2007). Other drugs (e.g., the atypical ziprasidone) do not increase BDNF directly but prevent stress from decreasing hippocampal BDNF. However, to the extent that any effective prophylactic treatment does prevent episodes of mania or depression, it would hypothetically prevent the decreases in BDNF, which would have otherwise occurred with each episode. Thus, in addition to considering a drug's negative side effects, we need to inform patients about their potential benefits, so that they will be able to make a more informed decision about the risk–benefit ratio for staying on long-term drug treatment in both recurrent unipolar depression and BD. Not only will effective treatment prevent episodes, with all their deleterious effects on behavior, social, and occupational function, but it may ameliorate some of the fundamental neurobiological alterations of the illness or prevent their progressive worsening.

IMPLICATIONS FOR A NEW LEVEL OF CLINICAL THERAPEUTICS

Attempting to lessen the magnitude of stress responsivity becomes a fundamental therapeutic goal not only for pharmacotherapy but also for psychotherapy. In animal models of depression, the ability to respond actively to a stressor can make the difference between developing learned helplessness or being protected from it. Similarly, teaching stress coping skills may provide buffering of the negative effects of stress in patients. If stressors cannot be avoided, which they usually cannot, they can be dealt with more effectively, with greater anticipatory preparation and equinamity, blunting their most negative psychological and neurochemical effects.

Having some control over the stressor can mitigate many of its adverse effects (Baratta et al., 2007). In the learned helplessness paradigm two sets of rats get exposed to identical amounts of foot shock stress. However, one is able to press a lever to terminate the inescapable shock, while the yoked-control animal receives the same shock but has no lever to press and passively has to wait for the shock to be terminated (as determined by the unknown actions of the first animal). Only the yoked-control animal develops learned helpless depressive-like behaviors, altered neurochemistry, and suppression of immune function.

Maier and colleagues have discovered that the medial prefrontal cortex is crucial to the protective effects of control over the termination of the shock stress (Amat, Paul, Watkins, & Maier, 2008; Christianson et al., 2008; Christianson, Thompson, Watkins, & Maier, 2008). If the medial prefrontal cortex is lesioned or temporarily rendered dysfunctional by a local anesthetic infusion, then even the animal that actively terminates the shock nevertheless develops the helpless depressive-like behavior. This suggests that it is not merely the actions of terminating the shock, but knowledge or awareness of the efficacy of the animals' actions that is protective.

Not only do these data give new insights into the crucial neural substrates of self-efficacy and control over unavoidable stressors, but point to a further difficulty for the clinically depressed patient. The dorsolateral and medial prefrontal cortexes are often hypoactive in depression, whereas the amygdala and nucleus accumbens are overactive (Ketter et al., 2001; Post, Speer, & Leverich, 2003; Post & Kauer-Sant'Anna, in press). The depressed patient may be less able to summon the required cortically based coping mechanisms. Moreover, the medial prefrontal cortex is also a critical substrate for extinction of old habits, suggesting that new learning that punishment or reward contingencies have shifted in a more positive direction may also be deficient and contribute to the perseveration of depression behaviors even when alternative strategies are readily available.

Moreover, while the prefrontal cortex normally exerts inhibitory control over the amygdala, and neural activity measured with positron emission tomography in these two parts of the brain are inversely correlated in normal volunteers, in patients with BD the cortex and amygdala and many nearby structures are abnormally positively hyperconnected (Benson et al., 2008). This altered pattern of regional neural associativity or connectivity could be associated with a lack of cortical inhibition of more primitive structures involved in emotion regulation. Such lack of normal modulation could account for exaggerated mood and behavior swings seen in BD. Thus, utilizing methods to bring the prefrontal cortex back online may be of special therapeutic value. These could include not only pharmacological interventions, but also psychotherapeutic ones (as discussed below) and physiological ones, such as high-frequency repetitive transcranial magnetic stimulation (rTMS) (Post & Speer, 2007).

Throughout the first portion of this chapter, we have emphasized the importance of the early institution and long-term maintenance of pharmacoprophylaxis in a dual attempt to ward off recurrent episodes of depression and mania and blunt their toxic neurobiological consequences. There are also a wide range of effective psychotherapeutic maneuvers that directly address each of the target points, wherein environmental stressors interacting with genetics, mediate processes of illness vulnerability, onset, and recurrence as well as the acquisition and relapse into substance abuse comorbidities.

Because extreme adversities of early childhood appear to be a vulnerability factor for early-onset bipolar illness in those otherwise predisposed, attempts at primary prophylaxis become critically important. Providing a safe and loving environment for each child is an easily conceptualized goal, but one that is difficult to engender across the general population. There has recently been a marked increase in the incidence of substance abuse and, concomitant with this, an increased incidence of documented physical and sexual abuse in the general North American population (Taddei, 2008). Because parental unipolar and bipolar affective disorders are themselves substantial risk factors for increased abuse of substances, and depressive episodes are associated with a high incidence of irritability and outright anger attacks, optimal treatment of parents becomes important in helping to ensure early healthy developmental trajectories of their offspring. Data from Weissman and colleagues (2006) show that in the Sequenced Treatment Alternatives for Recovery from Depression study, children of mothers treated with serotonin reuptake inhibitors who achieved remission of their depression had a lower rate of psychopathology compared with children of mothers who were treated, but remained symptomatic (although the effect sizes were modest).

A modicum of data even suggests that stress as well as the use of substances during pregnancy can affect a child's later behavioral responsivity and psychopathological development postnatally. During pregnancy and immediately thereafter, women with bipolar illness are at a much higher risk than the general population for the development of pre- and postpartum depression, mania, and psychosis. The postpartum period becomes a critical one for extra support, particularly if the mother has been recently ill. If there is an intact family and, preferably, an intact extended family, supportive resources may be available directly from the individuals in the household. Increasingly in the United States and elsewhere, multigenerational families have ceased to exist, and many households are headed by single parents. Single parenthood is a risk factor for depression, especially in the absence of social supports (Brown & Harris, 1978). Single parents, then, should receive extra psychosocial support during periods of illness and especially when infants and youngsters are in the household. Examples of this kind of support include mutual support groups, child care, extrafamilial supports, and financial aid.

Disappointingly, few such mechanisms are readily available for such needed support, and home visits by nurses and other medical practitioners are rarely offered. One possible ancillary solution to this problem would be for advocacy groups to develop not only the peer support programs that they are beginning to enact but to take this to the next level, as modeled by Alcoholics Anonymous. In that organization, a sponsor is specifically appointed and available to the individual on a 24-hour basis if a relapse is impending. Similarly, this sponsor or a related person from a support system could be available for the depressed, manic, or euthymic mother who is at her wit's end and in need of a time-out.

Counseling about enhancing and active modeling of physical contact between the infant and the mother with a postpartum depression, as well as other types of psychosocial support for both the mother and the infant could be extremely valuable. It has been repeatedly demonstrated that a series of weekly home visits by nurses for children at high risk for externalizing disorders and depression results in a much enhanced outcome, even many years later, as regards, for example, completion of high school, avoiding legal complications, and having decreased amounts of psychiatric symptoms and disorders (Cicchetti, Rogosch, & Toth, 2000; Eckenrode et al., 2001; Olds et al., 1999).

These strong data on primary prevention, particularly in high-risk families or those with depression and other psychiatric illnesses, need to be immediately extrapolated to parents with BDs in whom the needs may be even greater. Low parental warmth, family chaos, and high levels of expressed emotion have all been shown to be risk factors for delayed recovery and earlier recurrence among children with bipolar illness in naturalistic treatment (Geller et al., 2002, 2004; Miklowitz, Biuckians, & Richards, 2006).

Management of the young child with ADHD or other externalizing disorders, including oppositional defiant disorder or conduct disorder, is difficult enough even for a well parent with extreme equanimity. If the parent is depressed or manic, these difficulties are multiplied. If the child has childhood-onset bipolar illness, maintaining a safe and quiet home environment can be an extraordinary struggle for any parent, particularly one who is suffering from an affective disorder.

Studies of Hinshaw (2004) show that parents who accept and adopt enhanced positive communication strategies may see positive outcomes of their children's externalizing disorders. Likewise, Simoneau and colleagues (1999) found that adult patients with BD whose families improved in communication skills following treatment showed a greater trajectory of improvement over 1 year. Even in the absence of such data in youth with bipolar illness, clinicians and other care providers should take the position that similar support around family communication is essential.

This type of work is now being emphasized in many different psychotherapeutic approaches to either the "explosive child" (Greene, 1998) or to the child with BD. Family and psychotherapeutic support is more readily conceptualized in the family where the child already has a diagnosed externalizing disorder. In cases involving a child at high risk wherein the parent or parents are ill with an affective disorder, mechanisms for primary prophylaxis for the child are few. If the child has not yet been identified as a patient with a bona fide diagnosis, it may be difficult to generate such preventive approaches without a sea change toward greater attention to prevention in psychiatry and in DSM-V or its subsequent iterations. One approach capitalizes on methods from family-focused treatment (psychoeducation, communication skills training, and problem-solving skills training) for families of youth who are genetically at risk for BD and show subsyndromal mood swings (Miklowitz & Chang, 2008).

As noted, children and adults with childhood adversities (in the form of neglect or verbal, physical, or sexual abuse) not only appear to be sensitized to episodes being generated with subsequent stressors as adults but also are vulnerable to the accumulation of an increased number of negative life events compared with others without childhood adversity. This increased proneness for stressor accumulation combined with stress sensitization yields an individual with dual mechanisms for higher vulnerability to adversities later in life. A parental history of suicide attempt is a major risk factor for a child to make an attempt, and similarly a parental history of abuse or PTSD is a risk factor for the child acquiring these difficulties (Brent et al., 2002; Mann et al., 2005). Given these very high odds ratios in the population without regard to a bipolar diagnosis, acting preventively on the occurrence of these variables in parents with a bipolar diagnosis would appear even more justified.

Miklowitz and colleagues (2007) have demonstrated that any one of three types of focused psychotherapies for the treatment of patients with BD in the depressed phase is more effective than treatment as usual. There are now more than 19 controlled studies indicating that interpersonal, family, cognitive-behavioral, and psychoeducational techniques for bipolar illness are more effective on a variety of treatment outcome measures than conventional treatment without specific psychotherapeutic techniques (Miklowitz, 2008; Miklowitz et al., 2007; Scott & Colom, 2005; Vieta et al., 2005).

Although it has not yet been possible to identify which type of psychotherapy is best for which individual, many of the psychotherapeutic approaches have ingredients in common, including better management of stressful life experiences; enhancing communication in the work, social, and family environments; problem solving; learning emotional self-regulation techniques; recognizing and revising distorted cognitions; tuning in to better management of sleep and circadian-induced dysrhythms; better monitoring and recognition of early symptomatology suggesting an impending relapse; and enhancing communication with the physician about procedures to follow in attempts to abort the occurrence of a full-blown episode (Post & Leverich, 2008).

Table 12.2 lists the numerous essential components of an effective psychoeducational program. Each is critical to the maintenance of the long-term health of the individual. These include:

1. A fundamental understanding of the recurrent course of the illness and need for sustained intervention. This understanding sets up the entire course of clinical therapeutics and compliance with pharmacotherapy regimens.

2. In conjunction with this is the importance of building a treatment team, as spelled out in detail in Miklowitz's (2002) book, *The Bipolar Disorder Survival Guide: What You and Your Family Need to Know.* In contrast to the psychoanalytic exclusive focus on the individual patient to the exclusion of others, building a treatment team with family members and all available resources can be lifesaving for the patient with BD.

TABLE 12.2. Points for Psychoeducational Approaches to Bipolar Illness: Essential Ingredients to Long-Term Prophylaxis

1. The new conceptualization of bipolar disorder is that it is a complex brain disorder involving deficits and dysregulation of both neurons and glia, which can progress if not treated appropriately.
2. It is a highly recurrent disorder, and vulnerability to recurrences does not dissipate even with long-term stability but may even accumulate with recurrence of episodes, stressors, or use of substances of abuse.
3. The illness should be closely monitored, preferably with mood ratings on a daily basis. In this fashion, minor symptom breakthroughs can be readily recognized and treated expeditiously so that they do not lead to the occurrence of full-blown episodes.
4. Recruitment of a support team within or outside of the family is extraordinarily helpful.
   a. Utilizing this team, one should conduct "fire drills" for what procedures will be followed in case of minor or major symptom breakthroughs.
   b. Patients and the treatment team should understand that while manias can ruin family and employment ties and opportunities, they can also be associated with decrements in brain protective factors and increases in substances that are toxic to glia and neurons and thus further increase vulnerability to illness.
   c. The case is even clearer with recurrent bipolar depressions in which numbers of episodes are related to the degree of cognitive dysfunction, and if one has more than four bipolar (or unipolar) depressions, this doubles the rate of incidence of late-life dementia.
5. Each patient and the members of the support team should become familiar with the earliest symptoms of a manic or depressive relapse for a given individual so that they can help in the acquisition of further treatment.
6. Depressions are associated with drops in BDNF in association with the severity of symptomatology, and this could provide the explanation for progressively increasing vulnerability to episode recurrences as well as to cognitive decline.
7. In recurrent unipolar depression, antidepressant treatment appears to protect the brain and prevent decreases in hippocampal volume that would ordinarily occur with age in untreated depression.
8. Lithium increases the amount of gray matter in brain, and valproate (like lithium) also increases BDNF and Bcl-2, which are neuroprotective factors.
9. Thus, effective treatment may protect the brain.

Note. BDNF, brain-derived neurotrophic factor.

3. Establishing a careful monitoring system can also help in the delineation of the completeness of pharmacotherapeutic responsiveness and allow earlier intervention for symptomatic breakthroughs as well as help to clarify the role of stress life events and effective coping mechanisms in an individual illness course (Leverich & Post, 1996, 1998). Encouragement from the clinician and family members to maintain this record is of considerable import.

4. Patients and family members should review the earliest signs of prior depressions and manias so that these can be recognized before they become even more problematic. Establishing some of the specific guidelines for such an early warning system with the physician is of added usefulness. For example, the numbers of hours of sleep loss that should lead to a designated pharmacotherapeutic augmentation or a call to the physician should be made explicit.

5. In patients with rapidly progressing manic episodes or life-threatening descents into suicidal depression, establishing the specific procedures for physician contact, emergency room visit, and potential hospitalization should be clarified and rehearsed. In this fashion, each member of the treatment team who participated in such a "fire drill" can assist in the process should it be needed.

6. The psychoeducational program should provide good background information on the nature and actions of psychopharmacological treatments as well as the dangers of use and abuse of alcohol and other substances. Recognizing and dealing in advance with the high risks for engaging in substance abuse, particularly in teenagers and young adults, may help avoid multiple secondary complications.

7. For the adolescent with active depressive or manic illness, explaining the dangers of marijuana use (doubling the rate of psychosis) and alcohol abuse (further dysregulating serotonergic and glutamatergic mechanisms, leading to increased reactivity during each bout of alcohol withdrawal) and focusing on the seductive aspects of cocaine (the initial benign mood elevation and euphoria that can rapidly evolve into increasing dysphoria and paranoia) deserve careful attention. Moreover, explicit instructions, role-playing, and practice regarding how to approach friends who are drinking and using other substances so as to avoid being seduced into these difficulties are of extreme importance.

8. The recognition that stressors may not only be involved in the precipitation or re-precipitation of new episodes of affective illness but may, as well, trigger relapse into addictive behavior in someone who has remained abstinent should also lead to practice of specific mechanisms for anticipating conditional cues and ameliorating the impact of stressors.

9. Psychotherapeutic approaches to compliance with medications (Basco & Rush, 2007; Colom & Lam, 2005) are also an essential part of any type of ongoing psychosocial therapy. One should anticipate that patients may miss some of their medications. Inquire about this in a nonpejorative fashion, and discuss ways of avoiding this in the future. Utilizing once-daily or at most twice-daily dosing of medicines is particularly helpful: Noncompliance is directly proportional to the number of times medications are required to be taken over the course of the day. Linking medications to specific events or time frames can also be helpful, as can the utilization of pillboxes and other reminder techniques.

10. Developing effective communication techniques among family members may also be of extraordinary importance, as noted previously. Not only can high levels of expressed emotion, anger attacks, and aggressive interactions precipitate episodes, but they obviously preclude the level of sustained psychosocial support often required for the recovering or tenuously mood-stabilized individual. Moreover, family conflicts can precipitate medication nonadherence or discontinuation. Thus, enhancing the protective effects of the family can be critical to the success of a medication plan.

Ross Greene (1998), in his book on the explosive child, emphasizes the importance of avoiding repeated confrontations that lead to explosive outbursts and other "meltdowns." In this regard, he suggests placing most of a child's life events and behaviors into the third of three baskets: A, B, and C. Most behaviors should go in basket C, in which the behavior of the child is essentially ignored (e.g., distracting others during dinner). Basket B involves behaviors that can be negotiated (e.g., the time a child can watch TV); relatively few behaviors belong in this basket until the child's neuropsychological development and degree of mood stabilization make this possible. Very few things go into basket A, which is an uncompromising set of rules that must be followed because they are related to the safety of the child (e.g., avoiding weapons or toxic substances).

Greene points out that such a redistribution of parental reactions to most of the child's behaviors and life events is not an easy task and requires considerable psychotherapeutic support, working through, and practice. An essential ingredient is the fundamental understanding that the child is not always in good control of his or her own behavioral reactivity, and what appears to be intentional, provocative, malicious behavior may be better viewed as part of the neurodevelopmental and psychopathological expressions of psychiatric disorders. (Note: Greene usually avoids describing kids as bipolar.)

Other techniques emphasized by Miklowitz (2002), Miklowitz and George (2008), Fristad and Goldberg-Arnold (2003), and Pavuluri and colleagues (2004) in their family-centered therapies include:

1. Educating all members of the family about the disorder and how to recognize incipient episodes.
2. Assisting patients and family members to distinguish ongoing personality attributes (e.g., an explosive or reactive temperament) from the onset of new episodes.
3. Learning communication strategies for cooling down or exiting provocative interpersonal interchanges.
4. Assisting family members to learn self-soothing strategies such as meditation or relaxation.

As we more precisely define the neurocognitive deficits associated with different ages and stages of the development of BD, more specific remedial techniques may be forthcoming. As noted previously, it is now widely acknowledged that faulty recognition of facial emotions not only is prominent in adults (e.g., Bozikas, Tonia, Fokas, Karavatos, & Kosmidis, 2006) but exists in young children at the outset of their illness (Rich et al., 2008). Practicing ways of tuning into this process of facial emotion recognition better, or finding ways of circumventing the difficulty deserve consideration.

In adults the recognized deficits in executive functioning that may persist into the euthymic interval also require specific attention. Instructions should be given not only verbally but also in written or graphic form so that multimodal and repeated input may help reinforce new learning.

Some of the specific practice techniques of cognitive-behavioral therapy also deserve comment. As some abnormal behavioral processes become overlearned, they may migrate from initial encoding in the representational memory system involving the amygdala and hippocampus to habit memory, encoded by multiple repetitions in the striatum and elsewhere (Mishkin & Appenzeller, 1987). Insight and volition may be useful in dealing with many elements encoded in representational memory but of little use in more ingrained patterns of behavior involved in the habit motor system. The difficulty of reversing elements of memory encoded in the habit system is illustrated by patients who can clearly be desensitized and habituated to craving for cocaine upon stressor or drug cue presentation but continue to have autonomic hyperreactivity of which they may or may not be aware (O'Brien, Childress, McLellan, & Ehrman, 1993). Repeated passive presentation of information is not as effective in learning new material as a process that involves repeated recall and active practice of the material. Cognitive-behavioral approaches to symptom and stress reduction that emphasize homework and practice may thus be more efficient ways of achieving new learning than merely having repeated informational or acquisition trials. An example would be facilitating learning with recall and writing down answers or practicing solutions rather than just reexposure to the material to be learned.

The automaticity that develops with substance abuse behavior or the occurrence of affective episodes after many repetitions may require very different psychotherapeutic and psychopharmacological approaches from when these events occur very early in the course of illness. Moreover, stressful life events may catch the patient largely unaware of the connection to the affective response. Such an occurrence is recognized in the phenomenon of "funereal mania," when an event that may otherwise evoke sadness and mourning instead results in a manic episode (Ambelas, 1979; Krishnan, Swartz, Larson, & Santoliquido, 1984). Such clinical vignettes are now supported by the epidemiological data of Kessing, Agerbo, and Mortensen (2004), who reported increased incidence of manic onsets in individuals experiencing the death of a loved one, particularly the mother by way of suicide. Although the exact neuropsychological and neurobiological mechanisms for such events have not yet been adequately elucidated, discussion of the possible impact of stressful life events may have merit in its own right, even if specific therapeutic practice and techniques are not engendered. Discussion of a possible range of actions (e.g., sticking with sleep–wake habits even when events conspire to change them) may make anticipated stressful life events less pernicious.

Specific elements of the practice of the psychotherapeutic approaches used in the STEP-BD therapies have not yet been attached to specific outcomes. Miklowitz and colleagues (2007), as noted previously, found that this variety of approaches resulted in a quicker time to recovery from a depression and a longer interval before the next episode. Specifying the critical components of the therapeutic pro-

---

RANDOMIZED TRIALS OF PSYCHOTHERAPY

Sixteen of 18 randomized controlled clinical trials of a focused psychotherapy for BD are positive. Adjunctive psychoeducation and/or psychotherapy over the short term is a necessity and over the long term highly desirable.

---

cess may lead to an increasingly refined and targeted psychotherapeutic approach to some of the unique peculiarities of bipolar illness.

Interpersonal therapy or family treatment may be most productive after the end of an acute episode, while cognitive-behavioral therapy may be best when used during recovery. Psychoeducation should be revised as a function of the stage of illness with a shift from managing acute episodes to a major emphasis on relapse prevention and achieving and maintaining remission.

CONCLUSIONS

The revolution in molecular genetics promised to reveal new mechanisms for the pathophysiology and treatment of bipolar illness. This hope has not yet been realized, and the field now recognizes that multiple genes, each of small effect, are likely involved in this and other complex psychiatric illnesses. As such, we can expect the elucidation of multiple gene × environmental interactions. Not only do early stressful life events sensitize one to the likelihood of adult stressful life events engendering a depressive episode, but this may be more or less likely depending on whether one inherits relatively common gene variants.

As noted previously, the val-66-val allele of proBDNF may be associated with early-onset and rapid-cycling bipolar illness, whereas the less well-functioning val-66-met allele is associated with cognitive deficits (Post, 2007). A recent unreplicated report suggested that those with the val-met variant are much more likely to make a serious suicide attempt than those with the better functioning alleles (Kim et al., 2007). Thus, we can postulate that not only will common SNPs and other genetic variants in the population yield patients who are more or less stress responsive, but also that this lesser to greater degree of vulnerability will be directly altered by the environmental context of stressful life events, depending on their quality, quantity, and timing. Not only are environmental events currently more subject to avoidance, amelioration, or therapeutic intervention than are genetic vulnerabilities, but also the degree of psychosocial support received may do much to blunt the effects of stressors.

We noted previously that some psychopharmacological agents block the effects of stressors in decreasing BDNF in the hippocampus. In this arena, too, we look for powerful psychotherapeutic and pharmacotherapeutic synergies in attempting to modify stress reactivity and its impact on the course of bipolar illness and its comorbidities.

It is perhaps paradoxical, but in this fashion the molecular genetics revolution has reemphasized the critical nature of psychosocial stress in the course of unipolar and bipolar recurrent affective disorders and given us new psychological and pharmacological leverage for dealing with it and related adversities. Genetic vulnerability and resilience are set down in unaltered DNA sequences, but what genes get turned on and off and expressed in different developmental trajectories and in response to stressors is an extraordinarily plastic process. For example, Pasco-Rakic (personal communication, December 1998) estimates that an adolescent primate prunes back 100,000 synapses/second in its brain in attempting to replace many excitatory synaptic connections with inhibitory ones and prepare the brain for a new set of adult tasks and learning and memory challenges. Our vulnerability and resilience to a variety of stressors, even in those otherwise highly genetically predisposed to bipolar illness, offer a multitude of opportunities for pharmacological and psychotherapeutic intervention (Roth et al., 2009).

Many of the basic pathophysiological mechanisms for how episodes, stresses, and substances of abuse affect the brain, and how these effects can be prevented or ameliorated, have been preliminarily outlined. Given this rich set of new information, it remains for the U.S. and other health care systems to adapt to the complex requirements of the treatment of bipolar illness and its comorbidities and begin to deliver appropriate therapeutic approaches to the illness in a much more concerted fashion.

We have talked about the importance of a paradigm shift in the conception of bipolar illness and its treatment. Such a new view will certainly be helpful at the level of individuals and their treatment by physicians and other clinicians, but what is strongly needed is a public health paradigm shift that would involve more comprehensive and sustained care for psychiatric illness in general and bipolar illness in particular. Given the complexity of the brain, with its 12 billion neurons and four times that many glial cells all rapidly rearranging themselves neuroanatomically, physiologically, and biochemically throughout one's life and in response to life events, one can only begin to appreciate its adaptive, maladaptive, and restorative processes.

With this viewpoint, one could readily make the argument that the psychiatric disorders are much more complex than those, for example, of the neurological disorders wherein there are often localized, highly selective, and well-recognized deficits, as seen in dopamine neurons in Parkinson's disease and in striatal neurons of Huntington's disease or even in the focal cell death involved in a stroke syndrome. The cellular processes involved in psychiatric disorder are subtler, more widespread, and heterosynaptic, but no less real. The extraordinary plasticity of the brain toward either psychopathological or resilience mechanisms deserves not only wonderment but increased funding for research and medical coverage for treatment.

Without such a public health revelation and revision, it is likely that many children and adults with bipolar illness will remain underserved and under-treated despite the many powerful psychotherapeutic and pharmacotherapeutic tools already available (Post, 2002, 2009; Post & Leverich, 2008). Given this current state of affairs, we can only wish each patient, family member, and treating physician and clinician the very best success with the multiple tools already in the therapeutic armamentarium. We hope that some of the information and concepts outlined in this chapter will not only help individual patients better deal with the complexities of the illness and enhance their treatment but also help in the ultimate achievement of a better public awareness and programs for enhancing research and treatment.

REFERENCES

Alonso, M., Bekinschtein, P., Cammarota, M., Vianna, M. R., Izquierdo, I., & Medina, J. H. (2005). Endogenous BDNF is required for long-term memory formation in the rat parietal cortex. *Learning and Memory, 12,* 504–510.

Altshuler, L. L., Bartzokis, G., Grieder, T., Curran, J., Jimenez, T., Leight, K., et al. (2000). An MRI study of temporal lobe structures in men with bipolar disorder or schizophrenia. *Biological Psychiatry, 15,* 147–162.

Amat, J., Paul, E., Watkins, L. R., & Maier, S. F. (2008). Activation of the ventral medial prefrontal cortex during an uncontrollable stressor reproduces both the immediate and long-term protective effects of behavioral control. *Neuroscience, 154,* 1178–1186.

Ambelas, A. (1979). Psychologically stressful events in the precipitation of manic episodes. *British Journal of Psychiatry, 135,* 15–21.

Andreazza, A. C., Kauer-Sant'Anna, M., Frey, B. N., Bond, D. J., Kapczinski, F., Young, L. T., et al. (2008). Oxidative stress markers in bipolar disorder: A meta-analysis. *Journal of Affective Disorders, 111,* 135–144.

Baratta, M. V., Christianson, J. P., Gomez, D. M., Zarza, C. M., Amat, J., Masini, C. V., et al. (2007). Controllable versus uncontrollable stressors bi-directionally modulate conditioned but not innate fear. *Neuroscience, 146,* 1495–1503.

Basco, M. R., & Rush, A. J. (1996). *Cognitive-behavioral therapy for bipolar disorder.* New York: Guilford Press.

Benson, B. E., Willis, M. W., Ketter, T. A., Speer, A., Kimbrell, T. A., George, M. S., et al. (2008). Interregional cerebral metabolic associativity during a continuous performance task (Part II): Differential alterations in bipolar and unipolar disorders. *Psychiatry Research, 164,* 30–47.

Bekinschtein, P., Cammarota, M., Igaz, L. M., Bevilaqua, L. R., Izquierdo, I., & Medina, J. H. (2007). Persistence of long-term memory storage requires a late protein synthesis- and BDNF-dependent phase in the hippocampus. *Neuron, 53,* 261–277.

Berk, M., Copolov, D. L., Dean, O., Lu, K., Jeavons, S., Schapkaitz, I., et al. (2008). N-acetyl cysteine for depressive symptoms in bipolar disorder—A double-blind randomized placebo-controlled trial. *Biological Psychiatry, 15,* 468–475.

Berton, O., McClung, C. A., DiLeone, R. J., Krishnan, V., Renthal, W., Russo, S. J., et al. (2006). Essential role of BDNF in the mesolimbic-dopamine pathway in social defeat stress. *Science, 311,* 864–868.

Birmaher, B., Axelson, D., Strober, M., Gill, M. K., Valeri, S., Chiapetta, L., et al. (2006). Clinical course of children and adolescents with bipolar spectrum disorders. *Archives of General Psychiatry, 63*, 175–183.

Blumberg, H. P., Kaufman, J., Martin, A., Whiteman, R., Zhang, J. H, Gore, J. C., et al. (2003). Amygdala and hippocampal volumes in adolescents and adults with bipolar disorder. *Archives of General Psychiatry, 60*, 1201–1208.

Bozikas, V. P., Tonia, T., Fokas, K., Karavatos, A., & Kosmidis, M. H. (2006). Impaired emotion processing in remitted patients with bipolar disorder. *Journal of Affective Disorders, 91*, 53–56.

Bredy, T. W., Wu, H., Crego, C., Zellhoefer, J., Sun, Y. E., & Barad, M. (2007). Histone modifications around individual BDNF gene promoters in prefrontal cortex are associated with extinction of conditioned fear. *Learning and Memory, 14*, 268–276.

Brent, D. A., Oquenda, M., Birmaher, B., Greenhill, L., Kolko, D., Stanley, B., et al. (2002). Familial pathways to early-onset suicide attempt: Risk for suicidal behavior in offspring of mood-disordered suicide attempters. *Archives of General Psychiatry, 59*, 801–807.

Brown, G., & Harris, T. (1978). *Social origins of depression: A study of psychiatric disorder in women.* New York: Free Press.

Brown, G. R., McBride, L., Bauer, M. S., & Williford, W. O. (2005). Impact of childhood abuse on the course of bipolar disorder. A replication study in U.S. veterans. *Journal of Affective Disorders, 89*, 57–67.

Calabrese, J. R., Muzina, D. J., Kemp, D. E., Sachs, G. S., Frye, M. A., Thompson, T. R., et al. (2006). Predictors of bipolar disorder risk among patients currently treated for major depression. *Medscape General Medicine, 15*, 38.

Carlson, G. A., & Meyer, S. E. (2006). Phenomenology and diagnosis of bipolar disorder in children, adolescents, and adults: Complexities and developmental issues. *Development and Psychopathology, 18*, 939–969.

Caspi, A., Sugden, K., Moffitt, T. E., Taylor, A., Craig, I. W., Harrington, H., et al. (2003). Influence of life stress on depression: Moderation by a polymorphism in the 5-HTT gene. *Science, 301*, 386–389.

Champagne, F., & Meaney, M. J. (2001). Like mother, like daughter: Evidence for non-genomic transmission of parental behavior and stress responsivity. *Progress in Brain Research, 133*, 287–302.

Champagne, F. A., & Meaney, M. J. (2006). Stress during gestation alters postpartum maternal care and the development of the offspring in a rodent model. *Biological Psychiatry, 15*, 1227–1235.

Chang, K., Steiner, H., Dienes, K., Adleman, N., & Ketter, T. (2003). Bipolar offspring: A window into bipolar disorder evolution. *Biological Psychiatry, 53*, 945–951.

Christianson, J. P., Paul, E. D., Irani, M., Thompson, B. M., Kubala, K. H., Yirmiya, R., et al. (2008). The role of prior stressor controllability and the dorsal raphe nucleus in sucrose preference and social exploration. *Behavioural Brain Research, 193*, 87–93.

Christianson, J. P., Thompson, B. M., Watkins, L. R., & Maier, S. F. (2008). Medial prefrontal cortical activation modulates the impact of controllable and uncontrollable stressor exposure on a social exploration test of anxiety in the rat. *Stress, 12*(5), 445–450.

Cicchetti, D., Rogosch, F. A., & Sturge-Apple, M. L. (2007). Interactions of child maltreatment and serotonin transporter and monoamine oxidase A polymorphisms: Depressive symptomatology among adolescents from low socioeconomic status backgrounds. *Development and Psychopathology, 19*, 1161–1180.

Cicchetti, D., Rogosch, F. A., & Toth, S. L. (2000). The efficacy of toddler–parent psychotherapy for fostering cognitive development in offspring of depressed mothers. *Journal of Abnormal Child Psychology, 28*, 135–148.

Coe, C. L., Kramer, M., Czeh, B., Gould, E., Reeves, A. J., Kirschbaum, C., et al. (2003). Pre-natal stress diminishes neurogenesis in the dentate gyrus of juvenile rhesus monkeys. *Biological Psychiatry, 54*, 1025–1034.

Colom, F., & Lam, D. (2005). Psychoeducation: Improving outcomes in bipolar disorder. *European Psychiatry, 20*, 359–364.

Comings, D. E. (1995). *The gene bomb.* Duarte, CA: Hope Press.

Covington, H. E., III, & Miczek, K. A. (2001). Repeated social-defeat stress, cocaine or mor-phine. Effects on behavioral sensitization and intravenous cocaine self-administration "binges." *Psychopharmacology (Berl), 158*, 388–398.

Cunha, A. B., Frey, B. N., Andreazza, A. C., Goi, J. D., Rosa, A. R., Gonçalves, C. A., et al. (2006). Serum brain-derived neurotrophic factor is decreased in bipolar disorder during depressive and manic episodes. *Neuroscience Letters, 8*, 215–219.

DelBello, M. P., Adler, C. M., Whitsel, R. M., Stanford, K. E., & Strakowski, S. M. (2007). A 12-week single-blind trial of quetiapine for the treatment of mood symptoms in ado-lescents at high risk for developing bipolar I disorder. *Journal of Clinical Psychiatry, 68*, 789–795.

Dienes, K. A., Hammen, C., Henry, R. M., Cohen, A. N., & Daley, S. E. (2006). The stress sen-sitization hypothesis: Understanding the course of bipolar disorder. *Journal of Affective Disorders, 95*, 43–49.

Diler, R. S., Uguz, S., Seydaoglu, G., & Avci, A. (2008). Mania profile in a community sample of prepubertal children in Turkey. *Bipolar Disorders, 10*, 546–553.

Duman, R. S., & Monteggia, L. M. (2006). A neurotrophic model for stress-related mood dis-orders. *Biological Psychiatry, 59*, 1116–1127.

Eckenrode, J., Zielinski, D., Smith, E., Marcynyszyn, L. A., Henderson, C. R., Jr., Kitzman, H., et al. (2001). Child maltreatment and the early onset of problem behaviors: Can a program of nurse home visitation break the link? *Development and Psychopathology, 13*, 873–890.

Egan, M. F., Kojima, M., Callicott, J. H., Goldberg, T. E., Kolachana, B. S., Bertolini, A., et al. (2003). The BDNF val66met polymorphism affects activity-dependent secretion of BDNF and human memory and hippocampal function. *Cell, 112*, 257–269.

Eisch, A. J., Bolanos, C. A., de Wit, J., Simonak, R. D., Pudiak, C. M., Barrot, M., et al. (2003). Brain-derived neurotrophic factor in the ventral midbrain-nucleus accumbens pathway: A role in depression. *Biological Psychiatry, 54*, 994–1005.

Eley, T. C., Liang, H., Plomin, R., Sham, P., Sterne, A., Williamson, R., et al. (2004). Parental familial vulnerability, family environment, and their interactions as predictors of depres-sive symptoms in adolescents. *Journal of the American Academy of Child and Adolescent Psychiatry, 43*, 298–306.

Emsley, R., Chiliza, B., & Schoeman, R. (2008). Predictors of long-term outcome in schizo-phrenia. *Current Opinions in Psychiatry, 21*, 173–177.

Fleck, D. E., Arndt, S., DelBello, M. P., & Strakowski, S. M. (2006). Concurrent tracking of alcohol use and bipolar disorder symptoms. *Bipolar Disorders, 8*, 338–344.

Findling, R. L., McNamara, N. K., Stansbrey, R., Gracious, B. L., Whipkey, R. E., Demeter, C. A., et al. (2006). Combination lithium and divalproex sodium in pediatric bipolar symp-tom re-stabilization. *Journal of the American Academy of Child and Adolescent Psychiatry, 45*, 142–148.

Findling, R. L., McNamara, N. K., Youngstrom, E. A., Stansbrey, R., Gracious, B. L., Reed, M. D., et al. (2005). Double-blind 18-month trial of lithium versus divalproex maintenance treatment in pediatric bipolar disorder. *Journal of the American Academy of Child and Adolescent Psychiatry, 44*, 409–417.

Francis, D. D., Caldji, C., Champagne, F., Plotsky, P. M., & Meaney, M. J. (1999). The role of corticotrophin-releasing factor–norepinephrine systems in mediating the effects of early experience on the developments of behavioral and endocrine responses to stress. *Biological Psychiatry, 46*, 1153–1166.

Francis, D., Diorio, J., Liu, D., & Meaney, M. J. (1999). Nongenomic transmission across generations of maternal behavior and stress responses in the rat. *Science, 296*, 1155–1158.

Fristad, M. A., & Goldberg-Arnold, J. S. (2003). *Raising a moody child: How to cope with depression and bipolar disorder.* New York: Guilford Press.

Garno, J. L., Goldberg, J. F., Ramirez, P. M., & Ritzler, B. A. (2005). Impact of childhood abuse on the clinical course of bipolar disorder. *British Journal of Psychiatry, 186*, 121–125.

Geller, B., Craney, J. L., Bolhofner, K., Nickelsburg, M. J., Williams, M., & Zimerman, B. (2002). Two-year prospective follow-up of children with a prepubertal and early adolescent bipolar disorder phenotype. *American Journal of Psychiatry, 159*, 927–933.

Geller, B., Tillman, R., Craney, J. L., & Bolhofner, K. (2004). Four-year prospective outcome and natural history of mania in children with a prepubertal and early adolescent bipolar disorder phenotype. *Archives of General Psychiatry, 61*, 459–467.

Gershon, E. S., Hamovit, J. H., Guroff, J. J., & Nurnberger, J. I. (1987). Birth-cohort changes in manic and depressive disorders in relatives of bipolar and schizoaffective patients. *Archives General Psychiatry, 44*, 314–319.

Gomez-Pinilla, F., & Vaynman, S. (2005). A "deficient environment" in prenatal life may compromise systems important for cognitive function by affecting BDNF in the hippocampus. *Experimental Neurology, 192*, 235–243.

Gotlib, I. H., Lewinsohn, P. M., & Seeley, J. R. (1998). Consequences of depression during adolescence: Marital status and marital functioning in early adulthood. *Journal of Abnormal Psychology, 107*, 686–690.

Greene, R. W. (1998). *The explosive child: A new approach for understanding and parenting easily frustrated, chronically inflexible children.* New York: HarperCollins.

Hinshaw, S. P. (2004). Parental mental disorder and children's functioning: Silence and communication, stigma and resilience. *Journal of Clinical Child and Adolescent Psychology, 33*, 400–411.

Kalivas, P. W., Lalumiere, R. T., Knackstedt, L., & Shen, H. (2008). Glutamate transmission in addiction. *Neuropharmacology, 56*, 169–173.

Kalivas, P. W., & Stewart, J. (1991). Dopamine transmission in the initiation and expression of drug- and stress-induced sensitization of motor activity. *Brain Research. Brain Research Review, 16*, 223–244.

Kalivas, P. W., & Volkow, N. D. (2005). The neural basis of addiction: A pathology of motivation and choice. *American Journal of Psychiatry, 162*, 1403–1413.

Kapczinski, F., Vieta, E., Andreazza, A. C., Frey, B. N., Gomes, F. A., Tramontina, J., et al. (2008). Allostatic load in bipolar disorder: Implications for pathophysiology and treatment. *Neuroscience and Biobehavioral Reviews, 32*, 675–692.

Karege, F., Perret, G., Bondolfi, G., Schwald, M., Bertschy, G., & Aubry, J. M. (2002). Decreased serum brain-derived neurotrophic factor levels in major depressed patients. *Psychiatry Research, 109*, 143–148.

Kauer-Sant'Anna, M., Tramontina, J., Andreazza, A. C., Cereser, K., da Costa, S., Santin, A., et al. (2007). Traumatic life events in bipolar disorder: Impact on BDNF levels and psychopathology. *Bipolar Disorders, 9*(Suppl. 1), 128–135.

Kendler, K. S., Thornton, L. M., & Gardner, C. O. (2000). Stressful life events and previous episodes in the etiology of major depression in women: An evaluation of the "kindling" hypothesis. *American Journal of Psychiatry, 157*, 1243–1251.

Kendler, K. S., Thornton, L. M., & Gardner, C. O. (2001). Genetic risk, number of previous depressive episodes, and stressful life events in predicting onset of major depression. *American Journal of Psychiatry, 158,* 582–586.

Kessing, L. V., Agerbo, E. , & Mortensen, P. B. (2004). Major stressful life events and other risk factors for first admission with mania. *Bipolar Disorders, 6,* 122–129.

Kessing, L. V., & Andersen, P. K. (2003). Does the risk of developing dementia increase with the number of episodes in patients with depressive disorder and in patients with bipolar disorder? *Journal of Neurology, Neurosurgery and Psychiatry, 75,* 1662–1666.

Kessing, L. V., Andersen, P. K., Mortensen, P. B., & Bolwig, T. G. (1998). Recurrence in affective disorder: I. Case register study. *British Journal of Psychiatry, 172,* 23–28.

Ketter, T. A., Kimbrell, T. A., George, M. S., Dunn, R. T., Speer, A. M., Benson, B. E., et al. (2001). Effects of mood state, illness subtype, and course on cerebral glucose metabolism in bipolar disorders. *Biological Psychiatry, 49,* 97–109.

Kim, J.-M., Stewart, R., Kim, S.-W., Yang, S.-J., Shin, I.-S., Kim, Y.-H., et al. (2007). Interactions between life stressors and susceptibility genes (5-HTTLPR and BDNF) on depression in Korean elders. *Biological Psychiatry, 62,* 423–428.

Korte, M., Carroll, P., Wolf, E., Brem, G., Thoenen, H., & Bonhoeffer, T. (1995). Hippocampal long-term potentiation is impaired in mice lacking brain-derived neurotrophic factor. *Proceedings of the National Academy of Sciences USA, 92,* 8856–8860.

Kowatch, R. A., Fristad, M., Birmaher, B., Wagner, K. D., Findling, R. L., Hellander, M., et al. (2005). Treatment guidelines for children and adolescents with bipolar disorder. *Journal of the American Academy of Child and Adolescent Psychiatry, 44,* 213–235.

Kraepelin, E. (1921). *Manic-depressive insanity and paranoia.* Edinburgh, UK: E.S. Livingstone.

Krishnan, R., Swartz, M. S., Larson, M. J., & Santoliquido, G. (1984). Funeral mania in recurrent bipolar affective disorders: Reports of three cases. *Journal of Clinical Psychiatry, 45,* 310–311.

Lang, U. E., Hellweg, R., Seifert, F., Schubert, F., & Gallinat, J. (2007). Correlation between serum brain-derived neurotrophic factor level and an in vivo marker of cortical integrity. *Biological Psychiatry, 62, 530–535.*

Lange, K. J., & McInnis, M. G. (2002). Studies of anticipation in bipolar affective disorder. *CNS Spectrums, 7,* 196–202.

Leverich, G. S., Altshuler, L. L., Frye, M. A., Suppes, T., Keck, P. E., McElroy, S. L., et al. (2003). Factors associated with suicide attempts in 648 patients with bipolar disorder in the Stanley Foundation Bipolar Network. *Journal of Clinical Psychiatry, 64,* 506–515.

Leverich, G. S., McElroy, S. L., Suppes, T., Keck, P. E., Jr., Denicoff, K. D., Nolen, W. A., et al. (2002). Early physical and sexual abuse associated with an adverse course of bipolar illness. *Biological Psychiatry, 51,* 288–297.

Leverich, G. S., Perez, S., Luckenbaugh, D. A., & Post, R. M. (2002). Early psychosocial stressors: relationship to suicidality and course of bipolar illness. *Clinical Neuroscience Research, 2,* 161–170.

Leverich, G. S., & Post, R. M. (1996). Life charting the course of bipolar disorder. *Current Reviews of Mood and Anxiety Disorders, 1,* 48–61.

Leverich, G. S., & Post, R. M. (1998). Life charting of affective disorders. *CNS Spectrums, 3,* 21–37.

Leverich, G. S., & Post, R. M. (2006). Course of bipolar illness after history of childhood trauma. *The Lancet, 367,* 1040–1042.

Leverich, G. S., Post, R. M., Keck, P. E., Jr., Altshuler, L. L., Frye, M. A., Kupka, R. W., et al. (2007). The poor prognosis of childhood-onset bipolar disorder. *Journal of Pediatrics, 150*(5), 485–490.

Maguire, E. A., Spiers, H. J., Good, C. D., Hartley, T., Frackowiak, R. S., & Burgess, N. (2003).

Navigation expertise and the human hippocampus: A structural brain imaging analysis. *Hippocampus, 13,* 250–259.

Mann, J. J., Bartinger, J., Oquendo, M. A., Currier, D., Li, S., & Brent, D. A. (2005). Family history of suicidal behavior and mood disorders in probands with mood disorders. *American Journal of Psychiatry, 162,* 1672–1679.

Mares, P., Lindovský, J., Slamberová, R., & Kubová, H. (2007). Effects of a GABA-B receptor agonist baclofen on cortical epileptic afterdischarges in rats. *Epileptic Disorders, 9,* S44–S51.

Martinowich, K., Hattori, D., Wu, H., Fouse, S., He, F., Hu, Y., et al. (2003). DNA methylation-related chromatin remodeling in activity-dependent BDNF gene regulation. *Science, 301,* 793–795.

McElroy, S. A. L., Altshuler, L. L., Suppes, T., Keck, P. E., Frye, M. A., Denicoff, K. D., et al. (2001). Axis I psychiatric comorbidity and its relationship to historical illness variables in 288 patients with bipolar disorder. *American Journal of Psychiatry, 158,* 420–426.

McEwen, B. S. (2003). Early life influences on life-long patterns of behavior and health. *Mental Retardation and Developmental Disabilities Research Review, 9,* 149–154.

Miklowitz, D. J. (2002). *The bipolar disorder survival guide: What you and your family need to know.* New York: Guilford Press.

Miklowitz, D. J. (2008). Adjunctive psychotherapy for bipolar disorder: State of the evidence. *American Journal of Psychiatry, 165*(11), 1408–1419.

Miklowitz, D. J., Biuckians, A., & Richards, J. A. (2006). Early-onset bipolar disorder: a family treatment perspective. *Development and Psychopathology, 18, 1247–1265.*

Miklowitz, D. J., & Chang, K. D. (2008). Prevention of bipolar disorder in at-risk children: Theoretical assumptions and empirical foundations. *Development and Psychopathology, 20,* 881–897.

Miklowitz, D. J., & George, E. L. (2008). *The bipolar teen: What you can do to help your child and your family.* New York: Guilford Press.

Miklowitz, D. J., Otto, M. W., Frank, E., Reilly-Harrington, N. A., Wisniewski, S. R., Kogan, J. N., et al. (2007). Psychosocial treatments for bipolar depression: A 1-year randomized trial from the Systematic Treatment Enhancement Program. *Archives of General Psychiatry, 64,* 419–427.

Mishkin, M., & Appenzeller, T. (1987). The anatomy of memory. *Scientific American, 256,* 80–89.

Moreno, C., Laje, G., Blanco, C., Jiang, H., Schmidt, A. B., & Olfson, M. (2007). National trends in the outpatient diagnosis and treatment of bipolar disorder in youth. *Archives of General Psychiatry, 64,* 1032–1039.

Nestler, E. J., & Carlezon, W. A., Jr. (2006). The mesolimbic dopamine reward circuit in depression. *Biological Psychiatry, 59,* 1151–1159.

Nierenberg, A. A. (2009). The long tale of the short arm of the promoter region for the gene that encodes the serotonin uptake protein. *CNS Spectrums, 14*(9), 462–463.

O'Brien, C. P., Childress, A. R., McLellan, A. T., & Ehrman, R. (1993). Developing treatments that address classical conditioning. *NIDA Research Monograph, 35,* 71–91.

Olds, D. L., Henderson, C. R., Jr., Kitzman, H. J., Eckenrode, J. J., Cole, R. E., & Tatelbaum, R. C. (1999). Prenatal and infancy home visitation by nurses: Recent findings. *Future Child, 9,* 44–51.

Pavuluri, M. N., Graczyk, P. A., Henry, D. B., Carbray, J. A., Hendenreich, J., & Miklowitz, D. J. (2004). Child- and family-focused cognitive-behavioral therapy for pediatric bipolar disorder: Development and preliminary results. *Journal of the American Academy of Child and Adolescent Psychiatry, 43,* 528–537.

Perlis, R. H., Miyahara, S., Marangell, L. B., Wisniewski, S. R., Ostacher, M., DelBello, M. P., et al. (2004). Long-term implications of early onset in bipolar disorder: Data from the first 1000 participants in the systematic treatment enhancement program for bipolar disorder (STEP-BDNF). *Biological Psychiatry, 55,* 875–881.

Plotsky, P. M., Thrivikraman, K. V., Nemeroff, C. B., Caldji, C., Sharma, S., & Meaney, M. J. (2005). Long-term consequences of neonatal rearing on central corticotropin-releasing factor systems in adult male rat offspring. *Neuropsychopharmacology, 30,* 2192–2204.

Post, R. M. (1992). Transduction of psychosocial stress into the neurobiology of recurrent affective disorder. *American Journal of Psychiatry, 149,* 999–1010.

Post, R. M. (2002). Preface and overview. *Clinical Neuroscience Research, 2, 122–126.*

Post, R. M. (2004). The status of the sensitization/kindling hypothesis of bipolar disorder. *Current Psychosis and Therapeutics Reports, 2,* 135–141.

Post, R. M. (2007). Role of BDNF in bipolar and unipolar disorder: Clinical and theoretical implications. *Journal of Psychiatric Research, 41,* 979–990.

Post, R. M. (2009). Childhood-onset bipolar disorder: The perfect storm. *Psychiatric Annals, 39*(10), 879–886.

Post, R. M., & Kauer-Sant'Anna, M. (in press). An introduction to the neurobiology of bipolar illness onset, recurrence, and progression. In L. N. Yatham & V. Kusumakar (Eds.), *Bipolar disorder: A clinician's guide to treatment management* (2nd ed.). New York: Routledge.

Post, R. M., & Leverich, G. S. (2006). The role of psychosocial stress in the onset and progression of bipolar disorder and its comorbidities: The need for earlier and alternative modes of therapeutic intervention. *Development and Psychopathology, 18,* 1181–1211.

Post, R. M., & Leverich, G. S. (2008) *Treatment of bipolar illness: A case book for clinicians and patients.* New York: Norton.

Post, R. M., Leverich, G. S., Kupka, R., Keck, P., McElroy, S., Altshuler, L., et al. (in press). Early onset bipolar disorder and treatment delay are risk factors for poor outcome in adulthood. *Journal of Clinical Psychology.*

Post, R. M., Luckenbaugh, D. A., Leverich, G. S., Altshuler, L. L., Frye, M. A., Suppes, T., et al. (2008). Incidence of childhood-onset bipolar illness in the USA and Europe. *British Journal of Psychiatry, 192,* 150–151.

Post, R. M., & Post, S. L. W. (2004). Molecular and cellular developmental vulnerabilities to the onset of affective disorders in children and adolescents: some implications for therapeutics. In H. Steiner (Ed.), *Handbook of mental health interventions in children and adolescents* (pp. 140–192). New York: Jossey-Bass.

Post, R. M., & Speer, A. M. (2007). rTMS and related somatic therapies: Prospects for the future. In R. H. Belmaker & M. S. George (Eds.), *TMS in clinical psychiatry* (pp. 225–255). Washington, DC: American Psychiatric Press.

Post, R. M., Speer, A. M., Hough, C. J., & Xing, G. (2003). Neurobiology of bipolar illness: Implications for future study and therapeutics. *Annals of Clinical Psychiatry, 15,* 85–94.

Post, R. M., Speer, A. M., & Leverich, G. S. (2003). Bipolar illness: Which critical treatment issues need study? *Clinical Applications in Bipolar Disorder, 2,* 24–30.

Post, R. M., & Wozniak, J. (2009). Survey of expert treatment approaches for children with bipolar disorder–not otherwise specified and bipolar-I presentations. *Psychiatric Annals, 39*(10), 887–895.

Reichart, C. G., Wals, M., Hillegers, M. H., Ormel, J., Nolen, W. A., & Verhulst, F. C. (2004). Psychopathology in the adolescent offspring of bipolar parents. *Journal of Affective Disorders, 78,* 67–71.

Rich, B. A., Grimley, M. E., Schmajuk, M., Blair, K. S., Blair, R. J., & Leibenluft, E. (2008), Face emotion labeling deficits in children with bipolar disorder and severe mood dysregulation. *Development and Psychopathology, 20,* 529–546.

Rich, B. A., Vinton, D. T., Roberson-Nay, R., Hommer, R. E., Berghorst, L. H., McClure, E. B., et al. (2006). Limbic hyperactivation during processing of neutral facial expressions in children with bipolar disorder. *Proceedings of the National Academy of Sciences USA, 103,* 8900–8905.

Roceri, M., Cirulli, F., Pessina, C., Peretto, P., Racagni, G., & Riva, M. A. (2004). Postnatal repeated maternal deprivation produces age-dependent changes of brain-derived neurotrophic factor expression in selected rat brain regions. *Biological Psychiatry, 55,* 708–714.

Roth, T. L., Lubin, F. D., Funk, A. J., & Sweatt, J. D. (2009). Lasting epigenetic influence of early-life adversity on the BDNF gene. *Biological Psychiatry, 65*(9), 760–769.

Schretlen, D. J., Cascella, N. G., Meyer, S. M., Kingery, L. R., Testa, M., Munro, C. A., et al. (2007). Neuropsychological functioning in bipolar disorder and schizophrenia. *Biological Psychiatry, 62,* 179–186.

Scott, J., & Colom, F. (2005). Psychosocial treatments for bipolar disorders. *Psychiatric Clinics of North America, 28,* 371–384.

Shimizu, E., Hashimoto, K., Watanabe, H., Komatsu, N., Okamura, N., Koike, K., et al. (2003). Serum brain-derived neurotrophic factor (BDNF) levels in schizophrenia are indistinguishable from controls. *Neuroscience Letters, 351,* 111–114.

Simoneau, T. L., Miklowitz, D. J., Richards, J. A., Saleem, R., & George, E. L. (1999). Bipolar disorder and family communication: Effect of a psychoeducational treatment program. *Journal of Abnormal Psychology, 108,* 588–597.

Smith, M. A., Makino, S., Kvetnansky, R., & Post, R. M. (1995). Stress and glucocorticoids affect the expression of brain derived neurotrophic factor and neurotrophin-3 mRNAs in the hippocampus. *Journal of Neuroscience, 15,* 1768–1777.

Sonne, S. C., Brady, K. T., & Morton, W. A. (1994). Substance abuse and bipolar disorder. *Journal of Nervous and Mental Disease, 182,* 349–352.

Soutullo, C. A., Chang, K. D., Díez-Suárez, A., Figueroa-Quintana, A., Escamilla-Canales, I., Rapado-Castro, M., et al. (2005). Bipolar disorder in children and adolescents: International perspective on epidemiology and phenomenology. *Bipolar Disorders, 7,* 497–506.

Strakowski, S. M., DelBello, M. P., Fleck, D. A., & Arndt, S. (2000). The impact of substance abuse on the course of bipolar disorder. *Biological Psychiatry, 48,* 477–485.

Strakowski, S. M., DelBello, M. P., Sax, K. W., Zimmerman, M. E., Shear, P. K., Hawkins, J. M., et al. (1999). Brain magnetic resonance imaging of structural abnormalities in bipolar disorder. *Archives of General Psychiatry, 56,* 254–260.

Taddei, J. (2008). *Emotional abuse is most common form of 'violence,' students say.* Retrieved October 9, 2009, from *www.bloomberg.com/apps/news?pid=20601202&sid=aeI8WccR5iMI &refer=healthcare.*

Taylor, S. E., Way, B. M., Welch, W. T., Hilmert, C. J., Lehman, B. J., & Eisenberger, N. I. (2006). Early family environment, current adversity, the serotonin transporter promoter polymorphism, and depressive symptomatology. *Biological Psychiatry, 60*(7), 671–676.

Torres, I. J., Boudreau, V. G., & Yatham, L. N. (2007). Neuropsychological functioning in euthymic bipolar disorder: A meta-analysis. *Acta Psychiatrica Scandinavica, Supplement 434,* 17–26.

Tsankova, N. M., Berton, O., Renthal, W., Kumar, A., Neve, R. L., & Nestler, E. J. (2006). Sustained hippocampal chromatin regulation in a mouse model of depression and antidepressant action. *Nature Neurosciences, 9,* 519–525.

Vieta, E., Pacchiarotti, I., Scott, J., Sanchez-Moreno, J., Di Marzo, S., & Colom, F. (2005). Evidence-based research on the efficacy of psychologic interventions in bipolar disorders: A critical review. *Current Psychiatry Reports, 7,* 449–455.

Weissman, M. M., Bland, R., Joyce, P. R., Newman, S., Wells, J. E., & Wittchen, H. U. (1993).

Sex differences in rates of depression: Cross-national perspectives. *Journal of Affective Disorders, 29,* 77–84.

Weissman, M. M., Pilowsky, D. J., Wickramaratne, P. J., Talati, A., Wisniewski, S. R., Fava, M., et al. (2006). STAR*D-Child Team. Remissions in maternal depression and child psychopathology: A STAR*D-child report. *Journal of the American Medical Association, 295,* 1389–1398.

Wilens, T. E., Biederman, J., Kwon, A., Ditterline, J., Forkner, P., Moore, H., et al. (2004). Risk of substance use disorders in adolescents with bipolar disorder. *Journal of the American Academy of Child and Adolescent Psychiatry, 43,* 1380–1386.

Zhang, L.-X., Levine, S., Dent, G., Zhan, Y., Xing, G., Okimoto, D., et al. (2002). Maternal deprivation increases cell death in the infant rat brain. *Development and Brain Research, 133,* 1–11.

Zhou, W., & Kalivas, P. W. (2008). N-acetylcysteine reduces extinction responding and induces enduring reductions in cue- and heroin-induced drug-seeking. *Biological Psychiatry, 63,* 338–340.

PART IV

TREATMENT

Developmental Considerations in the Pharmacological Treatment of Youth with Bipolar Disorder

Robert A. Kowatch, Jeffrey R. Strawn,
and Melissa P. DelBello

Children and adolescents with bipolar disorder (BD) can be difficult to treat with psychotropic medications because of developmental changes in biological and psychological systems (Cicchetti & Rogosch, 2002; Spear, 2000) and developmental differences in bipolar symptom expression, disease course and comorbid disorders (e.g., attention-deficit/hyperactivity disorder [ADHD] and oppositional defiant disorder). Children with BD may first present with symptoms of a major depressive episode or ADHD and are often treated with medications that can potentially exacerbate illness course, such as antidepressants and psychostimulants. In the past, there were few well-controlled studies to guide treatment in this population. There are now several large, well-controlled treatment studies of psychotropic medications in children and adolescents with BD. However, developmental differences in medication response and dosing between children and adolescents versus adults with BD add to the complexity of treating this population.

In this article, we review developmental differences among children, adolescents, and adults in terms of general physiology, metabolic factors, disease course and presentation, and specific differences in pharmacological treatment responses. Additionally, we examine pharmacological treatment studies of children and adolescents with BD and discuss preliminary data examining the effectiveness of pharmacological interventions for treating children and adolescents who are at familial risk for BD.

GENERAL PHYSIOLOGICAL DIFFERENCES

It can be easy to forget that children and adolescents are not just small adults. There are significant differences between children and adults in drug pharmacokinetics, pharmacodynamics, efficacy, and safety (Bartelink, Rademaker, Schobben, & van den Anker, 2006). Pharmacokinetics is how a drug is metabolized or cleared in the body, whereas pharmacodynamics explains what effects a drug has in the body. Pharmacokinetics includes the study of the mechanisms of absorption and distribution of an administered drug, the rate at which a drug action begins and the duration of the effect, the chemical changes of the substance in the body (e.g., by enzymes), and the effects and routes of excretion of the metabolites of the drug.

Children have proportionally larger livers and kidneys, more body water, less fat, and less plasma albumin, which means that some medications are distributed differently than in adults while others are cleared more rapidly (Tosyali & Greenhill, 1998). The P450 enzymatic system in the liver is responsible for the clearance of several psychotropics, including the selective serotonin reuptake inhibitor (SSRI) antidepressants and several atypical antipsychotics (e.g., aripiprazole is metabolized by P450 2D6) (Black, O'Kane, & Mrazek, 2007). The P450 cytochrome system is encoded by 59 functional genes that code for 18 enzymes that mature in early childhood (Hines, 2008). Six different P450 isozymes— CYP1A2, CYP2C19, CYP2C9, CYP2D6, CYP2E1, and CYP3A4—that play important roles in drug metabolism have been identified. There can be interindividual variability in how well a drug is metabolized by the P450 system, owing to genetic polymorphisms. Sometimes these variations are ethnically determined. The majority of people are intermediate or extensive metabolizers for most of the P450 isoenzymes. Among individuals who are "ultrarapid" or "poor metabolizers," adjustments may have to be made to drugs metabolized by the particular P450 isoenzyme.

DEVELOPMENTAL DIFFERENCES IN NEUROBIOLOGY

BD is characterized by disturbances in mood regulation (Goodwin & Ghaemi, 1998), behavior (West et al., 1996), cognition (Shear, DelBello, Lee Rosenberg, & Strakowski, 2002), social skills (Geller, Bolhofner, et al., 2000), and vegetative functions like sleep, appetite, and circadian rhythms (Post, Speer, Hough, & Xing, 2003). The neurobiological basis of BD involves a range of disturbances in noradrenergic, serotonergic, dopaminergic, cholinergic, gamma-aminobutyric acid (GABA)–ergic, glutaminergic, and other neurotransmitter systems (Zarate, Singh, & Manji, 2006). Evidence from neuroanatomical, neurophysiological, neurochemical, and behavioral studies in humans and animals supports the view that specific neuroendocrine, neurotransmitter, and intracellular signaling systems are dysregulated in BD (Martinowich, Schloesser, & Manji, 2009). More recently, genetic association studies have identified numerous genes that confer vulnerability to the disorder, many of which are known to function in the signaling pathways identified as relevant to the etiology of BD (Newberg, Catapano, Zarate, & Manji, 2008).

Several authors have developed models of the functional networks thought to be involved in the mood and cognitive dysregulation of patients with mood disorders. These include the limbic-cortical model of Mayberg (1997), the frontotemporal model of Blumberg and colleagues (2004), the ventral/dorsal system of Philips (2006), and the anterior limbic network of Adler, DelBello, and Strakowski (2006). Each of these models involves the amygdala, hippocampus, prefrontal and orbitofrontal cortex, and parts of the striatum. It is increasingly being recognized that for BD multiple areas of the brain are involved in several different cortical, subcortical, and limbic networks (Haldane & Frangou, 2004). These models are reviewed in detail in Fleck and colleagues' Chapter 9 (this volume) on neuroimaging.

DEVELOPMENTAL DIFFERENCES IN PHENOMENOLOGY

Children and adolescents with BD present differently than adults with BD (see Diler, Birmaher, & Miklowitz, Chapter 5, and Youngstrom, Chapter 3, this volume). However, whether these differences are due to developmental differences in symptom expression or differences in underlying etiologies of pediatric- versus adult-onset BD remains unclear (Bowring & Kovacs, 1992; Wozniak, Biederman, & Richards, 2001). Symptoms of BD in children and adolescents may also be difficult to establish because of the variability of symptom expression depending on the context and phase of the illness and the mood and behavioral effects of psychotropic medications.

Several recent studies have highlighted developmental differences in the phenomenology and clinical course between children and adolescents versus adults with BD (Findling et al., 2001; Geller, Tillman, Craney, & Bolhofner, 2004; Geller et al., 2000; Wozniak & Biederman, 1997). Typically, children and adolescents with BD have severe mood dysregulation characterized by four to eight severe mood swings per day (Geller et al., 2002). This affective dysregulation often leads to disruptive and aggressive behaviors (Isaac, 1992, 1995; Wozniak et al., 1995). Additionally, children with BD commonly present with mixed (co-occurring mania and depression) episodes and psychotic symptoms (Kowatch & DelBello, 2006; Tillman & Geller, 2003).

PHARMACOLOGICAL INTERVENTIONS

Mood Stabilizers

Lithium

Lithium is the oldest mood stabilizer and has significant data supporting its use for BD in adults (Cade, 1949; Geddes, Burgess, Hawton, Jamison, & Goodwin, 2004). A review of adult placebo-controlled studies revealed an effect size of 0.40 (95% confidence interval [CI]: 0.28–0.53) and an overall number needed to treat of six (95% CI: 4–13) for lithium in the treatment of acute mania in adults (Storosum et al., 2007). Lithium is the only mood stabilizer approved by the U.S. Food and Drug Administration (FDA) for use in the treatment of mania in adolescents (ages 12–18 years).

There have been six, older "controlled" trials of lithium in children and adolescents with BD. Of these six studies, four (Delong & Nieman, 1983; Gram & Rafaelsen, 1972; Lena, 1979; McKnew et al., 1981) used a crossover design, which is not ideal for assessing outcome in an illness whose inherent nature is to wax and wane. The average number of subjects in each of these older studies was 18 and response rates ranged from 33 to 80%, reflecting the heterogeneity of the sample and the differences among study designs. Several open-label studies suggest that approximately 40–50% of manic children and adolescents with BD will improve symptomatically with lithium monotherapy (Findling et al., 2003; Kowatch et al., 2000; Youngerman & Canino, 1978).

In the first prospective, placebo-controlled trial of lithium in children and adolescents with BDs and comorbid substance abuse, subjects treated with lithium for 6 weeks showed a significant improvement in global assessment of functioning (46% response rate in the lithium-treated group vs. 8% in the placebo group; Geller, Cooper, Sun, et al., 1998). There was also a statistically significant decrease in positive urine toxicology screens following lithium treatment. The study was limited by its small sample size ($n = 25$). Furthermore, not all of these subjects met full criteria for bipolar I disorder, some were "bipolar with predictors," and no specific mania rating scales were used.

In an open, prospective study of 100 adolescents 12 to 18 years of age with an acute manic episode treated with lithium, 63 met response criteria and 26 achieved remission of manic symptoms at a 4-week assessment (Kafantaris, Coletti, Dicker, Padula, & Kane, 2003). Prominent depressive features, age at first mood episode, severity of mania, and comorbidity with ADHD did not distinguish lithium responders from nonresponders. Kafantaris and colleagues (2003) subsequently reported the results of a placebo-controlled, discontinuation study of lithium in adolescents with mania ($n = 40$, mean age, 15). During the first part of this study, subjects received open treatment with lithium at therapeutic serum levels (mean, 0.99 mEq/liter) for at least 4 weeks. Responders to lithium were then randomly assigned to continue or discontinue lithium during a 2-week double-blind, placebo-controlled phase. Fifty-eight percent of these subjects experienced a clinically significant symptom exacerbation during the 2-week double-blind phase. However, the slightly lower exacerbation rate in the group maintained on lithium (53%) versus the group switched to placebo (62%) did not reach statistical significance. This study did not appear to support a large effect for lithium continuation treatment of adolescents with acute mania, but with only a 2-week discontinuation period it is hard to draw definitive conclusions about efficacy. It is very possible that if the discontinuation period had been longer, a clear separation between the lithium and placebo groups would have been observed.

Kowatch, Findling, Scheffer, and Stanford (2007) presented the results of a large National Institute of Mental Health–funded controlled trial of lithium versus divalproex versus placebo in subjects ages 7 to 17 years with bipolar I disorder, the Pediatric Bipolar Collaborative Trial (PBC). In this double-blind trial, 153 outpatients between the ages of 7 and 17 (mean, 10.6 years) were randomized to treatment with lithium, divalproex, or placebo. The total trial length for each subject was 24 weeks. During the first 8 weeks, subjects were treated with lithium, divalproex, or placebo in a double-blind fashion; no other psychotropic medications were allowed other than short-term "rescue" agents. At the end of 8 weeks, divalproex demonstrated efficacy on both a priori outcome measures, whereas lithium did not. The response rates based on a Clinical Global Impression (CGI) improvement score of "1 or 2" (much or very much improved) were 54% for divalproex, 42% for lithium, and 29% for placebo. There was a definite trend toward efficacy for lithium, but it did not clearly separate from placebo on the primary outcome measures.

Based on the studies reviewed previously, it appears that lithium is a mood stabilizer with a moderate effect size in children and adolescents, similar to that found in adult lithium studies. However, lithium may cause renal, hematological, thyroid, and other endocrine changes that must be monitored. Common side effects of lithium that may be particularly problematic for children and adolescents include nausea, polyuria, polydipsia, tremor, acne, and weight gain.

Valproate

Valproic acid is a chemical compound that has found clinical use as an anticonvulsant and mood stabilizer. Related drugs include the sodium salts of valproic acid, sodium valproate, and divalproex sodium (Depakote), which consist of a compound of sodium valproate and valproic acid. For many years, valproate has been used to treat adults with mania. A review of the five controlled studies of valproate for the acute treatment of mania in adults showed an average response rate of 54%, demonstrating efficacy for valproate versus placebo (McElroy & Keck, 2000). In many of these studies, positive results were obtained even though patients were selected from a population previously refractory to lithium treatment and were characterized by rapid cycling, mixed affective states, and irritability.

Several case reports and open prospective trials have suggested the effectiveness of valproate for the treatment of children and adolescents with BD (Deltito,

Levitan, Damore, Hajal, & Zambenedetti, 1998; Kastner & Friedman, 1992; Kastner, Friedman, Plummer, Ruiz, & Henning, 1990; Papatheodorou & Kutcher, 1993; Papatheodorou, Kutcher, Katic, & Szalai, 1995; West & McElroy, 1995; West et al., 1994; Whittier, West, Galli, & Raute, 1995). Wagner and colleagues (2002) published the results of an open-label study of valproate in 40 children and adolescents (ages 7–19 years) with BD. In the open-label phase of this study, subjects were given 15 mg/kg of divalproex daily. The mean final dose was 17 mg/kg/day. Twenty-two subjects (55%) showed a greater than 50% improvement in Mania Rating Scale scores during the open phase of treatment.

A discontinuation trial of lithium and divalproex was conducted to determine whether divalproex was superior to lithium in the maintenance monotherapy of BD youth who had been previously stabilized on the combination of lithium and divalproex (Findling et al., 2005). Children with bipolar I or II disorder (n = 139) with a mean age of 10.8 ± 3.5 years were initially treated with lithium and divalproex for a mean duration of 10.7 weeks initially. Patients meeting remission criteria for 4 consecutive weeks were then randomized in a double-blind fashion to treatment with lithium (n = 30) or divalproex (n = 30) for up to 76 weeks. At the end of the study period, the lithium and divalproex treatment groups did not differ in survival time until emerging symptoms of relapse or until discontinuation for any reason. The authors concluded that lithium was not superior to divalproex as maintenance treatment in youth who had stabilized on combination lithium/divalproex pharmacotherapy. This trial also demonstrated that monotherapy was not sufficient for maintenance treatment of children and adolescents with BD.

Wagner and colleagues (2009) recently reported the results of an industry-funded, randomized, placebo-controlled, double-blind, multicenter study to evaluate the safety and efficacy of Depakote ER in the treatment of bipolar I disorder, manic or mixed episode, in children and adolescents. During this trial, 150 children ages 10–17 with a current clinical diagnosis of bipolar I disorder were enrolled at 20 study sites. Subjects were outpatients with a manic or mixed episode with a Young Mania Rating Scale (YMRS) score of 20 or higher at screening and baseline. Subjects were randomized in a 1:1 ratio to receive active study medication (250-mg and/or 500-mg tablets of Depakote ER) or matching placebo tablets. The duration of this study was 6 weeks, including a screening period lasting 3 to 14 days, a 4-week treatment period, and an optional 1-week taper period.

There were no statistically significant differences between the valproate and placebo arms on any of the efficacy variables. This trial may have been negative because of differences in the absorption and distribution of the extended-release formulation of valproate that was used. Moreover, the active treatment period of 4 weeks may not have been long enough to detect a drug–placebo difference. Alternatively, serum levels of divalproex may have been inadequate. In contrast to the results of the Wagner and colleagues (2009) trial, the PBC trial (discussed previously) found that valproate was superior to lithium over 8 weeks. The PBC trial used the immediate-release formulation of valproate; the acute treatment period was 8 weeks; and the mean serum levels of valproate were 100 ng/liter, as opposed to the Wagner and colleagues study, for which the mean level was 80 ng/liter.

Common side effects of valproate in children and adolescents include nausea, increased appetite, weight gain, sedation, thrombocytopenia (low blood platelets), transient hair loss, tremor, and vomiting. Rarely, pancreatitis (Sinclair, Berg, & Breault, 2004; Werlin & Fish, 2006) and liver failure (Ee et al., 2003; Konig et al., 1994; Treem, 1994) can occur in children treated with valproate. Fetal exposure to valproate is associated with an increased rate of neural tube defects (Ketter, Nasrallah, & Fagiolini, 2006). Valproate-induced hyperammonemia (abnormally high levels of blood ammonia) has been observed in children and adolescents treated with valproate (Carr & Shrewsbury, 2007; Raskind & El-Chaar, 2000). It can present as lethargy, disorientation, and reversible cognitive deficits, which may progress to marked sedation, coma, and even death. It is a transient and asymptomatic phenomenon but can become chronic if undetected.

There are increasing concerns about the association between valproate and polycystic ovarian syndrome (PCOS). PCOS is an endocrine disorder charac- terized by ovulatory dysfunction and hyperandrogenism, affecting between 3% and 5% of women who are not taking psychotropic medications (Rasgon, 2004). Common symptoms of PCOS include irregular or absent menstruation, lack of ovulation, weight gain, hirsutism, and acne. The initial reports of the associa- tion between PCOS and divalproex exposure were in women with epilepsy. The association was particularly strong if their exposure was during adolescence (Isojarvi, Laatikainen, Pakarinen, Juntunen, & Myllyla, 1993). In Joffe and col- leagues' (2006) report on adults with BD, there was a sevenfold increased risk of new-onset oligoamenorrhea with hyperandrogenism in women treated with valproate. The current recommendations are that females treated with valproate should have a baseline assessment of menstrual cycle patterns and should be con- tinually monitored for menstrual irregularities, weight gain, hirsutism, and acne during treatment (Buchsbaum et al., 1997). If symptoms of PCOS develop, referral to a pediatric endocrinologist should be considered.

Carbamazepine

Carbamazepine is an anticonvulsant agent structurally similar to imipramine that was first introduced in the United States in 1968 for the treatment of seizures. Two controlled studies of a long-acting preparation of carbamazepine in adults with BD demonstrated efficacy for carbamazepine as monotherapy for mania (Weisler, Cutler, Ballenger, Post, & Ketter, 2006). There have been no controlled studies of carbamazepine for the treatment of children and adolescents with BD; the major- ity of reports in the literature concern its use in children and adolescents with ADHD or conduct disorder (Cueva et al., 1996; Evans, Clay, & Gualtieri, 1987; Kafantaris et al., 1992; Puente, 1975). Pleak, Birmaher, Gavrilescu, Abichandani, and Williams (1988) reported the worsening of behavior in six of 20 children and adolescents treated with carbamazepine for ADHD and conduct disorder. There is not good evidence to support the use of carbamazepine as a first-line agent for children and adolescents with BD, and this drug's numerous P450 drug interactions make its clinical use difficult.

Carbamazepine should not be used in patients with a history of bone marrow depression, hypersensitivity to the drug, or known sensitivity to any of the tricyclic compounds. Common side effects of carbamazepine in children and adolescents include sedation, ataxia, dizziness, blurred vision, nausea, and vomiting. Uncommon side effects of carbamazepine include aplastic anemia and hyponatremia (low sodium). Serious and sometimes fatal dermatological reactions, notably Stevens–Johnson syndrome and toxic epidermal necrolysis have been reported in about one to six per 10,000 new users in countries with mainly Caucasian populations (Devi, George, Criton, Suja, & Sridevi, 2005; Keating & Blahunka, 1995). Carbamazepine can cause fetal harm and is, therefore, contraindicated during pregnancy (Ciraulo, Shader, Greenblatt, & Creelman, 1995).

Novel Antiepileptic Agents

Several new antiepileptic drugs have been developed for the treatment of epilepsy that may be useful for the treatment of BD, although the data are presently limited regarding the efficacy and tolerability of these agents for pediatric BD. Additionally, there have been several negative trials of these agents in adults with mania or mixed episodes (Bowden & Karren, 2006).

Lamotrigine

Lamotrigine (Lamictal) has a novel mechanism of action by blocking voltage-sensitive sodium channels and secondarily inhibiting the release of excitatory neurotransmitters, particularly glutamate and aspartate (Ketter, Wang, Becker, Nowakowska, & Yang, 2003). Lamotrigine also inhibits serotonin reuptake, suggesting that it might possess antidepressant properties. In 2003 the FDA approved lamotrigine for the long-term maintenance treatment of bipolar type I disorder in adults.

Several prospective studies in adults with BD suggest that lamotrigine may be beneficial for the treatment of mood (especially depressive) symptoms in BD (Bowden et al., 2003; Calabrese et al., 1999). Chang, Saxena, and Howe (2006) conducted an 8-week open-label trial of lamotrigine alone or as adjunctive therapy for the treatment of 20 adolescents ages 12–17 years (mean age, 15.8 years) with BD (I, II, and not otherwise specified), who were experiencing a depressive or mixed episode. The mean final dose was 131.6 mg/day. Eighty-four percent of these subjects were rated as much or very much improved on the CGI. Larger, placebo-controlled studies of lamotrigine in children and adolescents with BD are needed.

The most common side effects of lamotrigine are dizziness, tremor, somnolence, nausea, asthenia, and headache. Benign rashes develop in 12% of adult patients, typically within the first 8 weeks of lamotrigine therapy (Calabrese et al., 2002). Rarely, severe cutaneous reactions such as Stevens–Johnson syndrome and toxic epidermal necrolysis have been described. The risk of developing a serious rash is approximately three times greater in children and adolescents younger than 16 years compared with adults. Adolescent patients on oral contraceptives may require increased lamotrigine doses because estrogen induces the metabolism of lamotrigine. If the contraceptives are discontinued or the patient is postpartum, the dose of lamotrigine has to be decreased (Reimers, Helde, & Brodtkorb, 2005).

Alternative Mood Stabilizers

Gabapentin (Neurontin) is structurally similar to GABA, increases GABA release from glia, and may modulate sodium channels. Double-blind controlled studies of gabapentin as adjunctive therapy to lithium or valproate and as monotherapy suggest that it is no more effective than placebo for the treatment of mania in adults (Pande, Crockatt, Janney, Werth, & Tsaroucha, 2000). However, gabapentin may be useful in combination with other mood-stabilizing agents for the treatment of anxiety disorders in individuals with BD (Keck, Strawn, & McElroy, 2006).

Topiramate (Topamax) is a sulfamate-substituted monosaccharide, with several potential mechanisms of action, including blockade of voltage-gated sodium channels, antagonism of the kainate/AMPA subtype of glutamate receptor, enhancement of GABA activity, and carbonic anhydrase inhibition. The one double-blind placebo-controlled study of topiramate for children and adolescents with manic or mixed episodes associated with BD (ages 6–17 years, $n = 56$) was inconclusive because it was discontinued early when adult mania trials with topiramate failed to show efficacy (DelBello et al., 2005).

Wagner and colleagues (2006) have reported the results of a multicenter, industry-funded, controlled study of oxcarbazepine (Trileptal) in 116 youth with BD (mean age, 11.1 years). The difference in the primary outcome variable, change in YMRS mean scores, between the treatment and placebo groups was not statistically or clinically significant. Therefore, there is little evidence to support the use of oxcarbazepine for the treatment of children and adolescents with BD.

Summary

Both the traditional and novel mood stabilizers/antiepileptics may be effective in the treatment of children and adolescents with mood and behavior disorders. The evidence is strongest for lithium, somewhat strong for valproate, and weaker for the other agents.

Atypical Antipsychotics

The atypical antipsychotics are widely used in child, adolescent, and adult psychiatry. A recent meta-analysis of controlled atypical antipsychotic trials in adults with BD concluded that all of the five newer atypical antipsychotics (aripiprazole, olanzapine, quetiapine, risperidone, and ziprasidone) were superior to placebo for the treatment of mania in adults with BD (Perlis, Welge, Vornik, Hirschfeld, & Keck, 2006). All of the atypical antipsychotics (except clozapine, which is generic) have received FDA approval for the treatment of acute mania associated with BD in adults. Olanzapine, aripiprazole, and quetiapine have also received FDA approval as maintenance treatment for adults with BD.

There are now five large, well-designed, placebo-controlled studies that have studied the efficacy of atypical antipsychotics in children and adolescents with BD. Risperidone, olanzapine, and ziprasidone are indicated by the FDA for the short-term treatment of acute manic or mixed episodes associated with bipolar I in children and adolescents ages 10–17 years. Quetiapine is indicated for the treatment of bipolar mania in children and adolescents ages 10–17 years, and aripiprazole is indicated for the acute and maintenance treatment of manic and mixed episodes associated with bipolar I with or without psychotic features in pediatric patients 10–17 years of age.

Risperidone's efficacy for short-term treatment of mania in children and adolescents was demonstrated in a 3-week, randomized, double-blind, placebo-controlled, multicenter study of 169 patients ages 10–17 who were experiencing a manic or mixed episode of bipolar I disorder (Haas et al., 2009). Subjects were assigned to either low-dose, 0.5–2.5 mg/day, or high-dose, 3.0–6.0 mg/day, risperidone. In both active medication groups, treatment with risperidone significantly decreased the total YMRS score. No evidence of increased efficacy was observed at doses greater than 2.5 mg/day. Subjects in the high-dose group had significantly more extrapyramidal side effects than those in the low-dose group: 25% versus 5%.

A large industry-sponsored, double-blind, placebo-controlled study of olanzapine (Tohen et al., 2007) included 159 children and adolescents (ages 10–17 years) with BD who were randomized to placebo or olanzapine (1:2 ratio) for 3 weeks. There was a statistically significant greater reduction in manic symptoms in the olanzapine group compared with the placebo group. However, 42% of the children and adolescents gained 7% or more of their baseline body weight. Other side effects of olanzapine included lipid profile abnormalities and elevated prolactin levels.

There is an unpublished controlled trial of quetiapine in which 277 subjects with a bipolar I manic episode were assigned to quetiapine, 400 mg/day or 600 mg/day, or placebo in a double-blind trial for 3 weeks (DelBello, Findling, Earley, Acevedo, & Stankowski, 2007b). Both doses of quetiapine demonstrated efficacy compared with placebo. The most common adverse effects noted with quetiapine were somnolence, sedation, dizziness, and weight gain (1.7 kg).

There was also a large industry-supported multisite trial of aripiprazole in which 296 subjects with bipolar I mixed or manic episodes were randomized to aripiprazole or placebo for 4 weeks (Wagner et al., 2007). During this trial, subjects were randomized to either 10 mg/day or 30 mg/day of aripiprazole, or placebo in a 1:1:1 ratio. Both doses of aripiprazole demonstrated clinical and statistical superiority to placebo, with 45% in the low-dose group versus 64% in the high-dose group demonstrating a drop in their baseline YMRS scores of at least 50%. The most common adverse events reported during this trial were somnolence (23%), extrapyramidal disorder (18%), and fatigue (11%).

Last, ziprasidone was studied in a large multisite trial during which 238 pediatric subjects with bipolar I, manic or mixed, were randomized in a 2:1 ratio in a double-blind fashion to treatment with flexible-dose ziprasidone (80–160 mg/day) or placebo (DelBello, Findling, Wang, Gundapaneni, & Versavel, 2008). In the intent-to-treat analysis, ziprasidone demonstrated an effect that was clinically and statistically significant in children and adolescents with bipolar I disorder. No significant changes in mean body mass index scores or lipids, liver enzymes, or glucose levels were reported. Ziprasidone appears to be the only atypical antipsychotic that causes little or no weight gain in children and adolescents with BD.

Adverse Effects of Atypical Antipsychotics

The second-generation antipsychotics, although efficacious, may also cause significant side effects that must be recognized and managed effectively. These side effects include extrapyramidal effects, tardive dykinesia, obesity, hyperlipidemia, increased prolactin levels, and cardiac QTc changes (a measure of the time between the start of the Q wave and the end of the T wave in the heart's electrical cycle). Emerging evidence indicates that children and adolescents may be more susceptible to these side effects than adults, although the reasons are unclear (Correll, 2005).

EXTRAPYRAMIDAL SYMPTOMS

Drug-induced parkinsonism and akathisia are the most common extrapyramidal symptoms (EPS) in children and adolescents with BD who are treated with the atypical antipsychotics (Correll, 2008a). In a placebo-controlled trial of aripiprazole with 296 subjects with BD ages 10–17 years, Correll and colleagues (2007) reported a 10% rate of EPS in the groups treated with aripiprazole. Treatment-emergent EPS was also observed in the controlled trial of risperidone (Haas et al., 2009). In this risperidone study, EPS-related adverse events were associated with higher doses of risperidone, but none of the akathisia/EPS measures were thought to be "clinically significant."

In the 3-week trial of quetiapine sponsored by AstraZeneca for acute bipolar mania discussed previously, the frequency of EPS was relatively low and comparable to placebo (DelBello, Findling, Earley, Acevedo, & Stankowski, 2007a). No statistically significant differences in EPS were observed during 3 weeks of olanzapine treatment in adolescents with BD experiencing a manic or mixed episode

(Tohen et al., 2007). No changes in movement disorder scales were observed during 4 weeks of ziprasidone treatment in children/adolescents with BD (manic or mixed state) (DelBello et al., 2008).

Following the emergence of extrapyramidal symptoms, attempts to reduce the antipsychotic dose may be a reasonable first-line intervention. In addition, anticholinergics (e.g., benztropine, diphenhydramine) and propranolol are often effective in treating these symptoms, although these agents may have their own side effects

TARDIVE DYSKINESIA

Tardive dyskinesia is characterized by involuntary, repetitive movements and is caused by long-term or high-dose use of dopamine antagonists, usually antipsychotics. The risk of tardive dyskinesia is thought to be lower with atypical antipsychotics compared with first-generation antipsychotics in both pediatric and adult populations (Correll & Carlson, 2006). At present, short-term trials and one meta-analysis of atypical antipsychotic trials (> 11 months duration, subjects < 18 years) in the child and adolescent population suggest a low annual risk for tardive dyskinesia of 0.4% (Correll & Kane, 2007). However, large prospective, long-term trials of second-generation antipsychotics are necessary before the actual risk of tardive dyskinesia in this population can be more accurately known.

Current retrospective analyses of adolescents treated with antipsychotics suggest that the risk factors for tardive dyskinesia include early age of antipsychotic use, medication nonadherence, and concomitant use of antiparkinsonian agents (McDermid, Hood, Bockus, & D'Alessandro, 1998). However, antiparkinsonian use may serve as a surrogate for the presence of EPS, which in adults may be associated with tardive dyskinesia, although this relationship is likely quite complex (Barnes & McPhillips, 1998). Kumra and colleagues (1998) examined a cohort of children and adolescents at the National Institute of Mental Health with early-onset psychotic spectrum disorders who were treated with either first-line or atypical antipsychotics. They observed a number of factors to be associated with the combined entity "withdrawal dyskinesia/tardive dyskinesia," including lower premorbid functioning and greater positive symptoms at baseline.

To minimize the risk of development of tardive dyskinesia, clinicians should always use the lowest effective dose of antipsychotic agent, routinely monitoring patients with standardized assessments for abnormal involuntary movement scales, regularly review risks and benefits with parents and patients, and regularly evaluate the indication and need for antipsychotic therapy.

NEUROLEPTIC MALIGNANT SYNDROME

The neuroleptic malignant syndrome (NMS) is a serious neurological disorder often caused by antipsychotic drugs, including atypical antipsychotics. It generally presents with muscle rigidity, fever, autonomic instability, and cognitive changes such as delirium and is associated with elevated creatine phosphokinase or other evidence of muscle injury. However, relatively little is known about NMS in children and adolescents, although at least one recent review of pediatric NMS cases (Croarkin, Emslie, & Mayes, 2008) suggests that many of its essential features (e.g., hyperthermia and severe muscular rigidity) are retained in children.

WEIGHT GAIN AND GLUCOSE METABOLISM

Obesity is becoming endemic among children and adolescents in most Western countries (Coffey, Wilkinson, Weiner, Ritchie, & Aque, 1993). The term *obesity* refers to children with body mass index (BMI) greater than the 95th percentile for age and sex, and the term *overweight* refers to children with a BMI between the 85th and 95th percentiles for age and sex. Increased appetite and the resultant weight gain, and possible obesity, are some the major side effects of the atypical antipsychotics (Correll, 2005).

As with studies of olanzapine in adults with BD, olanzapine in adolescents with BD resulted in weight increases of 3.7 ± 2.8 kg over a 3-week period (Tohen et al., 2007). Forty-two percent of patients in the olanzapine-treated group had a change in body weight from baseline greater than 7% compared with 2% among patients receiving placebo (Tohen et al., 2007).

In children and adolescents experiencing a manic episode who were treated with aripiprazole, weight gain was observed during a 4-week period but "relative to the normal rate of growth in this patient population, there was no clinically significant weight gain" (Wagner et al., 2007). Increases in body weight for children and adolescents with BD experiencing a manic episode and treated with either 400 or 600 mg of quetiapine were clinically significant. Potentially important changes in glucose metabolism were also observed (DelBello et al., 2007a). Preliminary reports from this trial noted greater than 7% increases in weight in 14.5% of subjects treated with 400 mg/day and in 9.9% of patients treated with 600 mg/day (mean increase of 1.7 kg in both groups).

In a similar placebo-controlled study of risperidone (0.5–2.5 mg/day or 3–6 mg/day), weight increases of 1.9 kg and 1.4 kg were observed over 3 weeks in the 1.5–2.5 mg/day group and in the 3–6 mg/day group, respectively (Haas et al., 2009). Finally, no clinically significant changes in BMI scores were noted during a 4-week course of ziprasidone treatment nor were there changes in glucose values (DelBello et al., 2007a).

Important strategies to help patients manage the weight gain associated with psychotropics are to emphasize diet and exercise with restriction of high-carbohydrate-content foods, soda, and fast foods as much as possible. Another tactic for weight gain is a trial of metformin, an agent indicated for the management of type II diabetes. Metformin decreases hepatic glucose production, decreases intestinal absorption of glucose, and improves insulin sensitivity by increasing peripheral glucose uptake and utilization. Klein, Cottingham, Sorter, Barton, and Morrison (2006) studied 39 patients with mood and psychotic disorders, ages 10–17 years, whose weight had increased by more than 10% during less than 1 year of olanzapine, risperidone, or quetiapine therapy. This was a 16-week double-blind, placebo-controlled trial during which body weight, BMI, and waist circumference were measured regularly, as were fasting insulin and glucose levels. They reported that weight was stabilized in subjects receiving metformin, whereas those receiving placebo continued to gain weight (0.31 kg/week). The investigators concluded that metformin therapy is safe and effective in reversing atypical induced weight gain, decreasing insulin sensitivity, and normalizing glucose metabolism in children and adolescents treated with atypical antipsychotics.

HYPERLIPIDEMIA

Many patients treated with atypical antipsychotics who gain weight will also develop hyperlipidemia, an elevation of blood lipids. Tohen and colleagues (2007), in their double-blind, placebo-controlled trial of olanzapine, noted increases in total cholesterol, low-density lipoprotein, high-density lipoprotein, and triglycerides over a 3-week period in 13- to 17-year-olds experiencing manic or mixed episodes . Changes in serum lipids and glucose were not clinically significant in a study of aripiprazole-treated children and adolescents experiencing an acute manic episode during a 30-week period (Correll et al., 2007). Finally, quetiapine-treated acutely manic children and adolescents were found to have clinically important shifts in lipid metabolism (DelBello et al., 2008), while ziprasidone-treated patients did not experience these effects during 4 weeks of treatment (DelBello et al., 2008)

CHANGES IN SERUM PROLACTIN LEVELS

In the risperidone-controlled trial discussed previously, the mean changes in baseline prolactin levels were 41 ng/liter for males and 59 ng/liter for females (Pandina, DelBello, et al., 2007), values two to three times greater than normal. Results of the double-blind, placebo-controlled trial of olanzapine in adolescents with acute manic or mixed episodes suggest a very high incidence of hyperprolactinemia (26% of females, 63% of males) (Tohen et al., 2007). Decreases in serum prolactin were observed in children and adolescents with BD who were treated with aripiprazole for 30 weeks (Correll et al., 2007). The relative tendency of atypical antipsychotics to cause hyperprolactinemia is roughly as follows: risperidone/paliperidone > olanzapine > ziprasidone > quetiapine > clozapine > aripiprazole (Correll, 2008a).

Elevated prolactin concentrations may have a number of deleterious effects in the developing child or adolescent, including gynecomastia, oligomenorrhea, and amenorrhea (Correll, 2008b) and may sometimes cause migraine headaches. The long-term effects of this elevation on growth and sexual maturation have not been fully evaluated, but there is a concern that long-term hyperprolactinemia may alter patients' reproductive function (Jamison, 1989). Patients who develop any of these side effects should be switched to another atypical antipsychotic that does not increase serum prolactin levels. Interventions should focus on dose reduction and switching to another atypical antipsychotic.

PROLONGATION OF THE CARDIAC QTC INTERVAL

All of the atypical antipsychotics have the potential to cause the QTc interval (see prior discussion) to increase, with ziprasidone being the one most often reported to cause QTc prolongation (Blair, Scahill, State, & Martin, 2005). There have been several case reports of significant QTc prolongations in children and adolescents treated with ziprasidone (Blair et al., 2005; Malone, Delaney, Hyman, & Cater, 2007). In the large controlled trial of ziprasidone discussed previously, ziprasidone-induced QTc prolongation was not clinically significant and did not lead to any adverse events for the majority of patients (Malone et al., 2007). However, patients enrolled in clinical trials are screened very carefully, and those with any preexisting medical abnormalities are typically excluded, thus limiting the generalizability of these findings to real-world patients. Until additional information is known about the cardiac effects of atypical antipsychotics in children and adolescents, it is good clinical practice to perform a careful history; review symptoms and physical exam, looking for any history of palpitations, shortness of breath, or syncope; and obtain a baseline resting electrocardiogram if indicated by history, review of systems, or physical exam.

Combination Treatment Strategies

Kafantaris, Coletti, Dicker, Padula, and Kane (2001) evaluated acutely manic adolescents with psychotic features following treatment with lithium to assess whether adjunctive antipsychotics are necessary to stabilize psychotic mania. Antipsychotics were gradually tapered and discontinued after 4 weeks of therapeutic lithium levels in patients whose psychotic symptoms resolved. These patients were maintained with lithium monotherapy for up to 4 weeks. Significant improvement was seen in 64% of the sample with psychotic features after 4 weeks of combination treatment. However, 43% did not maintain their response after discontinuation of the antipsychotic medication, suggesting that greater than 4 weeks of antipsychotic treatment is required for some adolescents with psychotic mania. Variables associated with successful discontinuation of antipsychotic medication were first episode status, shorter duration of psychosis, and presence of thought disorder at baseline (Kafantaris et al., 2001).

One study found that the combination of mood stabilizers and atypical antipsychotics is more effective than mood stabilizer alone for adolescent mania (Del-Bello, Schwiers, Rosenberg, & Strakowski, 2002). A 6-month open trial compared the efficacy of two combination therapies for manic or mixed episodes of pediatric BD (Pavuluri et al., 2004). This study examined divalproex and risperidone versus lithium and risperidone in 37 subjects ages 5–18 years with a mixed or manic episode. Response rates based on a 50% or greater decrease from baseline in YMRS score were 80% for the divalproex/risperidone group and 82.4% for the lithium/risperidone group; both combination treatments were well tolerated. Results of this open trial suggest that either treatment strategy may be used for adolescents with mania, although the findings must be confirmed in randomized designs.

BIPOLAR DEPRESSION: A DEVELOPMENTAL PERSPECTIVE

Adolescents with BD whose index episode is major depression are more likely to experience a poorer outcome compared with those with an index episode of mania or mixed mania (Strober et al., 1995). Despite the severe morbidity and mortality associated with bipolar depression, there are limited data regarding the treatment of depression in children and adolescents with BD.

Treatment of bipolar depression can be complicated because of the often necessary use of combinations of medications, including antidepressants, that may induce mania, hypomania, or rapid cycling (Compton & Nemeroff, 2000). A retrospective study assessing treatment of depressed children and adolescents with BD suggests that SSRIs may be effective for acute bipolar depression, but these agents may be associated with mood destabilization and exacerbation of manic symptoms (Biederman, Mick, Spencer, Wilens, & Faraone, 2000). Specifically, in this study depressive symptoms were 6.7 times more likely to improve when subjects received an SSRI. However, SSRIs were associated with a threefold greater probability of relapse of manic symptomatology. In patients with active manic symptoms, the concomitant use of SSRIs with mood stabilizer treatment did not significantly inhibit the improvement of manic symptoms associated with mood stabilizer treatment (Biederman et al., 2000). Thus, further studies of antidepressants in combination with mood stabilizers or atypical antipsychotics are needed. Antidepressant medications should be used with caution in children and adolescents with BD because of the potential risk for increased mood instability and for the emergence of suicidal ideation.

As previously described, there have been two recent prospective, open-label studies assessing lithium and lamotrigine for bipolar depression in adolescents (Chang et al., 2006; Patel et al., 2006). Methodological differences between the studies make it difficult to compare their results. Specifically, Chang and colleagues (2006) included adolescents with depression or mixed episodes and bipolar type I or II disorder, and lamotrigine was used as monotherapy or adjunctive to other medication. In contrast, Patel and colleagues (2006) included only adolescents with bipolar type I disorder with depression, and lithium was used as monotherapy. Nonetheless, these studies suggest that both medications may be useful for depression associated with BD in adolescents.

Recent placebo-controlled studies suggest that atypical antipsychotics, specifically quetiapine and olanzapine, are useful for the treatment of depression in adults with BD (Calabrese, Elhaj, Gajwani, & Gao, 2005). In contrast, a double-blind, placebo-controlled study revealed that quetiapine may be no more effective than placebo for depression associated with BD in adolescents, although the response rate to placebo in this study was large and the sample was small ($n = 32$) (DelBello et al., 2009).

MAINTENANCE TREATMENT: A DEVELOPMENTAL PERSPECTIVE

In addition to the treatment of acute affective episodes, lithium may also be useful for the prevention of recurrent affective episodes in children and adolescents with BD. One early maintenance treatment study for pediatric BD (Strober, Morrell, Lampert, & Burroughs, 1990) prospectively evaluated 37 adolescents whose mood had been stabilized with lithium while hospitalized. After 18 months of follow-up, 35% of these patients discontinued lithium, and 92% of these subsequently relapsed compared with 38% of those who were lithium compliant, supporting the potential utility of lithium for maintenance treatment for adolescent BD.

Findling and colleagues (2006) published the results of an open trial of lithium combined with divalproex. The participants ($n = 38$; mean age, 10.5 years) had initially responded to lithium combined with divalproex but had relapsed during monotherapy with either medication. All were treated with lithium and divalproex as outpatients for 8 weeks. Eighty-nine percent of subjects responded to restabilization with this combination. On the basis of these findings, the authors concluded that youth who had initially responded to a combination of lithium with divalproex may be effectively restabilized on this combination if they relapse during maintenance monotherapy with either medication.

CO-OCCURRING PSYCHIATRIC DISORDERS: DEVELOPMENTAL CONSIDERATIONS

Children and adolescents with BD commonly present with co-occurring psychiatric disorders (Pavuluri, Birmaher, & Naylor, 2005), the most common of which is ADHD. Treatment of children with BD and co-occurring ADHD requires stabilization with a traditional mood stabilizer or an atypical antipsychotic as a necessary prerequisite to initiating stimulant medications (Biederman et al., 1999). However, controlled studies are lacking to support this common clinical practice. A randomized, controlled trial of 40 bipolar children and adolescents with ADHD demonstrated that low-dose mixed-salts amphetamine is effective and well tolerated for the treatment of comorbid ADHD symptoms following mood stabilization with divalproex (Scheffer, Kowatch, Carmody, & Rush, 2005). Sustained-release psychostimulants may be more effective at reducing rebound symptoms in children and adolescents with BD than immediate-release formulations of stimulant mediations.

Disruptive behavior disorders also commonly co-occur in children and adolescents with BD. One study suggested that divalproex may be effective to treat aggressive symptoms associated with BD in adolescents (DelBello, Adler, & Strakowski, 2004). Additionally, in a post hoc analysis of a controlled, prospective study, quetiapine was found to reduce aggression in adolescents with BD with co-occurring disruptive behavior disorders (Barzman, DelBello, Adler, Stanford, & Strakowski, 2006), suggesting that in the subset of youth with BD and co-occurring disruptive behavior disorders atypical antipsychotics may be warranted.

Up to 40% of adolescents with BD have co-occurring substance use disorders (Wilens et al., 2004). Despite this high co-occurrence, there has been only one small treatment study of adolescents with BD with substance use disorders, which suggested that lithium may be more effective than placebo (Geller, Cooper, Sun, et al., 1998). Results from recent studies suggest that topiramate may be useful for the treatment of disorders related to poor impulse control in adults, including alcohol dependence (Johnson et al., 2003), binge eating (McElroy et al., 2003, 2004), and bulimia nervosa (Hoopes et al., 2003). Alternatively, children and adolescents who are earlier in their illness course may respond differently than older patients, who typically have a history of multiple treatment failures. Specifically, the relationship between acute affective episodes and cellular stress has been well documented (Manji & Zarate, 2002). Stress-induced cortisol elevation results in excessive neuronal glutamate release that typically occurs following a major stressor (e.g., onset of an illness). Therefore, youth with BD who are closer to illness onset may be more likely than adults, who are further along in illness course, to respond to medications that block acute glutaminergic release. Indeed, topiramate inhibits the excitatory effects of glutaminergic receptors. These findings highlight the importance of evaluating new treatment options for BD in age-specific controlled trials.

EARLY INTERVENTION

The most common period of BD onset is during adolescence (Perlis et al., 2004). Therefore, children and adolescents are the ideal populations in which to identify those at risk for developing BD before illness onset and establish effective early intervention or prevention strategies (Perlis et al., 2004). Although children and adolescents of parents with BD are at an increased risk for developing BD, prodromal manifestations of BD are only beginning to be identified (Birmaher et al., 2006; DelBello & Geller, 2001). To determine prodromal manifestations of BD, longitudinal studies are needed to establish who will develop the fully syndromal illness. The Course and Outcome of Bipolar Youth study (Birmaher et al., 2006; see Diler et al., Chapter 5, this volume) is a notable step in the direction of clarifying prodromal states that predict the onset of bipolar I or II disorder.

On the basis of data suggesting that offspring of parents with BD have an elevated risk for developing ADHD and other mood disorders (e.g., major depressive disorder and cyclothymia), investigators have begun to examine whether early intervention treatment with mood stabilizers or atypical antipsychotics is effective. In a double-blind, controlled study, Geller, Cooper, Zimerman, and colleagues (1998) determined that lithium was no more effective than placebo for the treatment of adolescents with major depressive disorder and at familial risk for BD. More recently, there have been several investigations of divalproex for the treatment of mood symptoms in children at familial risk for BD. Among 23 children who did not have bipolar I disorder but were diagnosed with mood symptoms/syndromes and had a parent with BD, Chang and colleagues (2003) found a significant reduction in mood symptoms and improvement in overall functioning following treatment with divalproex . Similarly, Findling and colleagues (2003) reported that children with mood symptoms and a multigenerational family history of BD had a significant reduction in mood symptoms when treated with divalproex compared with placebo; however, there was no statistically significant group difference between those with and without a multigenerational family history.

In a recently completed 12-week study (DelBello, Adler, et al., 2007), adolescents (n = 20; mean age, 14.7 years) with a mood disorder other than bipolar I and a parent with BD were initiated on 100 mg quetiapine and titrated to 400 mg by day 4 (mean, 460 mg/day). The YMRS and Children's Depression Rating Scale—Revised scores decreased significantly from baseline at all time points (all p < .001). The most common side effects were somnolence (n = 11 [55%]), headache (n = 5 [25%]), musculoskeletal pain (n = 5 [25%]), and dyspepsia (n = 5 [25%]). The findings suggest that quetiapine may be useful for the treatment of early manifestations of bipolar I disorder in those at familial risk; however, placebo-controlled studies are needed. Additionally, whether these adolescents would have progressed to develop bipolar I disorder remains unknown.

CONCLUSIONS

Because of the high rate of co-occurring disorders, the shorter illness duration, and the greater susceptibility to side effects among children and adolescents with BD compared with adults with BD, additional age-specific efficacy and tolerability studies are needed to determine optimal pharmacological interventions for this population. Although there are now several large well-controlled studies demonstrating effective and well-tolerated treatment options for manic or mixed episodes associated with pediatric BD, there are few pharmacological intervention studies of the depressive pole of the disorder.

Other important issues that have yet to be explored: Why do so many pediatric patients with BD who present with the same symptoms respond so differently to the same medications (multifinality)? Alternatively, why do patients with BD with different initial symptoms sometimes respond well to the same medication (equifinality)? Are there any sex differences in response to medications or sensitivity to side effects? Does a family history of BD help a clinician choose medications? Are there any risk/protective factors that bode poorly/well for response to pharmacotherapy? These are all areas for future research.

Establishing evidence-based maintenance treatment strategies for BD, especially for youth with commonly co-occurring psychiatric disorders, is another area for future investigation. Nonetheless, over the past decade, there has been considerable progress in developing rational treatment strategies for children and adolescents with bipolar illness.

REFERENCES

Adler, C. M., DelBello, M. P., & Strakowski, S. M. (2006). Brain network dysfunction in bipolar disorder. *CNS Spectrums, 11*(4), 312–320; quiz, 323–314.

Barnes, T. R., & McPhillips, M. A. (1998). Novel antipsychotics, extrapyramidal side effects and tardive dyskinesia. *International Clinical Psychopharmacology, 13*(Suppl. 3), S49–S57.

Bartelink, I. H., Rademaker, C. M., Schobben, A. F., & van den Anker, J. N. (2006). Guidelines on paediatric dosing on the basis of developmental physiology and pharmacokinetic considerations. *Clinical Pharmacokinetics, 45*(11), 1077–1097.

Barzman, D. H., DelBello, M. P., Adler, C. M., Stanford, K. E., & Strakowski, S. M. (2006). The efficacy and tolerability of quetiapine versus divalproex for the treatment of impulsivity and reactive aggression in adolescents with co-occurring bipolar disorder and disruptive behavior disorder(s). *Journal of Child and Adolescent Psychopharmacology, 16*(6), 665–670.

Biederman, J., Mick, E., Prince, J., Bostic, J. Q., Wilens, T. E., Spencer, T., et al. (1999). Systematic chart review of the pharmacologic treatment of comorbid attention deficit hyperactivity disorder in youth with bipolar disorder. *Journal of Child and Adolescent Psychopharmacology, 9*(4), 247–256.

Biederman, J., Mick, E., Spencer, T. J., Wilens, T. E., & Faraone, S. V. (2000). Therapeutic dilemmas in the pharmacotherapy of bipolar depression in the young. *Journal of Child and Adolescent Psychopharmacology, 10*(3), 185–192.

Birmaher, B., Axelson, D., Strober, M., Gill, M. K., Valeri, S., Chiappetta, L., et al. (2006). Clinical course of children and adolescents with bipolar spectrum disorders. *Archives of General Psychiatry, 63*(2), 175–183.

Black, J. L., III, O'Kane, D. J., & Mrazek, D. A. (2007). The impact of CYP allelic variation on antidepressant metabolism: A review. *Expert Opinion on Drug Metabolism and Toxicology, 3*(1), 21–31.

Blair, J., Scahill, L., State, M., & Martin, A. (2005). Electrocardiographic changes in children and adolescents treated with ziprasidone: A prospective study. *Journal of the American Academy of Child and Adolescent Psychiatry, 44*(1), 73–79.

Blumberg, H. P., Kaufman, J., Martin, A., Charney, D. S., Krystal, J. H., & Peterson, B. S. (2004). Significance of adolescent neurodevelopment for the neural circuitry of bipolar disorder. *Annals of the New York Academy of Sciences, 1021*, 376–383.

Bowden, C. L., Calabrese, J. R., Sachs, G., Yatham, L. N., Asghar, S. A., Hompland, M., et al.

(2003). A placebo-controlled 18-month trial of lamotrigine and lithium maintenance treatment in recently manic or hypomanic patients with bipolar I disorder. *Archives of General Psychiatry, 60*(4), 392–400.

Bowden, C. L., & Karren, N. U. (2006). Anticonvulsants in bipolar disorder. *Australia and New Zealand Journal of Psychiatry, 40*(5), 386–393.

Bowring, M. A., & Kovacs, M. (1992). Difficulties in diagnosing manic disorders among children and adolescents. *Journal of the American Academy of Child and Adolescent Psychiatry, 31*(4), 611–614.

Buchsbaum, M. S., Wu, J., Siegel, B. V., Hackett, E., Trenary, M., Abel, L., et al. (1997). Effect of sertraline on regional metabolic rate in patients with affective disorder. *Biological Psychiatry, 41*(1), 15–22.

Cade, J. F. (1949). Lithium salts in the treatment of psychotic excitement. *Medical Journal of Australia, 36*, 349–352.

Calabrese, J., Bowden, C., Sachs, G., Ascher, J., Monaghan, E., & Rudd, G. (1999). A double-blind placebo-controlled study of lamotrigine monotherapy in outpatients with bipolar I depression. *Journal of Clinical Psychiatry, 60*, 79–88.

Calabrese, J. R., Elhaj, O., Gajwani, P., & Gao, K. (2005). Clinical highlights in bipolar depression: Focus on atypical antipsychotics. *Journal of Clinical Psychiatry, 66*(Suppl. 5), 26–33.

Calabrese, J. R., Sullivan, J. R., Bowden, C. L., Suppes, T., Goldberg, J. F., Sachs, G. S., et al. (2002). Rash in multicenter trials of lamotrigine in mood disorders: Clinical relevance and management. *Journal of Clinical Psychiatry, 63*(11), 1012–1019.

Carr, R. B., & Shrewsbury, K. (2007). Hyperammonemia due to valproic acid in the psychiatric setting. *American Journal of Psychiatry, 164*(7), 1020–1027.

Chang, K., Saxena, K., & Howe, M. (2006). An open-label study of lamotrigine adjunct or monotherapy for the treatment of adolescents with bipolar depression. *Journal of the American Academy of Child and Adolescent Psychiatry, 45*(3), 298–304.

Chang, K. D., Dienes, K., Blasey, C., Adleman, N., Ketter, T., & Steiner, H. (2003). Divalproex monotherapy in the treatment of bipolar offspring with mood and behavioral disorders and at least mild affective symptoms. *Journal of Clinical Psychiatry, 64*(8), 936–942.

Cicchetti, D., & Rogosch, F. A. (2002). A developmental psychopathology perspective on adolescence. *Journal of Consulting and Clinical Psychology, 70*(1), 6–20.

Ciraulo, D. A., Shader, R. J., Greenblatt, D. J., & Creelman, W. L. (Eds.). (1995). *Drug interactions in psychiatry.* Baltimore: Williams & Wilkins.

Coffey, C. E., Wilkinson, W. E., Weiner, R. D., Ritchie, J. C., & Aque, M. (1993). The dexamethasone suppression test and quantitative cerebral anatomy in depression. *Biological Psychiatry, 33*(6), 442–449.

Compton, M. T., & Nemeroff, C. B. (2000). The treatment of bipolar depression. *Journal of Clinical Psychiatry, 61*(Suppl. 9), 57–67.

Correll, C. U. (2005). Metabolic side effects of second-generation antipsychotics in children and adolescents: A different story? *Journal of Clinical Psychiatry, 66*(10), 1331–1332.

Correll, C. U. (2008a). Antipsychotic use in children and adolescents: Minimizing adverse effects to maximize outcomes. *Journal of the American Academy of Child and Adolescent Psychiatry, 47*(1), 9–20.

Correll, C. U. (2008b). Effect of hyperprolactinemia during development in children and adolescents. *Journal of Clinical Psychiatry, 69*(8), e24.

Correll, C. U., & Carlson, H. E. (2006). Endocrine and metabolic adverse effects of psychotropic medications in children and adolescents. *Journal of the American Academy of Child and Adolescent Psychiatry, 45*(7), 771–791.

Correll, C. U., & Kane, J. M. (2007). One-year incidence rates of tardive dyskinesia in children and adolescents treated with second-generation antipsychotics: A systematic review. *Journal of Child and Adolescent Psychopharmacology, 17*(5), 647–656.

Correll, C. U., Nyilas, M., Ashfaque, S., Aurang, C., Jin, N., Marcus, R., et al. (2007). *Long-term safety and tolerability of aripiprazole in children (10–17 years) with bipolar disorder.* Paper presented at the American College of Neuropharmacology, Boca Raton, FL.

Croarkin, P. E., Emslie, G. J., & Mayes, T. L. (2008). Neuroleptic malignant syndrome associated with atypical antipsychotics in pediatric patients: A review of published cases. *Journal of Clinical Psychiatry, 69*(7), 1157–1165.

Cueva, J. E., Overall, J. E., Small, A. M., Armenteros, J. L., Perry, R., & Campbell, M. (1996). Carbamazepine in aggressive children with conduct disorder: A double-blind and placebo-controlled study. *Journal of the American Academy of Child and Adolescent Psychiatry, 35*(4), 480–490.

DelBello, M., Findling, R. L., Earley, W., Acevedo, L., & Stankowski, J. (2007a, December). *Efficacy of quetiapine in children and adolescent with bipolar mania: A 3-week, double-blind, randomized, placebo-controlled trial.* Paper presented at the meeting of the American College of Neuropharmacology, Boca Raton, FL.

DelBello, M., Findling, R. L., Earley, W., Acevedo, L., & Stankowski, J. (2007b, October). *Efficacy of quetiapine in children and adolescents with bipolar mania: A 3-week, double-blind, randomized, placebo-controlled trial.* Paper presented at the 54th Annual Meeting of the American Academy of Child and Adolescent Psychiatry, Boston.

DelBello, M., Findling, R. L., Wang, P., Gundapaneni, B., & Versavel, M. (2008). *Safety and efficacy of ziprasidone in pediatric bipolar disorder.* Paper presented at the 161st Annual Meeting of the American Psychiatric Association, Washington, DC.

DelBello, M. P., Adler, C., & Strakowski, S. M. (2004). Divalproex for the treatment of aggression associated with adolescent mania. *Journal of Child and Adolescent Psychopharmacology, 14*(2), 325–328.

DelBello, M. P., Adler, C. M., Whitsel, R. M., Stanford, K. E., & Strakowski, S. M. (2007). A 12-week single-blind trial of quetiapine for the treatment of mood symptoms in adolescents at high risk for developing bipolar I disorder. *Journal of Clinical Psychiatry, 68*(5), 789–795.

DelBello, M. P., Chang, K., Welge, J. A., Adler, C. M., Rana, M., Howe, M., et al. (2009). A double-blind, placebo-controlled pilot study of quetiapine for depressed adolescents with bipolar disorder. *Bipolar Disorders, 11*(5), 483–493.

DelBello, M. P., Findling, R. L., Kushner, S., Wang, D., Olson, W. H., Capece, J. A., et al. (2005). A pilot controlled trial of topiramate for mania in children and adolescents with bipolar disorder. *Journal of the American Academy of Child and Adolescent Psychiatry, 44*(6), 539–547.

DelBello, M. P., & Geller, B. (2001). Review of studies of child and adolescent offspring of bipolar parents. *Bipolar Disorders, 3*, 325–334.

DelBello, M. P., Schwiers, M. L., Rosenberg, H. L., & Strakowski, S. M. (2002). A double-blind, randomized, placebo-controlled study of quetiapine as adjunctive treatment for adolescent mania. *Journal of the American Academy of Child and Adolescent Psychiatry, 41*(10), 1216–1223.

Delong, G. R., & Nieman, M. A. (1983). Lithium-induced behavior changes in children with symptoms suggesting manic-depressive illness. *Psychopharmacology Bulletin, 19*(2), 258–265.

Deltito, J. A., Levitan, J., Damore, J., Hajal, F., & Zambenedetti, M. (1998). Naturalistic experience with the use of divalproex sodium on an in-patient unit for adolescent psychiatric patients. *Acta Psychiatrica Scandinavica, 97*(3), 236–240.

Devi, K., George, S., Criton, S., Suja, V., & Sridevi, P. K. (2005). Carbamazepine—The commonest cause of toxic epidermal necrolysis and Stevens-Johnson syndrome: A study of 7 years. *Indian Journal of Dermatology, Venereology and Leprology, 71*(5), 325–328.

Ee, L. C., Shepherd, R. W., Cleghorn, G. J., Lewindon, P. J., Fawcett, J., Strong, R. W., et al. (2003). Acute liver failure in children: A regional experience. *Journal of Paediatrics and Child Health, 39*(2), 107–110.

Evans, R. W., Clay, T. H., & Gualtieri, C. T. (1987). Carbamazepine in pediatric psychiatry. *Journal of the American Academy of Child and Adolescent Psychiatry, 26*(1), 2–8.

Findling, R. L., Gracious, B. L., McNamara, N. K., Youngstrom, E. A., Demeter, C. A., Branicky, L. A., et al. (2001). Rapid, continuous cycling and psychiatric co-morbidity in pediatric bipolar I disorder. *Bipolar Disorders, 3,* 202–210.

Findling, R. L., McNamara, N. K., Stansbrey, R., Gracious, B. L., Whipkey, R. E., Demeter, C. A., et al. (2006). Combination lithium and divalproex sodium in pediatric bipolar symptom re-stabilization. *Journal of the American Academy of Child and Adolescent Psychiatry, 45*(2), 142–148.

Findling, R. L., McNamara, N. K., Gracious, B. L., Youngstrom, E. A., Stansbrey, R. J., Reed, M. D., et al. (2003). Combination lithium and divalproex sodium in pediatric bipolarity. *Journal of the American Academy of Child and Adolescent Psychiatry, 42*(8), 895–901.

Findling, R. L., McNamara, N. K., Youngstrom, E. A., Stansbrey, R., Gracious, B. L., Reed, M. D., et al. (2005). Double-blind 18-month trial of lithium versus divalproex maintenance treatment in pediatric bipolar disorder. *Journal of the American Academy of Child and Adolescent Psychiatry, 44*(5), 409–417.

Geddes, J. R., Burgess, S., Hawton, K., Jamison, K., & Goodwin, G. M. (2004). Long-term lithium therapy for bipolar disorder: Systematic review and meta-analysis of randomized controlled trials. *American Journal of Psychiatry, 161*(2), 217–222.

Geller, B., Bolhofner, K., Craney, J., Williams, M., DelBello, M. P., & Gundersen, K. (2000). Psychosocial functioning in a prepubertal and early adolescent bipolar disorder phenotype. *Journal of the American Academy of Child and Adolescent Psychiatry, 39*(12), 1543–1548.

Geller, B., Cooper, T. B., Sun, K., Zimerman, M. A., Frazier, J., Williams, M., et al. (1998). Double-blind and placebo-controlled study of lithium for adolescent bipolar disorders with secondary substance dependency. *Journal of the American Academy of Child and Adolescent Psychiatry, 37*(2), 171–178.

Geller, B., Cooper, T. B., Zimerman, B., Frazier, J., Williams, M., Heath, J., et al. (1998). Lithium for prepubertal depressed children with family history predictors of future bipolarity: A double-blind, placebo-controlled study. *Journal of Affective Disorders, 51*(2), 165–175.

Geller, B., Tillman, R., Craney, J. L., & Bolhofner, K. (2004). Four-year prospective outcome and natural history of mania in children with a prepubertal and early adolescent bipolar disorder phenotype. *Archives of General Psychiatry, 61*(5), 459–467.

Geller, B., Zimerman, B., Williams, M., Bolhofner, K., Craney, J., DelBello, M., et al. (2000). Diagnostic characteristics of 93 cases of a prepubertal and early adolescent bipolar disorder phenotype by gender, puberty and comorbid attention deficit hyperactivity disorder. *Journal of Child and Adolescent Psychopharmacology, 10,* 157–164.

Geller, B., Zimerman, B., Williams, M., DelBello, M. P., Frazier, J., & Beringer, L. (2002). Phenomenology of prepubertal and early adolescent bipolar disorder: Examples of elated mood, grandiose behaviors, decreased need for sleep, racing thoughts and hypersexuality. *Journal of Child and Adolescent Psychopharmacology, 12*(1), 3–9.

Goodwin, F. K., & Ghaemi, S. N. (1998). Understanding manic-depressive illness. *Archives of General Psychiatry, 55*(1), 23–25.

Gram, L. F., & Rafaelsen, O. J. (1972). Lithium treatment of psychotic children and adolescents. A controlled clinical trial. *Acta Psychiatrica Scandinavica, 48*(3), 253–260.

Haas, M., DelBello, M. P., Pandina, G., Kushner, S., Van Hove, I., Augustyns, I., et al. (2009). Risperidone for the treatment of acute mania in children and adolescents with bipolar disorder: A randomized, double-blind, placebo-controlled study. *Bipolar Disorders, 11*(7), 687–700.

Haldane, M., & Frangou, S. (2004). New insights help define the pathophysiology of bipolar affective disorder: Neuroimaging and neuropathology findings. *Progress in Neuro-Psychopharmacology and Biological Psychiatry, 28*(6), 943–960.

Hines, R. N. (2008). The ontogeny of drug metabolism enzymes and implications for adverse drug events. *Pharmacology and Therapeutics, 118*(2), 250–267.

Hoopes, S. P., Reimherr, F. W., Hedges, D. W., Rosenthal, N. R., Kamin, M., Karim, R., et al. (2003). Treatment of bulimia nervosa with topiramate in a randomized, double-blind, placebo-controlled trial: Part 1. Improvement in binge and purge measures. *Journal of Clinical Psychiatry, 64*(11), 1335–1341.

Isaac, G. (1992). Misdiagnosed bipolar disorder in adolescents in a special educational school and treatment program. *Journal of Clinical Psychiatry, 53*(4), 133–136.

Isaac, G. (1995). Is bipolar disorder the most common diagnostic entity in hospitalized adolescents and children? *Adolescence, 30*(118), 273–276.

Isojarvi, J. I., Laatikainen, T. J., Pakarinen, A. J., Juntunen, K. T., & Myllyla, V. V. (1993). Polycystic ovaries and hyperandrogenism in women taking valproate for epilepsy. *New England Journal of Medicine, 329*(19), 1383–1388.

Jamison, K. R. (1989). Mood disorders and patterns of creativity in British writers and artists. *Psychiatry, 52*(2), 125–134.

Joffe, H., Cohen, L. S., Suppes, T., McLaughlin, W. L., Lavori, P., Adams, J. M., et al. (2006). Valproate is associated with new-onset oligoamenorrhea with hyperandrogenism in women with bipolar disorder. *Biological Psychiatry, 59*(11), 1078–1086.

Johnson, B. A., Ait-Daoud, N., Bowden, C. L., DiClemente, C. C., Roache, J. D., Lawson, K., et al. (2003). Oral topiramate for treatment of alcohol dependence: A randomised controlled trial. *Lancet, 361,* 1677–1685.

Kafantaris, V., Campbell, M., Padron-Gayol, M. V., Small, A. M., Locascio, J. J., & Rosenberg, C. R. (1992). Carbamazepine in hospitalized aggressive conduct disorder children: An open pilot study. *Psychopharmacology Bulletin, 28*(2), 193–199.

Kafantaris, V., Coletti, D. J., Dicker, R., Padula, G., & Kane, J. M. (2001). Adjunctive antipsychotic treatment of adolescents with bipolar psychosis. *Journal of the American Academy of Child and Adolescent Psychiatry, 40,* 1448–1456.

Kafantaris, V., Coletti, D. J., Dicker, R., Padula, G., & Kane, J. M. (2003). Lithium treatment of acute mania in adolescents: A large open trial. *Journal of the American Academy of Child and Adolescent Psychiatry, 42*(9), 1038–1045.

Kastner, T., & Friedman, D. L. (1992). Verapamil and valproic acid treatment of prolonged mania. *Journal of the American Academy of Child and Adolescent Psychiatry, 31*(2), 271–275.

Kastner, T., Friedman, D. L., Plummer, A. T., Ruiz, M. Q., & Henning, D. (1990). Valproic acid for the treatment of children with mental retardation and mood symptomatology. *Pediatrics, 86*(3), 467–472.

Keating, A., & Blahunka, P. (1995). Carbamazepine-induced Stevens-Johnson syndrome in a child. *Annals of Pharmacotherapy, 29*(5), 538–539.

Keck, P. E., Jr., Strawn, J. R., & McElroy, S. L. (2006). Pharmacologic treatment considerations in co-occurring bipolar and anxiety disorders. *Journal of Clinical Psychiatry, 67*(Suppl. 1), 8–15.

Ketter, T. A., Nasrallah, H. A., & Fagiolini, A. (2006). Mood stabilizers and atypical antipsychotics: Bimodal treatments for bipolar disorder. *Psychopharmacology Bulletin, 39*(1), 120–146.

Ketter, T. A., Wang, P. W., Becker, O. V., Nowakowska, C., & Yang, Y. S. (2003). The diverse roles of anticonvulsants in bipolar disorders. *Annals of Clinical Psychiatry, 15*(2), 95–108.

Klein, D. J., Cottingham, E. M., Sorter, M., Barton, B. A., & Morrison, J. A. (2006). A randomized, double-blind, placebo-controlled trial of metformin treatment of weight gain associated with initiation of atypical antipsychotic therapy in children and adolescents. *American Journal of Psychiatry, 163*(12), 2072–2079.

Konig, S. A., Siemes, H., Blaker, F., Boenigk, E., Gross-Selbeck, G., Hanefeld, F., et al. (1994). Severe hepatotoxicity during valproate therapy: An update and report of eight new fatalities. *Epilepsia, 35*(5), 1005–1015.

Kowatch, R., Findling, R., Scheffer, R., & Stanford, K. (2007, October). *Placebo controlled trial of divalproex versus lithium for bipolar disorder.* Paper presented at the 54th Annual Meeting of the American Academy of Child and Adolescent Psychiatry, Boston.

Kowatch, R. A., & DelBello, M. P. (2006). Pediatric bipolar disorder: Emerging diagnostic and treatment approaches. *Child and Adolescent Psychiatric Clinics of North America, 15*(1), 73–108.

Kowatch, R. A., Suppes, T., Carmody, T. J., Bucci, J. P., Hume, J. H., Kromelis, M., et al. (2000). Effect size of lithium, divalproex sodium and carbamazepine in children and adolescents with bipolar disorder. *Journal of the American Academy of Child and Adolescent Psychiatry, 39*(6), 713–720.

Kumra, S., Jacobsen, L. K., Lenane, M., Zahn, T. P., Wiggs, E., Alaghban-Rad, J., et al. (1998). "Multidimensionally impaired disorder": Is it a variant of very early-onset schizophrenia? *Journal of the American Academy of Child and Adolescent Psychiatry, 37,* 91–99.

Lena, B. (1979). Lithium in child and adolescent psychiatry. *Archives of General Psychiatry, 36*(8, Spec No), 854–855.

Malone, R. P., Delaney, M. A., Hyman, S. B., & Cater, J. R. (2007). Ziprasidone in adolescents with autism: An open-label pilot study. *Journal of Child and Adolescent Psychopharmacology, 17*(6), 779–790.

Manji, H. K., & Zarate, C. A. (2002). Molecular and cellular mechanisms underlying mood stabilization in bipolar disorder: Implications for the development of improved therapeutics. *Molecular Psychiatry, 7*(Suppl. 1), S1–S7.

Martinowich, K., Schloesser, R. J., & Manji, H. K. (2009). Bipolar disorder: From genes to behavior pathways. *Journal of Clinical Investigation, 119*(4), 726–736.

Mayberg, H. S. (1997). Limbic-cortical dysregulation: A proposed model of depression. *Journal of Neuropsychiatry and Clinical Neurosciences, 9*(3), 471–481.

McDermid, S. A., Hood, J., Bockus, S., & D'Alessandro, E. (1998). Adolescents on neuroleptic medication: Is this population at risk for tardive dyskinesia? *Canadian Journal of Psychiatry. Revue Canadienne de Psychiatrie, 43*(6), 629–631.

McElroy, S. L., Arnold, L. M., Shapira, N. A., Keck, P. E., Jr., Rosenthal, N. R., Karim, M. R., et al. (2003). Topiramate in the treatment of binge eating disorder associated with obesity: A randomized, placebo-controlled trial. *American Journal of Psychiatry, 160*(2), 255–261.

McElroy, S. L., & Keck, P. J. (2000). Pharmacologic agents for the treatment of acute bipolar mania. *Biological Psychiatry, 48,* 539–557.

McElroy, S. L., Shapira, N. A., Arnold, L. M., Keck, P. E., Rosenthal, N. R., Wu, S. C., et al. (2004). Topiramate in the long-term treatment of binge-eating disorder associated with obesity. *Journal of Clinical Psychiatry, 65*(11), 1463–1469.

McKnew, D. H., Cytryn, L., Buchsbaum, M. S., Hamovit, J., Lamour, M., Rapoport, J. L., et al.

(1981). Lithium in children of lithium-responding parents. *Psychiatric Research, 4*(2), 171–180.

Newberg, A. R., Catapano, L. A., Zarate, C. A., & Manji, H. K. (2008). Neurobiology of bipolar disorder. *Expert Review of Neurotherapeutics, 8*(1), 93–110.

Pande, A. C., Crockatt, J. G., Janney, C. A., Werth, J. L., & Tsaroucha, G. (2000). Gabapentin in bipolar disorder: A placebo-controlled trial of adjunctive therapy. *Bipolar Disorders, 2,* 249–255.

Pandina, G. J., Bossie, C. A., Youssef, E., Zhu, Y., & Dunbar, F. (2007). Risperidone improves behavioral symptoms in children with autism in a randomized, double-blind, placebo-controlled trial. *Journal of Autism and Developmental Disorders, 37*(2), 367–373.

Pandina, G. J., DelBello, M., Kushner, S., Van Hove, I., Augustynus, I., Kusumakar, V., et al. (2007, October). *Risperidone for the treatment of acute mania in bipolar youth.* Paper presented at the annual meeting of the American Academy of Child and Adolescent Psychiatry, Boston.

Papatheodorou, G., & Kutcher, S. P. (1993). Divalproex sodium treatment in late adolescent and young adult acute mania. *Psychopharmacology Bulletin, 29*(2), 213–219.

Papatheodorou, G., Kutcher, S. P., Katic, M., & Szalai, J. P. (1995). The efficacy and safety of divalproex sodium in the treatment of acute mania in adolescents and young adults: An open clinical trial. *Journal of Clinical Psychopharmacology, 15*(2), 110–116.

Patel, N. C., DelBello, M. P., Bryan, H. S., Adler, C. M., Kowatch, R. A., Stanford, K., et al. (2006). Open-label lithium for the treatment of adolescents with bipolar depression. *Journal of the American Academy of Child and Adolescent Psychiatry, 45*(3), 289–297.

Pavuluri, M. N., Birmaher, B., & Naylor, M. W. (2005). Pediatric bipolar disorder: A review of the past 10 years. *Journal of the American Academy of Child and Adolescent Psychiatry, 44*(9), 846–871.

Pavuluri, M. N., Henry, D. B., Carbray, J. A., Sampson, G., Naylor, M. W., & Janicak, P. G. (2004). Open-label prospective trial of risperidone in combination with lithium or divalproex sodium in pediatric mania. *Journal of Affective Disorders, 82*(Suppl. 1), S103–S111.

Perlis, R. H., Miyahara, S., Marangell, L. B., Wisniewski, S. R., Ostacher, M., DelBello, M. P., et al. (2004). Long-term implications of early onset in bipolar disorder: Data from the first 1000 participants in the Systematic Treatment Enhancement Program for Bipolar Disorder (STEP-BD). *Biological Psychiatry, 55*(9), 875–881.

Perlis, R. H., Welge, J. A., Vornik, L. A., Hirschfeld, R. M., & Keck, P. E. (2006). Atypical antipsychotics in the treatment of mania: A meta-analysis of randomized, placebo-controlled trials. *Journal of Clinical Psychiatry, 67*(4), 509–516.

Phillips, M. L. (2006). The neural basis of mood dysregulation in bipolar disorder. *Cognitive Neuropsychiatry, 11*(3), 233–249.

Pleak, R. R., Birmaher, B., Gavrilescu, A., Abichandani, C., & Williams, D. T. (1988). Mania and neuropsychiatric excitation following carbamazepine. *Journal of the American Academy of Child and Adolescent Psychiatry, 27*(4), 500–503.

Post, R. M., Speer, A. M., Hough, C. J., & Xing, G. (2003). Neurobiology of bipolar illness: Implications for future study and therapeutics. *Annals of Clinical Psychiatry, 15*(2), 85–94.

Puente, R. M. (1975). The use of carbamazepine in the treatment of behavioural disorders in children. In W. Birkmayer (Ed.), *Epileptic seizures–behaviour–pain* (pp. 243–252). Baltimore: University Park Press.

Rasgon, N. (2004). The relationship between polycystic ovary syndrome and antiepileptic drugs: A review of the evidence. *Journal of Clinical Psychopharmacology, 24*(3), 322–334.

Raskind, J. Y., & El-Chaar, G. M. (2000). The role of carnitine supplementation during valproic acid therapy. *Annals of Pharmacotherapy, 34*(5), 630–638.

Reimers, A., Helde, G., & Brodtkorb, E. (2005). Ethinyl estradiol, not progestogens, reduces lamotrigine serum concentrations. *Epilepsia, 46*(9), 1414–1417.

Scheffer, R., Kowatch, R., Carmody, T., & Rush, A. (2005). A randomized placebo-controlled trial of Adderall for symptoms of comorbid ADHD in pediatric bipolar disorder following mood stabilization with divalproex sodium. *American Journal of Psychiatry, 162,* 58–64.

Shear, P. K., DelBello, M. P., Lee Rosenberg, H., & Strakowski, S. M. (2002). Parental reports of executive dysfunction in adolescents with bipolar disorder. *Child Neuropsychology, 8*(4), 285–295.

Sinclair, D. B., Berg, M., & Breault, R. (2004). Valproic acid-induced pancreatitis in childhood epilepsy: Case series and review. *Journal of Child Neurology, 19*(7), 498–502.

Spear, L. P. (2002). Alcohol's effects on adolescents. *Alcohol Research and Health, 26*(4), 287–291.

Storosum, J. G., Wohlfarth, T., Schene, A., Elferink, A., van Zwieten, B. J., & van den Brink, W. (2007). Magnitude of effect of lithium in short-term efficacy studies of moderate to severe manic episode. *Bipolar Disorders, 9*(8), 793–798.

Strober, M., Morrell, W., Lampert, C., & Burroughs, J. (1990). Relapse following discontinuation of lithium maintenance therapy in adolescents with bipolar I illness: A naturalistic study. *American Journal of Psychiatry, 147*(4), 457–461.

Strober, M., Schmidt-Lackner, S., Freeman, R., Bower, S., Lampert, C., & DeAntonio, M. (1995). Recovery and relapse in adolescents with bipolar affective illness: A five-year naturalistic, prospective follow-up. *Journal of the American Academy of Child and Adolescent Psychiatry, 34*(6), 724–731.

Tillman, R., & Geller, B. (2003). Definitions of rapid, ultrarapid, and ultradian cycling and of episode duration in pediatric and adult bipolar disorders: A proposal to distinguish episodes from cycles. *Journal of Child and Adolescent Psychopharmacology, 13*(3), 267–271.

Tohen, M., Kryzhanovskaya, L., Carlson, G., DelBello, M., Wozniak, J., Kowatch, R., et al. (2007). Olanzapine versus placebo in the treatment of adolescents with bipolar mania. *American Journal of Psychiatry, 164*(10), 1547–1556.

Tosyali, M. C., & Greenhill, L. L. (1998). Child and adolescent psychopharmacology. Important developmental issues. *Pediatric Clinics of North America, 45*(5), 1021–1035, vii.

Treem, W. R. (1994). Inherited and acquired syndromes of hyperammonemia and encephalopathy in children. *Seminars in Liver Disease, 14*(3), 236–258.

Wagner, K. D., Nyilas, M., Forbes, R. A., Aurang, C., Van Beck, A., Jin, N, et al. (2007, December). *Acute efficacy of aripiprazole for the treatment of bipolar I disorder, mixed or manic, in pediatric patients.* Paper presented at the meeting of the American College of Neuropsychopharmacology, Boca Raton, FL.

Wagner, K. D., Kowatch, R. A., Emslie, G. J., Findling, R. L., Wilens, T. E., McCague, K., et al. (2006). A double-blind, randomized, placebo-controlled trial of oxcarbazepine in the treatment of bipolar disorder in children and adolescents. *American Journal of Psychiatry, 163*(7), 1179–1186.

Wagner, K. D., Redden, L., Kowatch, R. A., Wilens, T. E., Segal, S., Chang, K., et al. (2009). A double-blind, randomized, placebo-controlled trial of divalproex extended-release in the treatment of bipolar disorder in children and adolescents. *Journal of the American Academy of Child and Adolescent Psychiatry, 48*(5), 519–532.

Wagner, K. D., Weller, E. B., Carlson, G. A., Sachs, G., Biederman, J., Frazier, J. A., et al. (2002). An open-label trial of divalproex in children and adolescents with bipolar disorder. *Journal of the American Academy of Child and Adolescent Psychiatry, 41*(10), 1224–1230.

Weisler, R. H., Cutler, A. J., Ballenger, J. C., Post, R. M., & Ketter, T. A. (2006). The use of antiepileptic drugs in bipolar disorders: A review based on evidence from controlled trials. *CNS Spectrums, 11*(10), 788–799.

Werlin, S. L., & Fish, D. L. (2006). The spectrum of valproic acid-associated pancreatitis. *Pediatrics, 118*(4), 1660–1663.

West, K., & McElroy, S. L. (1995). Oral loading doses in the valproate treatment of adolescents with mixed bipolar disorder. *Journal of Child and Adolescent Psychopharmacology, 5*, 225–231.

West, S. A., Keck, P. E., Jr., McElroy, S. L., Strakowski, S. M., Minnery, K. L., McConville, B. J., et al. (1994). Open trial of valproate in the treatment of adolescent mania. *Journal of Child and Adolescent Psychopharmacology, 4*, 263–267.

West, S. A., Strakowski, S. M., Sax, K. W., McElroy, S. L., Keck, P. E., Jr., & McConville, B. J. (1996). Phenomenology and comorbidity of adolescents hospitalized for the treatment of acute mania. *Biological Psychiatry, 39*(6), 458–460.

Whittier, M. C., West, S. A., Galli, V. B., & Raute, N. J. (1995). Valproic acid for dysphoric mania in a mentally retarded adolescent. *Journal of Clinical Psychiatry, 56*(12), 590–591.

Wilens, T. E., Biederman, J., Kwon, A., Ditterline, J., Forkner, P., Moore, H., et al. (2004). Risk of substance use disorders in adolescents with bipolar disorder. *Journal of the American Academy of Child and Adolescent Psychiatry, 43*(11), 1380–1386.

Wozniak, J., & Biederman, J. (1997). Childhood mania: Insights into diagnostic and treatment issues. *Journal of the Association for Academic Minority Physicians, 8*(4), 78–84.

Wozniak, J., Biederman, J., Kiely, K., Ablon, J. S., Faraone, S. V., Mundy, E., et al. (1995). Mania-like symptoms suggestive of childhood-onset bipolar disorder in clinically referred children. *Journal of the American Academy of Child and Adolescent Psychiatry, 34*(7), 867–876.

Wozniak, J., Biederman, J., & Richards, J. A. (2001). Diagnostic and therapeutic dilemmas in the management of pediatric-onset bipolar disorder. *Journal of Clinical Psychiatry, 62*(Suppl. 14), 10–15.

Youngerman, J., & Canino, I. A. (1978). Lithium carbonate use in children and adolescents. A survey of the literature. *Archives of General Psychiatry, 35*(2), 216–224.

Zarate, C. A., Jr., Singh, J., & Manji, H. K. (2006). Cellular plasticity cascades: Targets for the development of novel therapeutics for bipolar disorder. *Biological Psychiatry, 59*(11), 1006–1020.

CHAPTER 14

Pharmacotherapy for Adults with Bipolar Depression

Michael E. Thase

After decades of relative inactivity, there has been a recent upsurge in research on the treatment of bipolar depression. There is little doubt that this trend is partly driven by the pharmaceutical industry: The first pharmacotherapy specifically indicated for bipolar depression—olanzapine–fluoxetine combination (OFC)—was approved by the U.S. Food and Drug Administration (FDA) in 2003, with the first monotherapy—quetiapine—approved in 2006. Nevertheless, it is also true that there was growing recognition that the existing therapies, particularly lithium and antidepressants, were not adequate for a substantial proportion of patients with bipolar depressive episodes (Thase, 2005). Moreover, data documenting the deleterious impact of the depressed phase of bipolar illness also have steadily emerged (Altshuler et al., 2006; Angst, 2004; Hirschfeld, Lewis, & Vornik, 2003; Judd et al., 2002; Kupka et al., 2007). Because it is now known that people with bipolar disorder (BD) spend on average between one-third (Judd et al., 2002; Kupka et al., 2007) to one-half (Judd et al., 2003) of their adult lives with depressive symptoms, it is incumbent on their clinicians to recognize and vigorously treat the depressive pole of the illness with the most appropriate therapies. In this chapter, the clinical issues that pertain to the diagnosis and pharmacotherapy of BD in adults are reviewed, with a particular focus on recent developments in the therapeutics of depressive episodes. This material is presented with reference to the major theme of this volume: the role of developmental continuities and discontinuities in the onset, diagnosis, course, and treatment of BD.

BACKGROUND: BIPOLAR DEPRESSION WAS UNDERRECOGNIZED IN PAST DECADES

Many people with bipolar affective disorder report that they were misdiagnosed early in the course of their illness. In a survey of the membership of the Depression and Bipolar Support Alliance, for example, approximately two-thirds of the respondents reported that they were initially received a psychiatric diagnosis other than BD, with about one-quarter reporting they had been misdiagnosed by four or more physicians (Hirschfeld et al., 2003). Because a depressive episode cannot usually be diagnosed as being part of a bipolar affective disorder unless the individual has already suffered from at least one hypomanic or manic episode (American Psychiatric Association, 2000) and, at least as often as not, the first lifetime bout of illness is a depressive episode (Goodwin & Jamison, 1990), it should not be surprising that the most common misdiagnosis was so-called unipolar depression. As such, some proportion of these misdiagnoses is inevitable. Nevertheless, among those who reported that they were misdiagnosed, there was an average lag of nearly 9 years between the onset of symptoms and subsequently obtaining the "correct" diagnosis (Hirschfeld et al., 2003). Reaching a correct diagnosis is not merely an academic exercise: Clinical management of bipolar depressive episodes differs from that for major depressive disorder (MDD) in several key ways, and for some a long delay in diagnosis will correspond to numerous courses of ineffective or inappropriate treatment, with mounting psychosocial consequences (Thase, 2005). This is particularly true when the initial episodes of illness occur during adolescence and young adult life, that is, a time in which a number of critical developmental tasks must be accomplished in order to emancipate from the family of origin, complete education or vocational training, initiate one's work career, and begin the processes of dating and courtship, which usually lead to establishing long-term intimate relationships (Cicchetti & Rogosch, 2002). Because secure employment and supportive relationships with family and friends convey substantial prognostic advantages, recognition of BD and initiating and maintaining appropriate treatments before these assets are irreparably damaged has vital clinical importance. Moreover, if the kindling hypothesis of bipolar illness is correct (Post, 2007; see Chapter 12, Post & Miklowitz, this volume), some of these individuals may have developed a more autonomous, highly recurrent, and potentially treatment-resistant form of illness long before they ever received a single course of therapy with lithium or another mood stabilizer.

One problem complicating recognition of BD is that the diagnostic criteria for hypomania may be too restrictive. For example, Akiskal and colleagues (2000) observed that some individuals experience mood swings that either are too short lived (i.e., durations of less than 1 week) or are characterized by too few symptoms to meet the formal syndromal definition of a hypomanic episode. They suggested that broadening the definition of hypomania to include briefer or less symptomatic episodes results in a large increase in the proportion of depressions that could be grouped within a broader spectrum of bipolar illness, increasing the proportion from about 10% of all cases of depression to up to 50%. It is further argued that many individuals are not able to distinguish these subtler, or "soft," hypomanias from their nature or usual self, and, as such, unless collateral informants are interviewed, they will go undetected in a diagnostic interview.

Although further longitudinal study is needed to determine the validity of this broad and inclusive definition, in the DSM-IV-TR (American Psychiatric Association, 2000) system such subsyndromal cases can be classified as the "not otherwise specified" form of BD. This diagnosis is often given to children and adolescents who show severe mood swings within the bipolar spectrum but who do not meet the formal criteria for bipolar I or II disorder (see Meyer & Carlson, Chapter 2; Youngstrom, Chapter 3; and Diler, Birmaher, and Miklowitz, Chapter 5, this volume).

Aside from uncovering a history of discrete mood swings through a careful interview of the person presenting for treatment and one or more significant others, there are several other clinical correlates of depressive episodes that are associated with a higher risk of bipolarity; these features include an early age of onset (i.e., before age 21), highly recurrent episodes, a seasonal pattern of recurrence, marked severity (including psychotic features), reverse neurovegetative features, significant psychomotor disturbance, and a multigenerational pedigree of affective illness (see Akiskal & Benazzi, 2005, or Thase, 2005, for more detailed discussions). Although none of these characteristics is truly pathognomonic for bipolar forms of depression, each one raises the index of suspicion, and the greater the number of characteristics, the higher the likelihood of BD. In addition to these clinical correlates, Akiskal (2005) has persuasively argued that identification of bipolar illness also can be enhanced by recognizing behavioral and temperamental indicators of bipolarity, such as tempestuosity, impulsivity, promiscuity, flamboyance in appearance or makeup preferences, or a history of driven accomplishment. As has been stated elsewhere in this volume, however, a singular behavioral phenotype can eventuate in a multifinality of outcomes, some that fall within the bipolar spectrum and some that do not (see Cicchetti, Chapter 1, this volume).

Because even the most astute clinician cannot correctly divine all cases early in the course of the illness, the realistic goal for practitioners is to recognize as high a proportion of these "occult" cases of BD as possible as early in the course of illness as possible. This is particularly relevant when evaluating older adolescents or younger adults who are presenting for treatment of a first or second lifetime depressive episode. The first task is to determine whether there is a history of mood swings or periods of unusual productivity, decreased need for sleep, or heightened energy and self-confidence. Because many individuals do not recognize such upward mood excursions as pathological, some past episodes of hypomania or nonpsychotic mania will be overlooked or simply not recalled when the history of illness is taken in the midst of a depressive episode. As noted, additional history should be obtained from family members whenever possible to minimize this risk.

As the popularity of the bipolar spectrum concept has grown, so too has the likelihood that some individuals will be diagnosed as suffering from BD without sufficient documentation or clinical justification. The results of one recent study (Zimmerman, Ruggero, Chelminski, & Young, 2008) suggest that this is not an uncommon occurrence. In fact, they found that less than half (43.5%) of a consecutive series of patients who reported a past diagnosis of BD actually met criteria for this diagnosis on the basis of the Structured Clinical Interview for DSM-IV.

ANTIDEPRESSANT RESPONSE AND THE EARLY RECOGNITION OF BIPOLAR DISORDER

Assuming that BD was not diagnosed at the initial evaluation, the next most likely opportunity to recognize the illness is during a course of antidepressant medication. This is particularly topical because the greater recognition of depression in adolescent and young adults over the past several decades led to a large increase in prescription of antidepressants. Of course, the emergence of a manic or clinically significant hypomanic episode during antidepressant therapy is essentially diagnostic of BD (Akiskal et al., 2003; Chun & Dunner, 2004). Nevertheless, it remains somewhat controversial whether or not someone who has only had manic or mixed episodes during antidepressant therapy should be diagnosed with BD (see, e.g., the formal criteria in the DSM-IV-TR). From my vantage point, patients who experience treatment-emergent affective switches (TEAS) during antidepressant therapy have BD. This view is supported by the clinical similarity of the characteristics of "spontaneous" and treatment-emergent hypomanic episodes (Akiskal et al., 2003; Chun & Dunner, 2004).

It is also a clinical challenge is to recognize individuals with mixed states among those who experience adverse behavioral outcomes during antidepressant therapy, such as worsening of insomnia, anxiety, irritability, or agitation. Some experts have suggested that the emergence of suicidal ideation or behaviors following the initiation of antidepressant treatment may reflect the same process as in TEAS (Rihmer & Akiskal, 2006; Thase, 2006). This particular adverse response to antidepressant medication has only been documented to occur, at least in a proportion that exceeds the risk of placebo, in children, teenagers, and very young adults, demographic groups that are at high risk for the onset of bipolar illness. The hypothesis that the emergence of insomnia, irritability, suicidality, and agitation during antidepressant therapy reflect bipolar mixed states deserves careful longitudinal study. Whereas it is certain that some individuals who experience these adverse behavioral reactions during antidepressant therapy will develop BD, it is not clear whether the proportion is relatively low or high.

One caveat pertinent to this discussion is that the DSM-IV-TR does not have a code for classification of a mixed state in an individual with a diagnosis of bipolar II disorder. Because there is no doubt that this entity exists (see, e.g., Suppes, Mintz, et al., 2005), it is hoped that the revisions in the nomenclature that will be made is the DSM-V will formally recognize mixed hypomania in individuals with bipolar II disorder.

TREATMENT OF BIPOLAR DEPRESSION

When Should Bipolar Depression Be Treated with Antidepressants?

Whereas antidepressant medications are generally considered to be one of the cornerstones of treatment for individuals with MDD ("unipolar depression"), there is not a similarly strong consensus about the role of antidepressants for bipolar depressive episodes (American Psychiatric Association, 2002; Goodwin et al., 2008; Keck et al., 2004; Suppes, Dennehy, et al., 2005). In fact, expert opinion ranges from one clinical extreme ("Use antidepressants sparingly, if at all)" to the other ("Use antidepressants exactly as in the treatment of other depressions") (see, e.g., Keck et al., 2004). As I have discussed elsewhere in more detail (Thase, 2005), part of the reason for this lack of consensus is that the relevant evidence base is, to be blunt, embarrassingly inadequate: Only a small number of randomized, controlled trials (RCTs) of antidepressant therapy have been conducted in bipolar I depression (see, e.g., the systematic review of Gijsman, Geddes, Rendell, Nolen, & Goodwin, 2004). There are several reasons for this dearth of evidence, including the way that manufacturers of new drugs study and market their compounds (i.e., it is more lucrative to have an indication for MDD than bipolar depression) and difficulties in both design and implementation of RCTs that result from the complex nature of bipolar illness (e.g., high rates of comorbidity and the need for concomitant therapy with a mood stabilizer). Among the handful of properly controlled studies of antidepressant therapy of bipolar I depression that have been undertaken with so-called modern antidepressants, the findings of RCTs of fluoxetine (Cohn, Collins, Ashbrook, & Wernicke, 1989), bupropion (Sachs et al., 1994, 2007), moclobemide (Silverstone, 2001), and paroxetine (Nemeroff et al., 2001; Sachs et al., 2007) either failed to establish efficacy versus placebo (Nemeroff et al., 2001; Sachs et al., 2007) or did not document significant efficacy advantages compared with first-generation standards such as the tricyclic antidepressants (TCAs) imipramine or desipramine (Cohn et al., 1989; Nemeroff et al., 2001; Sachs et al., 1994; Silverstone, 2001). Because many experts consider the TCAs to be relatively contraindicated for bipolar I depression (see, e.g., Suppes, Dennehy, et al., 2005; Thase, 2005), this particular finding of therapeutic parity is hardly reassuring!

The study of Tohen and colleagues (2003), which contrasted both olanzapine alone and of OFC versus placebo, is arguably the most compelling study of a newer antidepressant in the published literature. In this trial, OFC was significantly more effective than olanzapine alone, which, in turn, was more effective than placebo. Importantly, the added therapeutic activity observed in the OFC arm was not at the cost of an increased risk of TEAS or a greater level of adverse events. In fact, the risk of TEAS in the OFC arm was no higher than that observed in the placebo arm.

By contrast, the results of the study of Sachs and colleagues (2007), which was conducted as part of the National Institute of Mental Health–funded Systematic Treatment Evaluation Program for Bipolar Disorder (STEP-BD) project, may well be the most discouraging with respect to the efficacy of antidepressants: Neither paroxetine nor bupropion was significantly more effective than placebo in patients with bipolar depression treated with mood stabilizers. Although it is true that "good" antidepressants often fail in contemporary studies (Thase, 2008), it is also true that the STEP-BD randomized bipolar depression pathway was not plagued by a high placebo response rate (i.e., the major reason RCTs of antidepressants fail to detect significant drug vs. placebo differences). One might then speculate that the STEP-BD study group was atypical in some way and, as such, more treatment resistant. However, a concurrent and largely overlapping study of bipolar depression conducted by the STEP-BD investigators demonstrated a significant effect for three different forms of focused psychotherapy compared with a minimal-contact control condition (Miklowitz et al., 2007). Thus, the failure of paroxetine and bupropion in the STEP-BD study could not be attributable to the patients being too refractory to treatment.

One factor that may influence antidepressant response in bipolar depression is the integrity of the thyroid axis. In fact, in a study of patients with bipolar type I depression conducted at the University of Pittsburgh (Cole et al., 2002), only the subset of patients with "better than average" thyroid function, as defined by an above-median free thyroxine index and a below-median thyroid-stimulating hormone level, were likely to benefit from adjunctive therapy with antidepressants. Whether this observation can translate into therapeutic action, namely by prescribing adjunctive thyroid hormone to patients with "below-average" thyroid function, remains to be tested. This study does, however, take a step in the direction of identifying moderators of drug response, which is rarely done in studies funded by the pharmaceutical industry.

In addition to concerns about limited efficacy, the major factor that has historically limited the use of antidepressants to treat bipolar I depressive episodes has been the risk of TEAS and concerns about inducing a pattern of rapid cycling (i.e., defined as a pattern of four or more discrete mood episodes within 1 year). Indeed, because rapid cycling was rare before the introduction of antidepressant medications, there is reason to believe that it is largely an iatrogenic phenomenon (Goodwin & Jamison, 1990). There is reasonable certainty that the TCAs are associated with an increased risk of TEAS (Gijseman et al., 2004; Joffe et al., 2002). When one looks at more recent RCTs, however, there is reason to believe that most of the newer antidepressants are not associated with a particularly high risk of TEAS when prescribed in combination with mood stabilizers (Bottlender, Rudolf, Strauss, & Möller, 2001; Nemeroff et al., 2001; Post et al., 2006; Sachs et al., 1994, 2007; Tohen et al., 2003; Vieta et al., 2002). In fact, among the newer antidepressants, only the serotonin–norepinephrine reuptake inhibitor venlafaxine appears to stand out with a relatively higher risk of TEAS compared to paroxetine (Vieta et al., 2002) and sertraline or bupropion (Post et al., 2006). Nevertheless, a relatively lower risk (compared with TCAs) in shorter term studies does not necessarily mean no risk across longer courses of therapy, and 44% of the first 500 patients to enter the STEP-BD study reported a history of at least one episode of mood switching or cycling during antidepressant treatment (Truman et al., 2007). Although Truman and colleagues found that the risk of switching was highest with TCAs, patients who had experienced at least one episode of TEAS also reported increased rates of switching with selective serotonin reuptake inhibitors (SSRIs) and bupropion.

There is even less consensus about the role of antidepressants for management of bipolar II depression than there is for bipolar I depression (American Psychiatric Association, 2002; Goodwin et al., 2008; Keck et al., 2004; Suppes, Dennehy, et al., 2005; Yatham et al., 2009). The disparate findings in the literature suggest that there is a least a subgroup of individuals with bipolar II depression who respond well to modern antidepressants alone (see, e.g., Amsterdam & Shults, 2008), and for these individuals, an approach to treatment that is similar to that recommended for recurrent MDD is reasonable. For others, particularly those with a history of TEAS and more frequent or severe episodes of hypomania, a management plan similar to that recommended for an individual with bipolar I depression would be more appropriate.

Selecting an Antidepressant: Clinical Considerations

If an antidepressant is judged to be clinically indicated and no particular medication has been established as the treatment of choice, which one should be chosen? For the past several decades the most widely chosen options have been the SSRIs and the norepinephrine–dopamine reuptake inhibitor bupropion (Keck et al., 2004; Thase, 2005). These particular choices reflect both the overall widespread use of these medications for treatment of unipolar depression as well as the evidence reviewed earlier that suggests that these medications are less likely to provoke TEAS than the tricyclics. Many clinicians have favored bupropion because this particular medication has a low incidence of sexual side effects and, among widely used antidepressants, the lowest likelihood of weight gain, which can be great advantages for the treatment of younger patients with bipolar depression, particularly when the medication is added to a regimen that includes mood stabilizers and/or second-generation antipsychotics. The SSRIs are perceived to have an advantage over bupropion in terms of treatment of comorbid anxiety symptoms, although this clinical observation has not been demonstrated in a prospective trial. Among the SSRIs, only fluoxetine and escitalopram are approved for treatment of depression in youth, although there has been some concern about the use of fluoxetine because of the long elimination half-life of its principal metabolite (norfluoxetine), which functionally precludes rapid cessation of therapy following a switch into a severe episode of mania (Thase, 2005).

A significant minority of patients with bipolar depression will not benefit from sequential trials of SSRIs and bupropion, and for these individuals with more treatment-resistant episodes, it can be challenging to select the next best option among the large number of other second-, third-, and fourth-line medications. There is no doubt about the efficacy of the monoamine oxidase inhibitors (MAOIs), even for treatment of more refractory depressive episodes (Thase, 2005), although the need to adhere to a low-tyramine diet to minimize the risk of hypertensive crises can be a turn-off for many younger patients.

When Effective, How Long Should an Antidepressant Be Continued?

After nearly 50 years of use, one might think that we would know the answer to the question, "When an antidepressant works for a patient with bipolar depression, how long should it be maintained?" Sadly, and in stark contrast to the state of the evidence in MDD, the answer is not known, and there are no properly controlled studies of maintenance phase treatment of bipolar depression with the newer antidepressants. What is clear is that there is a subset of patients with bipolar I depression who respond well to antidepressants in combination with mood stabilizers and who continue to do well on longer term therapy (see, e.g., Altshuler et al., 2009). The same appears to be true for a subset of patients with bipolar II depression treated with antidepressant monotherapy (Amsterdam & Shults, 2005; Amsterdam, Wang, Shwarz, & Shults, 2009). In my practice, I recommend maintenance therapy with adjunctive antidepressants for patients with BD who (1) have a clinical course dominated by depression, (2) have no history of TEAS, and (3) have had an unequivocal response to antidepressant therapy.

Although I do recommend longer term, adjunctive antidepressant therapy for some individuals with BD, I do not use the word "lifetime" in discussing this treatment plan for several reasons. First, and especially for younger patients who may have a life expectancy of 50, 60, or even 70 additional years, it is fair to say that we have no idea about what treatment discoveries the future holds. Although our current treatments only suppress or control episodes of illness, it is possible that truly curative interventions may be developed in our lifetime. Second, our evidence base, scant as it is, only covers relatively short periods of 1 or 2 years, not a lifetime. I, therefore, recommend using the term "indefinite" and suggest that decisions about whether or not to continue the adjunctive antidepressant be made on an every 6-month or 1-year basis, weighing both the perceived benefits of the treatments and the known costs, including later emerging or later reported side effects such as weight gain or sexual dysfunction.

What Are the Best Pharmacological Alternatives to Prescribing Antidepressants?

Conventional Mood Stabilizers

In U.S.-based practice guidelines, monotherapy with a mood stabilizer is widely endorsed as the first line of therapy for all but the most severe episodes of bipolar

I depression (American Psychiatric Association, 2002; Keck et al., 2004; Suppes, Dennehy, et al., 2005). Although there is no universally accepted definition of a mood stabilizer, one useful approach is to use this term to describe a medication that (1) is an effective, acute-phase treatment of manic and/or depressive episodes; (2) does not cause TEAS; and (3) conveys significant prophylaxis against subsequent episodes of mania and depression (Ketter & Calabrese, 2002). From this perspective, there is broad consensus that lithium, valproate, and carbamazepine should be classified as mood stabilizers.

There is a strong rational for recommending a "mood stabilizer first" strategy for most patients with bipolar I depression; although none of these medications are formally approved for this indication by the FDA, there is evidence that all of these compounds have some antidepressant effects, and when monotherapy with a mood stabilizer is effective, there is minimal (i.e., no different than placebo) risk of TEAS (American Psychiatric Association, 2002). Moreover, even if ineffective, therapy with a mood stabilizer, particularly lithium or valproate, will be recommended for prophylaxis against mania (Thase, 2005).

LITHIUM AND VALPROATE

Among the mood stabilizers, lithium arguably should be favored for treatment of bipolar depression because of evidence of reduction of suicidal behavior (Baldessarini, Tondo, & Hennen, 2003; Goodwin et al., 2003). The main limitation of lithium therapy is that it does not have especially robust or reliable antidepressant effects (Thase, 2005). Several other, developmentally relevant considerations might also weigh against picking lithium as the mood stabilizer of first choice. For example, among the mood stabilizers, lithium is the most notorious in terms of its use as a psychiatric drug, and some patients, particularly older adolescents and younger adults, will simply refuse to accept it because of its stigma. Stigmatization can be a powerful mediator of treatment nonadherence in younger psychiatric populations (Hinshaw & Cicchetti, 2000).

Other younger patients find the need for periodic blood tests, the cognitive and dermatological side effects, and tremor associated with lithium therapy to be vexing and will discontinue therapy relatively quickly. For women wanting to conceive during longer term lithium therapy, there is also some risk of birth defects, including congenital hypothyroidism and a relatively rare heart condition known as Epstein's anomaly (Cohen, Friedman, Jefferson, Johnson, & Weiner, 1994). The risks of teratogenicity are not so high so as to always preclude the use of lithium in pregnant women, however, and abrupt discontinuation of mood stabilizers is associated with a significant increase in recurrence risk (Viguera et al., 2007).

Lithium efficacy is not well established in older adults, and patients older than 60 tend to show increased sensitivity to a large number of side effects. In fact, it is not uncommon to see frank lithium toxicity at doses and blood levels that are normally considered to be "therapeutic." Sensitivity to side effects can sometimes can be managed by using extremely low-dose therapy (e.g., 150 mg twice/day). A decline in renal function associated with hypertension or some other chronic kidney disease may also preclude the use of lithium for treatment of a significant proportion of elders.

When lithium is contraindicated, has been poorly tolerated, or is simply refused because of stigma, valproate and carbamazepine provide useful alternatives for monotherapy for bipolar depression. In fact, following the FDA approval of valproate for acute treatment of mania in 1994, it rapidly supplanted lithium as the most widely prescribed antimanic therapy. In my experience, a substantial proportion of younger individuals who have found lithium to be unacceptable have been able to tolerate valproate therapy. This impression was partly confirmed by a recent pharmacoepidemiological study in which valproate therapy was found to have significantly greater "persistence" (i.e., patients were more likely to stay on therapy for longer periods of time) than lithium therapy, with the greatest difference among younger patients. Like lithium, valproate has antidepressant effects in bipolar depression (Davis, Bartolucci, & Petty, 2005), although efficacy has not been systematically evaluated and the benefits are likely to be modest for the average patient. However, unlike lithium, valproate has not shown the same magnitude of effect for reduction of the risk of suicide (Goodwin et al., 2003).

Carbamazepine also has significant antimanic effects, although it is the least well tolerated of the three conventional mood stabilizers (see, e.g., Baldessarini, Henk, Sklar, Chang, & Leahy, 2008) and is generally reserved for use in individuals who have either not responded to or not been able to tolerate both lithium and valproate (American Psychiatric Association, 2002). Many younger patients find this medication to be too sedating. Antidepressant effects have been suggested in small studies focusing on patients with unstable or rapid-cycling forms of BD (see Thase, 2005).

Perhaps the most relevant developmental considerations pertaining to valproate are its effects on female reproduction function, including menstrual irregularities, androgenization, and polycystic ovary syndrome (Joffe et al., 2006). Both valproate and carbamazepine are associated with an increased incidence of birth defects, particularly neural tube defects, and are relatively contraindicated for treatment during pregnancy. Because abrupt discontinuation of these medications during pregnancy can provoke rapid relapse (Viguera et al., 2007), it is best to plan for changes in medication before pregnancy.

LAMOTRIGINE

Unlike lithium, valproate, and carbamazepine, lamotrigine is not an effective acute-phase therapy for mania, and there is some controversy about whether or not it should be grouped with the conventional mood stabilizers. It was initially argued that lamotrigine met the definition because of its effects in bipolar depression (Ketter & Calabrese, 2002), and lamotrigine figured prominently in the recommendations of the last edition of the American Psychiatric Association practice guideline (2002). Whereas the initial studies of lamotrigine monotherapy yielded promising results (Calabrese et al., 1999; Frye et al., 2000), efficacy in bipolar depression subsequently was not confirmed by a series of adequately powered, multicenter RCTs (see Calabrese et al., 2008). In the face of what must have seemed to be an unending series of failed trials, the manufacturer ended the research program without obtaining an FDA indication for acute-phase therapy of bipolar depression. A meta-analysis of all available data determined that lamotrigine monotherapy did indeed have a statistically significant antidepressant effect, albeit a very modest one (i.e., about a 9% advantage in response/remission rates compared with placebo) (Geddes, Calabrese, & Goodwin, 2009).

Most recently, van der Loos and colleagues (2009) studied adjunctive lamotrigine therapy in a placebo-controlled trial of patients with bipolar I disorder treated with lithium salts. Adjunctive lamotrigine therapy was found to have a larger, more clinically significant antidepressant effect, with a 20% advantage in response rates compared with the group treated with lithium and placebo (i.e., 52% vs. 32%). Because many clinicians prefer to add lamotrigine to ongoing therapy with other mood stabilizers to ensure protection against subsequent manic episodes, the findings of this most recent study of combined therapy may help to explain the disconnect between the widespread use for treatment of bipolar depression and the discouraging results of the RCTs of lamotrigine monotherapy.

Two smaller studies of lamotrigine add-on therapy in antidepressant-resistant bipolar depression yielded less encouraging results. In the first, which was conducted as part of the STEP-BD research program (Nierenberg et al., 2006), lamotrigine augmentation was a significantly more effective treatment than risperidone augmentation in patients who had not responded to treatment with conventional mood stabilizers and standard antidepressants, although the recovery rates on both strategies were quite low (24% vs. 5%). Moreover, lamotrigine was not significantly more effective than augmentation with inositol (17%), which served as a sort of active placebo in this trial. In the second trial (Nolen et al., 2007), which was conducted as part of the series of studies by the Stanley Foundation Bipolar Network, 19 patients with bipolar depression who had not responded to therapy with mood stabilizers and standard antidepressants were randomized to treatment with either the MAOI tranylcypromine or lamotrigine. Five of the eight patients (62.5%) responded to tranylcypromine compared with only four of the 11 patients (36.4%) on lamotrigine augmentation. No patient experienced an episode of TEAS on tranylcypromine compared with two patients switching on lamotrigine. Thus, the therapeutic merit of lamotrigine is also somewhat relatively limited among patients with more difficult-to-treat bipolar depressive episodes.

Relapse prevention efficacy was demonstrated in the two pivotal studies of preventive lamotrigine therapy in bipolar I disorder, which documented significant prophylactic effects after stabilization of manic (Bowden et al., 2003) and depressive (Calabrese et al., 2003) episodes. Although a pooled analysis of these studies reported statistically significant prophylaxis against both poles of the ill-ness, the preventive effect for depressive relapse was approximately twice as large as prevention of mania (Goodwin et al., 2004).

It, therefore, appears likely that, like the conventional mood stabilizers, lam-otrigine has modest but clinically significant antidepressant efficacy. For patients with bipolar I disorder, its value may be greater in combination with a conven-tional mood stabilizer, particularly keeping in mind the relatively small effect for prophylaxis against mania. In practice, the utility of lamotrigine is further limited by the relatively slow initial titration schedule, which is necessary to minimize the risk of drug rashes and other dermatological allergic reactions that can be preludes to severe, life-threatening systemic reactions such as Stevens–Johnson syndrome.

On the plus side, lamotrigine has the most favorable overall tolerability pro-file of the mood stabilizers and, unlike most other medications approved for treat-ment of bipolar depression, is not associated with complaints of oversedation during treatment initiation or weight gain during longer term therapy. Because lamotrigine has been extensively studied for treatment of epilepsy in pediatric age groups, there is also considerable clinical experience about its safety and tolerabil-ity in children and adolescents. Morevover, lamotrigine is likely to have the lowest teratogenic potential among the mood stabilizers, which adds additional value as a potential longer term treatment for women of reproductive age.

Second-Generation Antipsychotics

Whereas the first generation of antipsychotic medications was well known to have strong antimanic effects, clinical experience indicated that this class of medica-tion was not useful for the treatment of bipolar depressive episodes. By contrast, early clinical experience following the introduction of clozapine suggested signifi-cant antidepressant effects for patients with BD with difficult-to-treat depressions (Thase, 2005). Given the established efficacy of the second-generation antipsy-chotics (SGAs) for acute-phase therapy for mania and subsequent prophylaxis, there was hope that at least some members of the SGA class could come to be considered as a new type of mood stabilizer, including the potential for use in bipolar depression as a monotherapy. Olanzapine was the first SGA to be stud-ied systematically for treatment of bipolar I depression. The initial publication described a pair of placebo-controlled trials of olanzapine monotherapy (Tohen et al., 2003). The investigators found a statistically significantly greater reduction in depressive symptoms in the group treated with active olanzapine compared with the placebo group, with approximately a 10% difference in response and remission rates (Tohen et al., 2003). However, whereas olanzapine had a modest antidepressant effect as a monotherapy, a much larger and more meaningful effect was observed among the patients who were treated with OFC. Of equal clinical importance, when compared with olanzapine monotherapy, the added antidepressant effect of OFC was not associated with any increase in risk of TEAS or any significant differences in tolerability.

Thus, OFC, a proprietary formulation that combined fixed doses of both drugs in a single capsule, became the first treatment to be approved by the FDA for treatment of bipolar I depression. Only one subsequent study has evaluated OFC therapy of bipolar I depression; this two-stage trial compared OFC with lamotrigine across acute (Brown et al., 2006) and continuation (Brown et al., 2009) phases of double-blind therapy. During the acute phase of the study, trends favoring OFC were found on the efficacy measures, with differences in tolerability consistently favoring the group that had been randomly assigned to lamotrigine monotherapy (Brown et al., 2006, 2009). There have been no controlled studies of OFC treatment of bipolar II depression, nor have there been any placebo-controlled studies of longer term therapy with OFC.

The efficacy of quetiapine in bipolar depression was initially established by two unequivocally positive studies (Calabrese et al., 2005; Thase et al., 2006). These studies, described by the acronyms BOLDER I and BOLDER II (BipOLar DEpRession), were large placebo-controlled trials of two doses of quetiapine, 300 and 600 mg per day. The BOLDER studies enrolled patients with bipolar I and bipolar II depressive episodes, including those with a history of rapid cycling. In both studies, both doses of quetiapine were comparably effective and generally had similar tolerability profiles. In the absence of a clear benefit for higher dose therapy, the lower dose is recommended as the usual therapeutic strategy. Like OFC, quetiapine therapy was not associated with TEAS, with a rate of affective switching that was, at the least, comparable to PBO group, even among patients with a history of rapid cycling (Calabrese et al., 2005; Thase et al., 2006).

Among the smaller subgroup of patients with bipolar II depression, which accounted for only about one-third of the study participants, the drug versus placebo difference was statistically significant in BOLDER II (Thase et al., 2006) but not in BOLDER I (Calabrese et al., 2005). A subsequent pooled analysis of the two studies confirmed a statistically significant effect in bipolar II depressive episodes, with an overall magnitude of effect approaching that observed in bipolar I depressive episodes (Suppes, Hirschfeld, Vieta, Raines, & Paulsson, 2008). On the basis of these findings, quetiapine became only the second treatment strategy, and the first monotherapy, to be approved by the FDA for treatment of bipolar I depression as well as the first medication to be approved for treatment of bipolar II depressive episodes.

Relapse prevention efficacy following treatment of bipolar I depressive episodes has been demonstrated in two placebo-controlled studies of adjunctive quetiapine therapy; all participants in these trials also were treated with lithium or valproate (Suppes, Vieta, Liu, Brecher, Paulsson, & Trial 127 Investigators, 2009; Vieta et al., 2008). Additional longer term studies of quetiapine monotherapy in patients with bipolar I and bipolar II depressive disorders are ongoing. No longer term, placebo-controlled studies of OFC have been undertaken in bipolar depression, although the results of one extension study were strongly suggestive of sustained therapeutic benefit (Corya et al., 2006).

The major drawbacks of longer term therapy with quetiapine or OFC are weight gain and associated metabolic risks such as dyslipidemia and glucose intolerance. Clinical experience and data from studies of longer term, preventive therapy of BD indicate that the risk of problematic weight gain or other metabolic complications are not inconsiderable, and over time approximately 25% of patients will experience at least one of these adverse effects (Corya et al., 2006; Suppes et al., 2009; Vieta et al., 2008). Although longer term data specifically evaluating the outcomes of younger patients with BD are not yet available, clinical experience suggests that youth may be particularly vulnerable to problematic weight gain and metabolic side effects. For this reason, clinicians sometimes opt to treat younger patients with other SGAs with a lower risk of weight gain, such as aripiprazole or ziprasidone. However, the antidepressant efficacy of these SGAs has not been established in controlled studies, and it cannot be assumed that they have the same therapeutic potential as OFC or quetiapine (see, e.g., Thase, Jonas, et al., 2008). It is also true that there is a small but not yet well-characterized risk of tardive dyskinesia associated with longer term treatment with the SGAs. Because older age is a well-established risk factor for tardive dyskinesia in antipsychotic therapy of schizophrenia, it is likely that this risk will also be significantly higher for older patients with BD. Thus, a longer term treatment plan that includes quetiapine or OFC for depression prophylaxis should include conscientious, ongoing monitoring for weight gain and metabolic consequences as well as development of movement disorders.

Other Therapeutic Options

A range of other therapeutic options are available for patients who are not responsive to conventional regimens, including mood stabilizers, antidepressants, and SGAs. As noted earlier, the focused psychotherapies studied in the STEP-BD randomized pathway were significantly effective in a patient group that obtained no objective benefit from adjunctive therapy with paroxetine or bupropion (Miklowitz et al., 2007). Although further studies of acute-phase therapy are needed and a scarcity of therapists who are well trained in these interventions is one real-world limitation that precludes broader availability of adjunctive psychotherapy of bipolar depression, it certainly seems like this is a viable alternative for patients who are not responding to conventional pharmacotherapies.

Several groups have conducted preliminary studies of the dopamine agonist pramipexole for treatment of bipolar depression (Goldberg, Burdick, & Endick, 2004; Zarate et al., 2004). The first study enrolled 22 patients with antidepressant-resistant bipolar depressive episodes taking concomitant mood stabilizers (15 with bipolar I and seven with bipolar II) (Goldberg et al., 2004). At the end of 6 weeks of double-blind adjunctive therapy, eight of 12 patients responded to active pramipexole compared with only two of 10 patients allocated to the adjunctive placebo group. In the second study, which was limited to patients with bipolar II depression, six of 10 patients treated with pramipexole responded to 6 weeks of double-blind therapy compared with only one of 11 patients allocated to placebo (Zarate et al., 2004). Pramipexole was reasonably well tolerated in both studies, with just two cases of TEAS. Pramipexole certainly warrants further study in bipolar depression.

Another medication with an "activating" pharmacological profile, modafinil, was studied as an adjunctive therapy for bipolar depression by investigators from the Stanley Foundation Bipolar Network (Frye et al., 2007). This study enrolled 85 patients (64 with bipolar II disorder) taking mood stabilizers; approximately 60% of the patients were receiving concomitant antidepressant medications. At week 6, the group receiving active modafinil had a 44% response rate with 23% for those allocated to augmentation with a placebo. A post hoc analysis suggested that modafinil therapy was effective in bipolar I but not bipolar II depressions.

CONCLUSIONS

The depressive phase of bipolar affective disorder can dominate the course of this illness and can have ruinous effects on affected people and their families. Often beginning in adolescence, a pattern of protracted or recurrent depressive episodes and poor response to conventional antidepressant medications can disrupt the normal transition to independent adult functioning and presage a lifelong pattern of chronicity and disability.

Standard approaches to treatment, including mood stabilizers such as lithium and valproate, either alone or in combination with antidepressants such as the SSRIs or bupropion, benefit a significant proportion of patients but are far from universally effective. A careful review of patients' past treatments and an in-depth assessment of their presenting signs and symptoms can provide important clues to treatment selection.

In recent years, there have been a number of important developments in the pharmacotherapy of bipolar depression, including both successes such as the FDA approval of the first medications specifically indicated for bipolar depression— OFC and quetiapine—and disappointments such as the failure of the registration program for lamotrigine for acute-phase treatment of bipolar depression and the poor performance of two widely used antidepressants, paroxetine and bupropion, in the STEP-BD study. Some novel compounds such as pramipexole and modafinil appear to hold promise, and development of effective medications that treat bipolar depression without causing TEAS or conveying significant metabolic side effects continues to be an extremely important area for new research.

Future pharmacological studies should attempt to identify moderators of response to various compounds. Given the variability in effect sizes for different agents across studies, and often within studies across different outcome measures, it is reasonable to hypothesize that there are subpopulations of patients with BD who respond better to one agent versus another. This chapter has considered one such moderator, bipolar I versus II status, and has given examples (e.g., modanafil) in which treatment response has been found to be more robust in patients with bipolar I disorder. There are many others variables that may help to explain drug response, including age at onset, the pattern and progression of episodes across different stages of the life cycle, premorbid social functioning, and the predominance of depressive versus manic symptoms.

Many of the same questions can be raised about psychotherapy in relation to premorbid variables such as childhood adversity or current psychosocial circumstances such as the presence or absence of a life event. Identifying moderators of response will be an important objective in the next generation of studies on the treatment of bipolar depression.

REFERENCES

Akiskal, H. S. (2005). Searching for behavioral indicators of bipolar II in patients presenting with major depressive episodes: The "red sign," the "rule of three" and other biographic signs of temperamental extravagance, activation and hypomania. *Journal of Affective Disorders, 84,* 279–290.

Akiskal, H. S., & Benazzi, F. (2005). Atypical depression: A variant of bipolar II or a bridge between unipolar and bipolar II? *Journal of Affective Disorders, 84,* 209–217.

Akiskal, H. S., Bourgeois, M. L., Angst, J., Post, R., Möller, H., & Hirschfeld, R. (2000). Re-evaluating the prevalence of and diagnostic composition within the broad clinical spectrum of bipolar disorders. *Journal of Affective Disorders, 59*(Suppl. 1), S5–S30.

Akiskal, H. S., Hantouche, E. G., Allilaire, J. F., Sechter, D., Bourgeois, M. L., Azorin, J. M., et al. (2003). Validating antidepressant-associated hypomania (bipolar III): A systematic comparison with spontaneous hypomania (bipolar II). *Journal of Affective Disorders, 73,* 65–74.

Altshuler, L. L., Post, R. M., Black, D. O., Keck, P. E., Jr., Nolen, W. A., Frye, M. A., et al. (2006). Subsyndromal depressive symptoms are associated with functional impairment in patients with bipolar disorder: Results of a large, multisite study. *Journal of Clinical Psychiatry, 67,* 1551–1560.

Altshuler, L. L., Post, R. M., Hellemann, G., Leverich, G. S., Nolen, W. A., Frye, M. A., et al. (2009). Impact of antidepressant continuation after acute positive or partial treatment response for bipolar depression: A blinded, randomized study. *Journal of Clinical Psychiatry, 70,* 450–457.

American Psychiatric Association. (2000). *Diagnostic and statistical manual of mental disorders* (4th ed., text rev.). Washington, DC: Author.

American Psychiatric Association. (2002). Practice guideline for the treatment of patients with bipolar disorder (revision). *American Journal of Psychiatry, 159*(4, Suppl.), 1–50.

Amsterdam, J. D., & Shults, J. (2005). Fluoxetine monotherapy of bipolar type II and bipolar NOS major depression: A double-blind, placebo-substitution, continuation study. *International Clinical Psychopharmacology, 20,* 257–264.

Amsterdam, J. D., & Shults, J. (2008). Comparison of short-term venlafaxine versus lithium monotherapy for bipolar II major depressive episode: A randomized open-label study. *Journal of Clinical Psychopharmacology, 28,* 171–181.

Amsterdam, J. D., Wang, C. H., Shwarz, M., & Shults, J. (2009). Venlafaxine versus lithium monotherapy of rapid and non-rapid cycling patients with bipolar II major depressive episode: A randomized, parallel group, open-label trial. *Journal of Affective Disorders, 112,* 219–230.

Angst, J. (2004). Bipolar disorder—A seriously underestimated health burden. *European Archives of Psychiatry and Clinical Neurosciences, 254,* 59–60.

Baldessarini, R., Henk, H., Sklar, A., Chang, J., & Leahy, L. (2008). Psychotropic medications for patients with bipolar disorder in the United States: Polytherapy and adherence. *Psychiatric Services, 59,* 1175–1183.

Baldessarini, R. J., Tondo, L., & Hennen, J. (2003). Lithium treatment and suicide risk in major affective disorders: Update and new findings. *Journal of Clinical Psychiatry, 64*(Suppl. 5), 44–52.

Bottlender, R., Rudolf, D., Strauss, A., & Möller, H. J. (2001). Mood stabilisers reduce the risk of developing antidepressant-induced maniform states in acute treatment of bipolar I depressed patients. *Journal of Affective Disorders, 63,* 79–83.

Bowden, C. L., Calabrese, J. R., Sachs, G., Yatham, L. N., Asghar, S. A., Hompland, M., et al. (2003). A placebo-controlled 18-month trial of lamotrigine and lithium maintenance treatment in recently manic or hypomanic patients with bipolar I disorder. *Archives of General Psychiatry, 60,* 392–400.

Brown, E., Dunner, D. L., McElroy, S. L., Keck, P. E., Adams, D. H., Degenhardt, E., et al. (2009). Olanzapine/fluoxetine combination vs. lamotrigine in the 6-month treatment of bipolar I depression. *International Journal of Neuropsychopharmacology, 12,* 773–782.

Brown, E. B., McElroy, S. L., Keck, P. E., Jr., Deldar, A., Adams, D. H., Tohen, M., et al. (2006). A 7-week, randomized, double-blind trial of olanzapine/fluoxetine combination versus lamotrigine in the treatment of bipolar I depression. *Journal of Clinical Psychiatry, 67,* 1025–1033.

Calabrese, J. R., Bowden, C. L., Sachs, G. S., Ascher, J. A., Monaghan, E., & Rudd, G. D. (1999). A double-blind placebo-controlled study of lamotrigine monotherapy in outpatients with bipolar I depression. Lamictal 602 Study Group. *Journal of Clinical Psychiatry, 60,* 79–88.

Calabrese, J. R., Bowden, C. L., Sachs, G., Yatham, L. N., Behnke, K., Mehtonen, O. P., et al. (2003). A placebo-controlled 18-month trial of lamotrigine and lithium maintenance treatment in recently depressed patients with bipolar I disorder. *Journal of Clinical Psychiatry, 64,* 1013–1024.

Calabrese, J. R., Huffman, R. F., White, R. L., Edwards, S., Thompson, T. R., Ascher, J. A., et al. (2008). Lamotrigine in the acute treatment of bipolar depression: Results of five double-blind, placebo-controlled clinical trials. *Bipolar Disorders, 10,* 323–333.

Calabrese, J. R., Keck, P. E., Jr., MacFadden, W., Minkwitz, M., Ketter, T. A., Weisler, R. H., et al. (2005). A randomized, double-blind, placebo-controlled trial of quetiapine in the treatment of bipolar I or II depression. *American Journal of Psychiatry, 162,* 1351–1360.

Chun, B. J., & Dunner, D. L. (2004). A review of antidepressant-induced hypomania in major depression: Suggestions for DSM-V. *Bipolar Disorders, 6,* 32–42.

Cicchetti, D., & Rogosch, F. A. (2002). A developmental psychopathology perspective on adolescence. *Journal of Consulting and Clinical Psychology, 7,* 6–20.

Cohen, L. S., Friedman, J. M., Jefferson, J. W., Johnson, E. M., & Weiner, M. L. (1994). A reevaluation of risk of in utero exposure to lithium. *Journal of the American Medical Association, 271,* 146–150.

Cohn, J. B., Collins, G., Ashbrook, E., & Wernicke, J. F. (1989). A comparison of fluoxetine, imipramine, and placebo in patients with bipolar depressive disorder. *International Clinical Psychopharmacology, 4,* 313–322.

Cole, D. P., Thase, M. E., Mallinger, A. G., Soares, J. C., Luther, J. F., Kupfer, D. J., et al. (2002). Slower treatment response in bipolar depression predicted by lower pretreatment thyroid function. *American Journal of Psychiatry, 159,* 116–121.

Corya, S. A., Perlis, R. H., Keck, P. E., Jr., Lin, D. Y., Case, M. G., Williamson, D. J., et al. (2006). A 24-week open-label extension study of olanzapine-fluoxetine combination and olanzapine monotherapy in the treatment of bipolar depression. *Journal of Clinical Psychiatry, 67,* 798–806.

Davis, L. L., Bartolucci, A., & Petty, F. (2005). Divalproex in the treatment of bipolar depression: A placebo-controlled study. *Journal of Affective Disorders, 85,* 259–266.

Frye, M. A., Grunze, H., Suppes, T., McElroy, S. L., Keck, P. E., Jr., Walden, J., et al. (2007). A placebo-controlled evaluation of adjunctive modafinil in the treatment of bipolar depression. *American Journal of Psychiatry, 164,* 1242–1249.

Frye, M. A., Ketter, T. A., Kimbrell, T. A., Dunn, R. T., Speer, A. M., Osuch, E. A., et al. (2000). A placebo-controlled study of lamotrigine and gabapentin monotherapy in refractory mood disorders. *Journal of Clinical Psychopharmacology, 20,* 607–614.

Geddes, J. R., Calabrese, J. R., & Goodwin, G. M. (2009). Lamotrigine for treatment of bipolar depression: Independent meta-analysis and meta-regression of individual patient data from five randomised trials. *British Journal of Psychiatry, 194,* 4–9.

Gijsman, H. J., Geddes, J. R., Rendell, J. M., Nolen, W. A., & Goodwin, G. M. (2004). Antidepressants for bipolar depression: A systematic review of randomized, controlled trials. *American Journal of Psychiatry, 161,* 1537–1547.

Goldberg, J. F., Burdick, K. E., & Endick, C. J. (2004). Preliminary randomized, double-blind, placebo-controlled trial of pramipexole added to mood stabilizers for treatment-resistant bipolar depression. *American Journal of Psychiatry, 161,* 564–566.

Goodwin, F. K., Fireman, B., Simon, G. E., Hunkeler, E. M., Lee, J., & Revicki, D. (2003). Suicide risk in bipolar disorder during treatment with lithium and divalproex. *Journal of the American Medical Association, 290,* 1467–1473.

Goodwin, F. K., & Jamison, K. R. (1990). *Manic-depressive illness.* London: Oxford University Press.

Goodwin, G. M., Anderson, I., Arango, C., Bowden, C. L., Henry, C., Mitchell, P. B., et al. (2008). ECNP consensus meeting. Bipolar depression. Nice, March 2007. *European Neuropsychopharmacology, 18,* 535–549.

Goodwin, G. M., Bowden, C. L., Calabrese, J. R., Grunze, H., Kasper, S., White, R., et al. (2004). A pooled analysis of 2 placebo-controlled 18-month trials of lamotrigine and lithium maintenance in bipolar I disorder. *Journal of Clinical Psychiatry, 65,* 432–441.

Hinshaw, S. P., & Cicchetti, D. (2000). Stigma and mental disorder: Conceptions of illness, public attitudes, personal disclosure, and social policy. *Development and Psychopathology, 12,* 555–598.

Hirschfeld, R. M., Lewis, L., & Vornik, L. A. (2003). Perceptions and impact of bipolar disorder: How far have we really come?: Results of the National Depressive and Manic-Depressive Association 2000 survey of individuals with bipolar disorder. *Journal of Clinical Psychiatry, 64,* 161–174.

Joffe, H., Cohen, L. S., Suppes, T., McLaughlin, W. L., Lavori, P., Adams, J. M., et al. (2006). Valproate is associated with new-onset oligoamenorrhea with hyperandrogenism in women with bipolar disorder. *Biological Psychiatry, 59,* 1078–1086.

Joffe, R. T., MacQueen, G. M., Marriott, M., Robb, J., Begin, H., & Young, L. T. (2002). Induction of mania and cycle acceleration in bipolar disorder: Effect of different classes of antidepressant. *Acta Psychiatrica Scandinavica, 105*, 427–430.

Judd, L. L., Akiskal, H. S., Schettler, P. J., Coryell, W., Endicott, J., Maser, J. D., et al. (2003). A prospective investigation of the natural history of the long-term weekly symptomatic status of bipolar II disorder. *Archives of General Psychiatry, 60*, 261–269.

Judd, L. L., Akiskal, H. S., Schettler, P. J., Endicott, J., Maser, J., Solomon, D. A., et al. (2002). The long-term natural history of the weekly symptomatic status of bipolar I disorder. *Archives of General Psychiatry, 59*, 530–537.

Keck, P. E., Perlis, R. H., Otto, M. W., Carpenter, D., Ross, R., & Docherty, J. P. (2004). The expert consensus guideline series. Treatment of bipolar disorder 2004. *Postgraduate Medicine Special Reports*, 1–119.

Ketter, T. A., & Calabrese, J. R. (2002). Stabilization of mood from below versus above baseline in bipolar disorder: A new nomenclature. *Journal of Clinical Psychiatry, 63*, 146–151.

Kupka, R. W., Altshuler, L. L., Nolen, W. A., Suppes, T., Luckenbaugh, D. A., Leverich, G. S., et al. (2007). Three times more days depressed than manic or hypomanic in both bipolar I and bipolar II disorder. *Bipolar Disorders, 9*, 531–535.

Miklowitz, D. J., Otto, M. W., Frank, E., Reilly-Harrington, N. A., Wisniewski, S. R., Kogan, J. N., et al. (2007). Psychosocial treatments for bipolar depression: A 1-year randomized trial from the Systematic Treatment Enhancement Program. *Archives of General Psychiatry, 64*, 419–426.

Nemeroff, C. B., Evans, D. L., Gyulai, L., Sachs, G. S., Bowden, C. L., Gergel, I. P., et al. (2001). Double-blind, placebo-controlled comparison of imipramine and paroxetine in the treatment of bipolar depression. *American Journal of Psychiatry, 158*, 906–912.

Nierenberg, A. A., Ostacher, M. J., Calabrese, J. R., Ketter, T. A., Marangell, L. B., Miklowitz, D. J., et al. (2006). Treatment-resistant bipolar depression: A STEP-BD equipoise randomized effectiveness trial of antidepressant augmentation with lamotrigine, inositol, or risperidone. *American Journal of Psychiatry, 163*(2), 210–216.

Nolen, W. A., Kupka, R. W., Hellemann, G., Frye, M. A., Altshuler, L. L., Leverich, G. S., et al. (2007). Tranylcypromine vs. lamotrigine in the treatment of refractory bipolar depression: A failed but clinically useful study. *Acta Psychiatrica Scandinavica, 115*, 360–365.

Post, R. M. (2007). Kindling and sensitization as models for affective episode recurrence, cyclicity, and tolerance phenomena. *Neuroscience and Biobehavioral Review, 31*, 858–873.

Post, R. M., Altshuler, L. L., Leverich, G. S., Frye, M. A., Nolen, W. A., Kupka, R. W., et al. (2006). Mood switch in bipolar depression: Comparison of adjunctive venlafaxine, bupropion and sertraline. *British Journal of Psychiatry, 189*, 124–131.

Rihmer, Z., & Akiskal, H. (2006). Do antidepressants t(h)reat(en) depressives?: Toward a clinically judicious formulation of the antidepressant-suicidality FDA advisory in light of declining national suicide statistics from many countries. *Journal of Affective Disorders, 94*, 3–13.

Sachs, G. S., Lafer, B., Stoll, A. L., Banov, M., Thibault, A. B., Tohen, M., et al. (1994). A double-blind trial of bupropion versus desipramine for bipolar depression. *Journal of Clinical Psychiatry, 55*, 391–393.

Sachs, G. S., Nierenberg, A. A., Calabrese, J. R., Marangell, L. B., Wisniewski, S. R., Gyulai, L., et al. (2007). Effectiveness of adjunctive antidepressant treatment for bipolar depression. *New England Journal of Medicine, 356*, 1711–1722.

Silverstone, T. (2001). Moclobemide vs. imipramine in bipolar depression: A multicentre double-blind clinical trial. *Acta Psychiatrica Scandinavica, 104*, 104–109.

Suppes, T., Dennehy, E. B., Hirschfeld, R. M., Altshuler, L. L., Bowden, C. L., Calabrese, J. R., et al. (2005). The Texas implementation of medication algorithms: Update to the algorithms for treatment of bipolar I disorder. *Journal of Clinical Psychiatry, 66*, 870–886.

Suppes, T., Hirschfeld, R. M., Vieta, E., Raines, S., & Paulsson, B. (2008). Quetiapine for the treatment of bipolar II depression: Analysis of data from two randomized, double-blind, placebo-controlled studies. *World Journal of Biological Psychiatry, 9*, 198–211.

Suppes, T., Mintz, J., McElroy, S. L., Altshuler, L. L., Kupka, R. W., Frye, M. A., et al. (2005). Mixed hypomania in 908 patients with bipolar disorder evaluated prospectively in the Stanley Foundation Bipolar Treatment Network: A sex-specific phenomenon. *Archives of General Psychiatry, 62*, 1089–1096.

Suppes, T., Vieta, E., Liu, S., Brecher, M., Paulsson, B., & Trial 127 Investigators. (2009). Maintenance treatment for patients with bipolar I disorder: Results from a North American study of quetiapine in combination with lithium or divalproex (trial 127). *American Journal of Psychiatry, 166*, 476–488.

Thase, M. E. (2005). Bipolar depression: Issues in diagnosis and treatment. *Harvard Review of Psychiatry, 13*, 257–271.

Thase, M. E. (2006). Bipolar depression: Diagnostic and treatment considerations. *Developmental Psychopathology, 18*, 1213–1230.

Thase, M. E. (2008). Do antidepressants really work?: A clinicians' guide to evaluating the evidence. *Current Psychiatry Reports, 10*, 487–494.

Thase, M. E., Jonas, A., Khan, A., Bowden, C. L., Wu, X., McQuade, R. D., et al. (2008). Aripiprazole monotherapy in nonpsychotic bipolar I depression: Results of 2 randomized, placebo-controlled studies. *Journal of Clinical Psychopharmacology, 28*, 13–20.

Thase, M. E., MacFadden, W., Weisler, R. H., Chang, W., Paulsson, B., Khan, A., et al. (2006). Efficacy of quetiapine monotherapy in bipolar I and II depression: A double-blind, placebo-controlled study (the BOLDER II study). *Journal of Clinical Psychopharmacology, 26*, 600–609.

Tohen, M., Vieta, E., Calabrese, J., Ketter, T. A., Sachs, G., Bowden, C., et al. (2003). Efficacy of olanzapine and olanzapine-fluoxetine combination in the treatment of bipolar I depression. *Archives of General Psychiatry, 60*, 1079–1088.

Truman, C. J., Goldberg, J. F., Ghaemi, S. N., Baldassano, C. F., Wisniewski, S. R., Dennehy, E. B., et al. (2007). Self-reported history of manic/hypomanic switch associated with antidepressant use: Data from the Systematic Treatment Enhancement Program for Bipolar Disorder (STEP-BD). *Journal of Clinical Psychiatry, 68*, 1472–1479.

van der Loos, M. L., Mulder, P. G., Hartong, E. G., Blom, M. B., Vergouwen, A. C., de Keyzer, H. J., et al. (2009). Efficacy and safety of lamotrigine as add-on treatment to lithium in bipolar depression: A multicenter, double-blind, placebo-controlled trial. *Journal of Clinical Psychiatry, 70*, 223–231.

Vieta, E., Martínez-Arán, A., Goikolea, J. M., Torrent, C., Colom, F., Benabarre, A., et al. (2002). A randomized trial comparing paroxetine and venlafaxine in the treatment of bipolar depressed patients taking mood stabilizers. *Journal of Clinical Psychiatry, 63*, 508–512.

Vieta, E., Suppes, T., Eggens, I., Persson, I., Paulsson, B., & Brecher, M. (2008). Efficacy and safety of quetiapine in combination with lithium or divalproex for maintenance of patients with bipolar I disorder (international trial 126). *Journal of Affective Disorders, 109*, 251–263.

Viguera, A. C., Whitfield, T., Baldessarini, R. J., Newport, D. J., Stowe, Z., Reminick, A., et al. (2007). Risk of recurrence in women with bipolar disorder during pregnancy: Prospective study of mood stabilizer discontinuation. *American Journal of Psychiatry, 164*, 1817–1824.

Yatham, L. N., Kennedy, S. H., Schaffer, A., Parikh, S. V., Beaulieu, S., O'Donovan, C., et al.

(2009). Canadian Network for Mood and Anxiety Treatments (CANMAT) and International Society for Bipolar Disorders (ISBD) collaborative update of CANMAT guidelines for the management of patients with bipolar disorder: Update 2009. *Bipolar Disorders, 11*, 225–255.

Zarate, C. A., Jr., Payne, J. L., Singh, J., Quiroz, J. A., Luckenbaugh, D. A., Denicoff, K. D., et al. (2004). Pramipexole for bipolar II depression: A placebo-controlled proof of concept study. *Biological Psychiatry, 56*, 54–60.

Zimmerman, M., Ruggero, C. J., Chelminski, I., & Young, D. (2008). Is bipolar disorder overdiagnosed? *Journal of Clinical Psychiatry, 69*, 935–940.

CHAPTER 15

Family-Based Approaches to Treating Bipolar Disorder in Adolescence

Family-Focused Therapy and Dialectical Behavior Therapy

David J. Miklowitz and Tina R. Goldstein

As other contributors to this volume have discussed, family relationships are key factors in the course and outcome of bipolar disorder (BD) across the life span. A "multiple-levels-of-analysis" approach (Cicchetti, Chapter 1, this volume) helps to place disturbed family processes in the complex causal chain leading to the expression of mood disorder symptoms in youth and adults. Specifically, the associations between mood problems and family relationships are bidirectional: Family factors can be risk factors for periods of mood instability in a vulnerable individual, and in turn mood instability affects the nature and quality of family life. The association between family factors and mood disturbances can also be attributed to underlying "third variable" causal mechanisms, including shared genetic or biological factors, sociocultural influences, and common environmental stressors (e.g., poverty, cramped living conditions, mental or medical illness in one or more family members). Moreover, family factors may reciprocally influence biological or socioenvironmental risk factors, such as when significant family conflict serves as a stressor that worsens underlying biological mechanisms (e.g., hypercortisolemia, abnormal thyroid functioning).

A variety of family environments can predate the onset of BD, although their causal relationship to the onset of the illness has not been established. Family conflict, criticism, sexual or physical abuse, emotional neglect, emotional overinvolvement, intense sibling rivalries, and other dimensions of family functioning have all been described in retrospective studies of BD (for a review, see Miklowitz, 2008). Thus, the concept of *equifinality* applies to the role of family factors in the onset of BD: Multiple disruptions to family life can predict the same outcome, the onset of BD. Likewise, among children or teens who develop BD, there is a wide dispersion of outcomes when considering the nature of family relationships (*multifinality*). When families attempt to cope with the disruption caused by the first onset of a son or daughter's illness, families may become disengaged, highly critical or rejecting, abusive, or overprotective; they may even dissolve as a direct result of their shame, guilt, or anger regarding the illness. Alternatively, family members may become more effective over time in their attempts to cope with the disorder: they may learn to distinguish behaviors that are controllable by the patient from those that are uncontrollable, to manage their own emotional and physical health, to deal with societal stigma, and to modulate their emotional reactions when in conflict with the individual with BD.

Families can also be risk or protective influences on the course of BD. The nature and direction of these influences can change over the course of one person's development. For example, an emotionally dysregulated child with a mild form of bipolar spectrum disorder may be less likely to "convert" to a more severe form of illness (i.e., bipolar I or II disorder) if he lives in a low-key, low-conflict, nurturing household versus a highly conflictual, emotionally tense household. A poor temperamental fit between himself and his primary caretaking parents may contribute to the earlier expression of biological and genetic vulnerabilities. After repeated mood episodes and other stressors, parent–offspring relationships that were once protective may become fraught with conflict and dysregulating to both parties. Less frequently, families may become highly interdependent as the illness progresses and it becomes more clear that the individual with BD cannot function independently. This type of adaptive emotional involvement may be protective for the patient but may come with emotional and physical costs to the relative (Fredman, Baucom, Miklowitz, & Stanton, 2008; Perlick, Hohenstein, Clarkin, Kaczynski, & Rosenheck, 2005).

In support of these developmental scenarios, high maternal warmth protected against later recurrences of pediatric BD in an 8-year follow-up study of children with bipolar I disorder (Geller, Tillman, Bolhofner, & Zimerman, 2008). Highly critical family environments were associated with less complete recovery from episodes among BD teens in another study (Miklowitz, Biuckians, & Richards, 2006). The relationship between emotional involvement/overinvolvement and the course of pediatric or adult BD is not as well understood (Fredman et al., 2008).

Of course, many of these same disturbances in family equilibrium (i.e., high levels of conflict, parental overprotectiveness) occur in the course of normal adolescent development. A major premise of this chapter is that family distress moderates the course of bipolar illness, even if its direct causal role in the onset of the disorder cannot be established. Thus, the same family processes may have different effects on people who are and are not genetically or biologically vulnerable to BD.

The second premise of this chapter is that involving the family in the treatment of BD is a vital feature of treatment across the age range. The assumptions of different models of family treatment vary depending on which risk and protective factors are considered central to recovery from the disorder. We discuss the rationale for including families in the treatment of children and adolescents with BD. Then we describe and provide empirical evidence for two forms of family intervention: family-focused therapy (FFT; Miklowitz, 2008), which is based on the literature on expressed emotion (see later discussion) as a risk factor for recurrences, and a model using dialectical behavior therapy (DBT; Goldstein, Axelson, Birmaher, & Brent, 2007), which is based on literature concerning the role of emotional dysregulation in BD and borderline personality disorder.

WHY IS THE FAMILY CONTEXT AN IMPORTANT TARGET OF A PSYCHOSOCIAL INTERVENTION?

The most practical reason to involve families in the outpatient treatment of teens with BD is that most adolescents reside with their biological parents and stepparents. The success of pharmacological and psychosocial treatments depends in part on whether the caretaking parents understand the diagnosis and agree with the treatment plan. It is difficult to dispense complicated medication regimens within chaotic family environments. Parental "buy-in" is essential to ensuring the child's adherence and to develop strategies for communicating with the physician about medical side effects. Parental buy-in is also essential for medically managing recurrent medical disorders such as juvenile-onset diabetes.

Second, family relationships are important predictors of the course of BD. Notably, high levels of relative-to-patient criticism, hostility, or emotional overinvolvement (high expressed emotion [EE]) are associated with poorer outcomes of the disorder over 1- to 2-year periods (Miklowitz et al., 2000, 2006; Miklowitz, Goldstein, Nuechterlein, Snyder, & Mintz, 1988; O'Connell, Mayo, Flatow, Cuthbertson, & O'Brien, 1991; Priebe, Wildgrube, & Muller-Oerlinghausen, 1989; Yan, Hammen, Cohen, Daley, & Henry, 2004). These studies encompass patients in different age groups (teens, young adults, and middle-aged adults), different family constellations (parent–offspring pairs and spousal pairings), and varying levels of chronicity.

Many contextual variables affect the strength of these relationships, among them (1) whether more than one member of the family has a mood disorder; (2) whether the affected offspring is a boy or girl; (3) the age and developmental stage of the child at the time of onset; (4) whether the biological family is intact or not; and (5) the presence or absence of comorbid disorders. In one of our studies, levels of parental EE-criticism were higher toward teenage girls than teenage boys. Moreover, there was an interaction between sex and age at onset in accounting for levels of parental EE-criticism: Parents were more critical toward adolescent-onset girls than childhood-onset girls. In contrast, parents were more critical of childhood-

---

KEY POINTS: WHY INCLUDE THE FAMILY IN TREATMENT?

- Childhood, adolescent, and young adult patients usually reside with their families of origin.
- The disorder has a significant impact on family relationships.
- The affective climate of family environments can affect the course of the illness and the success of medication treatments.
- Multiple members of the family are often affected by bipolar illness and its societal stigma.

---

onset boys than adolescent-onset boys. Girls in the sample were more depressed at the time of the EE assessment than boys. We interpreted this pattern of findings to suggest that parents were especially critical when girls reached pubescence, developed more internalizing symptoms (i.e., depression, pessimism, rumination, anxiety), and simultaneously pressed for more autonomy. In contrast, parents may become particularly disturbed by the externalizing behavior of boys, particularly those who have long-standing histories of ADHD or conduct problems predating the onset of their bipolar illness (Coville, Miklowitz, Taylor, & Low, 2008).

It is useful to compare these results with those of Silverthorne, Frick, and Reynolds (2001), who found that adolescent-onset conduct disorder in girls often phenomenologically resembles childhood-onset conduct disorder in boys (i.e., unemotional personality styles and poor impulse control). Thus, parental reactions to an episode of BD, or other childhood psychiatric disorders, must be understood in the context of gender and developmental differences in the illness presentation and course.

Finally, multiple members of a family are often diagnosed with BD. From a purely economic point of view, it makes sense to address the health issues of groups of individuals whenever possible. Issues of the stigma of mental illness often affect multiple members of the same family (Hinshaw & Cicchetti, 2000; Miklowitz, 2008; see also Hinshaw, Chapter 17, this volume). Family psychoeducation, which focuses on demystifying the nature of BD, clarifying the personal meanings that patients and relatives attach to the illness, and correcting misunderstandings of the causes of family members' behaviors, can do much to reduce the shame, guilt, and social isolation affecting families coping with the illness.

FAMILY-FOCUSED THERAPY

FFT is a BD-specific version of behavioral family therapy, a psychoeducational treatment for schizophrenia (Falloon, Boyd, & McGill, 1984). It was developed in the early 1980s as a way of treating young adult patients with BD who had had a manic episode and following hospitalization were discharged to their parents' home (Miklowitz & Goldstein, 1990). Subsequently, the model was extended to included older, married adults (Miklowitz et al., 2000) and adolescents and pre-adolescents with or at risk for the disorder (Miklowitz et al., 2006). Over time, the model has become less strictly behavioral and more oriented toward psycho-education, illness management, exploration of affect, and the addressing of family system imbalances related to coping with BD.

FFT consists of 21 hour-long sessions over 9 months (12 weekly, six biweekly, and three monthly), followed by maintenance sessions as needed. It has four major components: (1) an assessment phase, in which the diagnosis of BD is established, the nature of family problems are evaluated, and the family's current understand-ing of BD is clarified; (2) a psychoeducation phase, in which the nature, course, causes, treatment, and self-management of the disorder are discussed; (3) com-munication enhancement training, which includes role-playing and behavioral rehearsal of active listening skills, offering positive and constructive negative feed-back, and requesting changes in other family members' behaviors; and (4) prob-lem solving, which involves defining a set of current problems relevant to family life, generating solutions to each problem, evaluating the advantages and disad-vantages of each, and developing a solution-implementation plan that involves all family members. Each of these components of treatment is discussed in more detail as relevant to adolescent patients. The model for adults is structurally simi-lar, although the topical foci of communication and problem-solving sessions are somewhat different (see Miklowitz, 2008). For example, adults are more likely to focus on strategies to succeed on the job market; adolescents are usually more concerned with peer relationships or establishing autonomy from their parents.

There are seven objectives of FFT for adolescents. These are to assist the adolescent, parents, and siblings to (1) understand the nature, pattern, and biop-sychosocial context of the adolescent's recent mood episode or cycling pattern; (2) recognize the adolescent's vulnerability to the disease and develop plans to prevent future symptoms; (3) accept the necessity of ongoing medications; (4) distinguish the disorder from stable personality attributes or age-normative ado-lescent behaviors, usually by involving the family in a dialogue about what is and is not bipolar illness; (5) manage stressors or daily hassles that provoke swings of mood; (6) implement strategies for maintaining stability during euthymic periods (e.g., mood charting, sleep–wake cycle stabilization); and (7) promote a family environment whose communication and problem-solving practices enhance the adolescent's and parents' mood stability.

Stage 1: Psychoeducation

The psychoeducation module (sessions 1–9) gives adolescents, their parents, and siblings concrete, didactic information about the symptoms, differential diagno-sis, comorbidity, course, treatment, and self-management of BD. Handouts and self-guided homework (e.g., keeping a daily mood and sleep chart) accompany these topics. First, the clinician reviews the symptoms of BD and distinguishes them from symptoms of anxiety, psychosis, or disruptive behavior disorders. The clinician explains the interactive roles of genetic and biological vulnerability, stress, and coping in the disorder's onset; the role of risk factors (i.e., disruptions in sleep–wake rhythms, suddenly discontinuing medications, substance misuse, escalating family conflicts); and the role of protective factors (i.e., consistency with medications and pharmacotherapy visits, stable sleep–wake patterns, structured, low-conflict family routines). The impact of the disorder on family functioning is discussed.

Parents are more likely to express high levels of EE-criticism if they believe that the youth's aversive behaviors are the product of willful intention rather than uncontrollable factors, such as an illness (Miklowitz, Wendel, & Simoneau, 1998). Although the FFT clinician makes clear that BD is a genetically and biologically based illness, he or she also emphasizes that the youth is, to a large extent, responsible for the effects of his or her behavior on others (notably family members). This level of responsibility may depend on his or her age and severity of illness. We avoid referring to BD as a "brain disorder," knowing that this term marginalizes the patient and implies that we know more than we do about the nature of such inborn pathophysiologies. Importantly, "brain disorders" create a social stigma for the youth with the disorder because the term implies that the environment plays a relatively small role in his or her mood fluctuations (Hinshaw & Cicchetti, 2000). Furthermore, the term also implies that BD is in the same general category as neurological conditions such as Alzheimer's disease, Huntington's disease, or Parkinson's disease. Needless to say, such comparisons are not welcomed by youth or their family members.

Consistent with a multiple-levels-of-analysis approach, the clinician points to the interactions among stress, vulnerability, and risk and protective factors and the ways in which maximizing protection (e.g., by stabilizing sleep–wake cycles) and minimizing risk (e.g., by curtailing the destructiveness of family arguments) are likely to reduce the severity or frequency of mood episodes in vulnerable youth. The clinician avoids any implication of blame toward the parents, who are often suspicious of psychological explanations for psychiatric illnesses. There is a long and unfortunate history in psychiatry of blaming parents (particularly mothers) for causing major mental disorders in children. These theories have been discounted by research and by the community educational efforts of parent support groups such as the National Alliance on Mental Illness (Imber-Mintz, Liberman, Miklowitz, & Mintz, 1987).

A key component of psychoeducation is the "relapse drill," or the planning during periods of stability for medical or psychological intervention when the patient's moods start to deteriorate or he or she becomes suicidal. Families recall previous periods of mood instability and identify sequences consisting of *triggers*, *early warning signs of relapse*, and *palliative measures*. A prevention plan is developed (e.g., no suicide/no harm contracts, notifying the physician, reducing stress triggers at home, stabilizing sleep–wake rhythms). The plan is put into writing and presented for the participants in the next session.

Many parents in our studies suffer from mood disorders themselves. During psychoeducation and other phases of FFT, clinicians provide emotional support for parents and clinical referrals as appropriate (including pharmacotherapy). They teach parents to identify and cope with triggers for their own mood cycling (including high-intensity interactions with the offspring with BD) and emphasize communication strategies (discussed next) to help preserve marital relationships and relations with the affected and nonaffected offspring.

Stages 2 and 3: Communication and Problem-Solving Training

Sessions 10 to 15 are designed to reduce unproductive interactions among family members and improve the quality of exchanges. These sessions are guided by the assumption that aversive communication reflects distress in the family's attempts to cope with BD (Miklowitz et al., 1998). Communication training uses a role-playing format to teach adolescents and their family members four skills: expressing positive feelings, active listening, making positive requests for changes in one another's behaviors, and constructive negative feedback. The clinician first offers handouts listing the components of each skill (e.g., for active listening: making eye contact, paraphrasing) and models each skill for the family. Then participants practice the skills with each other, with coaching and shaping by the clinician. Communication training is done less formally with adolescents than adults, capitalizing as much as possible on spontaneous interactions. Homework assignments, in which the participants record their efforts to use each skill, facilitate generalization to the home setting.

The problem-solving module (sessions 16–21), in which families are taught to identify specific areas of disagreement, generate and evaluate solutions, and implement solutions, focuses on behavior management strategies the parents can use without interfering with the adolescent's normal developmental quest for independence. Participants list their most pressing problems and define each one (e.g., the adolescent does not get to school on time and conflict ensues). Then parents and adolescents generate two to three solution choices and are asked to evaluate the pros and cons of each. Next, the family conjointly chooses a best option or set of options and develops an implementation plan. Families practice problem solving between sessions using a self-guided homework sheet and report on their attempts in the next session. The difficulties families experience in agreeing on definitions of problems and suggesting or implementing solutions often reflect difficulties in establishing interpersonal boundaries during the period after a mood disorder episode.

Toward the end of FFT, maintenance sessions are scheduled as appropriate for up to 2 years. Maintenance sessions revisit the seven objectives of FFT: Has the family gained an understanding of the cyclic nature of the disorder? Is consistency of medication treatment in place? Has the family developed (and, where necessary, implemented) a relapse prevention plan? These sessions usually involve problem solving and rehearsal of communication skills.

Natalie, a 16-year-old, had a 7-year history of BD, including several depressive and mixed episodes and at least one suicide attempt. Her parents were most disturbed by her severe and seemingly abrupt attacks of rage, in which she would physically attack members of the family, destroy property, and impulsively harm herself. She described her internal state as "weird" and "different" during these times. She had difficulty pointing to a particular environmental trigger, except perhaps minor changes in the voice tone of other family members, responding to multiple requests from her parents, minor frustrations with her homework, and other common occurrences. Thus, stimuli that would evoke annoyance in most teenagers resulted in "knockdown, drag-out" fights, in which Natalie would rage for hours and sometimes assault other family members.

During psychoeducation, much effort was put into the relapse prevention drill. Natalie and her family constructed a mood "thermometer," in which they distinguished low, medium, and high levels of rage and how long each period was likely to last. She then described the different internal states associated with each and what would and would not help at each stage (e.g., her parents' tendency to point out her escalation was only helpful in the early stages; having them walk away and/or not verbally respond to her was more effective in later stages). The clinician drew parallels between Natalie's rages and the states of mind associated with epileptic seizures. Thinking about her rages as neural and cognitive events that were triggered by very ordinary environmental changes (rather than being expressions of "unconscious hatred," as her parents often thought) made her moods more acceptable and less threatening to her family members. Although Natalie continued to have rage reactions, these became few and far between, and were sometimes minimized by her own self-talk or her parents' measured responses to her.

Evidence for the Efficacy of Family-Focused Therapy among Adults with Bipolar Disorder

In BD adults, FFT has been tested in one open trial using a historical control group (Miklowitz & Goldstein, 1990; $n = 32$), two randomized trials focusing on relapse prevention (Miklowitz, George, Richards, Simoneau, & Suddath, 2003, $n = 101$; Rea et al., 2003, $n = 52$), and one multisite randomized trial involving stabilization of bipolar depressive episodes (Miklowitz, Otto, Frank, Reilly-Harrington, Wisniewski, et al., 2007; $n = 293$). Each of these trials established that, in patients with bipolar I and II disorders, adding FFT to pharmacotherapy led to longer delays before recurrences or shorter delays before recovery than was achieved with pharmacotherapy alone or pharmacotherapy with active clinical management. FFT was also associated with a decrease in the severity of depression symptoms in two of the studies (Miklowitz, George, et al., 2003; Miklowitz, Otto, Frank, Reilly-Harrington, Wisniewski, et al., 2007). Overall, FFT is associated with a 35–40% reduction in recurrence rates over 2 years and a 48% increase in recovery rates over 1 year.

One of these trials was the large-scale Systematic Treatment Enhancement Program for Bipolar Disorder, which tested the effectiveness of FFT, cognitive-behavioral therapy (CBT), and interpersonal therapy in comparison with a brief (three-session) psychoeducational treatment for 293 patients with bipolar I and II disorder in a depressive episode. Patients were treated with best evidence pharmacotherapy. All three intensive psychosocial treatments were superior to brief psychoeducation in hastening time to recovery from depression over 1 year. Time to recovery averaged 103 days in FFT, 112 days in CBT, 127 days in interpersonal therapy, and 146 days in brief psychoeducation (Miklowitz, Otto, Frank, Reilly-Harrington, Wisniewski, et al., 2007). Patients in intensive therapy (including FFT) also showed better overall psychosocial functioning, relationship functioning, and life satisfaction than those in brief psychoeducation (Miklowitz, Otto, Frank, Reilly-Harrington, Kogan, et al., 2007). The results did not suggest that one form of psychotherapy was better than the others, although each was superior to the control condition.

There are now preliminary data to indicate that certain variables moderate and mediate the impact of FFT on the symptomatic outcomes of bipolar adults. In a randomized trial at the University of California, Los Angeles (Rea et al., 2003), family treatment decreased the likelihood of relapse by threefold among patients with poor premorbid BD (those with low social and sexual adjustment during adolescence) in comparison with a comparably intensive individual therapy. The results were less impressive among patients with good premorbid adjustment. In two trials at the University of Colorado, one of adults (Kim & Miklowitz, 2004) and one of adolescents (Miklowitz et al., 2008, 2009; see below), FFT was more effective than brief psychoeducation in stabilizing depression and mania symptoms among patients in high-EE families.

In the Colorado trial, FFT was associated with an increase in the use of positive verbal and nonverbal communication in family interactions as measured at a pretreatment baseline and again at 9 months. Verbal interactions became slightly more negative if the family did not receive regular psychosocial treatment. Improvements in patient–relative interaction were correlated with symptomatic improvement of the patient over the 1-year interval (Simoneau, Miklowitz, Richards, Saleem, & George, 1999). Patients in FFT were also more consistent with their lithium and/or anticonvulsant regimens than patients who received a briefer (two-session) psychoeducational treatment; medication compliance, in turn, predicted the stabilization of mania symptoms over 2 years. Because of the design of the Colorado study, it was not possible to establish the direction of these associations (e.g., whether patients improved first and, therefore, communicated better with their relatives or the reverse).

These preliminary findings generate hypotheses for future trials about which subgroups of patients show greater or lesser responses to FFT and what family processes unfold as risk or protective mechanisms in the onset or course of the disorder. Future randomized trials could identify subgroups of patients who show similarities in symptoms or family processes (equifinality) and stratify groups before randomization based on these characteristics (Cicchetti & Rogosch, 1996). For example, it is possible that patients who develop the illness early and show social deficits during adolescence become unusually enmeshed with their families of origin. New episodes may then be triggered in part by negative interactions with parents. Children with early-onset BD appear to have particular problems reading the facial expressions of adults (see McClure-Tone, Chapter 11, this volume). These facial affect decoding problems may contribute to emotional dysregulation, which, in turn, may contribute to social dysfunction as well as difficulties in communicating or solving problems with family members. These processes, however, may be identifiable before beginning treatment and may be amenable to alteration through structured communication and problem-solving skills training.

FFT may be most effective when there is an obvious target for such interventions, such as (1) high marital or parent–offspring conflict, criticism, or hostility (including high-EE attitudes); (2) deficits in problem solving; (3) emotional overinvolvement or enmeshment; or (4) extreme difficulty when family members attempt to meet each others' practical and emotional needs (Heru, 2006). Table 15.1 describes some of the affective and cognitive communication variables we assess before commencing FFT. Although these variables are not inclusive, they

---

TABLE 15.1. Assessing the Family Environment of Patients with Bipolar Disorder

Research studies often use quite labor-intensive methods of assessing family environments, such as the Camberwell Family Interview system for rating expressed emotion (Vaughn & Leff, 1976) or the Categories for Coding Partner Interactions (Hahlweg et al., 1989). In general practice, clinicians often rely on clinical observations to guide treatment planning.

Among the *affective dimensions* that we have found most useful to assess prior to treatment are:

- *Criticism*: Frequent statements of annoyance, resentment, and dislike of specific behaviors expressed by family members (spouses, parents, siblings) toward the person with BD (e.g., "I resent the ridiculous hours he keeps"). The person with BD often counteracts the criticism with countercriticisms. Dyadic discussions frequently degenerate into "point–counterpoint" arguments, which escalate and become destructive.
- *Hostility*: The rejection of the "person" of the family member or all of his behavior (e.g., "I don't like anything about him").
- *Emotional overinvolvement*: Exaggerated overconcern, worry, excessive self-sacrifice, inappropriate protectiveness, or poor boundaries expressed by caretaking family members (e.g., "I can't sleep unless she sleeps"; "I've given up my favorite activities to make life easier for him").

Cognitive problems in communication can take many forms, including, but not limited to,

- *Poor problem solving*: Problems are not clearly operationalized; there is little agreement on the definition. The family or couple attempts to solve multiple problems simultaneously. Solutions generated by one family member are "shot down" by other members before they are discussed. No solutions to the original problem are chosen or the implementation plan is unstructured and vague.
- *Communication deviance*: Family communication is distorted, tangential, vague, unclear, or overtly thought disordered. Family members frequently seem to be talking about separate topics and do not acknowledge each others' statements. Ideas are expressed incompletely and participants jump from topic to topic. They occasionally use neologisms or odd turns of phrase that don't seem to be comprehended by others (e.g., "He'll never get over *that thing*"; "I wish you would just . . . whatever").

do provide targets for planning the content of family sessions and measuring the family's progress.

Application of Family-Focused Therapy to Patients with Juvenile-Onset Bipolar Disorder

There are only two clinical trials of FFT among pediatric patients with BD. In a two-site randomized trial (Miklowitz et al., 2008), we assigned 58 teenagers with bipolar I, bipolar II, or BD not otherwise specified (NOS) to FFT or a brief treatment (enhanced care) consisting of three family educational sessions. All adolescents received pharmacological treatment from study psychiatrists. Adolescents had had a fully syndromal or subsyndromal mood episode in the 3 months before randomization from which they had not yet recovered.

Over 2 years, the adolescents who received FFT and pharmacotherapy stabilized from their initial depression symptoms more quickly than those who received brief psychoeducation and pharmacotherapy. Furthermore, adolescents in FFT had less severe depressive symptoms, spent less time in depressive episodes, and spent more time remitted from depression symptoms over 2 years than those in the comparison treatment (Figure 15.1). The effects of FFT on mania symptoms were only statistically significant in the subgroup of youth with high EE families. Thus, FFT appears to be an effective treatment for teens who are coping with the initial phases of BD. The emphasis of FFT on improving the protective, buffering effects of family relationships may be more relevant to the course of depression than mania.

In an open trial of FFT in combination with individual CBT, West, Henry, and Pavuluri (2007) observed improvements in bipolar symptoms (mania, aggression,

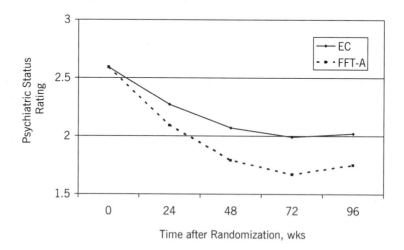

FIGURE 15.1. Levels of depression during and after treatment with family-focused therapy for adolescents (FFT-A) or enhanced care (EC). From Miklowitz et al. (2008). Copyright 2008 by the American Medical Association. Reprinted by permission.

KEY POINTS REGARDING FAMILY-FOCUSED TREATMENT FOR BIPOLAR DISORDER

- Multiple randomized trials suggest that FFT enhances medications in hastening recovery and delaying recurrences of BD among adults.
- One randomized trial finds that FFT and medication are more effective than brief psychoeducation and medication in stabilizing mood symptoms among adolescents with BD.
- Key mediating mechanisms may include improving family communication and enhancing medication adherence.

---

psychosis, depression) and global functioning among children (*n* = 34) ages 5–17 with BD. These improvements were observed immediately following the 12-session treatment and at 1, 2, and 3 years. Thus, data from controlled and uncontrolled trials suggest that FFT enhances symptom stabilization in childhood bipolar samples.

We are now examining FFT in a three-site randomized trial of 150 teens. This study should go much further in identifying the mediating and moderating processes relevant to the course of early-onset BD. We have also begun examining FFT as a preventive agent for children at risk for BD by virtue of having subsyndromal signs of mood disorder and a parent with bipolar I or II disorder (Miklowitz & Chang, 2008).

An ancillary study to the prevention study will examine changes in neural activation patterns among at-risk teens during a facial affect rating task. Evidence of perturbed neural development, and especially increased activation of the amygdala and decreased activation of the ventrolateral and dorsolateral prefrontal cortices during functional magnetic resonance imaging (fMRI) have been observed in children and adults with BD in response to emotional stimuli (Blumberg et al., 2003; Chang et al., 2004; Rich et al., 2006). Compared with healthy controls or children with attention-deficit/hyperactivity disorder, pediatric patients with BD are more likely to rate neutral faces as hostile and fear producing and to show greater activation of the amygdala, nucleus accumbens, and ventral prefrontal cortex on fMRI when doing so (Rich et al., 2006; see also McClure-Tone, Chapter 11, this volume). In the prevention study, we will examine changes in activation of these limbic and frontal-cortical structures from pre- to posttreatment in an FFT group (12 sessions) and a control group (one session) to determine whether changes in neural activation patterns predict levels of clinical improvement in these youth over 1 year of follow-up.

DIALECTICAL BEHAVIOR THERAPY

Another perspective on pediatric BD can be drawn from DBT (Linehan, 1993). DBT is an evidence-based psychotherapy originally developed for adults with borderline personality disorder that combines elements of psychoeducation and cognitive, behavioral, and mindfulness strategies. The main DBT target is emotional dysregulation, defined as high sensitivity to emotional stimuli, extreme emotional intensity, and a slow return to baseline emotional states.

Research indicates that emotion regulation processes are developmentally acquired and multiply determined by biological, psychological, and social processes. During adolescence, emotion regulatory processes undergo significant development, reorganization, and ultimately consolidation (Dahl & Spear, 2004). From a developmental standpoint, studies suggest that early difficulty with emotion regulation promotes later impairment, as the individual arrives at each progressive stage of development with inadequate resources to meet the challenges unique to the ensuing period (Cicchetti, Rogosch, & Toth, 1994). Thus, adolescence represents a critical window for intervention related to emotion regulation processes.

The study of normal adolescent development indicates that the ability to effectively modulate affect continues to develop into young adulthood. In comparison, youth with BD have been shown to experience significantly greater difficulty modulating a range of emotions (Birmaher et al., 2006), leading some to hypothesize that emotional dysregulation (characterized in terms of both valence and arousal) is the core clinical feature distinguishing pediatric BD from other classes of psychopathology in youth (Leibenluft, Charney, & Pine, 2003). Among adults with BD, difficulties with emotion regulation have been linked to impaired executive control associated with changes in the structure and function of the amygdala and prefrontal cortex (Green, Cahill, & Malhi, 2007). As discussed previously, increased activation of the amygdala and decreased activation of the ventromedial and dorsolateral prefrontal cortices have been observed in children with BD in response to emotional challenges, such as rating the emotion displayed on a face.

Given the vital importance of maximizing capacity for emotion regulation skills during adolescence, Goldstein and colleagues (2007) adapted DBT, a treatment targeting emotional dysregulation, for adolescents with BD. Additional high-priority treatment targets in DBT that are also associated with BD in adolescence include suicidal and nonsuicidal self-injurious behaviors (Goldstein et al., 2005; Lewinsohn, Klein, & Seeley, 1995), interpersonal deficits (Goldstein, Miklowitz, & Mullen, 2006), and treatment nonadherence (Coletti, Leigh, Gallelli, & Kafantaris, 2005), rendering DBT a face-valid approach to the psychosocial treatment of adolescents with BD.

Among adults with borderline personality disorder, DBT has been shown to reduce suicidal behaviors, hospitalizations, and anger, while improving social adjustment and treatment adherence relative to treatment as usual (Linehan, Tutek, Heard, & Armstrong, 1994). Miller, Rathus, Linehan, Wetzler, and Leigh (1997) adapted DBT for suicidal adolescents by incorporating age-appropriate language, decreasing treatment length, and involving family members in skills training groups. In a quasi-experimental design, adolescents receiving DBT had fewer psychiatric hospitalizations and greater treatment adherence than treatment-as-usual patients. DBT was also associated with decreases in depressive symptoms and suicidal ideation from pre- to posttreatment (Rathus & Miller, 2002). In light of this promising adaptation of DBT for adolescents and the seemingly good fit between the treatment targets in DBT and the clinical presentation of adolescents with BD, we describe here the DBT protocol for early-onset BD.

Treatment Structure

The DBT intervention for adolescents with BD is based on Miller and colleagues' (Miller, Rathus, Landsman, & Linehan, 2003; Miller, Rathus, & Linehan, 2006) intervention incorporating age-appropriate modifications for suicidal adolescents. DBT adapted for adolescents with BD is a yearlong treatment consisting of an acute treatment period (months 1–6; weekly 1-hour sessions) followed by a continuation phase of treatment (biweekly sessions months 7–10, monthly sessions months 10–12). Two treatment modalities are used: (1) family skills training (conducted with individual family units) and (2) individual therapy. This represents a modification from Miller's DBT treatment schedule for suicidal adolescents in which treatment spans 16 weeks, with a weekly skills group (2 hours/week) and individual therapy (1 hour/week). Given the cyclical nature of BD, extending the treatment period increases the opportunity for skills to be applied across mood states, which may increase the generalizability of skills. Furthermore, given that many adolescents with BD exhibit attentional and learning deficits, we found that abbreviating skills training sessions to 1 hour optimizes learning. In pilot studies, participants had difficulty focusing toward the end of longer sessions.

Miller, Rathus, and Linehan's (2006) DBT model for adolescents incorporates family members in skills training within a multifamily group format. Thus, not only do patients gain in vivo coaching from clinicians and family members, but family members gain skills for managing their own emotional reactions to the patient. Goldstein and colleagues (2007) elected to deliver family skills training to individual family units in order to maximize the DBT therapists' ability to address issues specific to each family and devote time to skills that addressed the areas of greatest need. To illustrate, during a pilot study, multiple individuals in one family unit struggled to understand and apply validation skills (i.e., the ability to communicate to another person that his or her feelings, thoughts, or actions make sense and are understandable in a particular situation). They had a difficult time parsing agreement from validation. By conducting skills training with the family unit (rather than in a multifamily group), the skills trainer had the flexibility to spend an additional session working on validation skills and relatively less time on another skill that had been of relative strength for individuals in this family unit.

Family Skills Training

A therapist referred to as the skills trainer works with the family unit. Although several skills are taught in both DBT family skills training sessions and FFT family sessions (i.e., psychoeducation, mood charting, problem solving and certain communication skills), it is the material taught in the DBT skills modules—mindfulness, distress tolerance, emotion regulation, interpersonal effectiveness, and walking the middle path (see Linehan, 1993, and Miller et al., 2006, for detailed descriptions of these modules)—that distinguish the content of the two treatments (Table 15.2). Furthermore, in DBT family skills sessions, skills trainers follow the DBT hierarchy of treatment targets in which the primary focus is on skills acquisition, strengthening, and generalization. In this way, skills trainers give very little direct attention to therapy-interfering behaviors (e.g., the teen doodling during skills training sessions) or in-session process issues (e.g., tension between two family members during skills training) except as they may apply to the specific skill being reviewed; these are addressed in individual DBT sessions. In FFT, psychoeducational content and process issues are usually balanced (see Miklowitz, 2008).

TAILORING SKILLS FOR BIPOLAR DISORDER

Skills trainers teach skills in a didactic fashion using handouts and homework assignments. In-session exercises, games, and activities provide family members

TABLE 15.2. Dialectical Behavior Therapy (DBT) Skills Modules and Their Associated Treatment Targets

Treatment target	DBT skills module
Confusion about bipolar disorder Lack of knowledge and/or misinformation about symptoms, causes, treatment, and course of illness	Psychoeducation
Confusion about self Limited ability to identify mood states as well as their associated vulnerabilities and triggers	Mindfulness
Impulsivity Tendency to act impulsively in order to decrease subjective distress without consideration of the consequences	Distress tolerance
Emotional instability Rapid, intense mood changes or steady negative emotional state	Emotion regulation
Interpersonal problems Difficulty keeping and maintaining relationships	Interpersonal effectiveness
Teenager and family dialectical dilemmas Inconsistent patterns of relating characterized by vacillation between extremes of thinking, feeling, and acting	Walking the middle path

Note. From Miller, Rathus, and Linehan (2006). Copyright 2006 by The Guilford Press. Adapted by permission.

with the opportunity to apply skills in a hands-on manner. Although DBT skills were expressly developed for individuals prone to emotional dysregulation, further adaptation for individuals with BD was necessary. One unique aspect of applying DBT to BD is that while the same skills can be effective for managing a range of mood states, the way each skill is *conceptualized* and *applied* may vary based on the individual's affective state. To illustrate, when introducing the mindfulness concept "states of mind," skills trainers explicitly discuss the experience of "emotional mind" associated with depressed, manic, mixed, and euthymic states. These distinctions help the teen and family members identify early warning signs of pending mood episodes and distinguish "normal" emotions from illness symptoms in a nonjudgmental fashion. Similarly, when reviewing vulnerabilities to "emotional mind," skills trainers lead the family in a discussion of cognitive and behavioral attributes of different mood states, highlighting differences and commonalities. One patient identified changes in his sleep–wake cycle as a common vulnerability to emotional mind: Too much sleep made him vulnerable to depression, whereas too little sleep made him vulnerable to hypomania.

Thus, for each skill taught, skills trainers encourage participants to discern which skills are most applicable and effective in various mood states. For example, when manic, the emotion regulation skill of building positive emotions by engaging in pleasant activities may escalate manic mood and behavior; when depressed, this skill may improve mood. To aid the teen in determining which skills to apply when, the clinician helps him or her to articulate a situation-specific goal. Once this goal is clearly defined, the therapist and family members help the patient determine which skills may help him or her attain it. When teaching skills, the skills trainer often poses the question, "When do you think you would need this skill the most?"

Adolescents commonly exhibit willfulness about behavior change. In DBT, commitment to change is conceptualized as a behavior that is expected to fluctuate throughout treatment. In DBT, the therapist uses specific commitment strategies to increase commitment to change (e.g., pros and cons, devil's advocate, highlighting freedom of choice in the absence of reasonable alternatives; see Linehan, 1993). These same strategies would also be useful in encouraging healthy adolescents to commit to health-related behavior changes (e.g., eating properly, keeping regular sleep schedules).

A 15-year-old girl diagnosed with bipolar I disorder found that, when depressed, she would isolate in her room and listen to depressing music, which would often precede incidents of self-injurious behavior. She was able to identify that when in this state her goal was to "feel less miserable." In a family session, she and her parents reviewed the list of pleasant activities designed to build positive emotions, and she circled five that she was willing to try when feeling miserable. She elected to try one of the activities from her list, taking a bubble bath, and that proved helpful as a distraction tool and a temporary mood elevator.

PSYCHOEDUCATION

Psychoeducation begins with socialization to DBT, including treatment agreements and guidelines. The skills trainer then orients the family to the DBT skills modules and discusses how each module applies to difficulties experienced by adolescents with BD and their family members.

The skills trainer invites a discussion on the meaning and relevance of dialectics: two concepts or ideas that appear to be opposite but can both be true at the same time. The skills trainer provides concrete examples of dialectics to the family (e.g., candy that can be both sweet and sour, a wedding that can be both happy and sad) and encourages family members to identify dialectics they notice in their lives. Dialectics are then put into the context of illness (e.g., during mixed states, individuals experience symptoms of mania and depression at the same time), relationships (e.g., there is always more than one way to see a situation and more than one way to solve a problem), and self-management (e.g., I am both tough and gentle). These discussions lay the foundation for adopting a dialectical approach in which things are not black and white, thus broadening options for problem solving and negotiating.

The skills trainer then conducts psychoeducation on early-onset BD. Topics include symptoms of BD in adolescence, treatments, and risk and protective factors. As in FFT, a key element of psychoeducation involves the presentation of a biopsychosocial model of the development and maintenance of BD. A unique aspect of psychoeducation in DBT compared with FFT is presentation and discussion of the three main components of emotional dysregulation: reactivity, intensity, and duration of affective response. Triggers for mood states are identified and revisited throughout the course of treatment as they pertain to skills use.

MINDFULNESS

Mindfulness skills help the adolescent use both rational and emotional input to make choices that are more balanced and less impulsive (Miller et al., 1997). In the mindfulness module, family members learn steps for increasing awareness and bringing attention fully to one object of focus. In this way, mindfulness skills help family members gain an increased sense of control over thoughts and emotions. Mindfulness skills may be especially helpful for parents and teens who become polarized when engaging in ineffective exchanges characterized by emotional extremes; in FFT, these would be characterized as high-EE, "point–counterpoint" struggles.

EMOTION REGULATION

The emotion regulation module provides concrete skills for managing the emotional intensity and lability characteristic of early-onset BD. Skills trainers teach family members to identify and label their emotions as well as the accompanying prompting events, experiences, and actions as a means of improving the ability to recognize when such skills are warranted. Participants learn skills to attend to self-care (e.g., proper sleep, nourishment, and exercise) and increase positive events in order to decrease vulnerability to dysregulated mood. Skills for changing an undesirable mood state are taught and practiced; for example, trainers teach family members to change emotions by "acting opposite" to the current emotion. To illustrate, Jon would frequently become very frustrated when playing online games with friends. His frustration would escalate to the point that he would yell, curse, throw things at the screen, and slam the keyboard down when he was not happy with the way the game was going. His parents and siblings found this behavior very disruptive to the household, and Jon would lose computer privileges as a result. Applying the steps in the "acting opposite to the current emotion" skill, Jon learned to (1) identify the emotion he was having (i.e., frustration) and ask himself if the emotion was justified (in his opinion, it was), (2) identify the associated action urge (i.e., yell, scream, throw things) and subsequently, (3) ask himself if he wanted to change the emotion and not go with the action urge. Jon clearly had motivation to change the emotion given its unwanted consequences. He learned to figure out the opposite action to the emotion urge. In this case, Jon would whisper rather than yell, speak kindly rather than curse, and gently handle his computer and keyboard as opposed to being aggressive. Jon's parents coached him to implement opposite action "all the way." In fact, in the beginning, Jon jokingly stroked his computer gently and said kind things when he was frustrated ("You are such a wonderful computer").

DISTRESS TOLERANCE

Skills in this module teach adolescents to tolerate and accept painful emotions and circumstances. First, family members work toward acceptance of the reality that life involves pain and unfairness, and that people cope more effectively with life's challenges (including having BD) by accepting pain rather than fighting against it. These skills are based on the premise that the impulsive, high-risk, and self-injurious behaviors common among adolescents with BD result in part from urges associated with intolerable emotions. Although high-risk or self-injurious behaviors may relieve or modify the emotion momentarily, they may also make the situation worse. Participants work toward increasing willingness to use coping skills to sit with unpleasant emotions. These skills can include breathing, distraction, and other self-soothing techniques.

INTERPERSONAL SKILLS

A central developmental task of adolescence includes the ability to build and negotiate interpersonal relationships. However, research indicates that adolescents with BD lag behind their healthy peers in terms of social skill development (Goldstein et al., 2006). These skills aim to help the teen become aware of interpersonal goals and apply skills to achieve these goals. Specific skills address themes prominent in navigating relationships during adolescence, including saying no to unwanted requests, coping with interpersonal conflict, asking for what you want, and maintaining self-respect in relationships. This module is similar to the communication enhancement training module of FFT, in which adolescents and parents rehearse skills such as active listening and making positive requests for change in another's behavior.

> Ann, age 16, frequently expressed her frustration during skills training sessions, reporting that "my parents never let me have *anything* I ask for." This was particularly problematic when Ann was hypomanic, during which time her requests increased dramatically; she would constantly seek to buy things, go out with friends, be driven somewhere by her parents, or ask favors from her parents or her sister. The perception that her parents *never* said yes to her would then contribute to her increased irritability and aggression when she was hypomanic. Ann would then behave in a hostile and impatient manner toward her family members. In turn, her parents asked, "Why should she have privileges when she treats us like that?" With practice using the interpersonal effectiveness skills "asking for what you want" and "maintaining relationships," Ann became more skillful when approaching her parents with requests. As a result, Ann was more effective when requesting things from her parents and, because they felt more respected, they were more likely to approve her requests. This contributed to improved mood regulation because Ann was less likely to become irritable and aggressive during hypomanic episodes.

WALKING THE MIDDLE PATH

Families learn principles of behaviorism (e.g., reinforcement, punishment) and gain practice applying these principles to shape one another's behavior. In addition, this module focuses on aiding family members in identifying dialectical dilemmas and patterns they encounter (e.g., vacillating between being very strict with rules and consequences at some times and being overly permissive at other times) and working toward a more balanced "middle path" approach.

Individual Therapy

In individual therapy sessions, the DBT therapist consults with the adolescent on ways to apply DBT skills he or she is learning in the skills training sessions to situations encountered in his or her daily life. The individual DBT therapist selects behaviors on which to focus based on the following priorities: (1) decreasing life-threatening behaviors, (2) decreasing therapy-interfering behaviors, (3) decreasing quality-of-life interfering behaviors, and (4) increasing behavioral skills. Patients complete diary cards on which they track mood, sleep, suicidality, and medication adherence daily as well as any other targeted behaviors tied to treatment goals. Adolescents also track daily use of DBT skills on the diary card and rate the helpfulness of the skills. Nonadherence with the diary card is considered therapy-interfering behavior and is targeted as a problem behavior in individual sessions using assessment, commitment, and dialectical strategies.

Adolescents apply problem-solving strategies in individual DBT in a manner similar to the FFT therapist. Behavioral chain analyses are undertaken for targeted problems (e.g., medication nonadherence) to understand the function of specific behaviors, identify constructive alternative solutions, and develop techniques for avoiding future problem behaviors. Like the family skills trainer, the individual DBT therapist is available to the adolescent by pager or cell phone for *in vivo* skills coaching.

Application of Dialectical Behavior Therapy to Adolescents with Bipolar Disorder

A recent treatment development trial demonstrated the feasibility and acceptability of this model of DBT for adolescents with BD (Goldstein et al., 2007). Ten adolescents (mean age, 16 years) with BD (bipolar I = 7, bipolar II = 2, BD NOS = 1) who met criteria for a syndromal mood episode within the prior 3 months were enrolled in open treatment with DBT. All were engaged in a pharmacotherapy regimen managed by a child psychiatrist.

Results indicate that DBT was highly feasible to administer to adolescent patients with BD and their families. Attendance at treatment was high: Over the 1-year treatment period, patients attended an average of 33 of 36 scheduled sessions. Posttreatment satisfaction questionnaires indicated that the intervention was acceptable and appropriate to participants' needs. Patients and parents reported that the frequency of visits and treatment length were acceptable. Patients and parents reported feeling highly satisfied with DBT as well as with the adolescents' clinical and psychosocial gains during treatment.

Patients exhibited significant improvement from pre- to posttreatment in suicidality, nonsuicidal self-injurious behavior, emotional dysregulation, and depressive symptoms (Figure 15.2). These data indicate that DBT may offer promise as an approach to the psychosocial treatment of adolescent BD, particularly for those who exhibit suicidal or self-injurious thoughts and behaviors as well as those who demonstrate significant difficulty with impulsivity and interpersonal relationships.

These findings are from a small open trial and, therefore, should be viewed as preliminary. Given that we do not have data from a comparison group, we cannot conclude that DBT was responsible for the observed improvement. That is, the improvements reported could be attributable to other factors, including the natural course of the illness over time, medications, or even nonspecific therapeutic elements like attention or support.

On the basis of promising preliminary findings, we are currently completing a larger open trial of DBT for adolescents with BD. In this trial, we aim to

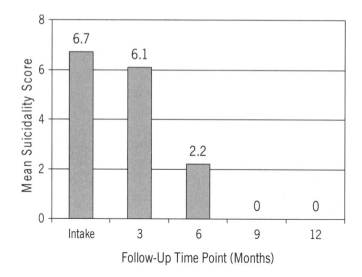

FIGURE 15.2. Changes in suicidality scores during a dialectical behavior therapy intervention (10 adolescents with bipolar disorder). Data from Goldstein, Axelson, Birmaher, and Brent (2007).

examine moderators of treatment response in order to better determine for whom this treatment approach holds most promise as well as mechanisms of change in DBT. Hypothesized predictors of positive treatment response for adolescents with BD in DBT include developmental stage (i.e., postpubertal participants), lesser psychiatric comorbidity, and history of suicidality or nonsuicidal self-injurious behavior. Mediators of treatment response in DBT may include skills generalization and use (measured via daily diary card ratings).

In this study, we aim to extend our understanding of emotional dysregulation in BD by using a multiple-levels-of-analysis approach to the evaluation of the DBT intervention. Specifically, participants are completing emotional laboratory tasks at baseline and again posttreatment, during which psychophysiological data are recorded. Participants complete an affective modification of the Continuous Performance Task while data on pupil dilation are collected (Siegle, Granholm, Ingram, & Matt, 2001). Pupil response is time-locked to presentation of emotional stimuli to permit fine-grained analyses of the magnitude and time course of neural responses during emotional processing. These biological data will be examined in relation to treatment-related outcomes. We hypothesize that data from the pupillometric assessment will correlate highly with clinical ratings of emotional dysregulation and will normalize with DBT treatment.

In addition to providing valuable information regarding abnormal affective processes in adolescents with mood disorder, we will also be able to compare these data with those of healthy adolescents to better understand the nature of affective processes in normal development. If the hypotheses of this ancillary study are

---

**KEY POINTS REGARDING DIALECTICAL BEHAVIOR THERAPY (DBT)
FOR ADOLESCENTS WITH BIPOLAR DISORDER**

- Multiple randomized trials suggest that DBT decreases depressive symptoms, suicidal behaviors, and hospitalizations and improves treatment adherence among adults with borderline personality disorder compared with treatment as usual.

- In a quasi-experimental design, suicidal adolescents receiving DBT had fewer psychiatric hospitalizations and greater treatment adherence than patients receiving treatment as usual.

- Data from an open treatment development trial of DBT for adolescents with BD support the feasibility and acceptability of the intervention as well as pre–post treatment improvements in depression, suicidality, and emotional dysregulation.

---

supported, a pupillary response measure may prove to be a useful marker of the development of emotional regulation skills.

CONCLUSIONS

BD relapses and remits within a familial/interpersonal context. The affective tone of this family context, whether it is supportive and nurturing versus highly conflictual and discordant, will affect whether patients have earlier recurrences, residual symptoms, psychosocial dysfunction, or adhere to a medication regimen. This chapter has examined family processes in BD at multiple levels of analysis. Many questions remain about the degree to which family processes, such as highly charged emotional interchanges between youth with BD and their parents, are best conceptualized as (1) "learned," habitual styles of relating, (2) unstable reactions to the stress of illness in a child, (3) the end product of genetically shared vulnerabilities to temperamental disturbances (e.g., a poor temperamental fit between child and parent), or (4) an interaction between these factors. Ongoing studies of neural activation during emotional challenge tasks in youth with BD and their first-degree relatives may shed light on these alternative explanations.

One way to address these challenging contextual factors is to combine pharmacotherapy with a family-based intervention. This chapter has described two treatment models for managing BD, especially in teens: FFT and DBT. Both emphasize the importance of family involvement as a protective influence in the course of the disorder, recognizing that families can also contribute to the overall liability to recurrence if relationships, especially those during the high-risk, postepisode period, are stressful and conflict ridden. Both treatments include psychoeducation about BD, including learning to identify early warning signs of recurrence and implement mood management skills.

Both FFT and DBT emphasize skills training as a means of enhancing day-to-day interpersonal functioning and problem solving. FFT emphasizes improvement in parent–offspring communication as a mediating variable in the pathways from treatment to the outcome of BD. DBT emphasizes emotional self-regulation in parents and offspring as mediating mechanisms. Both models acknowledge the feelings of shame, social rejection, and isolation often experienced by persons with BD and their caregivers and emphasize talking openly about the disorder within sessions, at home, and eventually with important people outside the family.

The two treatment models emphasize the importance of EE as a prognostic factor but conceptualize the genesis of these attitudes differently. The FFT model emphasizes the lack of communication and problem-solving skills as central to critical or hostile attitudes as well as the attribution among parents that the negative behaviors of the adolescent with BD are the product of willful opposition and hostile intention rather than illness. The DBT model views EE as reflecting the tendency for parents and teens to become polarized around common dialectical dilemmas that families face. Skills deficits in multiple arenas (i.e., mindfulness, emotion regulation, distress tolerance, interpersonal effectiveness) contribute to family members' difficulties moving toward a synthesis in resolving these dilemmas.

No studies have directly compared the outcomes of patients treated with FFT and DBT. What might be more significant than their relative efficacy, however, would be identifying the subgroups who might respond to each. For example, dual-parent families struggling with marital conflict or difficulty agreeing on parenting strategies might be well suited to the communication and problem-solving orientation of FFT. Some families may be unwilling to consider how less traditional skills in DBT, such as mindfulness, could be helpful. In contrast, a single mother of a teen exhibiting dangerous behaviors might respond less openly to practical, conjoint problem solving, which, in the past, led to no useful or enduring results. Instead, this parent might benefit from learning mindfulness skills to manage her own difficulties with emotion regulation and distress tolerance. Older adolescents may be more likely to benefit from the individual DBT therapy component than younger adolescents.

The format of the DBT treatment model raises the question of whether family skills training is enhanced by adjunctive individual sessions. In a nonrandomized study of adults with BD, Miklowitz, Richards, and colleagues (2003) combined FFT sessions with individual "interpersonal and social rhythm therapy" sessions in alternating weeks. Patients in this intensive combination treatment benefited in terms of longer periods of stability before depressive relapses and the severity of depressive symptoms relative to a treatment-as-usual comparison group. Thus, there are reasons to suspect that a synergy developed between the individual and family skills training; however, no randomly assigned comparison group of patients who received just the FFT or just the interpersonal sessions was available. Further tests of the DBT model should include "dismantling" designs to test the relative contribution of the individual component, the family component, and their synergy in stabilizing the short-term course of adolescent BD.

Family Therapy as Early Intervention for Children at Risk for Bipolar Disorder

The role of family and other psychosocial interventions in delaying or preventing the onset of BD is an important direction for future research (Miklowitz & Chang, 2008). The early signs of BD in genetically at-risk youth can include moderate to severe mood lability, sleep disturbance, outbursts of irritability and aggression, and impulsive suicidal gestures (Birmaher et al., 2006). Nonetheless, these early warning signs may portend a variety of diagnostic outcomes, depending on what risk or protective factors intervene (multifinality; Cicchetti & Rogosch, 2002). Little is known about the combination of risk and protective factors or the weighting of genetic, neurobiological, social, familial, or cultural factors at different phases of the life cycle that are most closely associated with the eventual onset of BD. Elucidating these developmental trajectories would inform the design of preventive interventions for BD, especially those interventions specifically targeting specific developmental phases. For example, preventive interventions for teens may need to take stronger account of peer relationships than interventions for school-age children.

Modern behavioral genetic approaches to psychiatric disorders examine the role of environmental variables while controlling for genetic factors, and the reverse. For example, Caspi and colleagues (2004) showed that, among identical twin pairs, the twin to whom the mother expressed less warmth and more emotional negativity was at greater risk for developing antisocial behavior than the twin to whom the mother expressed more warmth and less negativity. Examining parent–offspring interactions in sibling or twin pairs in which one has BD would help clarify how family stressors lead to differences in gene expression and elucidate one of many gene–environment pathways in the onset of BD.

Thus, longitudinal studies that elucidate the nature of genetic, biological, social, and cultural mechanisms in illness onset will inform the design of prevention studies. In parallel, preventive intervention studies will inform our understanding of the multiple causal pathways to illness onset. For example, if early intervention trials were to show that modifying family relationships or teaching emotion regulation skills delays the first onset of a manic episode, we will have evidence that these processes play causal rather than purely reactive roles in the pathways to BD among some youth. If treatment-associated changes in neurobiological risk markers (such as amygdalar volume) are associated with changes in the trajectory of mood symptoms, we can develop hypotheses about the causal primacy of these biological risk markers. The next phase of research on BD should address these developmental questions.

REFERENCES

Birmaher, B., Axelson, D., Strober, M., Gill, M. K., Valeri, S., Chiappetta, L., et al. (2006). Clinical course of children and adolescents with bipolar spectrum disorders. *Archives of General Psychiatry, 63*(2), 175–183.

Blumberg, H. P., Martin, A., Kaufman, J., Leung, H. C., Skudlarski, P., Lacadie, C., et al. (2003). Frontostriatal abnormalities in adolescents with bipolar disorder: Preliminary observations from functional MRI. *American Journal of Psychiatry, 160*(7), 1345–1347.

Caspi, A., Moffitt, T. E., Morgan, J., Rutter, M., Taylor, A., Arseneault, L., et al. (2004). Maternal expressed emotion predicts children's antisocial behavior problems: Using monozygotic-twin differences to identify environmental effects on behavioral development. *Developmental Psychology, 40*, 149–161.

Chang, K., Adleman, N. E., Dienes, K., Simeonova, D. J., Menon, V., & Reiss, A. (2004). Anomalous prefrontal-subcortical activation in familial pediatric bipolar disorder: A functional magnetic resonance imaging investigation. *Archives of General Psychiatry, 61*(8), 781–792.

Cicchetti, D. (2008). A multiple levels of analysis perspective on research in development and psychopathology. In T. Beauchaine & S. Hinshaw (Eds.), *Child and adolescent psychopathology* (pp. 27–57). Hoboken, NJ: Wiley.

Cicchetti, D., & Rogosch, F. A. (1996). Equifinality and multifinality in developmental psychopathology. *Development and Psychopathology, 8*, 597–600.

Cicchetti, D., & Rogosch, F. A. (2002). A developmental psychopathology perspective on adolescence. *Journal of Consulting and Clinical Psychology, 70*(1), 6–20.

Cicchetti, D., Rogosch, F. A., & Toth, S. L. (1994). A developmental psychopathology perspective on depression in children and adolescents. In W. M. Reynolds & H. F. Johnston (Eds.), *Handbook of depression in children and adolescents* (pp. 123–141). New York: Plenum Press.

Coletti, D. J., Leigh, E., Gallelli, K. A., & Kafantaris, V. (2005). Patterns of adherence to treatment in adolescents with bipolar disorder. *Journal of Child and Adolescent Psychopharmacology, 15*(6), 913–917.

Coville, A. L., Miklowitz, D. J., Taylor, D. O., & Low, K. (2008). Correlates of high expressed emotion attitudes among parents of bipolar adolescents. *Journal of Clinical Psychology, 64*(4), 438–449.

Dahl, R. E., & Spear, L. (2004). Adolescent brain development: A period of vulnerabilities and opportunities. Keynote address. *Annals of the New York Academy of Sciences, 1021*, 1–22.

Falloon, I. R. H., Boyd, J. L., & McGill, C. W. (1984). *Family care of schizophrenia: A problem-solving approach to the treatment of mental illness.* New York: Guilford Press.

Fredman, S. B., Baucom, D. H., Miklowitz, D. J., & Stanton, S. E. (2008). Observed emotional involvement and overinvolvement in families of bipolar patients. *Journal of Family Psychology, 22*(1), 71–79.

Geller, B., Tillman, R., Bolhofner, K., & Zimerman, B. (2008). Child bipolar I disorder: Prospective continuity with adult bipolar I disorder; characteristics of second and third episodes; predictors of 8-year outcome. *Archives of General Psychiatry, 65*(10), 1125–1133.

Goldstein, T. R., Axelson, D. A., Birmaher, B., & Brent, D. A. (2007). Dialectical behavior therapy for adolescents with bipolar disorder: A 1-year open trial. *Journal of the American Academy of Child and Adolescent Psychiatry, 46*(7), 820–830.

Goldstein, T. R., Birmaher, B., Axelson, D., Ryan, N. D., Strober, M. A., Gill, M. K., et al. (2005). History of suicide attempts in pediatric bipolar disorder: Factors associated with increased risk. *Bipolar Disorders, 7*(6), 525–535.

Goldstein, T. R., Miklowitz, D. J., & Mullen, K. (2006). Social skills knowledge and performance among adolescents with bipolar disorder. *Bipolar Disorders, 8*(4), 350–361.

Green, M. J., Cahill, C. M., & Malhi, G. S. (2007). The cognitive and neurophysiological basis of emotion dysregulation in bipolar disorder. *Journal of Affective Disorders, 103*, 29–42.

Hahlweg, K., Goldstein, M. J., Nuechterlein, K. H., Magana, A. B., Mintz, J., Doane, J. A., et al. (1989). Expressed emotion and patient-relative interaction in families of recent-onset schizophrenics. *Journal of Consulting and Clinical Psychology, 57*, 11–18.

Heru, A. M. (2006). Family psychiatry: From research to practice. *American Journal of Psychiatry, 163*(6), 962–968.

Hinshaw, S. P., & Cicchetti, D. (2000). Stigma and mental disorder: Conceptions of illness, public attitudes, personal disclosure, and social policy. *Development and Psychopathology, 12*(4), 555–598.

Imber-Mintz, L., Liberman, R. P., Miklowitz, D. J., & Mintz, J. (1987). Expressed emotion: A call for partnership among relatives, patients, and professionals. *Schizophrenia Bulletin, 13*(2), 227–235.

Kim, E. Y., & Miklowitz, D. J. (2004). Expressed emotion as a predictor of outcome among bipolar patients undergoing family therapy. *Journal of Affective Disorders, 82*, 343–352.

Leibenluft, E., Charney, D. S., & Pine, D. S. (2003). Researching the pathophysiology of pediatric bipolar disorder. *Biological Psychiatry, 53*, 1009–1020.

Lewinsohn, P. M., Klein, D. N., & Seeley, J. R. (1995). Bipolar disorders in a community sample of older adolescents: Prevalence, phenomenology, comorbidity, and course. *Journal of the American Academy of Child and Adolescent Psychiatry, 34*, 454–463.

Linehan, M. M. (1993). *Cognitive-behavioral treatment of borderline personality disorder.* New York: Guilford Press.

Linehan, M. M., Tutek, D. A., Heard, H. L., & Armstrong, H. E. (1994). Interpersonal outcome of cognitive behavioral treatment for chronically suicidal borderline patients. *American Journal of Psychiatry, 151*, 1771–1776.

Miklowitz, D. J. (2008). *Bipolar disorder: A family-focused treatment approach* (2nd ed.). New York: Guilford Press.

Miklowitz, D. J., Axelson, D. A., Birmaher, B., George, E. L., Taylor, D. O., Schneck, C. D., et al. (2008). Family-focused treatment for adolescents with bipolar disorder: Results of a 2-year randomized trial. *Archives of General Psychiatry, 65*(9), 1053–1061.

Miklowitz, D. J., Axelson, D. A., George, E. L., Taylor, D. O., Schneck, C. D., Sullivan, A. E., et al. (2009). Expressed emotion moderates the effects of family-focused treatment for bipolar adolescents. *Journal of the American Academy of Child and Adolescent Psychiatry, 48*, 643–651.

Miklowitz, D. J., Biuckians, A., & Richards, J. A. (2006). Early-onset bipolar disorder: A family treatment perspective. *Development and Psychopathology, 18*(4), 1247–1265.

Miklowitz, D. J., & Chang, K. D. (2008). Prevention of bipolar disorder in at-risk children: Theoretical assumptions and empirical foundations. *Development and Psychopathology, 20*(3), 881–897.

Miklowitz, D. J., George, E. L., Richards, J. A., Simoneau, T. L., & Suddath, R. L. (2003). A randomized study of family-focused psychoeducation and pharmacotherapy in the outpatient management of bipolar disorder. *Archives of General Psychiatry, 60*, 904–912.

Miklowitz, D. J., & Goldstein, M. J. (1990). Behavioral family treatment for patients with bipolar affective disorder. *Behavior Modification, 14*, 457–489.

Miklowitz, D. J., Goldstein, M. J., Nuechterlein, K. H., Snyder, K. S., & Mintz, J. (1988). Family factors and the course of bipolar affective disorder. *Archives of General Psychiatry, 45*, 225–231.

Miklowitz, D. J., Otto, M. W., Frank, E., Reilly-Harrington, N. A., Kogan, J. N., Sachs, G. S., et al. (2007). Intensive psychosocial intervention enhances functioning in patients with bipolar depression: Results from a 9-month randomized controlled trial *American Journal of Psychiatry, 164*(9), 1–8.

Miklowitz, D. J., Otto, M. W., Frank, E., Reilly-Harrington, N. A., Wisniewski, S. R., Kogan, J. N., et al. (2007). Psychosocial treatments for bipolar depression: A 1-year randomized trial from the Systematic Treatment Enhancement Program. *Archives of General Psychiatry, 64*, 419–427.

Miklowitz, D. J., Richards, J. A., George, E. L., Suddath, R. L., Frank, E., Powell, K., et al. (2003). Integrated family and individual therapy for bipolar disorder: Results of a treatment development study. *Journal of Clinical Psychiatry, 64*, 182–191.

Miklowitz, D. J., Simoneau, T. L., George, E. L., Richards, J. A., Kalbag, A., Sachs-Ericsson, N., et al. (2000). Family-focused treatment of bipolar disorder: 1-year effects of a psychoeducational program in conjunction with pharmacotherapy. *Biological Psychiatry, 48*, 582–592.

Miklowitz, D. J., Wendel, J. S., & Simoneau, T. L. (1998). Targeting dysfunctional family interactions and high expressed emotion in the psychosocial treatment of bipolar disorder. *In Session: Psychotherapy in Practice, 4*, 25–38.

Miller, A. L., Rathus, J. H., Landsman, M., & Linehan, M. M. (2003). *Dialectical behavior therapy: Multi-family skills training group*. Unpublished manuscript.

Miller, A. L., Rathus, J. H., & Linehan, M. M. (2006). *Dialectical behavior therapy with suicidal adolescents*. New York: Guilford Press.

Miller, A. L., Rathus, J. H., Linehan, M. M., Wetzler, S., & Leigh, E. (1997). Dialectical behavior therapy adapted for suicidal adolescents. *Journal of Practical Psychiatry and Behavioral Health, 3*, 78–86.

O'Connell, R. A., Mayo, J. A., Flatow, L., Cuthbertson, B., & O'Brien, B. E. (1991). Outcome of bipolar disorder on long-term treatment with lithium. *British Journal of Psychiatry, 159*, 123–129.

Perlick, D. A., Hohenstein, J. M., Clarkin, J. F., Kaczynski, R., & Rosenheck, R. A. (2005). Use of mental health and primary care services by caregivers of patients with bipolar disorder: A preliminary study. *Bipolar Disorders, 7*(2), 126–135.

Priebe, S., Wildgrube, C., & Muller-Oerlinghausen, B. (1989). Lithium prophylaxis and expressed emotion. *British Journal of Psychiatry, 154*, 396–399.

Rathus, J. H., & Miller, A. L. (2002). Dialectical behavior therapy adapted for suicidal adolescents. *Suicide and Life-Threatening Behavior, 32*, 146–157.

Rea, M. M., Tompson, M., Miklowitz, D. J., Goldstein, M. J., Hwang, S., & Mintz, J. (2003). Family focused treatment vs. individual treatment for bipolar disorder: Results of a randomized clinical trial. *Journal of Consulting and Clinical Psychology, 71*, 482–492.

Rich, B. A., Vinton, D. T., Roberson-Nay, R., Hommer, R. E., Berghorst, L. H., McClure, E. B., et al. (2006). Limbic hyperactivation during processing of neutral facial expressions in children with bipolar disorder. *Proceedings of the National Academy of Sciences USA, 103*(23), 8900–8905.

Siegle, G. J., Granholm, E., Ingram, R. E., & Matt, G. E. (2001). Pupillary and reaction time measures of sustained processing of negative information in depression. *Biological Psychiatry, 49*, 624–636.

Silverthorne, P., Frick, P. J., & Reynolds, R. (2001). Timing of onset and correlates of severe conduct problems in adjudicated girls and boys. *Journal of Psychopathology, 23*, 171–181.

Simoneau, T. L., Miklowitz, D. J., Richards, J. A., Saleem, R., & George, E. L. (1999). Bipolar disorder and family communication: Effects of a psychoeducational treatment program. *Journal of Abnormal Psychology, 108*, 588–597.

Vaughn, C. E., & Leff, J. P. (1976). The influence of family and social factors on the course of psychiatric illness: A comparison of schizophrenia and depressed neurotic patients. *British Journal of Psychiatry, 129*, 125–137.

West, A. E., Henry, D. B., & Pavuluri, M. N. (2007). Maintenance model of integrated psychosocial treatment in pediatric bipolar disorder: A pilot feasibility study. *Journal of the American Academy of Child and Adolescent Psychiatry, 46*(2), 205–212.

Yan, L. J., Hammen, C., Cohen, A. N., Daley, S. E., & Henry, R. M. (2004). Expressed emotion versus relationship quality variables in the prediction of recurrence in bipolar patients. *Journal of Affective Disorders, 83*, 199–206.

CHAPTER 16

Psychoeducational Psychotherapy for Children with Bipolar Disorder

Amy N. Mendenhall and Mary A. Fristad

Pediatric bipolar disorder (BD) can be extremely impairing for both the children and their families. The earlier the onset of symptoms and the longer the children are in episode, the less time they have for the "normal" developmental process. Parents report delayed social and cognitive functioning directly related to the amount of time in episode (Kowatch & Fristad, 2006). Affected youth often have difficulty getting along with peers and have few or no friends (Geller et al., 2000). Quackenbush, Kutcher, Robertson, and Boulos (1996) found that, before the onset of BD, adolescents were putting moderate to strong effort into school and many were in college preparatory courses. After onset of BD, however, these same youth were putting minimal effort into school, were having difficulty with math, and were unlikely to graduate. Children with BD often find themselves struggling to function successfully and in an age-appropriate manner with family, peers, and school.

Difficulties also occur for family members of youth diagnosed with BD because of unfamiliar responsibilities and strain. When asked to identify their primary needs, caregivers of individuals with serious psychiatric disorders identified the top three as (1) information about symptoms, (2) learning coping strategies, and (3) interacting with other caregivers and families in the same situation (Hatfield, 1979). A later study found that most families were not getting any of these needs met in their current treatment (Hatfield, 1983). Many parents report that they not only are struggling with their children's illness but are also in a struggle with their treatment providers (Mackinaw-Koons & Fristad, 2004). Additionally, parents often feel that treatment providers blame them or do not have the knowledge to treat their children. Overall, caregivers report struggling with stigma, isolation, financial strain, guilt, blame, physical illness, worry about the future, care for their high-needs child, advocating for their child at school, and exhaustion (Hellander, Sisson, & Fristad, 2003).

Youth are still dependent on their families; therefore, for treatment to be successful long term, interventions must occur at the family level (Kowatch et al., 2005). Treatment can help children and families learn about symptoms and coping mechanisms, increase treatment adherence, and decrease symptomatology. Literature on interventions for BD in adults, unipolar depression in children, and anger management for children suggests that two specific family-based treatment components may be critical in psychosocial treatment for youth with BD. These components are information sharing with family members and skill development in children and parents to manage symptoms, in part via improved family communication and problem solving (Lofthouse & Fristad, 2004). Through this process, the overall family climate may improve.

A developmental psychopathology perspective provides a theoretical framework for understanding the disorder and its treatment. The perspective utilizes a systems approach that relies on family, social, biological, and cultural factors to explain and predict the development of psychiatric illness. In line with this perspective, psychoeducational psychotherapy integrates methods to educate individuals with severe psychiatric disorders and their families, with the objective of increasing knowledge and changing attitudes about psychiatric disorders and its treatment (Lukens & McFarlane, 2004). The term *psychoeducation* has been applied to education and intervention efforts that vary widely in intensity. We have chosen to use the term *psychoeducational psychotherapy* to differentiate interventions that provide psychoeducation and therapy from simpler, short-term, educational efforts, which have also been termed "psychoeducation" by some in the field. Examples of short-term psychoeducation include providing information about an illness and its treatment to a patient through a brochure, book, television program, DVD, or website. In contrast, psychoeducational psychotherapy is a more intensive, longer term treatment that combines education with individual, group, and/or family therapy linked to the educational material provided. This approach integrates providing knowledge about mental illness with teaching strategies to address the unique challenges faced by an individual or family in coping with a disorder. Psychoeducational psychotherapy aids families in applying the knowledge gained to their real-life experiences.

This chapter explores the developmental psychopathology perspective on pediatric BD and psychoeducational psychotherapy. Specifically, three areas are reviewed. First, the developmental psychopathology perspective is explained in relation to BD. Second, psychoeducational psychotherapy is reviewed and its compatibility with a developmental psychopathology perspective for pediatric BD is considered. Finally, two formats of psychoeducational psychotherapy developed for and tested in youth with BD—multi-family psychoeducational psychotherapy (MF-PEP) and individual family psychoeducational psychotherapy (IF-PEP)—are described in detail.

A Developmental Psychopathology Perspective on Pediatric Bipolar Disorder

Developmental psychopathology is a perspective commonly used in psychology to explain the occurrence and course of behavioral and emotional disorders originating in childhood. The perspective provides a general template for understanding the processes underlying the emergence of psychopathology in children, how psychopathology changes over time, and how psychopathology is influenced by developmental context and the capacities of the child (Cicchetti & Richters, 1993). According to this perspective, an understanding of the child's history and past experiences is essential for decoding the child's current moods and behaviors, normal and abnormal. Even during ongoing changes and transformations, there is a coherence or predictability in development, both adaptive and maladaptive (Cicchetti & Toth, 1997). Developmental psychopathology relies on past and current family, social, biological, and cultural factors to explain and predict development.

Developmental psychopathologists believe a child's mood disorder symptoms and resulting impairment are a result of interactive influences that include genetic vulnerability, family distress, and life stress at different points of development (Cicchetti & Rogosch, 2002). The perspective can be used to consider the symptoms and impairment of BD over time in the context of various risk and protective factors in the social, emotional, cognitive, and biological developmental domains (Cicchetti & Rogosch, 2002; Miklowitz, 2004). Research from a developmental psychopathology perspective focuses on questions such as "What do we know about how the symptoms of BD emerge over time at different stages of development?"; "In what ways do treatments for BD need to be modified to take into account age, developmental stage, and phase of illness?"; and "What factors moderate response to treatment, and what might be some of the mediating mechanisms by which treatments operate?" (Miklowitz & Cicchetti, 2006).

In particular, the family environment of a child with BD plays a key role in this theoretical perspective and can vary considerably between families. For children in particular, the family environment can have a strong influence because families provide the primary source of structure, safety, guidance, and comfort. A protective family environment is characterized by caregivers who seek knowledge about the disorder, the likely effect of the disorder on their child, and guidance on managing symptoms (Miklowitz, Biuckians, & Richards, 2006). Additionally, families rely on outside resources such as treatment, family, and community supports. A high-risk family environment is characterized by members who engage in negative communication and have fluctuating boundaries. Negative family environments may prevent individuals suffering with mental illness from stabilizing and their families from advancing to the next developmental level (Simoneau, Miklowitz, & Saleem, 1998). Family environment is an especially important component of the developmental psychopathology perspective on youth with BD and, therefore, should play a prominent role in treatment.

Psychoeducational psychotherapy is an intervention closely aligned with the developmental psychopathology perspective of BD. The intervention content and format can be adapted for varying ages, to include parents and families, to address developmental issues and skills, and to target disorder-specific content such as symptoms, course, risk and protective factors, symptom management, and treatment.

PSYCHOEDUCATIONAL PSYCHOTHERAPY

History of Psychoeducational Psychotherapy

The passage and implementation of the Community Mental Health Act of 1963 contributed to the trend of deinstitutionalization and the development of psycho-educational interventions (Iodice & Wodarski, 1987). This act established a network of community mental health centers to decrease the number of individuals in public mental hospitals by moving them into community services. The deinstitutionalization of persons with mental illness led to incredible strain on both families and communities. Mental health facilities in the community struggled to provide services to more individuals than they had the resources to serve, often resulting in poor or no treatment (Iodice & Wodarski, 1987). Families struggled to care for their loved ones without sufficient education and training and fought against stigma and the reigning belief that blamed them for their loved one's psychiatric disorder (Miklowitz & Goldstein, 1997).

During this time of transition in the mental health system, psychoeducational interventions emerged when it became evident that knowledge about illness and treatment was needed not only by professionals but also by the individuals suffering with severe psychiatric disorders and their families. This recognition led to treatment efforts focused on educating and helping the ill individuals and their families manage symptoms. Since its development, psychoeducation has been used successfully in both the physical health and mental health fields for various illnesses and populations, including diabetes, chronic pulmonary disease, cancer, and asthma. The success of psychoeducation has led to recent national and international mandates to use psychoeducation for the treatment of schizophrenia and other mental illnesses. As success of psychoeducation has spread, the term "psychoeducation" has increasingly been used to refer to efforts that vary widely in intensity. As previously explained, we have chosen to use the term "psychoeducational psychotherapy" to differentiate interventions that provide psychoeducation and therapy from simpler, short-term educational efforts.

Clinical Description of Psychoeducational Psychotherapy

Psychoeducational psychotherapy is designed as a treatment that can stand alone or be adjunctive to medication or other treatments already in progress (Lofthouse & Fristad, 2004). Education is provided regarding diagnoses, course of illness, medication, other treatments, and symptom management. Psychoeducational psychotherapy can be delivered individually, in family sessions, or in multifamily groups. Individual psychoeducational psychotherapy consists of the diagnosed individual working one on one with a clinician to learn about diagnosis and possible treatments. Likewise, IF-PEP consists of the diagnosed family member and his or her family members working one on one with a clinician to learn more about a loved one's diagnosis and treatment. MF-PEP consists of multiple families with similar presenting problems following a standardized format of education. Table 16.1 provides a comparison of the advantages and disadvantages of MF-PEP and IF-PEP. Among adults with schizophrenia, McFarlane and colleagues (1995) found that the multifamily group format was more effective in reducing relapse rates and increasing functioning than either individual or family formats, but this comparison has not yet been tested in families of youth with mood disorders.

Although formats vary, psychoeducational interventions typically are outlined in a clinician's treatment manual and consist of sessions focused at least in part on providing education. Information is presented through formats such as lecture, discussion, video, role-playing, and homework assignments, and topics covered include diagnoses, symptom management, communication, medication,

TABLE 16.1. Comparison of Multi-Family Psychoeducational Psychotherapy and Individual-Family Psychoeducational Psychotherapy

MF-PEP	IF-PEP
Advantages	
Provides services to multiple families at once	Easy for an individual clinician to implement
Opportunity for families to develop social network of support	Limited space needed
	Gives the family privacy
Opportunity for families to identify with families who have similar struggles	Flexibility in scheduling
	Ability to tailor to individual family's needs
Opportunity to learn from other families' experiences	
Disadvantages	
May be difficult to recruit enough families for group	No opportunity to gain advice from other families
Lack of privacy and anonymity	Little opportunity for social support
Physical space needed for child and parent groups	Can only be provided to one family at a time
Multiple group leaders needed	Greater number of sessions takes more time commitment
Little flexibility to adapt content to individual needs	
Little flexibility in scheduling	
Complications with billing for two simultaneous services	

other treatments, and skill building. Psychoeducational interventions described in the literature have ranged from one to 20 sessions, each one lasting 1–2 hours. Psychoeducational psychotherapy can be easily adapted to a variety of settings, including schools, hospitals, mental health centers, and detention centers.

Psychoeducational Psychotherapy Research Findings: Adults

Psychoeducational psychotherapy was first developed for adults diagnosed with schizophrenia. Following a hospital discharge, Goldstein, Rodnick, Evans, May, and Steinberg (1978) provided adults with schizophrenia and their families with a program designed to help them understand the illness and its treatment and to prepare for future crises. This program was the first to combine neuroleptic medication and family intervention, and results revealed that the combined program was more effective than either separate intervention. Similarly, Hogarty, Anderson, Reiss, and Kornblith (1991) provided family psychoeducation to patients with schizophrenia who lived in family environments characterized by high expressed emotion (EE). After 2 years of treatment, the group of patients who received both family psychoeducation and medication had a lower relapse rate than the group who received medication only.

The effectiveness of these educational programs spurred a series of studies on the use of psychoeducational psychotherapy for schizophrenia, BD, and other adult mental health disorders. Following the success in treating schizophrenia, Miklowitz and Goldstein (1997) studied the similarities and differences in the relapse of schizophrenia and another severe psychiatric illness, BD. They developed a psychoeducational psychotherapy model for adults with BD that was similar to the one used for schizophrenia. This approach was called family-focused treatment (FFT) and was the first treatment for BD that combined medication and family intervention (Miklowitz & Goldstein, 1997). FFT is an adjunctive treatment of 21 sessions over a 9-month period with core treatment components of psychoeducation, communication skills, and problem solving. Three randomized controlled trials (RCTs) of FFT found lower relapse rates, lower mood symptoms, faster time to recovery, and better medication adherence for adults diagnosed with BD (Miklowitz, George, Richards, Simoneau, & Suddath, 2003; Miklowitz et al., 2007; Rea et al., 2003). A recent randomized trial found that FFT was also effective in improving the depressive symptoms of BD among adolescents (Miklowitz et al., 2008).

Research on psychoeducational psychotherapy for adults with BD has found reduced relapse rates in both group and individual family psychoeducation formats (Miklowitz & Goldstein, 1990; Reinares et al., 2008) and decreased EE status in families (Honig, Hofman, Rozendaal, & Deingemans, 1997). Although development of and research on psychoeducational interventions have been positive, little work has been done to translate these findings into community settings, and this gap is an important area for future study (Miklowitz & Hooley, 1998).

Psychoeducational Psychotherapy
for Children with Bipolar Disorder:
A Developmental Psychopathology Perspective

Psychoeducational psychotherapy is a viable treatment option for children with mental illness and their families. Education about specific disorders can help parents understand their children's experiences and how best to help them. Education about medications and side effects, other available treatments, and building a treatment team can promote treatment adherence and use of quality services. Studies have investigated the use of psychoeducational psychotherapy with numerous mental illnesses in youth, including anxiety disorder (Copping, Warling, Benner, & Woodside, 2001), behavioral disorders (Lopez, Toprac, Crismon, Boemer, & Baumgartner, 2005), BD (Fristad, 2006; Fristad, Verducci, Walters, & Young, 2009; Miklowitz et al., 2004, 2008; Pavuluri et al., 2004), depression (Sanford et al., 2006), and serious emotional and behavioral disturbance in general (Ruffolo, Kuhn, & Evans, 2005). The majority of these studies have been open studies rather than RCTs.

In particular, psychoeducational psychotherapy appears to be an appropriate intervention for BD in youth based on its adoption of many concepts central to the developmental psychopathology perspective of BD. The intervention has the ability to address both the developmental and the environmental contexts in order to reach positive child and family outcomes, including mood symptoms. The following sections summarize the developmental and contextual factors that psychoeducational psychotherapy addresses and explore some of these factors as potential treatment mediators of psychoeducational psychotherapy.

Developmental Context

As with any illness occurring in childhood, the developmental context of pediatric BD is an important consideration. The age or developmental stage of the children can have an impact on how BD presents and how it should be treated. If illness strikes in adulthood, patients have largely developed their sense of self, but the social-emotional and cognitive development of children and adolescents can be derailed as a result of illness. As a result, they either never develop skills or develop them later than same-aged peers. Youth suffering from BD often lag behind their peers developmentally as a function of the amount of time they have spent in episode. The longer children are in episode, the less time they have to develop successfully across all developmental milestones (Kowatch & Fristad, 2006).

For children who have been ill most of their lives, they and their family members may not even be able to distinguish personality traits from the illness (Fristad, Gavazzi, & Soldano, 1999). For example, parents may have difficulty recognizing that their child is not by nature whiny, lazy, and irritable but is actually suffering from depressive symptoms. Severely ill children often lag behind their peers in cognitive (Kowatch & Fristad, 2006) and social (Geller et al., 2000) skills, which can impair social interactions and friendships. Additionally, research has shown that BD can appear somewhat differently in children and adolescents. Adolescents tend to have more classic bipolar symptoms, whereas younger children are more likely to experience a more severe, treatment-resistant, continuous subtype (Geller & Luby, 1997).

Psychoeducational psychotherapy seeks to address these developmental issues in several ways. Children are taught age-appropriate affect regulation, problem-solving, social, and communication skills. When delivered in a multifamily group format, psychoeducational psychotherapy gives children an opportunity to interact with peers in a safe environment and to talk to other children who suffer with similar issues. The children also learn symptom management techniques, which helps them to function more successfully in settings such as at school, with peers, in their families, and in public. Helping children develop age-appropriate skills and symptom management techniques may increase their resilience in the future. Parents are taught communication, problem-solving, and symptom management skills to better help their children. Additionally, psychoeducational treatment is typically adapted to address the issues most pertinent to specific age groups. Having groups with a smaller age range also helps children relate to each other better. Separate groups may be run for different ages, and content may be presented differently in the groups to fit the cognitive and social-emotional levels of the children.

Environmental Context

Environmental factors can be risk or protective factors for the future course of pediatric BD. Youth are more dependent on their families than adults, so providing intervention and education at the family level is necessary for successful outcomes. In particular, families have influence on whether youth adhere to treatment. Between one-third and two-thirds of all youth in outpatient psychiatric clinics fail to keep their appointments (Brasic, Nadrich, & Kleinrock, 2001). The key to improving adherence may be in educating parents as well as the children about treatment and its importance. Most psychoeducational psychotherapy programs include parent sessions that provide information about medications and other types of services and treatment for children with mood disorders.

Several studies have found that a negative family environment can lead to negative child outcomes, including a slower course of recovery (Asarnow, Goldstein, Tompson, & Guthrie, 1993) and higher rates of child diagnosis (Schwartz, Dorer, Beardslee, Lavori, & Keller, 1990). In contrast, families in which the climate is supportive, open, and nonblaming can promote healthier interactions and practices, which can positively impact children's mental health. Psychoeducational psychotherapy teaches both parents and children about mood disorders, healthy communication practices, and symptom management in an attempt to improve understanding of the children's symptoms as well as overall family functioning.

The impact of mood disorders on caregivers and families can be enormous and undoubtedly contributes to the quality of family functioning and parents' ability to care for their children. Psychoeducational psychotherapy attempts to alleviate some of the stress and difficulties of caring for a child with mood disorders. This is done by focusing on the parents' feelings, struggles, and stress, which have often been neglected in pursuit of their children's treatment. The parents' own psychiatric disorder may also be influencing their children's functioning. Psychoeducational psychotherapy addresses these stresses not only by empowering parents with knowledge about their children's illness and treatment but also by promoting parent health and mental health and addressing parental needs. Parents are offered support, validation, and recognition of their own struggles (Fristad, Goldberg-Arnold, & Gavazzi, 2003).

Treatment Mediators

Because of the varied range of content presented in psychoeducational psychotherapy, several treatment mediators may ultimately impact children's mood stability. These potential mediators are specific factors that fall within the broader developmental and environmental contexts addressed in treatment. Developmental mediators may include social skills and hopelessness; environmental mediators may include expressed emotion, family concordance or agreement, knowledge of mood disorders, and quality of services utilized.

Children's Social Skills

Children and adolescents suffering from BD often have poor social skills, which can contribute to difficulty maintaining friendships and frequent teasing from peers (Geller et al., 2000). Dodge's social information processing model states that a social-behavioral response is based on encoding and interpreting information, forming social goals, deciding how to act, evaluating the effects and desirability of the actions, and enacting the chosen action (Dodge, Pettit, McClaskey, & Brown, 1986). One study found that adolescents with BD do not differ from controls on social skills knowledge but do significantly lag behind controls in social skills performance (Goldstein, Miklowitz, & Mullen, 2006). This finding suggests that whereas adolescents with BD have appropriate social skill knowledge, they have difficulty translating the knowledge into action, possibly as a result of deficits with one or more of the social information processing model components. Some programs, including MF-PEP and IF-PEP, target these components for children with BD through education about and practice of social and communication skills. As a result of treatment, improvement in social skills and relations may contribute to improvement of children's mood.

Hopelessness

A sense of hopelessness often pervades the thinking of children and adolescents who suffer from chronic illnesses such as BD. In adults with BD, research suggests that a negative cognitive style and dysfunctional attitudes may contribute to additional manic and depressive symptoms (Alloy, Reilly-Harrington, Fresco, Whitehouse, & Zechmeister, 1999). Even in remission, adults with BD maintain a negative problem-solving attitude and "hopelessness scars" (Joiner, Vohs, Rudd, Schmidt, & Pettit, 2003). A meta-analysis of 27 studies investigating the hopelessness theory in children and adolescents found that cognitive style is cross-sectionally associated with both self-reported and observer-rated clinical depression (Joiner & Wagner, 1995). A study of youth with an inpatient hospitalization found that a combination of negative cognitive style and negative life events leads to depressive symptoms (Joiner, 2000). The two formats of family psychoeducational psychotherapy described in this chapter both challenge negative assumptions using cognitive-behavioral techniques, with the expectation that decreasing hopelessness will improve children's mood symptom severity.

Expressed Emotion

EE refers to attitudes held by families regarding a family member who is mentally ill. EE can potentially contribute to the perpetuation of symptoms in the ill individual. EE is frequently studied as a treatment mediator or moderator of psychoeducational approaches. High EE refers to a critical, hostile, and overinvolved family environment, and low EE is characterized by low levels of these attributes. The concept of EE originated from a series of studies on relapse rates in adults with schizophrenia, which found that high EE among parents predicted relapse rates in adults with schizophrenia (Brown, Birley, & Wing, 1972; Brown, Carstairs, & Topping, 1958). Research has revealed that high EE also relates to poor outcomes for mood disorders in adults (Hooley, 1998; Koenig, Sachs-Ericsson, & Miklowitz, 1997; Miklowitz, Goldstein, Nuechterlein, Snyder, & Mintz, 1988; Simoneau et al., 1998) and adolescents (Miklowitz et al., 2006).

More recently, the impact of EE on youth suffering from mood disorders has been studied. In a series of reports investigating EE and its relation to childhood depression, Asarnow, Tompson, Hamilton, Goldstein, and Guthrie (1994) found that high EE in families of children with major depressive disorder is associated with a more insidious onset of the disorder (Asarnow, 1987) and a slower course of recovery (Asarnow et al., 1993). Schwartz and colleagues (1990) studied 273 high-risk mother–child pairs and found that high EE among parents was associated with three times the rate of children's diagnoses of major depression, substance abuse, and conduct disorder. When maternal criticism and paternal affective illness were present, the predicted rate of diagnosis for the adolescents was 62.3% compared with 6.5% when these factors were absent. Although the directionality of findings cannot be determined from this cross-sectional study, the association between high EE and relapse suggests that family-based interventions that teach family members about diagnoses and treatment and help to develop skills to manage symptoms may lower EE in some families in addition to decreasing symptom manifestations. Quite likely, a bidirectional relationship exists such that improvement in each area would enhance outcome in the other.

A meta-analysis of 27 adult studies found that, although EE is a general predictor of poor outcome, it can be modified (Butzlaff & Hooley, 1998). Psychoeducational psychotherapy targets EE through parent support and education (Hooley, 1998). It helps families adopt a strategy of problem-focused coping rather than emotion-focused coping, leading to improved family communication and symptom management (Sloper, 1999). Lowering EE through psychoeducational psychotherapy may lead to an improved course of illness for both the individual and his or her family. In a pilot study, parents who participated in MF-PEP reported gains in positive expressed emotion, whereas parents in a wait-list control group reported decreases in positive expressed emotion over time (Fristad, Goldberg-Arnold, & Gavazzi, 2003).

Family Concordance

Lack of concordance among caregivers or between the parent and child is relevant to family functioning and, therefore, potentially related to the child's symptom severity. Concordance can be measured by assessing how much caregivers agree with their child, their child's clinician, and their child's other caregiver about the needs of their child. A lack of agreement between caregivers in how they think about and respond to their child's problems has been linked to many negative outcomes, including higher rates of child problem behavior (Schoppe, Mangelsdorf, & Frosch, 2001), less positive child self-concepts (Lau & Pun, 1999), and lower levels of family problem solving (Vuchinich, Vuchinich, & Wood, 1993). Following a psychoeducational psychotherapy intervention, parents think about and respond to their child and his or her problems in a more uniform and positive manner (Fristad, Arnett, & Gavazzi, 1998).

Parent–child concordance is also related to family functioning. In outpatient treatment settings, one study found that 75% of the child, parent, and therapist triads began treatment without consensus on a single-focus problem, and nearly half of the triads failed to agree even on a broad problem area (Hawley & Weisz, 2003). Disagreement between parent and child on the primary focus of treatment may affect their ability to work toward and attain therapy goals (Yeh & Weisz, 2001). Parent–child concordance may also improve with family-based psychoeducational psychotherapy, such that following treatment, parental expectations of the child may become more similar, resulting in less familial/marital conflict. This healthier family climate may assist the child in managing symptoms and recovering from the current episode (Schock, Gavazzi, Fristad, & Goldberg-Arnold, 2002).

Knowledge of Mood Disorders and Treatment

The knowledge and beliefs carried by children and their families about mood disorders may directly impact children's impairment and functioning or indirectly impact functioning by changing other mediating variables such as the quality of treatment. Children with caregivers who perceive themselves as competent, knowledgeable, and efficacious function better than children of parents who feel less knowledgeable and empowered (Resendez, Quist, & Matshazi, 2000). Yeh and colleagues (2005) found that parents' beliefs about the etiology of their children's symptoms affected whether they sought services for their children. Similarly, Kerkorian, McKay, and Bannon (2006) found that parents' attitudes and beliefs about mental health treatment affected whether parents thought services were accessible to their children. Improving knowledge about mood disorders and treatment is one of the primary goals of psychoeducational psychotherapy, and the educational content is reflective of this goal with sessions about symptoms, medications and side effects, and other types of services and treatment. MF-PEP has been shown in a pilot study and in an RCT to increase parents' knowledge of mood disorders (Fristad, Goldberg-Arnold, & Gavazzi, 2003; Mendenhall, Fristad, & Early, 2009).

Quality of Other Services and Treatment

Research suggests that access and engagement in quality mental health services may be critical to positive outcomes (Weisz, Donenberg, Han, & Weiss, 1995). However, only one-quarter of children with impairing mental illness receive mental health services (Leaf et al., 1996), and it is unknown how many of those children are receiving high-quality services that meet their needs. Quality is the "degree to which health services for individuals and the population increase the likelihood of desired health outcomes and are consistent with current professional knowledge" (Lohr, 1990). The concept integrates several aspects of service utilization such as type and intensity of treatment, quality of relationship with the service provider, appropriateness of treatment for the problem, and whether the services have been shown to be effective for the specific diagnosis. Our family psychoeducational psychotherapy models seek to improve the quality of the other services by providing education about medications and treatments and building a treatment team. Examples of these other services or treatments include medication management, therapy, and school services. Improvement in the quality of the other services utilized may contribute to a reduction in mood symptom severity. For example, we found that MF-PEP leads parents to access higher quality services, and when children receive services appropriate for meeting their needs, symptom severity decreases (Mendenhall et al., 2009).

Summary

The complex, highly impairing nature of pediatric BD suggests that multifaceted treatment is necessary to improve mood symptom severity and global functioning. Treatment outcomes may be mediated by developmental factors such as the child's social skills and hopelessness or environmental factors such as EE, family concordance, quality of services utilized, and knowledge about mental illness and treatment. Psychoeducational programs in general tend to address many of these potentially mediating factors; in particular, the MF-PEP and IF-PEP interventions are designed to teach social skills and symptom management, provide hope and support, and improve knowledge about mood disorders and treatment. Psychoeducational psychotherapy programs designed for youth with BD are described next.

Psychoeducational Psychotherapy Research Findings: Children and Adolescents

Four main psychoeducational psychotherapy approaches have been developed for the treatment of BD in children and adolescents. Miklowitz and colleagues (2004) adapted FFT to create a program for adolescents ages 13–17 years with bipolar I disorder. The program is called family-focused treatment for adolescents and uses a manualized approach similar to FFT. The focus of the intervention is on psychoeducation, communication training, and problem solving. An open study with 20 adolescents and their families found a decreased level of symptoms up to 2 years later (Miklowitz et al., 2006). A multisite randomized controlled study of adolescents with BD (*n* = 58) found that FFT and medication were more effective than brief psychoeducation and medication in speeding recovery from depressive symptoms, decreasing the length of episodes, and improving the trajectory of depressive symptoms (Miklowitz et al., 2008).

Child- and family-focused cognitive-behavioral therapy (CFF-CBT), or the Rainbow Program, is the second psychoeducational psychotherapy approach developed for children ages 8–12 with BD (Pavuluri et al., 2004). Like the FFT model, treatment components include psychoeducation, family skill building, and problem solving. The Rainbow Program is an adjunctive treatment with 12 one-hour sessions. No randomized control study has yet been conducted on the Rainbow Program, but outcomes from a nonrandomized trial of 34 youth ages 5–17 were positive, with an initial decrease in symptoms and an increase in global functioning and treatment adherence (Pavuluri et al., 2004). Participation in the maintenance model of CFF-CBT was associated with positive impact on symptoms and functioning over a 3-year follow-up period (West, Henry, & Pavuluri, 2007).

MF-PEP and IF-PEP are two formats of psychoeductional psychotherapy for children with BD developed by Fristad and colleagues (Fristad & Goldberg-Arnold, 2003; see Table 16.1). MF-PEP is a psychoeducational approach designed for children with mood disorders between the ages of 8 and 12 and their parents. IF-PEP is an individualized version of MF-PEP for one-on-one use between a clinician and a family. The following section describes the MF-PEP and IF-PEP interventions, which have also been identified in past literature as Multi-Family Psychoeducation Groups and Individual Family Psychoeducation.

FAMILY PSYCHOEDUCATIONAL PSYCHOTHERAPY FOR CHILDREN WITH MOOD DISORDERS: MF-PEP AND IF-PEP

Our research group has conducted programmatic research to develop and empirically validate psychoeducational psychotherapy for children with BD. Efforts toward this end include (1) explicating the developmental adaptations necessary to adapt psychoeducation for families of children with mood disorders (Fristad, Gavazzi, Centolella, & Soldano, 1996); (2) developing therapeutic techniques to work with children with mood disorders (Fristad et al., 1999; Fristad, Davidson, & Leffler, 2006); (3) developing the manual-based MF-PEP and IF-PEP programs for families of children with BD (Fristad & Goldberg-Arnold, 2003; Goldberg-Arnold & Fristad, 2003); (4) developing and testing instruments for assessing variables relevant to this focus area (Davidson & Fristad, 2006; Gavazzi, Fristad, & Law, 1997; Sisson & Fristad, 2001); (5) implementing initial outcome studies (Fristad, Arnett, & Gavazzi, 1998; Fristad, Gavazzi, & Soldano, 1998); and (6) implementing RCTs of the programs, which are further described in this chapter (Fristad, Gavazzi, & Mackinaw-Koons, 2003; Fristad, Goldberg-Arnold, & Gavazzi, 2002, 2003).

The theoretical background and adaptations behind the development of our multifamily and individual family formats are summarized, and then a description of each intervention and its related research findings is provided. The primary outcome studied in the MF-PEP research is mood symptom severity rather than relapse, which is often used in adult literature. Children often have more chronic, unremitting symptoms and rapid cycling without periods of remission (Pavuluri, Birmaher, & Naylor, 2005). As a result, studies focusing on relapse in youth might find little significant change even if children are functionally improved, as evidenced by their decreased symptom severity. Additionally, a unified mood symptom severity measure that incorporates both depressive and manic symptoms is a more appropriate outcome because simply switching from one phase of illness to another does not represent improvement.

Theoretical Basis of MF-PEP and IF-PEP

The family-based psychoeducational psychotherapy interventions developed by our group integrate teaching families about their child's mood disorder and its treatment with training in cognitive-behavioral skills such as cognitive restructuring, mood monitoring, affect regulation skills, communication skills, and social problem-solving strategies (Fristad, Gavazzi, & Mackinaw-Koons, 2003). The guiding belief of MF-PEP and IF-PEP is that the three main components of education, support, and skill building will lead to a better understanding of the illness, which, in turn, will lead to better treatment adherence and less conflict in the family, at school, and among peers, which will lead to decreased child symptom severity and better outcomes for all.

In family psychoeducational psychotherapy, families are not blamed for the illness. Children learn how to separate themselves from their symptoms, and family members learn how to manage symptoms (Fristad et al., 1999). The intervention offers families support in their difficult role of raising children with BD by acknowledging the difficulties they face and then guiding families to seek new strategies to manage symptoms (Klaus & Fristad, 2005). In addition to learning about the illness and current treatment guidelines, parents learn symptom management techniques. These include recognizing when symptoms are interfering with the children's functioning, negative behaviors to avoid, the steps of problem solving, more effective communication strategies to use with the children, development of a safety plan, and determining how to adjust expectations. Symptom management techniques introduced to the children include building a "tool kit" of resources to use during difficult times, learning the connection among feelings, thoughts, and actions; developing effective problem-solving strategies; accurately reading nonverbal cues; and using positive communication strategies. Children may have varying preexisting levels of resiliency or developmental ability; MF-PEP and IF-PEP start at whatever level the children are at and build on it. The same techniques are used for children with varying abilities or comorbidities, but some children may need more support or scaffolding than others to be successful. This empowering and integrative approach aligns with the developmental psychopathology perspective on pediatric BD by including families in treatment, addressing developmental issues and skills, and including disorder-specific content.

Adaptation of Family Psychoeducation for Children with Mood Disorders

The first step in developing psychoeducational intervention for children was identifying the developmental and environmental adaptations necessary to adapt the available adult intervention models for youth with mood disorders (Fristad et al., 1996). Adult interventions considered in this adaptation included interventions for depressive disorder (Holder & Anderson, 1990), BD (Miklowitz & Goldstein, 1990), or any mood disorder (Clarkin, Haas, & Glick, 1988). These adaptations were necessary to ensure that MF-PEP appropriately addressed the differences in developmental abilities and context among children, adolescents, and adults. Adaptations included (1) clarifying for the children and family what is the mood disorder and what are the children's personal traits; (2) adding social skills training; (3) greater intensity of treatment and longer follow-up; (4) developmentally appropriate group content; (5) assessment and treatment of the parents for mood disorders; (6) emphasis on the importance of the home and family; and (7) addressing environmental issues, including peer relationships. These adaptations were initially tested in an open-label manner via outpatient groups (Fristad, Gavazzi, & Soldano, 1998) and a 90-minute psychoeducation workshop for parents of youth hospitalized for mental illness (Fristad, Arnett, & Gavazzi, 1998). Participants from the outpatient groups expressed satisfaction with the psychoeducation intervention, and data showed improvement in the family climate immediately following the outpatient group treatment and 4 months later (Fristad, Gavazzi, & Soldano, 1998). With the inpatient psychoeducation workshop, parents' understanding of mood disorders immediately increased (based on their completed Understanding Mood Disorders Questionnaire; Gavazzi et al., 1997). At a 4-month follow-up, parents reported increased positive EE and decreased negative EE in their homes (based on parent completion of the Expressed Emotion Adjective Checklist; Friedmann & Goldstein, 1993). Prior to the workshop, mothers had greater knowledge of mood disorders than did fathers, but afterward mothers' and fathers' knowledge was equal (Fristad, Arnett, & Gavazzi, 1998). These adaptations and pilot findings have been utilized in the further development and study of MF-PEP and IF-PEP.

Research Findings on MF-PEP

Small-Scale MF-PEP Randomized Controlled Trial

An RCT of 35 children (ages 8–11) with mood disorders and 47 of their parents was initially conducted on a six-session, 75-minutes/session format of MF-PEP (Fristad, Gavazzi, & Mackinaw-Koons, 2003; Fristad, Goldberg-Arnold, Gavazzi, 2003; Goldberg-Arnold, Fristad, & Gavazzi, 1999). Primary mood disorder diagnoses for the sample included major depressive disorder (n = 13 [37%]), dysthymic disorder (n = 6 [17%]), bipolar I disorder (n = 5 [14%]), and bipolar II disorder (n = 11 [32%]).

Eligible families were randomized by pairs to the immediate MF-PEP group (IMM; n = 18) or a 6-month wait-list control group (WLC; n = 17), and, regardless of treatment condition, all were encouraged to continue treatment as usual. Four assessments were conducted with all study participants: baseline (time 1), 2 months after study enrollment (post-MF-PEP for IMM; time 2), 6 months after study enrollment (pre-MF-PEP for WLC; time 3), and, for the WLC only, post-MF-PEP (time 4).

The IMM children reported a significant increase in perceived social support from their parents compared with WLC children and an increase in perceived social support from peers compared with WLC children, which was not statistically significant. Mood symptom severity did not decline significantly following the MF-PEP treatment, which may be a result of the small sample size or the use of the briefer version of the MF-PEP model. The IMM parents demonstrated significantly more knowledge than the WLC parents immediately after MF-PEP and at 6-month follow-up. Parents also reported significantly improved family interactions and ability to obtain appropriate services. Immediately after treatment, families most commonly reported increased knowledge as the outcome of the treatment, and fewer parents reported change in behavior or attitudes. Six months after treatment, parents still reported a gain of knowledge but also indicated improvement in family interactions and ability to obtain services.

A review of the MF-PEP treatment program was conducted after the completion of the small-scale MF-PEP RCT. Based on the feedback in the review, the following changes were made to MF-PEP: (1) The number of sessions was changed from six to eight to increase the amount of time available for practicing skill development; (2) session length was changed from 75 to 90 minutes to allow more time for discussion; and (3) utilization of family projects was increased to enhance learning and provide a method for sharing group content with non-attending family members. The current MF-PEP program is described next in further detail.

Description of MF-PEP

MF-PEP consists of eight highly formatted 90-minute sessions (Fristad, Gavazzi, & Mackinaw-Koons, 2003). Table 16.2 lists the weekly topic schedule for MF-PEP. Parents are given workbooks containing the materials presented in both the parent and child sessions. Children receive workbooks of the activities completed in their sessions as well as the projects they are expected to do between sessions. Sessions start with youth and parents together for a brief check-in; then the two groups break apart for separate lessons. At the end of each session, children rejoin their parents for a wrap-up. Parents and children receive projects to do at home between sessions to practice the skills learned in the group.

Large-Scale MF-PEP Randomized Controlled Trial

A larger National Institute of Mental Health–funded randomized controlled study of the efficacy of MF-PEP was conducted with a sample of 165 children with mood disorders and their families. Participants were recruited through presentations made by the MF-PEP principal investigator, local media, and a previously developed referral network of local mental health professionals. Recruitment of 15 families occurred every 3 months, resulting in 11 sets of 15 families. Within each set, seven families were randomized into an immediate treatment condition and eight were randomized into a 1-year WLC condition. Regardless of assigned condition, all families participated in follow-up assessments at 6, 12, and 18 months. The immediate treatment condition participated in MF-PEP between the baseline and 6-month follow-up assessments. The WLC condition participated in MF-PEP between the 12- and 18-month follow-up assessments. Regardless of treatment condition, families were encouraged to continue receiving treatment as usual

TABLE 16.2. The Weekly Topic Schedule for Multi-Family Psychoeducational Psychotherapy

Session	Parents' group	Children's group
1	Welcome to the group Overview of mood symptoms and mood disorders	Welcome to the group Overview of mood symptoms and mood disorders
2	Medications	Medications
3	Systems of care Treatment teams School services	Building a "tool kit" to manage symptoms
4	Mood disorders and the family Negative family cycles Review of first 4 weeks	Connection among thoughts, feelings, and actions Personal responsibility and choices
5	Learning and practicing problem-solving skills	Learning and practicing problem-solving skills
6	Learning and practicing communication skills	Learning and practicing nonverbal communication skills
7	Learning and practicing symptom management techniques	Learning and practicing verbal communication skills
8	Review of session topics Graduation	Review of session topics Graduation

(TAU) throughout the study. TAU refers to any treatment, such as medication or therapy, the child received other than the MF-PEP intervention.

Children's age range at study entry was 8–11 years (M = 9.9, SD = 1.3). A majority were male (73%) and white (91%). Most (70%) had a bipolar disorder spectrum diagnosis, and 30% had a depressive disorder. All had comorbid mental health diagnoses, including comorbid behavior disorder (97%) and comorbid anxiety disorder (68%).

Initial results suggest a mediated treatment relationship, as seen in the theoretical model in Figure 16.1 (Mendenhall et al., 2009). IMM parents reported significantly increased knowledge about mood disorders and changed beliefs about treatment for mood disorders compared with WLC parents over time, and these improvements were significantly related to improvement in the quality of other services utilized by these IMM families. Furthermore, IMM parents reported significantly higher quality of services utilized, and the higher quality of services utilized was significantly related to lower mood symptom severity in the children. This suggests that MF-PEP helps parents become better consumers

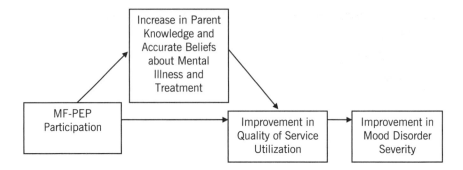

FIGURE 16.1. Theoretical relationship among multi-family psychoeducational psycho-therapy (MF-PEP), service utilization, and mood disorder severity.

of the mental health system, leading them to access higher quality services. Consequently, when children receive services appropriate for meeting their needs, symptom severity decreases. The success of MF-PEP suggests a state of equifinality; even though each family has a distinctively different history, they benefit from gaining the same knowledge and learning the same illness management strategies.

Individual Family Psychoeducational Psychotherapy

Description of IF-PEP

Several transportability issues emerged with the implementation of MF-PEP (Fristad, 2006). First, community-based treatment settings are often not conducive to group interventions, especially for children with low base rate diagnoses. There may not be enough children with severe mood disorders in these community settings to form a group of families to participate in MF-PEP. Second, some families are uncomfortable with sharing personal information in a group and would rather work privately with a clinician. In small, close-knit communities, families may worry about personal information being spread by group members to their workplaces or their children's schools. Third, families with a newly diagnosed child may want education immediately and prefer to not wait for the start of the next MF-PEP group. IF-PEP was developed as an individualized version of MF-PEP to address these transportability issues.

The original version of IF-PEP had sixteen 50-minute sessions, which alternated between parent-only sessions and child sessions, with parent check-in and check-out segments. Fifteen of the sessions focused on specific issues of BD, and the other session was an "in the bank" session for use at anytime to deal with crises or to review material. A Healthy Habits unit, which was not included as a specific unit in MF-PEP, was added to IF-PEP to address areas of importance for mood stabilization and for managing medication side effects and included sleep hygiene, eating practices, and exercise routines. These topics were discussed in MF-PEP but never as the primary focus of any particular session.

Small-Scale Wait-List Controlled Trial of IF-PEP

A pilot study of 20 children with BD and their parents was conducted to examine the efficacy of IF-PEP (Fristad, 2006). The majority of the children were male (85%) and white (90%). The children's primary diagnoses were bipolar I disorder (40%), bipolar II disorder (35%), and BD not otherwise specified (25%). Most of the youth had comorbid diagnoses; 95% had behavior disorders and 70% had anxiety disorders.

The families completed a baseline assessment, after which study eligibility was determined in a case review. Eligible participants were randomized into the immediate IF-PEP plus TAU condition or to a WLC plus TAU condition. The immediate group received the IF-PEP treatment following the baseline assessment and afterward completed follow-up assessments 6, 12, and 18 months after study entry. The WLC group received the IF-PEP treatment between the 12-month and 18-month follow-up assessments.

Results from this pilot study suggest positive outcomes for IF-PEP (Fristad, 2006). The children's mood symptom severity improved immediately following completion of treatment, with gains continuing to manifest 12 months later in the immediate treatment group. Although improvements were also observed in the WLC group, the rate of improvement was greater in the immediate treatment group. For the immediate treatment condition, families reported a significantly more positive change in family climate than the WLC condition. Treatment utilization by the families in both groups improved as well but to a nonsignificant degree. The improvements in mood severity, family climate, and treatment utilization were most pronounced for the immediate treatment group at 12-month follow-up, suggesting that changes resulting from IF-PEP may take longer than changes resulting from MF-PEP.

Expanded 24-Session IF-PEP

Following the pilot study, a review of the initial IF-PEP treatment program was conducted (Fristad, 2006). As with MF-PEP, several changes were made to IF-PEP. First, the number of IF-PEP sessions was increased from 16 to 24, which matches the amount of therapist face time that families receive in MF-PEP. The adapted IF-PEP has 20 scripted sessions and four in-the-bank sessions. New sessions include a review of symptoms and diagnoses for the parent and child, additional sessions to learn about mental health services and school services, Healthy Habits, a session for school professionals, and a session addressing sibling issues. Results of a pilot study on this extended 24-session IF-PEP program indicate that mood symptoms improved after treatment (Leffler, Klaus, & Fristad, in press), and that families find the session format acceptable (Davidson & Fristad, 2008).

Summary

Positive outcomes in the development and study of MF-PEP and IF-PEP suggest that the combination of education, support, and skill building is an effective blend for treating children with BD and their families. The interventions successfully target several potential mediating developmental and environmental factors that may impact treatment outcomes. Clinical trials indicate that family psychoeducational psychotherapy results in increased knowledge of mood disorders, improved treatment beliefs, enhanced family climate, improved treatment utilization, and decreased mood symptom severity. MF-PEP and IF-PEP each offer unique advantages and disadvantages. An empirical study comparing the cost-effectiveness, adherence to treatment, and improvement following treatment of the two approaches has not yet been conducted.

Psychoeducation and Translational Research

Once interventions have been shown to be efficacious, the next step is to test their effectiveness when implemented in a community setting. Unfortunately, the step of bridging the gap from RCTs of manualized psychotherapies to the use of manualized treatments in nonacademic mental health settings presents many challenges and often is not successfully accomplished (Kendall & Beidas, 2007). Two interrelated considerations for the successful translation of interventions for community settings are (1) community therapists' attitudes and experiences, which play a role in their willingness to implement an evidence-based treatment and refer children to it (Barlow, Levitt, & Bufka, 1999), and (2) working with practitioners to implement the program with "flexibility within fidelity" (Kendall & Beidas, 2007).

MF-PEP is currently being translated for broader use in the community. An effectiveness study is being conducted to evaluate whether MF-PEP outcomes are the same in community mental health settings as in a university medical center research setting for children with mood disorders and their families. The pilot study is evaluating child and family outcomes as well as perspectives from the children, families, treating therapists, and referring therapists about the dissemination and implementation of the intervention. The MF-PEP framework and components of the intervention are also being used to develop psychoeducational psychotherapy for youth with autism spectrum disorders.

CONCLUSIONS

The complexity of pediatric BD necessitates a treatment approach that addresses both the developmental and environmental contexts of the developmental psychopathology perspective. Psychoeducational psychotherapy addresses these important areas through education about symptoms and treatment; by training in social, communication, and problem-solving skills; and by providing encouragement and support. By addressing mediating factors such as children's social skill level, family climate, knowledge of mood disorders and treatment, and quality of treatments utilized, psychoeducational psychotherapy can lead to positive outcomes for children and their families.

Future directions for research in this area include investigation at multiple levels of analysis of other factors that may impact the effectiveness of IF-PEP and MF-PEP. Additional factors other than knowledge, quality of services, or symptoms may change in children and their families as a result of participation in psychoeducational psychotherapy. Further research may be able to uncover these mediating or moderating factors. For example, the ability of children or parents to form protective, supportive relationships outside the family may improve as they interact with other families in the safe, caring environment of MF-PEP. Parents' own mental health may stabilize as they become more knowledgeable about mental illness and the importance of self-care, which could lead to more effective parenting and lower expressed emotion in the home. As parents' acceptance of their child's illness increases with the intervention, their parenting styles may become more flexible and effective, and they may be better able to handle stigma and adversity. For the children, participation in the interventions may improve self-esteem and the ability to cope with highly critical environments as they learn more about their illness and how to manage it.

Many potential factors may moderate the impact of MF-PEP or IF-PEP. For example, families who are socially isolated prior to treatment may benefit more from the group dynamics of MF-PEP compared with families with an established social network. IF-PEP may be more appropriate for families in which contentious divorce issues are prominent. Also, the format of IF-PEP may be more beneficial for a child with a history of good friendships, whereas a child with more impaired social skills may benefit more from the social interactions available in MF-PEP.

Another step in testing these psychoeducational psychotherapy interventions may be to compare the individual family and multifamily formats with each other or with other forms of therapy using a design such as randomized parallel groups. This design may reveal that these approaches have different mediating mechanisms such as therapeutic relationship or group cohesiveness. Other forms of therapy that can be compared with psychoeducational psychotherapy are a basic short-term psychoeducation program, social skills groups, individual or group CBT, and pharmacotherapy. Regardless, promising psychoeducational psychotherapy interventions for youth with BD have been developed in research settings, but further efforts need to be made to test these interventions and translate them for use in community settings.

ACKNOWLEDGMENT

This chapter was written with the support of National Institute of Mental Health Grant Nos. R01MH061512 and R01MH073801.

REFERENCES

Alloy, L. B., Reilly-Harrington, N., Fresco, D. M., Whitehouse, W. G., & Zechmeister, J. S. (1999). Cognitive styles and life events in subsyndromal unipolar and bipolar disorders: Stability and prospective prediction of depressive and hypomanic mood swings. *Journal of Cognitive Psychotherapy, 13,* 21–40.

Asarnow, J. R., Goldstein, M. J., Tompson, M., & Guthrie, D. (1993). One-year outcomes of depressive disorders in child psychiatric in-patients: Evaluation of the prognostic power of a brief measure of expressed emotion. *Journal of Child Psychology and Psychiatry and Allied Disciplines, 34,* 129–137.

Asarnow, J. R., Tompson, M., Hamilton, E. B., Goldstein, M. J., & Guthrie, D. (1994). Family-expressed emotion, childhood-onset depression, and childhood-onset schizophrenia spectrum disorders: Is expressed emotion a nonspecific correlate of child psychopathology or a specific risk factor for depression? *Journal of Abnormal Child Psychology, 22,* 129–146.

Asarnow, R. F. (1987). The interaction between family transactions and individual differences in the attentional processes of schizophrenic patients. In K. Hahlweg & M. J. Goldstein (Eds.), *Understanding major mental disorder: The contribution of family interaction research* (pp. 91–102). New York: Family Process Press.

Barlow, D. H., Levitt, J. T., & Bufka, L. F. (1999). The dissemination of empirically supported treatments: A view to the future. *Behaviour Research and Therapy, 37,* S147–S162.

Brasic, J., Nadrich, R., & Kleinrock, S. (2001). Do families comply with child and adolescent psychopharmacology? *Child and Adolescent Psychopharmacology News, 6*(2), 6–10.

Brown, G. W., Birley, J. L., & Wing, J. K. (1972). Influence of family life on course of schizophrenic disorders: A replication. *British Journal of Psychiatry, 121,* 241–258.

Brown, G. W., Carstairs, G. M., & Topping, G. (1958). Post hospital adjustment of chronic mental patients. *Lancet, ii,* 685–689.

Butzlaff, R. L., & Hooley, J. M. (1998). Expressed emotion and psychiatric relapse: A meta-analysis. *Archives of General Psychiatry, 55,* 547–552.

Cicchetti, D., & Richters, J. E. (1993). Developmental considerations in the investigation of conduct disorder. *Development and Psychopathology, 5,* 331–344.

Cicchetti, D., & Rogosch, F. A. (2002). A developmental psychopathology perspective on adolescence. *Journal of Consulting and Clinical Psychology, 70,* 6–20.

Cicchetti, D., & Toth, S. L. (1997). Transactional ecological systems in developmental psychopathology. In S. S. Luthar, J. A. Burack, D. Cicchetti, & J. R. Weisz (Eds.), *Developmental psychopathology: Perspectives on adjustment, risk, and disorder* (pp. 317–349). Cambridge, UK: Cambridge University Press.

Clarkin, J. F., Haas, G. L., & Glick, I. D. (1988). *Affective disorders and the family: Assessment and treatment.* New York: Guilford Press.

Copping, V. E., Warling, D. L., Benner, D. G., & Woodside, D. W. (2001). A child trauma treatment pilot study. *Journal of Child and Family Studies, 10,* 467–475.

Davidson, K. H., & Fristad, M. A. (2008). Psychoeducation psychotherapy. In B. Geller & M. P. DelBello (Eds.), *Treatment of bipolar disorder in children and adolescents* (pp. 184–204). New York: Guilford Press.

Dodge, K. A., Pettit, G. S., McClaskey, C. L., & Brown, M. (1986). Social competence in children. *Monographs of the Society for Research in Child Development, 51,* 1–85.

Friedmann, M. S., & Goldstein, M. J. (1993). Relatives' awareness of their own expressed emotion as measured by a self-report adjective checklist. *Family Process, 32,* 459–471.

Fristad, M. A. (2006). Psychoeducational treatment for school-aged children with bipolar disorder. *Development and Psychopathology, 18,* 1289–1306.

Fristad, M. A., Arnett, M. M., & Gavazzi, S. M. (1998). The impact of psychoeducational workshops on families of mood-disordered children. *Family Therapy, 25*, 151–159.

Fristad, M. A., Davidson, K. H., & Leffler, J. M. (2006). Thinking–feeling–doing: A therapeutic technique for children with bipolar disorder and their parents. *Journal of Family Psychotherapy, 18*(4), 81–103.

Fristad, M. A., Gavazzi, S. M., Centolella, D. M., & Soldano, K. W. (1996). Psychoeducation: A promising intervention strategy for families of children and adolescents with mood disorders. *Contemporary Family Therapy, 18*, 371–384.

Fristad, M. A., Gavazzi, S. M., & Mackinaw-Koons, B. (2003). Family psychoeducation: An adjunctive intervention for children with bipolar disorder. *Biological Psychiatry, 53*, 1000–1008.

Fristad, M. A., Gavazzi, S. M., & Soldano, K. W. (1998). Multi-family psychoeducation groups for childhood mood disorders: Program description and preliminary data. *Contemporary Family Therapy, 20*, 385–402.

Fristad, M. A., Gavazzi, S. M., & Soldano, K. W. (1999). Naming the enemy: Learning to differentiate mood disorder "symptoms" from the "self" that experiences them. *Journal of Family Psychotherapy, 10*, 81–88.

Fristad, M. A., & Goldberg-Arnold, J. S. (2003). Family interventions for early-onset bipolar disorder. In B. Geller & M.P. DelBello (Eds.), *Bipolar disorder in childhood and early adolescence* (pp. 295–313). New York: Guilford Press.

Fristad, M. A., Goldberg-Arnold, J. S., & Gavazzi, S. M. (2003). Multifamily psychoeducation groups (MFPG) in the treatment of children with mood disorders. *Journal of Marital and Family Therapy, 29*, 491–504.

Fistad, M. A., Goldberg-Arnold, J. S., & Gavazzi, S. M. (2002). Multifamily psychoeducation groups (MFPG) for families of children with bipolar disorder. *Bipolar Disorders, 4*(4), 254–262.

Fristad, M. A., Verducci, J. S., Walters, K., & Young, M. E. (2009). Impact of multi-family psychoeducational psychotherapy in treating children aged 8 to 12 with mood disorders. *Archives of General Psychiatry, 66*(9), 1013–1021.

Gavazzi, S. M., Fristad, M. A., & Law, J. C. (1997). The Understanding Mood Disorders Questionnaire. *Psychological Reports, 81*(1), 172–174.

Geller, B., Bolhofner, K., Craney, J., Williams, M., DelBello, M. P., & Gundersen, K. (2000). Psychosocial functioning in a prepubertal and early adolescent bipolar disorder phenotype. *Journal of the American Academy of Child and Adolescent Psychiatry, 39*, 1543–1548.

Geller, B., & Luby, J. (1997). Child and adolescent bipolar disorder: A review of the past 10 years. *Journal of the American Academy of Child and Adolescent Psychiatry, 36*, 1168–1176.

Goldberg-Arnold, J. S., & Fristad, M. A. (2003). Psychotherapy for children with bipolar disorder. In B. Geller & M. P. DelBello (Eds.), *Bipolar disorder in childhood and early adolescence* (pp. 272–294). New York: Guilford Press.

Goldberg-Arnold, J. S., Fristad, M. A., & Gavazzi, S. M. (1999). Family psychoeducation: Giving caregivers what they want and need. *Family Relations, 48*, 411–417.

Goldstein, M. J., Rodnick, E. H., Evans, J. R., May, P. R., & Steinberg, M. (1978). Drug and family therapy in the aftercare of acute schizophrenics. *Archives of General Psychiatry, 35*, 1169–1177.

Goldstein, T. R., Miklowitz, D. J., & Mullen, K. L. (2006). Social skills knowledge and performance among adolescents with bipolar disorder. *Bipolar Disorders, 8*(4), 350–361.

Hatfield, A. B. (1983). What families want of family therapists. In W. R. McFarlane (Ed.), *Family therapy in schizophrenia* (pp. 41–65). New York: Guilford Press.

Hatfield, A. B. (1979). Help-seeking behavior in families of schizophrenics. *American Journal of Community Psychology, 7*(5), 563–569.

Hawley, K. M., & Weisz, J. R. (2003). Child, parent and therapist (dis)agreement on target problems in outpatient therapy: The therapist's dilemma and its implications. *Journal of Consulting and Clinical Psychology, 71*(1), 62–70.

Hellander, M., Sisson, D. P., & Fristad, M. A. (2003). Internet support for parents of children with early-onset bipolar disorder. In B. Geller & M. P. DelBello (Eds.), *Bipolar disorder in childhood and early adolescence* (pp. 314–329). New York: Guilford Press.

Hogarty, G. E., Anderson, C. M., Reiss, D. J., & Kornblith, S. J. (1991). Family psychoeducation, social skills training, and maintenance chemotherapy in the aftercare treatment of schizophrenia: II. Two-year effects of a controlled study on relapse and adjustment. *Archives of General Psychiatry, 48,* 340–347.

Holder, D., & Anderson, C. (1990). Psychoeducational family intervention for depressed patients and their families. In G. I. Keitner (Ed.), *Depression and families: Impact and treatment* (pp. 159–184). Washington, DC: American Psychiatric Press.

Honig, A., Hofman, A., Rozendaal, N., & Deingemans, P. (1997). Psychoeducation in bipolar disorder: Effect on expressed emotion. *Psychiatry Research, 72,* 17–22.

Hooley, J. M. (1998). Expressed emotion and psychiatric illness: From empirical data to clinical practice. *Behavior Therapy, 29,* 631–646.

Iodice, J. D., & Wodarski, J. S. (1987). Aftercare treatment for schizophrenics living at home. *Social Work, 32*(2), 122–128.

Joiner, T. E. (2000). A test of the hopelessness theory of depression in youth psychiatric inpatients. *Journal of Clinical Child Psychology, 29,* 167–176.

Joiner, T. E., Vohs, K. D., Rudd, M. D., Schmidt, N. B., & Pettit, J. W. (2003). Problem-solving and cognitive scars in mood and anxiety disorders: The sting of mania. *Journal of Social and Clinical Psychology, 22,* 192–212.

Joiner, T. E., & Wagner, K. D. (1995). Attribution style and depression in children and adolescents: A meta-analytic review. *Clinical Psychology Review, 15,* 777–798.

Kendall, P., & Beidas, R. (2007). Smoothing the trail for dissemination of evidence-based practices for youth: Flexibility within fidelity. *Professional Psychology: Research and Practice, 28,* 13–20.

Kerkorian, D., McKay, M., & Bannon, W. M. (2006). Seeking help a second time: Parents'/caregivers' characterizations of previous experiences with mental health services for their children and perceptions of barriers to future use. *American Journal of Orthopsychiatry, 76*(2), 161–166.

Klaus, N., & Fristad, M. A. (2005). Family psychoeducation as a valuable adjunctive intervention for children with bipolar disorder. *Directions in Psychiatry, 25,* 217–230.

Koenig, J. E., Sachs-Ericsson, N., & Miklowitz, D. J. (1997). How do psychiatric patients experience interactions with their relatives? *Journal of Family Psychology, 11,* 251–256.

Kowatch, R. A., & Fristad, M. A. (2006). Bipolar disorders. In M. Hersen, J. C. Thomas, & R. T. Ammerman (Eds.), *Comprehensive handbook of personality and psychopathology: Child psychopathology* (pp. 217–232). Hoboken, NJ: Wiley.

Kowatch, R. A., Fristad, M. A., Birmaher, B., Wagner, K. D., Findling, R., Hellander, M., et al. (2005). Treatment guidelines for children and adolescents with bipolar disorder. *Journal of the American Academy of Child and Adolescent Psychiatry, 44,* 213–235.

Lau, S., & Pun, K.-L. (1999). Parental evaluations and their agreement: Relationship with children's self-concepts. *Social Behavior and Personality, 27*(6), 639–650.

Leaf, P. J., Alegria, M., Cohen, P., Goodman, S. H., Horwitz, S. M., Hoven, C. W., et al. (1996). Mental health service use in the community and schools: Results from the four community MECA study. *Journal of the American Academy of Child and Adolescent Psychiatry,* *35,* 889–897.

Leffler, J. M., Klaus, N. M., & Fristad, M. A. (in press). Adaptation and extension of individual-family psychoeducational psychotherapy (IF-PEP) for children with bipolar disorder: A case study. *Journal of Family Psychotherapy.*

Lofthouse, N., & Fristad, M. (2004). Psychosocial interventions for children with early-onset bipolar spectrum disorder. *Clinical Child and Family Psychology Review, 7,* 71–88.

Lohr, K. N. (1990). *Medicare: A strategy for quality assurance.* Washington, DC: National Academy Press.

Lopez, M. A., Toprac, M. G., Crismon, M. L., Boemer, C., & Baumgartner, J. (2005). A psychoeducational program for children with ADHD or depression and their families: Results from the CMAP feasibility study. *Community Mental Health Journal, 41,* 51–66.

Lukens, E. P., & McFarlane, W. R. (2004). Psychoeducation as evidence-based practice: Considerations for practice, research and policy. *Brief Treatment and Crisis Intervention, 4,* 205–225.

Mackinaw-Koons, B., & Fristad, M. A. (2004). Children with bipolar disorder: How to break down barriers and work effectively together. *Professional Psychology: Research and Practice, 35,* 481–484.

McFarlane, W. R., Lukens, E., Link, B., Dushay, R., Deakins, S. A., Newmark, M., et al. (1995). Multiple-family groups and psychoeducation in the treatment of schizophrenia. *Archives of General Psychiatry, 52,* 679–687.

Mendenhall, A. N., Fristad, M. A., & Early, T. J. (2009). Factors influencing service utilization and mood symptom severity in children with mood disorders: Effects of multifamily psychoeducation groups (MFPG). *Journal of Consulting and Clinical Psychology, 77,* 463–473.

Miklowitz, D. J. (2004). The role of family systems in severe and recurrent psychiatric disorders: A developmental psychopathology view. *Development and Psychopathology, 16,* 667–688.

Miklowitz, D. J., Axelson, D. A., Birmaher, B., George, E. L., Taylor, D. O., Schneck, C. D., et al. (2008). Family-focused treatment for adolescents with bipolar disorder: Results of a 2-year randomized trial. *Archives of General Psychiatry, 65*(9), 1053–1061.

Miklowitz, D. J., Biuckians, A., & Richards, J. A. (2006). Early-onset bipolar disorder: A family treatment perspective. *Development and Psychopathology, 18,* 1247–1265.

Miklowitz, D. J., & Cicchetti, D. (2006). Toward a life span developmental psychopathology perspective on bipolar disorder. *Development and Psychopathology, 18,* 935–938.

Miklowitz, D. J., George, E. L., Axelson, D. A., Kim, E. Y., Birmaher, B., Schneck, C., et al. (2004). Family-focused treatment for adolescents with bipolar disorder. *Journal of Affective Disorders, 82S,* S113–S128.

Miklowitz, D. J., George, E. L., Richards, J. A., Simoneau, T. L., & Suddath, R. L. (2003). A randomized study of family-focused psychoeducation and pharmacotherapy in the outpatient management of bipolar disorder. *Archives of General Psychiatry, 60,* 904–912.

Miklowitz, D. J., & Goldstein, M. J. (1990). Behavioral family treatment for patients with bipolar affective disorder. *Behavior Modification, 14,* 457–489.

Miklowitz, D. J., & Goldstein, M. J. (1997). *Bipolar disorder: A family-focused treatment approach.* New York: Guilford Press.

Miklowitz, D. J., Goldstein, M. J., Nuechterlein, K. H., Snyder, K. S., & Mintz, J. (1988). Family factors and course of bipolar affective disorder. *Archives of General Psychiatry, 45,* 225–231.

Miklowitz, D. J., & Hooley, J. M. (1998). Developing family psychoeducational treatment for patients with bipolar and other severe psychiatric disorders: A pathway from basic research to clinical trials. *Journal of Marital and Family Therapy, 24*, 419–435.

Miklowitz, D. J., Otto, M. W., Frank, E., Reilly-Harrington, N. A., Wisniewski, S. R., Kogan, J. N., et al. (2007). Psychosocial treatments for bipolar depression: A 1-year randomized trial from the Systematic Treatment Enhancement Program. *Archives of General Psychiatry, 64*(4), 419–427.

Pavuluri, M. N., Birmaher, B., & Naylor, M. W. (2005). Pediatric bipolar disorder: A review of the past 10 years. *Journal of the American Academy of Child and Adolescent Psychiatry, 44*, 846–871.

Pavuluri, M. N., Graczyk, P. A., Henry, D. B., Carbray, J. A., Heidenreich, J., & Miklowitz, D. J. (2004). Child- and family-focused cognitive-behavioral therapy for pediatric bipolar disorder: Development and preliminary results. *Journal of the American Academy of Child and Adolescent Psychiatry, 43*, 528–537.

Quackenbush, D., Kutcher, S., Robertson, H. A., & Boulos, C. (1996). Premorbid and post-morbid school functioning in bipolar adolescents: Description and suggested academic interventions. *Canadian Journal of Psychiatry, 41*(1), 16–22.

Rea, M. M., Tompson, M. C., Miklowitz, D. J., Goldstein, M. J., Hwang, S., & Mintz, J. (2003). Family-focused treatment versus individual treatment for bipolar disorder: Results of a randomized clinical trial. *Journal of Consulting and Clinical Psychology, 71*(3), 482–492.

Reinares, M., Colom, F., Sánchez-Moreno, J., Torrent, C., Martínez-Arán, A., Comes, M., et al. (2008). Impact of caregiver group psychoeducation on the course and outcome of bipolar patients in remission: A randomized controlled trial. *Bipolar Disorders, 10*(4), 511–519.

Resendez, M. G., Quist, R. M., & Matshazi, D. G. M. (2000). A longitudinal analysis of family empowerment and client outcomes. *Journal of Child and Family Studies, 9*(4), 449–460.

Ruffolo, M. C., Kuhn, M. T., & Evans, M. E. (2005). Support, empowerment, and education: A study of multifamily group psychoeducation. *Journal of Emotional and Behavioral Disorders, 13*, 200–212.

Sanford, M., Boyle, M., McCleary, L., Miller, J., Steele, M., Duku, E., et al. (2006). A pilot study of adjunctive family psychoeducation in adolescent major depression: Feasibility and treatment effect. *Journal of the American Academy of Child and Adolescent Psychiatry, 45*, 386–395.

Schock, A. M., Gavazzi, S. M., Fristad, M. A., & Goldberg-Arnold, J. S. (2002). The role of father participation in the treatment of childhood mood disorders. *Family Relations: Interdisciplinary Journal of Applied Family Studies, 51*, 230–237.

Schoppe, S. J., Mangelsdorf, S. C., & Frosch, C. A. (2001). Coparenting, family process, and family structure: Implications for preschoolers' externalizing behavior problems. *Journal of Family Psychology, 15*, 526–545.

Schwartz, C. E., Dorer, D. J., Beardslee, W. R., Lavori, P. W., & Keller, M. B. (1990). Maternal expressed emotion and paternal affective disorder: Risk for childhood depressive disorder, substance abuse or conduct disorder. *Journal of Psychiatric Research, 24*, 231–250.

Simoneau, T. L., Miklowitz, D. J., & Saleem, R. (1998). Expressed emotion and interactional patterns in the families of bipolar patients. *Journal of Abnormal Psychology, 107*, 497–507.

Sisson, D. P., & Fristad, M. A. (2001). A survey of stress and support for parents of children with early-onset bipolar disorder. *Bipolar Disorders, 3*, 58.

Sloper, P. (1999). Models of service support for parents of disabled children. What do we know? What do we need to know? *Child: Care, Health, and Development, 25*, 85–99.

Vuchinich, S., Vuchinich, R., & Wood, B. (1993). The interparental relationship and family problem solving with preadolescent males. *Child Development, 64*, 1389–1400.

Weisz, J. R., Donenberg, G. R., Han, S. S., & Weiss, B. (1995). Bridging the gap between laboratory and clinic in child and adolescent psychotherapy. *Journal of Consulting and Clinical
Psychology, 63*, 688–701.

West, A. E., Henry, D. B., & Pavuluri, M. N. (2007). Maintenance model of integrated psychosocial treatment in pediatric bipolar disorder: A pilot feasibility study. *Journal of the
American Academy of Child and Adolescent Psychiatry, 46*(2), 205–212.

Yeh, M., McCabe, K., Hough, R., Lau, A., Fakhry, F., & Garland, A. (2005). Why bother with
beliefs?: Examining relationships between race/ethnicity, parental beliefs about causes of
child problems and mental health service use. *Journal of Consulting and Clinical Psychology, 73*, 800–807.

Yeh, M., & Weisz, J. R. (2001). Why are we here at the clinic?: Parent–child (dis)agreement on
referral problems at outpatient treatment entry. *Journal of Consulting and Clinical Psychology, 69*, 1018–1025.

PART V

A First-Person Account

CHAPTER 17

Growing Up in a Family
with Bipolar Disorder

Personal Experience, Developmental Lessons,
and Overcoming Stigma

Stephen P. Hinshaw

M y aims in this chapter are, by design, different from those in the other, more research-based entries in this volume. Whereas the preceding chapters utilize the best of current science to inform readers about assessment, diagnosis, etiology, and mechanisms related to bipolar disorder, as well as evidence-based prevention and treatment strategies, this chapter focuses on personal and family experience. Specifically, I describe the life of my father, a philosopher, who had his first episode of severe, lifelong bipolar disorder at age 16—misdiagnosed for the next 40 years as schizophrenia—and of my emerging reactions to both the silence that surrounded my childhood with regard to his condition and the disclosures he began to make to me as I attained young adulthood. All of these issues are described at book length elsewhere (Hinshaw, 2002; see also Hinshaw, 2004), so my goal here is to provide a cogent yet vivid summary. In addition, I hope to illuminate a number of themes related to the narrative of my father's life and to my growing up in a home with this level of psychopathology. Most of these issues (e.g., multiple risk factors for bipolar disorder, implications of adolescent-onset conditions for ultimate self-concept, effects on the family system, the importance of accurate diagnosis, the possibility of resilience, silence and communication within family systems, and stigma) have major developmental undercurrents. My ultimate hope is that the current qualitative material can help the next generation of investigators and clinicians to address key developmental questions related to etiology, maintenance, prevention, and treatment of the important, fascinating, and devastating condition known as bipolar disorder.

In all, this work is related to my growing conviction that the more that people in the mental health professions—clinicians, teachers, and scientists alike—tell their personal and family experiences of mental illness and relate raw clinical narrative material with evidence-based discovery, the less the entire topic will be infused with silence, suffering, and stigma and the greater the chances for a fundamental shift in public attitudes and responses (see Hinshaw, 2008a). Indeed, narrative accounts can convey to scholars and scientists a sense of the right questions to ask in future investigations of mechanisms, developmental course, and intervention; they can also inform policymakers of directions for key future initiatives related to bipolar disorder in particular and mental illness in general. So, with the objective of "telling my story" in the service of pressing for ever more accurate science and ever more responsive intervention, I begin my narrative.

A SINGULAR LIFE

Early Years

My father, Virgil Hinshaw, Jr., was born in November 1919, the fourth of four boys, in the town of LaGrange, Illinois, outside of Chicago. His father, Virgil Sr., was chairman of the Prohibition National Party of the United States from 1912 to 1924, whose greatest achievement—the passage of the 18th Amendment (the Prohibition Amendment)—occurred in the year of my father's birth. His wife, my father's mother, Eva Piltz Hinshaw, was a missionary. The three older brothers were between 1½ to 7 years older than Junior, as he was known. The family was quite religious, with a strong sense of Quaker ideals; they were a dedicated and active group.

Before he turned 3½, however, my father lost his beloved mother, who died in 1923 during surgery for an ovarian tumor. Distraught, my grandfather moved his group of four boys out West, finally settling in Pasadena, California. His letters at the time (he was an inveterate letter writer throughout his life) commented on his own sadness at seeing the attempts of the older boys at night to console his smallest son, little Junior, who tearfully grieved for his mother.

My grandfather remarried several years later, and his second wife was also a missionary. They had two more boys, my father's half-brothers. Among the six boys, however, my dad's stepmother singled Junior out for special treatment, in the form of both strong praise for his academic, athletic, and church-related accomplishments and special punishment for even minor infractions. In fact, as my father wrote in his personal journals many years later, he came to realize that her treatment of him became abusive. For example, he was made to wait, for an hour or two, in her room for the switchings and strappings that she administered with respect to his having violated even small household rules. She sometimes eased his subsequent pain by massaging him with oil, a practice that came to take on a sexual flavor as he neared adolescence. I comment later on my father's (1) early loss of his mother and (2) abusive treatment at the hands of his stepmother as potential risk factors for his subsequent serious mood disturbance, exacerbating his undoubted genetic vulnerability (i.e., several clear cases of depression and bipolar disorder, as well as suicides, exist through several generations of my paternal family). Certainly, his memories of waiting for severe punishment suffused his mind, and he wrote many years later that this experience was quite similar to the feelings he had when he was committed to mental hospitals: The sense of waiting for degradation and for deserved punishments over something he must have done wrong, knowing that the punishment would be extremely severe.

Adolescence and Young Adulthood

The home was a center of intellectual, athletic, and political activity. The six boys were a verbal and competitive group. Prohibition-oriented international leaders sometimes visited the family home in Pasadena during the early-to-mid 1930s, particularly once the U.S. experiment in Prohibition ended, discussing policies related to alcohol as well as the international political scene, increasingly marked by world depression and the growth of fascism in Europe. My father, a precocious student and a follower of history, began to take to heed of these discussions, wondering about the gravity of the world situation. Still, he played sports (football, shot put), studied hard, and took to heart his Sunday school and church lessons. He was popular, intelligent, and hard working.

At age 16, however, during the summer before his junior year in high school, he became preoccupied by thoughts of world domination by the Nazis and other fascist groups, the words of the international visitors resonating in his mind. At the end of the summer, he began a period of several days essentially without sleep, with growing agitation and grandiosity. He quickly became convinced of two ideas: first, that he could fly; and second, that his flight would send a message to world leaders that Hitler and fascism must be stopped. In clinical language, he escalated from experiencing ideas of reference (specialized meanings attributed to everyday events) to frank delusions, which had both paranoid and grandiose flavors. Fueled by his agitation, activity, obsessionality, and lack of sleep, he was fast escalating through the stages of a severe manic episode (Carlson & Goodwin, 1973), which was tinged with depressive themes.

On a September morning, following a night of wandering the streets, he returned to the family home (fortunately, a low-slung bungalow), ascended to the roof, and jumped, again with the delusional belief that his flight would send the all-important message of stopping fascism to world leaders. He crashed to the walkway below, emerging with a broken wrist but no other physical injuries.

He was taken to the huge Los Angeles County Hospital by his startled family, who had emerged from the house, wondering where he had been. Two weeks later, he was sent to a nearby public mental hospital in Norwalk, where he was treated by being chained to his bed, with a diagnosis of schizophrenia. Intriguingly, one psychiatrist gave a presumptive diagnosis of manic-depressive psychosis, but the consensus diagnosis was schizophrenia, as it was for much of the past century in the United States for any patients displaying psychotic symptoms (for discussion of these diagnostic practices, see Hinshaw, 2002).

He remained there for nearly 6 months, initially with delusions of grandeur ("celestial voices singing all night long," as he wrote in his journal years later) but subsequently with far more paranoid ideas, such as the belief that the hospital food was poisoned. As a result, during the fall he plummeted from a weight of nearly 180 to 121 pounds, becoming so malnourished that his life was threatened. The superintendent called in my grandfather to speak of the strong probability that his son would not pull through; the staff was convinced that he would starve to death.

Somehow, however, with no medication and no psychological treatment, my father regained his rationality and began to eat. He longed to be released in time for Christmas, but his symptoms were still severe. Several months later, he emerged with a return to euthymic, rational functioning. At that point, in March, he was released to start 11th grade, half a year late, without any pharmacological treatment (no true psychotropic medications existed at that time), any psychotherapy, or any psychoeducational discharge plans. Yet by June he had earned straight As for the entire academic year, making up quickly for lost time.

His family scarcely knew what to believe: How could their beloved, athletic, talented son and brother have plunged so quickly into madness, in the form of schizophrenia, and have come so near death—and then recovered, apparently in full, with almost equal speed? My father's next older brother, Robert, who had seen Junior sprawled on the walkway beneath the family home, told me decades later that he had decided then and there to go into the mental health professions, subsequently becoming both a psychologist and psychiatrist and assisting my father through a number of subsequent, severe episodes. The next oldest, Randall, who became an internationally renowned economist, was a source of comfort and compassion to my father for many years to come.

Back at home and proceeding with his high school and junior college career as though the 6-month span were a nightmare, my father was class valedictorian and entered Stanford University, where he received a bachelor's degree in philosophy and psychology. He was clearly attracted to "big ideas" about the mind and the world as well as the hidden mechanisms underlying our species' mysterious existence in the universe. Although the United States had now entered World War II, my father did not join the military, a joint consequence of the family's Quaker, pacifist leanings and his 4-F classification resulting from his lengthy bout with mental illness. He went on to earn a master's degree in philosophy at Iowa and then a doctorate in philosophy at Princeton University, sole-authoring several erudite publications related to epistemology and theory of knowledge during his graduate school days.

He had incredible experiences at Princeton. Early in his career he attended weekly, one-on-one meetings with the visiting Bertrand Russell for a term, and he later came to know Albert Einstein, contributing a chapter on Einstein's social and moral philosophy to an edited volume on the great physicist. Yet despite his strong academic accomplishments and heady company, shortly after completing his dissertation in early 1945, my father again ended up in a mental hospital following another period of agitation, paranoia, and psychosis. The loss of his girlfriend appeared to be a real trigger. Furthermore, the completion of a doctorate, which would usually be thought of as a positive event, may have signaled the transition to adult responsibilities and, therefore, served as an instigating event as well (for a review of the effects of psychosocial stressors on illness course, see Johnson, 2005).

This time he was hospitalized at the infamous Philadelphia State Hospital, known as Byberry and soon to become the subject of the late 1940s book and film, *The Snake Pit*. It was considered to be the worst mental hospital in the United States (Grob, 1994). While there, my father was beaten by fellow inmates. Sometime in the late spring, his older brother Randall, working as an economist for the government in Washington, DC, got a gas ration card and headed to Philadelphia to take his beloved brother out of the hospital on a day pass for a drive.

Reporting to me over 40 years later, Randall said that Virgil immediately shocked him by translating the road signs into German. "What are you doing, Junior?" he asked. "I'm being held in a concentration camp in Europe," my father immediately replied, stating that they should soon return, lest the guards notice. Startled, Randall tried to convince him otherwise, but to no avail. Although my father's statement reveals a clear delusion, perhaps he knew at some level that Hitler's avowed goals were to rid the earth not only of Jews but also of gay and lesbian individuals, Gypsies, those with mental retardation, and those suffering from mental illness. Moreover, the conditions at Philadelphia State were truly horrendous; the conditions he described were all too real.

By the summer my father again fully recovered—his chief treatment had been several rounds of insulin coma therapy—and he was released by late July. He returned to California to work and apply for academic positions. With his strong academic record, he received a number of offers and accepted a position at Ohio State University, moving to Columbus in 1946, beginning a career of 49 years that spanned the titles of instructor, assistant professor, associate professor, and full professor. He had been trained in modern philosophical methods, such as formal logic, but was widely knowledgeable about all aspects of the field. He became known as a brilliant scholar and galvanizing teacher.

Professorship, Marriage, Family—and Severe Episodes

He met my mother, a graduate student in history, on a blind date; they fell in love, getting married in 1950. As my mother later told me, however, her husband-to-be disclosed extremely little about his history of episodes, stating only that he had

"had some problems" in high school and at Princeton. In those days of silence and stigma, he said no more than he deemed necessary about a diagnosis of schizophrenia and having been warehoused in mental hospitals.

It was during her pregnancies with me and then my sister, in the early 1950s, that my mother learned firsthand about her husband's condition. When I was born, my father was symptomatic but at least present; when my sister was born, he was in a mental hospital. Indeed, during that decade he experienced several severe bouts of full mania, with the "mixed" features of manic-level energy, paranoia, grandiosity, irrationality, and sporadic bouts of extremely irritable, depressive mood. He was hospitalized not only in Columbus but also in California, with his brother Robert periodically needing to come to the Midwest and escort my father back to facilities out West. Only his tenured status at Ohio State allowed him to retain his professorship once he returned to campus, many months after an episode had begun.

He received Thorazine as early as 1954, the year of its introduction into the United States, one of the first patients in this country to be prescribed this, the first antipsychotic medication. He also received electroconvulsive therapy, in a day and age of long-pulse, bilateral currents. Some of these latter treatments led to severe memory loss, as my mother recounted to me years later: She recalled helping her disoriented husband, back home from the hospital, as he struggled to remember the names of the neighbors, despite his superior academic abilities and qualifications. Indeed, through her heroic efforts (performed with almost no support from the mental health system), the family remained intact.

Yet between episodes, my father was caring and loving at home, showing patience and sensitivity. Here is a remembrance I have from my kindergarten year, exemplifying some of my father's key qualities (Hinshaw, 2002, pp. 52–53):

> At age five, however, I have a . . . worry . . . about a fact that I have learned. I cannot now recall where I learned of this fact—perhaps on television, perhaps in a book or almanac. It must be true, given that I had seen or heard it, but I cannot seem to comprehend it.
>
> I walk downstairs to the basement of our first house, the colonial-style home across the river from campus. My father's study is there, always cool and musty in its basement location. His books—the many books on philosophy, history, arts, math—line the walls. The books give a reddish-brown tint to the room, smelling faintly of the dampness of the basement. They signify, to me, how much there is to learn. Although the study has a makeshift feel, with cinderblocks serving as many of the bookshelves, it is my father's sanctuary.
>
> He is reading, writing notes on a yellow legal pad, using his fountain pen, his elegant strokes filling the page. I ask to interrupt, as the fact I have learned is bothering me. Ever patient, he smiles at me and asks what I need.
>
> I tell him that I can't understand something I've heard and read. He must sense the puzzlement on my face. "What could that be?" he gently inquires.
>
> "Well, it says that Russia is the biggest country on earth in land"—by this, I mean in area—"and I think that this must be right. But they also say that

China has more people than Russia, a bigger population. Is that really true? How could it be?" Clearly, the concept is beyond my comprehension.

My father explains that yes, it is actually true. He begins to discuss how more people could crowd together in a smaller area. I can't quite hear his explanation, however, because another, even more pressing question has now entered my mind, which I must ask before he has finished.

"If it's true," I interrupt, "then how many more people live in China than Russia?" I am searching for some way to quantify this incredible state of affairs.

"A great many more," my father replies, pausing for me to take this in.

I think for a while, then dare to ask the most puzzling question of all: "Could there be a *hundred* more people living in China than in Russia?"

With infinite patience and without a hint of bemusement, he responds gently: "Son, I know that this will be hard to believe, but there are actually *more* than 100 more people living in China than Russia."

My amazement has peaked, and I try to absorb this onslaught of information.

Overall, it is a blatant stereotype to contend that people with severe mental illness are never fit to be parents. This vignette is one of many that reflect my father's patience and sensitivity. Laws that deny parental rights to individuals with mental illnesses are not only discriminatory but also potentially extremely counterproductive for the entire family (see Hinshaw, 2007).

What did my sister and I know of any of the difficult events of this time period? Nothing, because my father's doctors had told him quite clearly during the 1950s: "Never tell your children about mental illness—they can't understand." So my parents did their best to hide the worst of my father's destructive episodes. And when he was away, nothing was said. During my third-grade year, for example, my father was hospitalized in the West for a period of 1 year. I recall asking my mother where Daddy was, but all she could say was that "Daddy is resting in California." With no more information forthcoming, I learned not to ask any more questions. One day during the summer before fourth grade, without fanfare or any special notice, he returned, and life resumed pretty much as it had before—my sister's and my work at school and playing sports and my Dad's return to the classroom. By now, however, my mother had returned for additional graduate education and resumed a career. As she later told me, no one knew when the next episode might come. As noted in later sections of this chapter, evidence now documents the value of clear communication within families in which a parent has a mood disorder.

Going against Medical Advice: Disclosure

During the 1960s, following my father's longest episode, he was free of severe mood swings for some years. With hindsight, I can recall periods of flatness and low energy, as well as periods of excitement and energy but without disappearances for hospitalization. I still knew nothing about my Dad's history and psychological functioning.

Through middle school and junior high school, I became immersed in my studies and in various sports, fueling my denial of my Dad's prior absences and the hints, from certain behavior patterns, of his underlying problems. Yet I had also become interested in psychology. I did not realize, as I headed East for college, that my father was making a monumental decision: To go against medical advice and begin to tell me of his life. So during my first spring break back in Columbus, he called me into his study one afternoon, closed the door, and initiated our first open talk—of Pasadena, world fascism, mental hospitalization, and his diagnosis of schizophrenia. For the next 25 years, until his passing, we continued our discussions several times per year.

I had a host of emotions as he started his disclosures: sadness, concern, and fright, to be sure, but also a sense that I was at last hearing the truth and that I had always been waiting to hear what had really happened during those silences and those absences. Even so, my college years were a mixture of new learning and real anxiety. I worried, for example, about staying up too late: Would 1, like my father, not be able to shut off my thinking? Would I go crazy, needing to be sent to a mental hospital? Periodically during adolescence, I had severe migraine headaches (a history I share with my father and many other relatives); when the pain was unrelenting, I would vomit uncontrollably. I now came to believe that the only way I could deal with the fears of not sleeping and relaxing, and the deeper fears of what might lie underneath my controlled life, was to make myself physically sick to my stomach, recapitulating the relief from a migraine. It took a number of years before I realized that I could simply let go and relax and that sleep would come without resorting to such self-punishment.

At the same time, I continued my growing interest in psychology. I volunteered as a Big Brother to two young boys, themselves brothers, throughout college; I taught in a Massachusetts prison; and I became part of a community mental health center therapeutic team, making home visits to an adolescent who had not spoken outside the family home and working with the psychiatrist, psychologist, and social worker who were the team's professionals. After graduation, when I directed a residential camp for developmentally delayed children in New Hampshire and coordinated a school program in Boston for youth who could not "make it" in Boston public school classrooms, I continued to read more about severe mental illness and came to the conclusion that my father did not have schizophrenia but rather manic-depressive illness, or bipolar disorder. Visiting my uncle Robert out in California, who had dedicated his life to mental health after experiencing his brother's near demise, I triggered the generation of a new diagnosis 40 years after my father's initial misdiagnosis. In short order, his doctor back in Ohio initiated treatment with lithium rather than antipsychotic medications, which he had been receiving for over 20 years.

Despite this rediagnosis (and despite his intensive reading about bipolar disorder), my father's self-image remained, at a deep level, fixated as that of a flawed "psychotic," an inmate of mental hospitals. As we continued our discussions and he began to show me his most intimate journals, I came to realize that he still felt as he had when a boy, waiting for the inevitable punishments at the hands of his stepmother for real or imagined misdeeds. As I discuss later, when adolescence is shaken by severe mental illness of psychotic proportions that is accompanied by punitive, inhumane treatment, deep alterations in one's core identity are bound to ensue.

My Own Adulthood—and My Father's Final Years

Pursuing a doctorate in clinical psychology at the University of California, Los Angeles (UCLA), I continued to add to my knowledge of psychopathology, psychopharmacology, research design, and child behavior disorders. As an intern at UCLA's Neuropsychiatric Institute, I took a rotation in the Affective Disorders Clinic, directed by Kay Redfield Jamison, who supervised me and with whom I have continued important contact over the years. Through her erudite seminars, I came to learn of the history of misdiagnosis of many thousands of Americans during the 20th century as well as the shift in thinking related to the viability of bipolar disorder as a diagnostic category. Although I began to sense that my father's story had broad implications, I had internalized the stance of silence imposed on my family years earlier, telling almost no one about my father's life and tribulations. I simply didn't know how to talk about it and feared the responses of anyone I might tell.

Gradually, however, as a post-doc and assistant professor, I opened up to the idea of talking with more and more people (and eventually a far wider audience) about my Dad's story as well as my own. I also decided to have children, something I thought during my 20s that I should simply not do, given my nascent knowledge of the heritability of bipolar disorder and my still-rampant fears of family "contamination."

As a progressive, Parkinson-like illness came to take over my father's later years, we talked even more deeply and he showed me all of his most personal journals and writings. Finally, in the last year of his life, I secured his blessing in writing an account of his experiences. In the years following his death in 1995 at the age of 75, I worked and reworked my manuscript about his life and became further interested in disclosure, narrative, and stigma, supplementing my more "mainstream" interests in developmental psychopathology, clinical trials, and longitudinal studies of youth with attention problems and related disorders. Today I find that my teaching, research, clinical supervision, and general interests are far more integrated than ever before, given that my disclosure (as well as the resultant connections with many thousands of people interested in the topic) has deepened my sense of commitment to and love of the entire field of psychology. In many respects, my passion for my work has only intensified as I have come to understand more clearly the deep roots of my interests in children, development, and mental illness.

Given space limitations, there is much that I have had to omit about my father's life and my responses to it. In the remaining sections of this chapter, I hope to illuminate a number of themes and lessons related to this brief narrative, beginning with key developmental processes and issues and concluding with several core themes related to developmental psychopathology, including diagnostic accuracy, resilience, family experiences of mental illness, and stigma. In so doing, I will add some additional details of events that both my father and I experienced.

DEVELOPMENTAL CONSIDERATIONS

In this section I deal with several interrelated questions: What are the important developmental themes and issues exemplified by my father's life with bipolar illness, including potential risk factors for his psychiatric problems, the role of his severe psychoses and brutal hospitalizations on his adult-self image, and his abilities as a parent? What are the parallel developmental themes related to my having grown up in the family I did—in utter silence—only to learn of key issues related to my father's condition after I had left home? How do the concepts of internalization and parentification fit into this picture? What are the consequences of having a genetic legacy of serious mental illness for a child in such a family, and how can individuals in such families and homes deal with the risk and the promise of "loaded" family histories? These queries and more inform the following pages.

Issues Related to the Individual with Bipolar Disorder

Risk Factors

Although it is abundantly clear that individual case studies often include idiosyncratic, uncontrolled variables that may not apply to other cases or that might be spurious, my father's life history may still prove heuristic. It certainly exemplifies the truism that multiple risk variables are at work in serious instances of psychopathology (e.g., Goodwin & Jamison, 2007). In the first place, many members of my father's family have shown high professional attainment in terms of academic, artistic, and business success; yet many others, across multiple generations, have evidenced high risk for psychiatric illness in terms of mood, anxiety, and eating disorders. (In my stepgrandmother's side of the family, schizophrenia-spectrum conditions are more prevalent; see Hinshaw, 2002, 2004.) Yet at this point the field still does not know the precise genetic risks for bipolar disorder, and it is a major mistake to think that there is a single gene responsible for any of the major psychiatric conditions (Kendler, 2005). Thus, despite the strongly heritable nature of manic-depressive illness (see Goodwin & Jamison, 2007), the surge of research in gene × environment interplay across many areas of psychiatric disturbance (see reviews in Beauchaine, Hinshaw, & Gatzke-Kopp, 2008; Rutter, Moffitt, &

Caspi, 2006) suggests that there may well be environmental factors that moderate (via gene × environment interaction) and mediate (via gene–environment correlation) the undoubted genetic vulnerability for this condition (Goodwin & Jamison, 2007).

Related to such factors, in my father's case I can point to the loss of his mother when he was 3 years of age and the abusive treatment he received at the hands of his stepmother. First, early loss of a parent is certainly a risk factor for later mood disturbance, but even more important is the quality of the caregiving that exists following the loss (e.g., Maier & Lachman, 2000). Second, maltreatment has clearly been established as a risk factor for a variety of negative outcomes, mediated by such processes as neurobiological insult, hostile attribution biases, and decreased emotion recognition and emotion regulatory capabilities (see Cicchetti & Valentino, 2006). In terms of bipolar disorder per se, there is no compelling evidence that maltreatment is a sole causal factor, yet the presence of abuse in persons with vulnerability to bipolar illness predicts a particularly pernicious course (Post, Leverich, Xing, & Weiss, 2001; see also Garno, Goldberg, Ramirez, & Ritzler, 2005; Neria, Bromet, Carlson, & Naz, 2005). At the very least, whether or not it propelled the episodes themselves, my father's experiences of waiting for severe, imminent punishments shaped his worldview about expected degradation for moral flaws—and contributed to his view that something he had done wrong must have led to his hospitalizations.

Several key concepts from developmental psychopathology are relevant to this discussion. The search for causal factors for bipolar disorder forces consideration of *multiple levels of analysis*, ranging from molecular processes at the level of genes and neurons to mechanisms more related to personal, family-related, and social factors (see Cicchetti, 2008). Indeed, the "holy grail" for much current work in psychopathology involves understanding the linkages between and among genes, gene products, temperament and other building blocks of personality, child-rearing and other socialization practices, self-organization, peer relationships, neighborhood and community-level processes, and transmission of cultural beliefs—to name several of the most salient levels—in creating both normal-range and disordered functioning. My father's experiences also bring to life core constructs pertinent to developmental trajectories, including *multifinality*, the branching into differentiated outcomes from similar initial conditions or risk factors, and *equifinality*, the progression into a similar outcome from variegated vulnerabilities, pathways, or trajectories (Cicchetti, 2006; Hinshaw, 2008c). That is, family history and genetic vulnerability may or may not yield frank psychopathology, depending on a host of mitigating (or exacerbating) psychobiological and psychosocial influences; and it is extremely likely that a variety of processes may lead to the outcome of bipolar spectrum disorders in different individuals. The more the field gains understanding of psychopathology, the more we come to realize that (1) the categories of disturbance to which people are assigned are not static entities but rather dynamic conceptualizations and (2) reciprocal, transactional processes as well as variegated developmental trajectories characterize normal as well as atypical functioning (Hinshaw, 2008b, 2008c; Jensen, Hoagwood, & Zitner, 2006).

Implications of Adolescent Pathology for Self-Perceptions and Ultimate Self-Image

By all indications, my father's premorbid adjustment as a child and early adolescent was healthy. He was an intelligent, athletic, and spiritually minded boy who thrived in school and on the playing field even if he was succumbing to severe punishments at home and even if he was, at times, a bit tempestuous and headstrong. For example, he wrote in his journals about a time in first grade when he was confronted with a substitute teacher. He had been acting "smart" in the classroom, leading the teacher to call attention to his brash attitude. Climbing high on top of a desk, he quickly retorted: "Well, if you don't like my attitude, how about my altitude?" Unfortunately, the school reported this incident to my father's family, leading to a severe punishment from his stepmother.

Still, nothing led him or his family to prepare for his monumental escalation through the stages of mania at age 16, replete with grandiosity, paranoia, and psychosis and resulting in a devastating hospitalization—and the near loss of his life from jumping from the roof of his home and his refusal to eat for many weeks while hospitalized. It is difficult to imagine how individuals and family members alike readjust to such drastic changes of behavior and overall functioning. In addition, all members of the family system must now contend with a psychiatric label, the stigma of being a "mental patient," and the shift to viewing the individual in question as carrying a deep and fundamental flaw lying at the core of his or her being.

Note that there is major debate today about the nature of child-onset bipolar disorder and its chronic, ultrarapid, or ultradian cycling nature (Blader & Carlson, 2008; Geller et al., 1998; see also other chapters in the current volume). In cases with childhood onset, which often include impulsive, aggressive, and emotionally dysregulated symptoms from an early age, identity may well form around themes of chronic instability and the need for special education or restrictive placements. Yet in the case of the more classic presentation that my father displayed, with mid- to late-adolescent onset following a childhood and adolescence marked by high functioning, the contrasts between such strong performance and utter devastation are likely to present a huge challenge for the maintenance of any stability of subsequent self-perceptions.

Overall, given the major adolescent task of consolidating a core identity, which is linked to a number of underlying cognitive, emotional, and social processes (Harter, 2006), the repercussions of a major breakdown of contact with reality—and of dehumanizing, punitive "treatment" in the back ward of a mental hospital—can only be expected to be devastating during this phase of life. Even after my father returned to high levels of functioning between episodes, he retained a belief that his core self was flawed, tainted, and deserving of punishment. And even in his latter years, with his newly gained diagnosis of bipolar disorder replacing his four-decade-old label of schizophrenia, he viewed himself as "a psychotic," an individual whose foundation was forever eroded by his delusions, his sense of difference, his underlying despair at ever being able to communicate his experiences, and his treatment as subhuman by fellow inmates and staff (Hinshaw, 2002). All of the "book learning" he undertook at this late phase of his life regarding the biological, heritable nature of bipolar disorder did little to sway this fundamental self-perception. As for the treatments we currently administer and develop for the future, it will be essential that youth are given humane and compassionate care, with the best of evidence-based medicine and therapy, so that the overwhelming emotions they experience as a result of their bipolar condition are not magnified by a sense of difference, unworthiness, and hopelessness related to negative experiences in treatment. Social support, especially from interactions with others who have been through and successfully coped with bipolar disorder, could well be a major countervailing force along these lines.

Issues for Spouses and Family Members

Family members are the unsung heroes in a large proportion of cases of severe mental illness. Typically vilified by mental health professionals, who believed until recent decades that families were the causal agents for mental disorder in terms of faulty parenting and socialization practices, relatives must cope with shame, financial hardship, time away from work, demeaning responses from professionals, and other types of severe burden (Lefley, 1989; Struening et al., 2001; Wahl, 1999; see also Hinshaw, 2007). But we often don't consider the lengths to which family members must go in order to cope with the incomprehensibility of serious mental illness (for a compelling volume, see Tessler & Gamache, 2000; for recent evidence on family burden in relation to bipolar disorder, see Perlick et al., 2007).

As an example, in the late 1950s, when I was about 4 years of age and my sister not quite 3, an incident occurred on an autumn evening. Quoting from *The Years of Silence Are Past*, the book I wrote about my father's life:

> My mother has seen the signs before, over the past few years: A particular glint in her husband's eye, a too-ready smile, a penchant for nonstop talking, a different level of energy. A sure sign is his playing, at volumes far too loud, religious choral music on the phonograph. At these times it feels to her that a chemical change is overtaking him, although she gets nowhere when she tries to tell any doctors of this intuition. She knows what is bound to ensue with him: grand plans, sleeplessness, irritability, increasing irrationality, and paranoia, soon followed by utter disorganization. On some occasions, he has required hospitalization, and she is left with taking care of the household and the children, having to "cover" in front of friends and relatives. No one has really dwelled on it, but the term schizophrenia has floated in the air. When his episodes are over, however, they are really over, as mysteriously as they had begun. He acts

as though nothing has happened, without discussion. Silence lingers between the couple.

Back to the fall evening: The hour is getting late, as it is now after 10:00 P.M. A popular variety show is on the television, broadcast from Cincinnati, 100 miles away from Columbus. An attractive female singer is singing on a variety show. My father has seen her on this program before, but tonight it is different: He has become obsessed with her. He believes, in fact, that her lyrics are communicating messages to him. He needs to see her, to continue the communication in person. It is urgent.

For a week or more, his behavior has been escalating, increasingly energetic, enthusiastic, bombastic. My mother's worry increases daily: Where will it stop this time?

Growing even more excited and agitated with the show, my father contends that they must drive to Cincinnati to find the singer, so that he can respond to her messages. The idea takes complete hold of him; he can't let it go.

My mother is terrified: to Cincinnati, in the car, at this time of night? She knows better than to try and talk him out of such a plan when he has reached this state, as his anger will escalate. So should she let him drive off—and perhaps learn of a fatal accident the next day, given his growing impatience and irrationality? Or should she accompany him to Cincinnati . . . but then what of the children? There is no reasoning with him; he must leave. Thinking fast, she decides to go along, fighting her terror that the children may awaken in the night with no one to look after them.

One last thought: Could she call anyone at this late hour? Even if she did, what would she say? And there's no opportunity to wait for someone to arrive, given her husband's impatience and force. What can she do? Maybe her presence will somehow contain him.

They head for the family car, a 1956 Ford Victoria with a strong engine, and tear off in a southwesterly direction. The interstate highway system does not yet exist, and the roads are mostly two-lane highways. Yet he drives frightfully fast, possessed of his need. At speeds of over 90 miles per hour, they fly through the night. Does she dare allow herself too many thoughts of the children, asleep at home?

Somehow they arrive in Cincinnati after 11:30 P.M., managing to find the TV station from which the show had originated, its huge broadcasting tower providing a beacon. Almost as if in a dream—but if this is a dream, it's fast becoming a nightmare—my father insists on leaving the car to enter the station and find the singer. My mother fears for an ugly confrontation at the front desk. Fortunately, the hour is late enough that the gates are locked.

She struggles to maintain composure, concentrating on reining him in. Will he try to jump the fence? She talks simply and rationally, convincing him that the singer has left and that there is no use in staying. His internal struggle is apparent, but finally he relents, suddenly eager to return home. They roar back onto the highway. She can't believe the speedometer. What if a highway patrolman were to pull them over, with her husband in his state? Will there be a physical confrontation? Will they end up in jail? What will happen when the children awaken?

Luck is with them, however, and they make it back to Columbus safely by the wee hours of the morning, racing over the rolling hills of Southern Ohio as they flatten out into the farmland plains of Central Ohio. She can't believe it; they are back in the driveway at home. Heart in her throat, she rushes upstairs to find the two children still asleep in their beds, oblivious to the disruption and absence. Her heart begins to slow, but the terror hasn't left. How long can this last? she wonders, relieved, terrified, wishing for some rest. What is next? (Hinshaw, 2002, pp. 10–13)

How can we understand the terror that my mother felt—indeed, the terror and utter confusion that far too many parents, spouses, and offspring experience in the wake of irrational symptoms and impossible situations? What was the correct choice: to leave her children and try to head off her husband's demise, or to stay with my sister and me and learn, the following day, that her husband would never return? If we can appreciate the additional complexities that arise when no viable communication exists within a family and when professionals encourage silence, then we are forced to realize that the types of family burden experienced in relation to mental illness are multiplied immeasurably when shame and stigma are added to the mix (Hinshaw, 2007; see also further discussion of stigma later in the chapter).

In the case of bipolar disorder, despite the strong heritability of this condition, evidence reveals that family attitudes, including conflict and hostile emotion, are related to negative outcomes (Du Rochler Schuldich, Youngstrom, Calabrese, & Findling, 2008; Kim & Miklowitz, 2004; see also Simoneau, Miklowitz, & Saleem, 1998). Clearly, genetic vulnerability can be exacerbated by difficult family reactions, which are understandable given the severity of the symptoms and impairments related to this condition. Thus, as explained in the section on family intervention, procedures that can help increase understanding and communication and reduce conflict may well be helpful for optimal prognosis.

Parenting Abilities of Individuals with Serious Mental Illness

Less than a year after the incident just described, when I was in kindergarten and my father was again well, he showed great sensitivity as I pondered my 5-year-old questions about geography and populations (see earlier excerpt). When I was in fourth grade, following his return from a year away, he comforted me at night when I could not sleep, coming from my parents' bedroom to tell me that my fears of illness and dying could be remedied by the miracles of modern medicine (indeed, perhaps he wondered whether similar miracles could ever help his own mental problems). He immediately soothed me by stating that I would probably live to be 100 years of age because of such medical miracles; the number of 100, which had figured so prominently in my kindergarten amazement over the populations of Russia and China, seemed once again mysterious and healing. And in high school, he intervened with sensitivity and impact during a critical period when I believed I had made a terrible decision that caused me great despair.

In short, it is a myth to believe that individuals with severe mental illness cannot be sensitive, caring parents. Certainly, during the throes of psychosis or in the depths of a suicidal depression—or when substance abuse is added to the mix, as it so often is with mood disorders—parenting is inevitably compromised, and children require protection and adequate caregiving from the alternate parent or other supports. Yet the assumption that a diagnosis of bipolar disorder automatically disqualifies an adult from any rights to being a parent, or that "mentally ill parents" are, by definition, unable to provide support to their children, is simply false. (For a review of restrictive and discriminatory state legislation related to child custody as well as other domains, see Corrigan, Markowitz, & Watson, 2004; Corrigan et al., 2005.) It is essential to break stereotypes, which are themselves a key component of stigmatizing responses, and tell the real-life stories, both good and bad, about what mental illness is really like, and the ways in which individuals and families who cope with mental disorder can maintain a number of important life roles, especially when the condition is recognized and when adequate treatment and support are forthcoming (Hinshaw, 2007).

The Child in a "Bipolar Family System"

Several important questions from a family perspective are as follows: How did I respond to my Dad's episodes (which were almost entirely hidden from me) and from the doctor-ordered silence about his absences and hospitalizations? What are the consequences if a child does, in fact, witness disruptive, psychotic behavior? As a late adolescent, how did I integrate my new knowledge about his life into my identity, my sense of myself and my family, and my life goals?

Silence, Internalization, and Parentification

My father's doctors, operating via the ignorance and stigma of the time, clearly believed that keeping a child in silence about parental disruption and parental absences related to mental disorder would be optimal, given that children "can't understand mental illness," in their words. But what are the consequences of silence? When children realize that conflict is occurring but have no real explanation for it, they are likely to blame themselves, internalizing the conflict and disruption (see review in Hinshaw, 2004). On the face of it, this strategy seems maladaptive, even self-destructive. Yet it may be far better to hold oneself responsible for negative events than to either blame the person on whom one depends for love and support or, alternatively, to believe that the world is simply a cruel, heartless, random place.

As for me, I adopted a typically midwestern style of silent coping, using academics and athletics as means of keeping myself focused. Nonetheless, I was lonely, and there was simply no one to talk with about my fears, doubts, and insecurities. In addition, even as a child I had a high need for control and carried a strong sense of responsibility. I had become somewhat parentified, meaning that I took on an adult-style identity, although not to the extent of some youth from highly chaotic families or who have been sexually abused, who are prone to behave essentially in adult, parental roles from early ages (for discussion, see Byng-Hall, 2008; Peris & Emery, 2005).

In terms of my denial and my family's silence: Even during high school, when it had become quite clear that my father was in partial hospitalization during my senior year, my involvement in sports and studies essentially blinded me to this fact. So when he began his revelations to me once I was at Harvard and returning home for vacations, his words were the truth that I had always needed to hear. Over the many years since that time, I have gradually been able to relinquish some of my tight control and come to terms with being part of a family with both high promise and high risk.

Responses to Disclosure

Still, as noted in the beginning narrative of this chapter, his words engendered considerable anxiety in me during my college days. I now had a secret myself and one that I dared not tell roommates, teammates, or girlfriends. What would it mean to say that my father was a mental patient, with schizophrenia—and that I may well be at risk myself? Silence breeds silence, and I kept private my father's conversations with me.

Most striking were the fears that I would have at night, especially the fear that if I stayed up too late and couldn't sleep, I might lose control of my mind. Although I was learning psychology, the knowledge base I got in college with respect to clinical psychology was thin indeed with respect to modern differential diagnosis of schizophrenia versus bipolar disorder. And the academic learning I was doing was no match for the gnawing sense I had that my own hold on control and rationality could be tenuous. It took more than a year beyond college to come to terms with the fact that I didn't need to punish myself through induced vomiting to be able to relax enough to rest and sleep.

My volunteer work and my subsequent work as a camp director and therapeutic school coordinator provided me with real motivation to go to graduate school in clinical psychology and learn more directly about mental illness as well as a number of important related topics, most notably developmental psychology, research methods, and psychopharmacology. Maybe, I hoped, I could truly understand the causes of severe mental illness and better approaches to treatment than my father had experienced for most of his life. It is clear, with hindsight, that the roots of my deep commitment to clinical psychology and developmental psychopathology had emanated, in large part, from my experiences in my family of origin.

Also, through a committed relationship, I realized that my fears about having children were becoming replaced by a sense of deeply wanting to be a father. This change in attitude took time, however. In the wake of serious family mental illness, I have found that fundamental alterations in deeply entrenched responses of fear and overcontrol come quite slowly.

I have long had a major dose of survivor guilt. That is, I ask myself why I have made it through my life relatively unscathed. I do carry a certain level of emotional intensity: a real energy and a sense at other times that things are extremely bleak. After two significant losses, as well, I have experienced serious depression. But I have a sense of stability underneath, and despite my earlier fears, I have never become psychotic or experienced life in a mental hospital. Rather, I have been blessed with key talents, I have a sense of purpose in my life, and I continue to have wonderful family and professional experiences. Yet why should this be the case when so many relatives have truly suffered, some permanently? For example, two of my first cousins—each the first-born son of my father's half-brothers—have severe mental disorders, with one having committed suicide at age 30 secondary to schizoaffective disorder and the other now having completed four consecutive decades of chronic, debilitating schizophrenia. Even in my immediate family, my mother has suffered from severe rheumatoid arthritis for over 30 years, doubtless triggered at least in part from the unimaginable stress of having to contend with my father's episodes and absences throughout her family life.

So I often carry a sense of wonderment, befuddlement, and unease about having never had to contend with such debilitating problems while so many around me have struggled so greatly. Although it has not limited me in terms of family or career pursuits, at times I have felt burdened by my sense of having pulled through. Indeed, this sense has gnawed at me, as I try to understand the "luck of the genetic draw," perseverance, or some combination of the two that has permitted me to be where I am. Certainly, others with personal or family histories of serious mental disorder grapple with similar issues (Hinshaw, 2008a; Jamison, 1995).

Intergenerational Transmission

A related worry concerns the risk for mental illness in future generations of my family. As noted, I was convinced during my 20s that I should never have children of my own, but that fear dissipated as I matured. I now have two wonderful sons and an equally wonderful stepson. What does the future hold for them? The oldest clearly has seasonal mood issues, present since high school. Yet a combination of medication, athletics, a strong sense of humor, and hard work at maintaining social networks has made a huge difference. The youngest is an exuberant 5 years of age, with many of the characteristics of his grandfather, who died years before he was born. His wonderful qualities predominate, but does any of his precocity and intensity foreshadow deeper problems as he grows up?

My current struggle is to be watchful but not overinvolved, with enough flexibility to follow and be guided by each boy's temperamental "lead." How much, I continue to wonder, is my reflex to become vigilant (or overvigilant) an attempt to deal with the gaps I experienced as a child when my dad simply wasn't there versus a "prudent" monitoring of potential risk for serious mood disturbance, with all of the attendant impairment and misery it can create? What I now realize is that if crises occur, my family and I will be armed with awareness and the ability to quickly mobilize allies and interventions.

This entire topic is linked with the blending, in many "bipolar families," of creativity and productivity with despair and disorder (e.g., Jamison, 1993; Richards, Kinney, Lunde, Benet, & Merzel, 1988). Indeed, when genetic screening for risk for psychiatric conditions like bipolar disorder emerges as a viable enterprise, societies should think long and hard before emerging with any future plans to eliminate such genetic propensity. Lessening or eliminating any "bipolar risk" from the gene pool may well lead to a marked reduction in important genetic variability across our species, with the potential for squelching a range of important traits and features that are productive and adaptive.

ADDITIONAL ISSUES

My father's life, along with my experiences in the family system in which I grew up, reveals several additional themes and issues that I believe to be of major scientific and clinical importance. For more detail regarding the following themes, see Hinshaw (2002, 2004, 2006, 2007, 2008b).

Accurate Diagnosis and Evidence-Based, Responsive Treatment

Back in the 1930s, during and after my father's initial episode, it may not have really mattered whether his diagnosis was schizophrenia, manic-depressive illness, or any other condition: There were no viable treatments for any categories of mental illness. Hence, accurate diagnosis may have served only an administrative or strictly nosological function. Today, however, with a growing array of pharmacological and psychosocial treatment modalities of proven effectiveness—and many more of still-questioned validity awaiting clinical trials—accurate diagnosis indeed matters to the extent that specific treatments for different conditions have been documented (for bipolar disorder, see Keck & McElroy, 2007; Miklowitz & Craighead, 2007). Thus, rather than serving as a dehumanizing label, an accurate diagnosis may well point to treatment modalities that can not only ease symptomatology but also curtail suicidality and enhance overall functioning.

Still, there are major questions throughout the field of psychopathology as to whether the diagnostic categories currently in existence are actually valid. Indeed, there is no evidence that all individuals diagnosed with, for example, schizophrenia, bipolar disorder, attention-deficit/hyperactivity disorder (ADHD), or any other category of pathology have underlying similarities, given what we know about multiple risk factors, equifinality, and the sheer diversity of clinical presentations and underlying mechanisms (Jensen et al., 2006). Furthermore, there is increasing recognition that both psychotropic medications and key psychosocial interventions (e.g., cognitive therapy, interpersonal therapy, many types of family intervention) exert "transdiagnostic" effects, meaning that they may address fundamental dimensions of neural, behavioral, or emotional functioning that transcend any given diagnostic entity (e.g., Harvey, Watkins, Mansell, & Shafran, 2004). In short, the field cannot rest on its laurels because it is highly likely that the diagnostic nomenclature currently in use (DSM-IV; see American Psychiatric Association, 2000) will be supplanted in the coming decades with a fundamentally different approach.

These points are particularly salient with respect to the growing tendency for children and adolescents to receive diagnoses of bipolar disorder, despite major uncertainties about the validity of many such diagnostic decisions (Blader & Carlson, 2008), as well as an evidentiary base, for a multiplicity of mood-stabilizing and second-generation antipsychotic medications, that is growing slowly in relation to the numbers of youth who are prescribed these medications. A core challenge for the years ahead will be to balance the urgent clinical needs of a large number of children and adolescents who have serious emotional and behavioral disturbance with appropriate caution regarding (1) "jumping on the diagnostic bandwagon" and (2) the practice of polypharmacy in the absence of sound evidence-based intervention. Clinicians and research investigators will need to forge important new linkages in order to contend with the serious pathology exhibited by troublingly large proportions of children and adolescents, with major efforts required to achieve the important goal of enrolling youth in clinical trials of treatment efficacy and effectiveness as well as developmental investigations related to long-term outcomes (Hinshaw et al., 2004).

Finally, treatments must be responsive to the needs of the patient and family in question. Bipolar disorder often produces frightening, hope-depriving symptoms, frequently leading to confusion, disruption, despair, and hopelessness for all involved. Although pharmacological treatments are clearly indicated for nearly everyone with manic-depressive symptomatology, they need to be supplemented with psychoeducation, family involvement, and various forms of psychological therapy to motivate problem-solving and emotion regulation (see Miklowitz & Craighead, 2007). Clinicians need to show sensitivity to the huge tumult caused by bipolar symptomatology and to be responsive to the befuddlement, anger, shame, and confusion that are so clearly linked to the condition in patients as well as family members. My father's experience of being warehoused, in an era of both ignorance about the disorder and lack of respect for the dignity of patients, provides a tragic lesson for all who are concerned with mental health. In the current era of major closures of public mental hospitals (more than 550,000 Americans were institutionalized in such facilities in 1955 vs. fewer than 50,000 today), the challenge is to ensure that adequate community care and community supports are available.

Resilience

Can individuals at high risk for psychopathology, or even those who have exhibited clinical-level symptomatology, recover and thrive? More generally, are there systematic means of understanding how a subgroup of those with vulnerabilities for poor outcomes can overcome the odds and show positive trajectories? The study of resilience is concerned with just such issues (for reviews, see Luthar, 2006; Luthar, Cicchetti, & Becker, 2000; Masten, Burt, & Coatsworth, 2006).

My father provides a telling example, given that, despite devastating episodes and horrendous experiences in treatment, he maintained his ability to be a caring parent and was able to keep his teaching and research interests alive. Moreover, he maintained a philosophical attitude throughout his life. For instance, in the last years of his life, he told me that he would not have traded any of his life experiences, even those that had resulted in his hospitalizations, given his belief that he had learned and benefited from all such experiences. Among the potential factors related to his resilient functioning, several come readily to mind: his sense of humor; his strong religious faith, which coexisted with his scientific and philosophical interests; his strong work ethic and sense of responsibility; the tenure system (which enabled him to hold on to his job, even when severe episodes hit); his incredibly supportive wife (my mother); and his continuous desire to search for deeper meanings in life, which doubtless helped him to overcome the trauma and shame related to many of his episodes. Clearly, it is not the case that individuals experiencing serious mental illness are necessarily doomed to limited, sterile, impaired lives.

Initially, resilience was viewed as an all-or-none, "you-have-it-or-you-don't" kind of phenomenon (indeed, it was formerly termed "invulnerability" or "invincibility"; see Anthony, 1974). Investigators of resilience now view it as a set of processes that may promote strength and competence in different areas of functioning, distinguishing at least three levels of protective factors for those at high risk: intraindividual, dyadic/relational, and community/systemic. In terms of individual factors, evidence now exists that resilience may, in fact, be partly heritable; in other words, there are genes that confer "protection" for some individuals in high-risk contexts (see Kim-Cohen, Moffitt, Caspi, & Taylor, 2004). Solid evidence exists as well that strong interpersonal relationships are perhaps the key protective factors that vulnerable individuals may encounter (Luthar & Brown, 2007). Yet in the account of potential factors for my father, the only variable in the "community/systemic" category had to do with the tenure system. Indeed, given the institutional abandonment that he received, as well as the community/societal stance that essentially shunned and isolated those with mental illness, I cannot think of other systems-level factors that helped him. As noted later in the section on stigma, a key challenge is to institute attitudes and practices in schools, in the workplace, in the marketplace, and in our general culture that promote openness, knowledge, and tolerance of many forms of deviance, including mental illness. This is not to say that aberrant, psychotic behavior should be accepted; indeed, as emphasized later, access to treatment is a necessary part of resilience-fostering practices.

The construct of resilience has come under challenge (see Luthar et al., 2000). Indeed, many so-called protective factors are essentially the polar opposites of risk factors, calling into question the contention that resilience constitutes a distinct set of processes. Also, debate exists about whether one needs to have experienced vulnerabilities or high-risk circumstances in order to show resilient functioning. Still, focus on this concept is of enormous benefit because it not only removes the field from a nearly exclusive focus on negative outcomes and pathology but also reveals that normal and disordered functioning are not as separate as one might believe. In other words, most forms of mental disorder involve the interspersing of healthy with less healthy functioning; symptoms wax and wane (particularly in the case of bipolar illness); and understanding the factors that promote strength and recovery goes hand in hand with the discovery of risk processes (see Cic-chetti, 2006; Hinshaw, 2007). In short, stereotypes of mental disorder as chronic, hopeless, and unrelentingly negative not only are untrue, but they also fly in the face of a wealth of evidence related to protective processes and the potential for rehabilitation and recovery.

Silence and Communication in Family Systems

Despite the strong heritability of bipolar disorder, important research reveals that family processes are important for outcome (e.g., Miklowitz, 2004; for related evidence regarding the importance of family socialization regarding another highly heritable condition, ADHD, see Hinshaw et al., 2000). My focus here is not to review the many potential family factors that could be related to outcome in bipolar disorder but rather to address the particular stance that my family took, namely, on doctor's orders, to remain silent about my father's illness and absences.

As discussed earlier, such a stance is likely to promote internalization among children, who are prone to blame themselves rather than those on whom they count for love and protection. William Beardslee has examined this aspect of family communication in relation to parental mood disorders (both depression and bipolar disorder), emerging with a provocative and important brand of fam-ily treatment. In brief, his argument begins with the statistic that having a parent with a mood disorder provides a substantial risk for the offspring's parallel risk for mood disturbance. Indeed, people who have a parent with major depression have a 60% chance of experiencing major depression themselves before the age of 30, a substantially increased risk over the base rate (Beardslee, Versage, & Glad-stone, 1998). Yet the mediating factors in this regard are not exclusively genetic (particularly in the case of unipolar depression): A large number of variables, including insecurity of attachment bonds, parental irritability and/or withdrawal, the modeling of emotion dysregulation, harsh or lax parenting, interparental con-flict, and many more, increase the risk for mood disturbance in the children who live in such families (Goodman & Gotlib, 2002).

A factor of core interest to Beardslee is precisely the one under discussion: namely the shame and silence that all too often prevent any family discussion of the parent's condition. Parents are typically ashamed of their behavior patterns and diagnoses, lacking any viable means of discussing their own situations with their children. Thus, a core goal for this family therapy approach is to prevent the child's self-blame for family disruptions, erratic discipline, and the parent's suffering, which, in combination with other risk factors, serves to increase the probability that offspring will develop adjustment problems or mood disorders themselves. To combat this tendency, parents work with the therapist, initially without the children present, to form a plan for a series of family meetings in which the parents engage the child directly in discussions of the parent's mood disturbance. In other words, the parents begin to create a narrative, in language the child can understand, to promote understanding of Mom's irritable behavior or Dad's absences (or whatever the particulars) to prevent self-blame on the part of the offspring and to encourage a far more open style of communication. The therapist provides ample support for the parents as they construct their story, modeling and shaping direct and sensitive communication to the child (see Beardslee, 2002).

Other objectives are addressed in this family intervention, including motivation for the affectively disordered parents to receive evidence-based treatment for their condition and provision of other forms of family support. Still, a major factor that distinguishes it from other approaches is the emphasis on creating a narrative to end the typical stance of silence and shame. Importantly, controlled evidence reveals that this approach promotes better adjustment in the offspring immediately following the therapy, with effects on behavior and attitude changes in parents and youth up to 4½ years after treatment ends (Beardslee, Wright, Gladstone, & Forbes, 2007). In short, family intervention focused on promoting communication rather than silence may provide assistance in breaking an intergenerational cycle of mood disturbance (for an additional, evidence-based approach to the family treatment of bipolar disorder, see Miklowitz, 2008; see discussion in other chapters in this volume).

To conclude this section, what eventuated with respect to our own family's silence once I became an adult? My father's conversations about his life took place with me, not his wife (nor with my sister); indeed, he did not engage my mother in such parallel disclosure, perhaps because of the shame he felt when recalling his history of embarrassing, hostile, or out-of-control behavior that had sometimes required her to secure intervention for him. It may have also been difficult for him to be as open with females as with males, given the loss of his mother and the treatment he received at the hands of his stepmother. Thus, silence continued between them about key aspects of his life and their relationship.

Late in my father's life, and now in my role as a professor at Berkeley, I decided to write about his story, as noted earlier; and I talked about my intentions with my mother. She was not pleased, however, telling me that, although it would be fine with her if my observations appeared in academic journals, she did not want a story that was private, personal, and shameful to her to be widely known. I was, therefore, confronted with a dilemma: Do I continue to write about my father's experiences (and my own), risking a rift with my mother, who had single-handedly kept the family together throughout my childhood, or acquiesce to her legitimate wish for privacy and her sense that continued silence was the optimal approach?

Truly conflicted, I persevered, trying to let her know of the importance of my writing about his life and receiving real support from my wife, Kelly, who let me know that my mother would come to understand the intent behind my desire to tell the narrative. Once the book was published, my mother was still unhappy, although perhaps resigned; our communication was tense. Yet not long after its publication, she called me and asked for additional copies, noting that her book-reading group back in Ohio, which included some of her childhood friends, had selected it. She told me that even these close friends hadn't known all of what the family had encountered decades earlier or of the heroic efforts on my mother's part to negotiate the sometimes chaotic experiences related to my father's episodes. They praised her courage and strength, providing invaluable support for her many years after the fact. Soon thereafter, my mother wondered out loud to me why the book had not received more reviews in mainstream newspapers and magazines! In short, she now realized that her role had been validated and that silence had not been the best option.

Although I had not known it at the time I pressed the issue with my mother, I now see that breaking the family silence was optimal for everyone, albeit initially painful. The hope is that removing the general shame and silence surrounding mental illness will facilitate openness, recovery, and access to services at broader levels as well.

Stigma

The previous section provides an appropriate transition into what many consider to be the major issue in the entire field of mental health: the stigma that still enshrouds mental illness (e.g., Hinshaw, 2007; Sartorius, 1998, 1999; U.S. Department of Health and Human Services, 1999). A term from ancient Greece denoting a literal mark of shame (i.e., a mark or brand placed on a traitor or slave), stigma currently signifies deep psychological degradation related to being a member of a devalued outgroup (Goffman, 1963). A host of research evidence reveals that mental illness—both the constituent behaviors and the labels used to designate mental disturbance—is one of the most stigmatized attributes an individual can have (for reviews, see Corrigan, 2005b; Link & Phelan, 2001; Thornicroft, 2006).

Although even a cursory summary is not possible in the confines of the current chapter, several points are quite clear. First, humans may be predisposed, at the level of natural selection, to reject and stigmatize other people who signal threat, contagion, or major social norm violations (Kurzban & Leary, 2001). Even so, stigma is not inevitable; through individual effort and social programs, stereotyping and prejudice can be overcome. Second, some of the characteristics of severe mental illness may convey the very signals leading to castigation; thus, it is not completely surprising that mentally disordered behavior has received extreme levels of stigmatization, discrimination, exclusion, and even annihilation across cultures and across history (Hinshaw, 2007). Stigma is revealed today in the desire for social distance from persons with mental illness, discriminatory behaviors and legal restrictions, and in unconscious, implicit attitudes of fear and negativity (Stier & Hinshaw, 2007).

Third, the stereotyping and prejudice directed toward individuals with disturbed behaviors or a mental illness label are likely to produce self-stigma for recipients, leading to greatly reduced life opportunities, self-castigation, decisions to conceal a history of mental illness, and either failure to enter treatment or premature cessation of treatment (Link & Phelan, 2001; Sirey et al., 2001). Fourth, individuals with hidden or concealable stigmas (such as a history of mental illness) are prone to considerable anxiety and conflict over the revelation of such stigmatized attributes, adding to intrapersonal conflict and interpersonal trouble (Quinn, 2006). Fifth, despite the large increases in knowledge about mental illness in contemporary society, paralleling the major scientific and clinical advances that have taken place in recent decades, levels of stigmatization are not showing parallel reductions, related to fears of dangerousness as well as rampant media stereotypes (Phelan & Link, 1998; Phelan, Link, & Pescosolido, 2000). Sixth, mental health professionals may be inadvertent promoters of stigmatizing attitudes, given the tendency for "us versus them" attitudes and beliefs that healers and scientists must be objective and without flaw (see Hinshaw, 2008a; Wahl, 1999). In short, the stigmatization that still surrounds mental illness adds a huge level of hopelessness, shame, and societal loss to the considerable impairment and burden that attends to mental illness itself (Hinshaw, 2007; Prince et al., 2007).

My father's experience reveals considerable stigma. He was an inmate of state hospitals, which were originally designed in the mid-1800s as humanitarian, medical-model alternatives to poorhouses or (for youth) orphanages but which soon deteriorated into large, decrepit "total institutions" (Goffman, 1961; Grob, 1994), intentionally built far from urban centers. Moreover, he was ashamed to tell his own wife about his experiences, he had to "cover" when back from mental hospitals about the experiences he had undergone, and he continued to believe that his episodes and treatments constituted punishments for wrong thoughts or behaviors he had committed. Until he revealed to me his secrets, his main communication about his life events had been through his own thoughts and journal entries. At one point when he was in his 60s, during one of our conversations, he told me that at times he had wished he had cancer or some physical illness, anything real, he said, not what the world considered to be an imaginary, "mental" affliction.

Stigma affects families as well. My father's stance of silence, prescribed by his psychiatrist, isolated our family from receiving needed support and help. Goffman (1963) introduced the notion of "courtesy stigma" to indicate that the stereotyping, prejudice, and discrimination surrounding persons with devalued traits often extend to their associates, including family members. The taint associated with a severe mental illness and with involuntary psychiatric hospitalization doubtless extended to our entire family. For data on the stigma linked to caregivers of individuals with bipolar disorder, see Gonzalez and colleagues (2007).

Would it have made a difference had my father been told, during or following his initial episode, that he had bipolar disorder, a biochemically based illness with substantial heritability? In other words, would at least some of his lifelong shame have been mitigated had he—in fact, had all of society—been presented with a biogenetic attribution for his mental illness? One of the fundamental tenets of attribution theory, in fact, is that attributions of negative behaviors or characteristics to uncontrollable factors—those over which the person had no volitional input—should reduce blame and foster instead empathy and compassion (Weiner, Perry, & Magnusson, 1988). Indeed, a major aspect of many antistigma campaigns is to portray mental disorder as a genetically caused brain disease (e.g., Johnson, 1989), under the assumption that adoption of this view will dissuade the public from the view that mental disorders are results of faulty parenting or moral weakness, thereby serving to reduce stigma.

With regard to mental illness, however, the picture regarding attribution theory is not nearly so straightforward. In fact, experimental evidence reveals that biological/genetic ascriptions for mentally disturbed behavior may actually *increase* punitive responses and promote social distance toward both individuals and relatives (who are presumably tainted by the shared genes). For relevant research, with complex findings, see Mehta and Farina (1997); Phelan (2005); Phelan, Cruz-Rojas, and Reiff (2002); and Read and Harre (2001). Indeed, when the behaviors are as threatening and devalued as those constituting the core symptoms of severe mental illness, the belief that the behavior patterns are caused by faulty genes may fuel views of the permanence of the affliction and the fundamental subhumanity of the individual in question (Hinshaw, 2007). At the very least, attributing severe mental illness in reductionistic fashion to biogenetic causes is far from a panacea (Haslam, 2000).

Combating a phenomenon as complex as the stigmatization of mental illness will require multifaceted strategies (for a review, see Hinshaw, 2007). (1) Discriminatory laws must be repealed, and policies that deny equitable compensation for treatment of mental illness must give way to "parity." At the same time, deinstitutionalization must be matched by adequate funding of community-based services, treatments, and advocacy. (2) Media images of mental illness, which are hugely negative and stereotypic (see Wahl, 1995), need to be replaced by accurate, humane portrayals that convey the truth about mental disorders, neither glorifying nor demonizing it. (3) Mental health professionals need to adopt a new set of attitudes about those whom they treat, given that recipients of care often view the individuals from whom they receive services as conveying a number of highly stigmatizing attitudes and responses (e. g., Wahl, 1999; see also Hinshaw, 2008a). For example, a removed, distanced therapeutic stance may actually increase the patient's sense of being different or judged; jokes about "psychos" or other pejorative terms are extremely demeaning. (4) Increased public knowledge of mental illness is important but it is far from sufficient: Contact with persons with mental disorder, under conditions of equity and informality, is required to break down barriers and increase empathy (for data on the "contact hypothesis" for reducing prejudice and stigma, see Pettigrew & Tropp, 2000). (5) Family members need to receive education, support, and admiration; along these lines, self-help and advocacy groups serve an essential role. (6) Individual treatment is also part of stigma reduction, in order to reduce threatening symptoms and enhance the person's capabilities for independence and employment. Indeed, the situation is different from that of reducing racial prejudice: In that arena, societal attitudes are the sole locus of intervention, given that ethnic/racial status is a fixed characteristic of the individual in question. But mental illnesses are, in fact, dysfunctions—albeit dysfunctions reflecting complex, transactional, multilevel processes rather than simple, unidimensional causal forces. Thus, individual intervention for the person with a mental disorder, which requires policies of universal health coverage along with parity for mental health benefits, is a necessary component of any overall plan to reduce stigmatization.

In short, stigma reduction will require both access to evidence-based treatment and societal acceptance of a diversity of behavioral and emotional styles. Given the shocking waste of human potential and the real despair for families and individuals produced by mental disorder as well as its stigmatization, all of society stands to gain from intensive efforts toward reduction of prejudice and discrimination and toward assurance that treatment can be utilized (Corrigan, 2005a; Hinshaw, 2007).

Conclusion

Narratives help us construct the world and ourselves (Ochs & Capps, 2001). My father's life with bipolar disorder, replete with disruption, terror, and stigma but also filled with deep humanity and compassion, conveys a number of essential themes and lessons for those interested in the development of bipolar disorder, its accurate diagnosis and responsive treatment, implications for self-worth, family shame and silence, and consideration of just what it will take to understand and treat this virulent form of psychopathology. There is no substitute for vigorous, precise science related to (1) risk and causal factors and (2) treatment development and dissemination, but narrative accounts can help to inform future generations of scientists, clinicians, and policymakers of the core issues that need to be pursued. Families bear much of the burden of mental illness; my fervent hope is that acknowledgment of the kinds of struggles and triumphs of family members will prove valuable for all those concerned with easing the burden of mental disorder. There is no doubting that it is a time of enormous challenge and enormous opportunity with respect to multiple fronts in the battle against mental illness, particularly bipolar disorder, and I believe that narrative accounts and scientific progress go hand in hand.

REFERENCES

American Psychiatric Association. (2000). *Diagnostic and statistical manual of mental disorders* (4th ed., text rev.). Washington, DC: Author.

Anthony, E. J. (1974). Introduction: The syndrome of the psychologically invulnerable child. In E. J. Anthony & C. Koupernik (Eds.), *The child in his family: Children at psychiatric risk* (Vol. 3, pp. 3–10). New York: Wiley.

Beardslee, W. R. (2002). *Out of the darkened room: When a parent is depressed: protecting the children and strengthening the family.* Boston: Little, Brown.

Beardslee, W. R., Versage, E. M., & Gladstone, T. G. (1998). Children of affectively ill parents: A review of the last 10 years. *Journal of the American Academy of Child and Adolescent Psychiatry, 37,* 1134–1141.

Beardslee, W. R., Wright, E. J., Gladstone, T. R., & Forbes, P. (2007). Long-term effects from a randomized trial of two public-health preventive interventions. *Journal of Family Psychology, 21,* 703–713.

Beauchaine, T. P., Hinshaw, S. P., & Gatzke-Kopp, L. (2008). Genetic and environmental influences on behavior. In T. P. Beauchaine & S. P. Hinshaw (Eds.), *Child and adolescent psychopathology* (pp. 58–90). Hoboken, NJ: Wiley.

Blader, J. C., & Carlson, G. A. (2008). Bipolar disorder. In T. P. Beauchaine & S. P. Hinshaw (Eds.), *Child and adolescent psychopathology* (pp. 543–574). Hoboken, NJ: Wiley.

Byng-Hall, J. (2008). The significance of children fulfilling parental roles: Implications for family therapy. *Journal of Family Therapy, 30,* 142–162.

Carlson, G. A., & Goodwin, F. K. (1973). The stages of mania: A longitudinal analysis of the manic episode. *Archives of General Psychiatry, 28,* 221–228.

Cicchetti, D. (2006). Development and psychopathology. In D. Cicchetti & D. J. Cohen (Eds.), *Developmental psychopathology: Vol. 1. Theory and method* (2nd ed., pp. 1–23). Hoboken, NJ: Wiley.

Cicchetti, D. (2008). A multiple-levels-of-analysis perspective on research in development and psychopathology. In T. P. Beauchaine & S. P. Hinshaw (Eds.), *Child and adolescent psychopathology* (pp. 27–57). Hoboken, NJ: Wiley.

Cicchetti, D., & Valentino, K. (2006). An ecological-transactional perspective on child maltreatment: Failure of the average expectable environment and its influence on child development. In D. Cicchetti & D. J. Cohen (Eds.), *Developmental psychopathology: Vol. 3. Risk, disorder, and adaptation* (2nd ed., pp. 129–201). Hoboken, NJ: Wiley.

Corrigan, P. W. (2005a). Mental illness stigma as social injustice: Yet another dream to be achieved. In P. W. Corrigan (Ed.), *On the stigma of mental illness: Practical strategies for research and social change* (pp. 315–320). Washington, DC: American Psychological Association.

Corrigan, P. W. (Ed.). (2005b). *On the stigma of mental illness: Practical strategies for research and social change.* Washington, DC: American Psychological Association.

Corrigan, P. W., Markowitz, F. E., & Watson, A. (2004). Structural levels of mental illness stigma and discrimination. *Schizophrenia Bulletin, 30,* 481–491.

Corrigan, P. W., Watson, A. C., Heyrman, M. L., Warpinski, A., Gracia, G., Slopen, N., et al. (2005). Structural stigma in state legislation. *Psychiatric Services, 56,* 557–563.

Du Rochler Schuldich, T. D., Youngstrom, E. A., Calabrese, J. R., & Findling, R. L. (2008). The role of family functioning in bipolar disorder in families. *Journal of Abnormal Child Psychology, 36,* 849–863.

Garno, J. L., Goldberg, J. F., Ramirez, P. M., & Ritzler, B. A. (2005). Impact of childhood abuse on the clinical course of bipolar disorder. *British Journal of Psychiatry, 186,* 121–125.

Geller, B., Williams, M., Zimmerman, B., Frazier, J., Beringer, L., & Warner, K. L. (1998). Pre-pubertal and early adolescent bipolarity differentiate from ADHD by manic symptoms, grandiose delusions, ultra-rapid or ultradian cycling. *Journal of Affective Disorders, 51*, 81–91.

Goffman, E. (1961). *Asylums: Essays on the social situations of mental patients and other inmates.* New York: Doubleday.

Goffman, E. (1963). *Stigma: Notes on the management of spoiled identity.* Englewood Cliffs, NJ: Prentice Hall.

Gonzalez, J., Perlick, D., Miklowitz, D. J., Kaczynski, R., Hernandez, M., Rosenheck, R. A., et al. (2007). Factors associated with stigma among the caregivers of patients with bipolar disorder. *Psychiatric Services, 58*, 41–48.

Goodman, S. H., & Gotlib, I. H. (Eds.). (2002). *Children of depressed parents: Mechanisms of risk and implications for treatment.* Washington, DC: American Psychological Association.

Goodwin, F. K., & Jamison, K. R. (2007). *Manic-depressive illness: Bipolar disorders and recurrent depression* (2nd ed.). New York: Oxford University Press.

Grob, G. N. (1994). *The mad among us: A history of care of America's mentally ill.* New York: Free Press.

Harter, S. (2006). Self-processes and developmental psychopathology. In D. Cicchetti & D. J. Cohen (Eds.), *Developmental psychopathology: Vol. 1. Theory and method* (2nd ed., pp. 370–418). Hoboken, NJ: Wiley.

Harvey, A. G., Watkins, E., Mansell, W., & Shafran, R. (2004). *Cognitive behavioural processes across psychological disorders: A transdiagnostic approach to research and treatment.* Oxford, UK: Oxford University Press.

Haslam, N. (2000). Psychiatric categories as natural kinds: Essentialist thinking about mental disorder. *Social Research, 67*, 1031–1058.

Hinshaw, S. P. (2002). *The years of silence are past: My father's life with bipolar disorder.* New York: Cambridge University Press.

Hinshaw, S. P. (2004). Parental mental disorder and children's functioning: Silence and communication, stigma, and resilience. *Journal of Clinical Child and Adolescent Psychology, 33*, 400–411.

Hinshaw, S. P. (2006). Stigma and mental illness: Developmental issues. In D. Cicchetti & D. J. Cohen (Eds.), *Developmental psychopathology: Vol. 3. Risk, disorder, and adaptation* (2nd ed., pp. 841–881). New York: Wiley.

Hinshaw, S. P. (2007). *The mark of shame: Stigma of mental illness and an agenda for change.* New York: Oxford University Press.

Hinshaw, S. P. (Ed.). (2008a). *Breaking the silence: Mental health professionals disclose their personal and family experiences of mental illness.* New York: Oxford University Press.

Hinshaw, S. P. (2008b). Closing thoughts: The power of narrative. In S. P. Hinshaw (Ed.), *Breaking the silence: Mental health professionals disclose their personal and family experiences of mental illness* (pp. 347–360). New York: Oxford University Press.

Hinshaw, S. P. (2008c). Developmental psychopathology as a scientific discipline: Relevance to behavioral and emotional disorders of childhood and adolescence. In T. P. Beauchaine & S. P. Hinshaw (Eds.), *Child and adolescent psychopathology* (pp. 3–26). Hoboken, NJ: Wiley.

Hinshaw, S. P., Hoagwood, K., Jensen, P. S., Kratochvil, C., Bickman, L., Clarke, G., et al. (2004). AACAP 2001 Research Forum: Challenges and recommendations regarding recruitment and retention of participants in research investigations. *Journal of the American Academy of Child and Adolescent Psychiatry, 43*, 1037–1045.

Hinshaw, S. P., Owens, E. B., Wells, K. C., Kraemer, H. C., Abikoff, H. B., Arnold, L. E., et al. (2000). Family processes and treatment outcome in the MTA: Negative/ineffective parenting practices in relation to multimodal treatment. *Journal of Abnormal Child Psychology*, 28, 555–568.

Jamison, K. R. (1993). *Touched with fire: Manic–depressive illness and the artistic temperament.* New York: Free Press.

Jamison, K. R. (1995). *An unquiet mind: A memoir of moods and madness.* New York: Free Press.

Jensen, P. S., Hoagwood, K., & Zitner, L. (2006). What's in a name? Problems versus prospects in current diagnostic approaches. In D. Cicchetti & D. J. Cohen (Eds.), *Developmental psychopathology: Vol. 1. Theory and method* (2nd ed., pp. 24–40). Hoboken, NJ: Wiley.

Johnson, D. L. (1989). Schizophrenia as a brain disease: Implications for psychologists and families. *American Psychologist*, 44, 553–555.

Johnson, S. L. (2005). Life events in bipolar disorder: Towards more specific models. *Clinical Psychology Review*, 25, 1008–1027.

Keck, P. E., & McElroy, S. L. (2007). Pharmacological treatments for bipolar disorder. In P. E. Nathan & J. M. Gorman (Eds.), *A guide to treatments that work* (3rd ed., pp. 323–350). New York: Oxford University Press.

Kendler, K. A. (2005). "A gene for . . . ": The nature of gene action in psychiatric disorders. *American Journal of Psychiatry*, 162, 1243–1252.

Kim, E. Y., & Miklowitz, D. J. (2004). Expressed emotion as a predictor of outcome among bipolar patients undergoing family therapy. *Journal of Affective Disorders*, 82, 343–352.

Kim-Cohen, J., Moffitt, T. E., Caspi, A., & Taylor, A. (2004). Genetic and environmental processes in young children's resilience and vulnerability to socioeconomic deprivation. *Child Development*, 75, 651–668.

Kurzban, R., & Leary, M. R. (2001). Evolutionary origins of stigmatization: The functions of social exclusion. *Psychological Bulletin*, 127, 187–208.

Lefley, H. P. (1989). Family burden and family stigma in major mental illness. *American Psychologist*, 44, 556–560.

Link, B. G., & Phelan, J. C. (2001). Conceptualizing stigma. *Annual Review of Sociology*, 27, 363–385.

Luthar, S. S. (2006). Resilience in development: A synthesis of research across five decades. In D. Cicchetti & D. J. Cohen (Eds.), *Developmental psychopathology: Vol. 3. Risk, disorder, and adaptation* (2nd ed., pp. 739–795). New York: Wiley.

Luthar, S. S., & Brown, P. J. (2007). Maximizing resilience through diverse levels of inquiry: Prevailing paradigms, possibilities, and priorities. *Development and Psychopathology*, 19, 931–955.

Luthar, S. S., Cicchetti, D., & Becker, B. (2000). The construct of resilience: A critical evaluation and guide for future work. *Child Development*, 71, 543–562.

Maier, E., & Lachman, M. E. (2000). Consequences of early parental loss and separation for well-being in midlife. *International Journal of Behavioral Development*, 24, 183–189.

Masten, A. S., Burt, K. B., & Coatsworth, J. D. (2006). Competence and psychopathology in development. In D. Cicchetti & D. J. Cohen (Eds.), *Developmental psychopathology: Vol. 3. Risk, disorder, and adaptation* (2nd ed., pp. 696–738). New York: Wiley.

Mehta, S., & Farina, A. (1997). Is being "sick" really better?: Effect of the disease view of mental disorder on stigma. *Journal of Social and Clinical Psychology*, 16, 405–419.

Miklowitz, D. J. (2004). The role of family systems in severe and recurrent psychiatric disorders: A developmental psychopathology view. *Development and Psychopathology*, 16, 667–688.

Miklowitz, D. J. (2008). *Bipolar disorder: A family-focused treatment approach* (2nd ed.). New York: Guilford Press.

Miklowitz, D. J., & Craighead, W. E. (2007). Psychosocial treatments for bipolar disorder. In P. E. Nathan & J. M. Gorman (Eds.), *A guide to treatments that work* (3rd ed., pp. 309–322). New York: Oxford University Press.

Neria, Y., Bromet, E. J., Carlson, G. A., & Naz, B. (2005). Assaultive trauma and illness course in psychotic bipolar disorder: Findings from the Suffolk County mental health project. *Acta Psychiatrica Scandinavica, 111,* 380–383.

Ochs, E., & Capps, L. (2001). *Living narrative: Creating lives in everyday storytelling.* Cambridge, MA: Harvard University Press.

Peris, T. S., & Emery, R. E. (2005). Redefining the parent–child relationship following divorce: Examining the risk for boundary dissolution. *Journal of Emotional Abuse, 5,* 169–189.

Perlick, D. A., Rosenheck, R. A., Miklowitz, D. J., Chessick, C., Wolff, N., Kaczynski, R., et al. (2007). Prevalence and correlates of burden in caregivers of bipolar patients enrolled in the Systematic Treatment Enhancement Program for Bipolar Disorder. *Bipolar Disorders, 9,* 262–273.

Pettigrew, T. F., & Tropp, L. R. (2000). Does intergroup contact reduce prejudice?: Recent meta-analytic findings. In S. Oskamp (Ed.), *Reducing prejudice and discrimination: The Claremont Symposium on Applied Social Psychology* (pp. 93–114). Mahwah, NJ: Erlbaum.

Phelan, J. C. (2005). Geneticization of deviant behavior and consequences for stigma: The case of mental illness. *Journal of Health and Social Behavior, 46,* 307–322.

Phelan, J. C., Cruz-Rojas, R., & Reiff, M. (2002). Genes and stigma: The connection between perceived genetic etiology and attitudes and beliefs about mental illness. *Psychiatric Rehabilitation Skills, 6,* 159–185.

Phelan, J. C., & Link, B. G. (1998). The growing belief that people with mental illness are violent: The role of the dangerousness criterion for civil commitment. *Social Psychiatry and Psychiatric Epidemiology, 33*(Suppl. 1), S7–S12.

Phelan, J. C., Link, B. G., & Pescosolido, B. A. (2000). Public conceptions of mental illness in the 1950's and 1960's: What is mental illness and is it to be feared? *Journal of Health and Social Behavior, 41,* 188–207.

Post, R. M., Leverich, G. S., Xing, G., & Weiss, S. R. B. (2001). Developmental vulnerabilities to the onset and course of bipolar disorder. *Development and Psychopathology, 13,* 581–598.

Prince, M., Patel, V., Saxena, S., Maj, M., Maselko, J., Phillips, M. R., et al. (2007). No health without mental health. *Lancet, 370,* 859–877.

Quinn, D. M. (2006). Concealable versus conspicuous stigmatized identities. In S. Levin & C. Van Laar (Eds.), *Stigma and group inequality: Social psychological approaches* (pp. 83–103). Mahwah, NJ: Erlbaum.

Read, J., & Harre, N. (2001). The role of biological and genetic causal beliefs in the stigmatization of "mental patients." *Journal of Mental Health, 10,* 223–235.

Richards, R. L., Kinney, D. C., Lunde, I., Benet, M., & Merzel, A. P. (1988). Creativity in manic-depressives, cyclothymes, their normal relatives, and control subjects. *Journal of Abnormal Psychology, 97,* 281–288.

Rutter, M., Moffitt, T. E., & Caspi, A. (2006). Gene–environment interplay and psychopathology: Multiple varieties but real effects. *Journal of Child Psychology and Psychiatry, 47,* 226–261.

Sartorius, N. (1998). Stigma: What can psychiatrists do about it? *Lancet, 352,* 1058–1059.

Sartorius, N. (1999). One of the last obstacles to better mental health care: The stigma of mental illness. In J. Guimon, W. Fischer, & N. Sartorius (Eds.), *The image of madness: The public facing mental illness and psychiatric treatment* (pp. 138–142). Basel, Switzerland: Karger.

Simoneau, T. L., Miklowitz, D. J., & Saleem, R. (1998). Expressed emotion and the interactional patterns in the families of bipolar patients. *Journal of Abnormal Psychology, 107,* 497–507.

Sirey, J. A., Bruce, M. L., Alexopoulos, G., Perlick, D., Raue, P., Friedman, S., J., et al. (2001). Perceived stigma as a predictor of treatment discontinuation in young and older outpatients with depression. *American Journal of Psychiatry, 158,* 479–481.

Stier, A., & Hinshaw, S. P. (2007). Explicit and implicit stigma against individuals with mental illness. *Australian Psychologist, 42,* 106–117.

Struening, E. L., Perlick, D. A., Link, B. G., Hellman, F. G., Herman, D., & Sirey, J. A. (2001). The extent to which caregivers believe most people devalue consumers and their families. *Psychiatric Services, 52,* 1633–1638.

Tessler, R., & Gamache, G. (2000). *Family experiences with mental illness.* Westport, CT: Auburn House.

Thornicroft, G. (2006). *Shunned: Discrimination against people with mental illness.* Oxford, UK: Oxford University Press.

U.S. Department of Health and Human Services. (1999). *Mental health: A report of the surgeon general.* Rockville, MD: Author.

Wahl, O. F. (1995). *Media madness: Public images of mental illness.* New Brunswick, NJ: Rutgers University Press.

Wahl, O. F. (1999). *Telling is risky business: Mental health consumers confront stigma.* New Brunswick, NJ: Rutgers University Press.

Weiner, B., Perry, R. P., & Magnusson, J. (1988). An attributional analysis of reactions to stigmas. *Journal of Personality and Social Psychology, 55,* 738–748.

Index